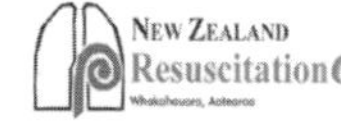

Advanced Life Support for Adults

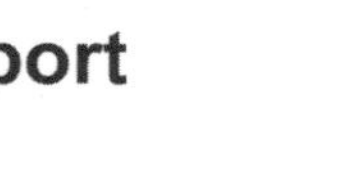

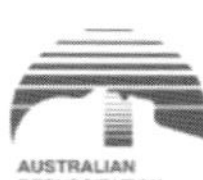

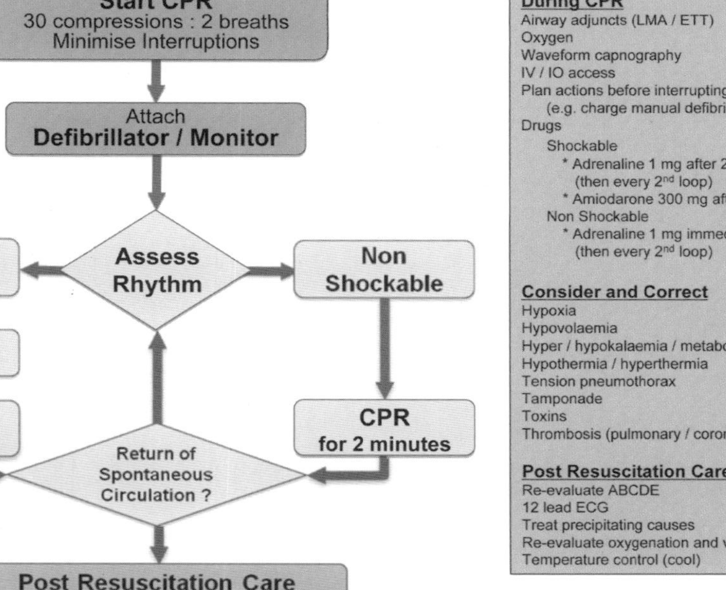

During CPR

Airway adjuncts (LMA / ETT)
Oxygen
Waveform capnography
IV / IO access
Plan actions before interrupting compressions
(e.g. charge manual defibrillator)
Drugs
Shockable
* Adrenaline 1 mg after 2nd shock (then every 2nd loop)
* Amiodarone 300 mg after 3rd shock
Non Shockable
* Adrenaline 1 mg immediately (then every 2nd loop)

Consider and Correct

Hypoxia
Hypovolaemia
Hyper / hypokalaemia / metabolic disorders
Hypothermia / hyperthermia
Tension pneumothorax
Tamponade
Toxins
Thrombosis (pulmonary / coronary)

Post Resuscitation Care

Re-evaluate ABCDE
12 lead ECG
Treat precipitating causes
Re-evaluate oxygenation and ventilation
Temperature control (cool)

December 2010

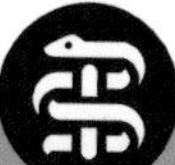

Quick reference

Compiled by Fiona Chow

Editorial Comment

This is a quick guide only. For more detail, please refer to the relevant chapter or to the index.

1 Cardiorespiratory arrest algorithms

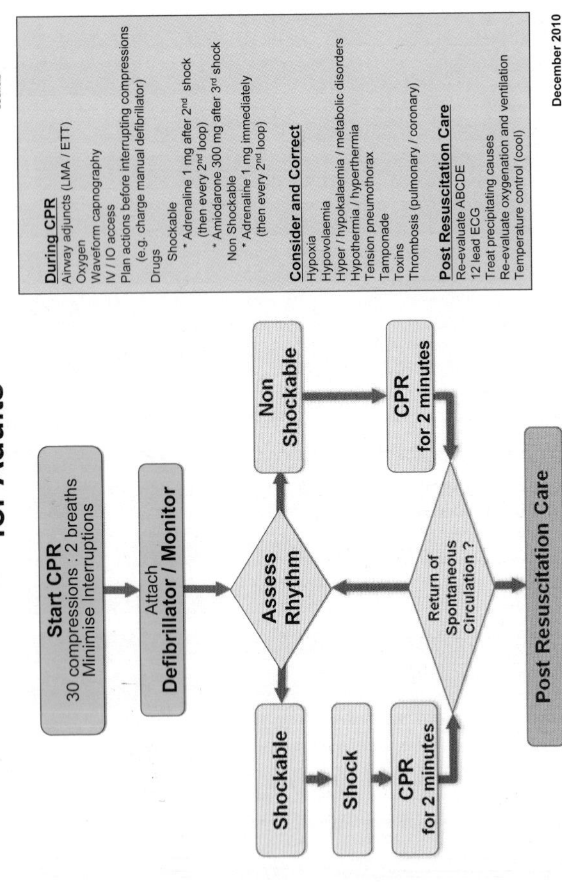

Figure 1.1 Adult cardiorespiratory arrest algorithm
Reproduced with permission from the Australian Resuscitation Guidelines. Online. Available: www.resus.org.au/public/arc_adult_cardiorespiratory_arrest.pdf (accessed 2 July 2012)

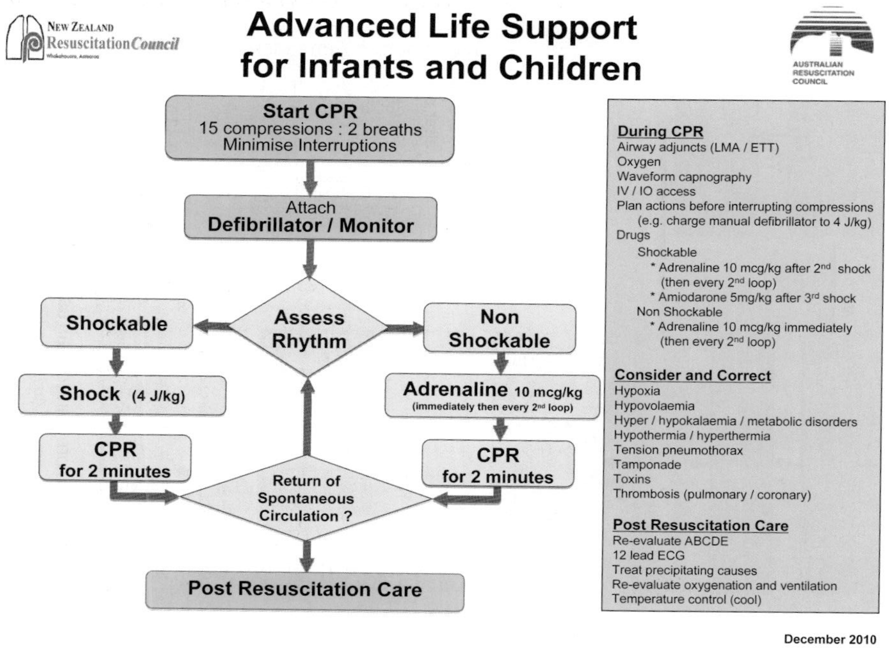

New Zealand Resuscitation Council
Advanced Life Support for Infants and Children
Australian Resuscitation Council
Start CPR
15 compressions : 2 breaths
Minimise Interruptions
Attach Defibrillator / Monitor
Assess Rhythm
Shockable
Shock (4 J/kg)
CPR for 2 minutes
Non Shockable
Adrenaline 10 mcg/kg (immediately then every 2nd loop)
CPR for 2 minutes
Return of Spontaneous Circulation ?
Post Resuscitation Care
During CPR
Airway adjuncts (LMA / ETT)
Oxygen
Waveform capnography
IV / IO access
Plan actions before interrupting compressions (e.g. charge manual defibrillator to 4 J/kg)
Drugs
Shockable
* Adrenaline 10 mcg/kg after 2nd shock (then every 2nd loop)
* Amiodarone 5mg/kg after 3rd shock
Non Shockable
* Adrenaline 10 mcg/kg immediately (then every 2nd loop)
Consider and Correct
Hypoxia
Hypovolaemia
Hyper / hypokalaemia / metabolic disorders
Hypothermia / hyperthermia
Tension pneumothorax
Tamponade
Toxins
Thrombosis (pulmonary / coronary)
Post Resuscitation Care
Re-evaluate ABCDE
12 lead ECG
Treat precipitating causes
Re-evaluate oxygenation and ventilation
Temperature control (cool)
December 2010

Figure 1.2 Paediatric cardiorespiratory arrest algorithm
Reproduced with permission from the Australian Resuscitation Council Guidelines. Online. Available: www.resus.org.au/public/arc_paediatric_cardiorespiratory_arrest.pdf (accessed 2 July 2012)

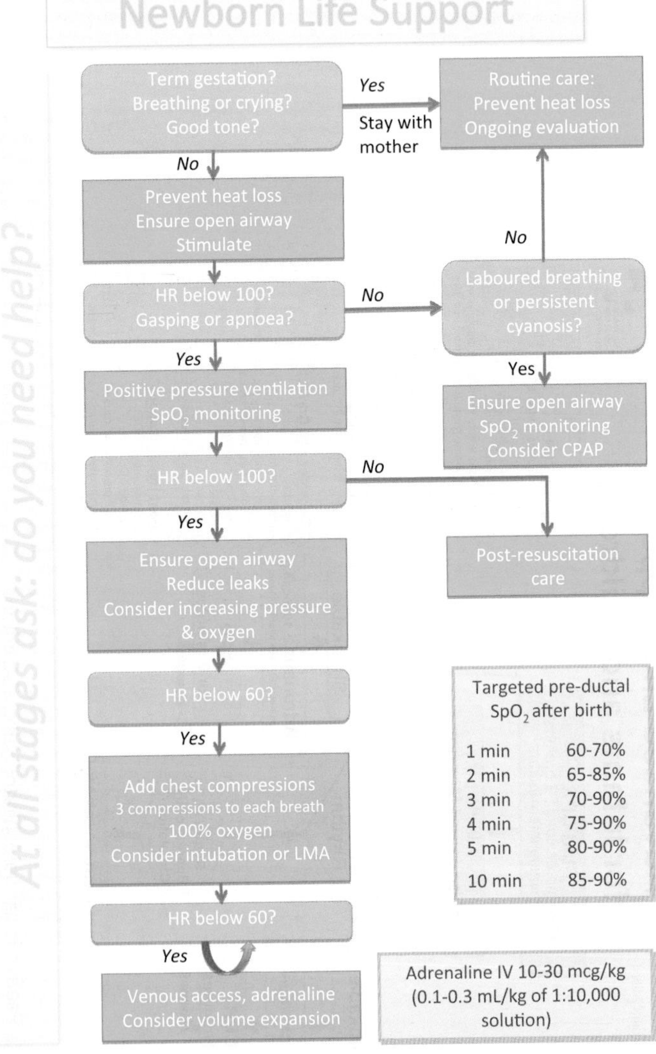

Figure 1.3 Neonatal cardiorespiratory arrest algorithm
Reproduced with permission from the Australian Resuscitation Council Guidelines. Online. Available: www.resus.org.au/public/arc_neonatal_flowchart.pdf (accessed 2 July 2012)

2 Cardiac arrest drugs

The following tables have been adapted from the Australian Resuscitation Council Guidelines.

Drugs routinely used in ADULT cardiac arrest

Drug	Dose	Indications
Adrenaline	1 mg IV repeat every 2nd loop during CPR	VF/VT Asystole/PEA
Amiodarone	300 mg IV Additional dose of 150 mg IV can be considered that may then be followed by infusion of 15 mg/kg over 24 h	VF/VT

Other drugs to consider in ADULT cardiac arrest

Drug	Dose	Indications
Calcium	5–10 mL IV of 10% calcium chloride	Hyperkalaemia Hypercalcaemia OD of calcium channel blockers
Magnesium	5 mmol IV can be repeated once, then followed with infusion (20 mmol over 4 h)	Torsades de pointes Cardiac arrest associated with digoxin toxicity VF/VT refractory to defibrillation and adrenaline Hypokalaemia Hypomagnesaemia
Potassium	5 mmol IV	Persistent VF due to hypokalaemia
Lignocaine	1 mg/kg IV	VF/VT where amiodarone cannot be used
Sodium bicarbonate	1 mmol/kg	Hyperkalaemia Treatment of documented metabolic acidosis Tricyclic antidepressant OD Prolonged arrest (> 15 min)

Drugs able to be given via endotracheal tube (ETT)

— Lignocaine
— Adrenaline
— Atropine
— Naloxone

Dilution with 0.9% may give better absorption.

If unable to gain intravenous access, consider intraosseous (IO) access.

2

Drugs routinely used in PAEDIATRIC cardiac arrest

Drug	Dose and route of administration
Adrenaline	10 microg/kg IV/IO = 0.1 mL/kg of 1:10,000 (max single dose = 1 mg) 100 microg/kg via ETT
Amiodarone	5 mg/kg IV/IO over 3–5 min
Defibrillation	4 joules/kg

Other drugs to consider in PAEDIATRIC cardiac arrest

Drug	Dose and route of administration
Atropine	20 microg/kg IV/IO (max 600 microg) 30 microg/kg via ETT
Calcium chloride 10% Calcium gluconate 10%	0.2 mL/kg IV/IO 0.7 mL/kg IV/IO
Glucose (dextrose)	0.25 g/kg IV/IO = 0.5 mL/kg of 50% dextrose (via CVC only) = 2.5 mL/kg of 10% dextrose IV/IO
Lignocaine (only if amiodarone is unavailable)	1 mg/kg IV
Magnesium sulfate 50% (= 2 mmol/L)	0.1–0.2 mmol/kg IV/IO bolus 0.3 mmol/kg infusion over 4 h
Potassium	0.03–0.07 mmol/kg IV/IO slow injection
Sodium bicarbonate (8.4%)	0.5–1 mmol/kg IV/IO

3 Miscellaneous drugs—adults

3

Miscellaneous drugs used in ADULTS

Drug	Dose and route of administration
Acetylcysteine	Initially 150 mg/kg IV over 15 min; then 50 mg/kg IV over 4 h; then 100 mg/kg IV over 16 h
Adenosine	Initially 6 mg IV (rapid bolus); if still unsuccessful within 1–2 min give 12 mg IV (rapid bolus) (follow with a rapid saline flush)
Adrenaline	
For cardiac arrest	1 mg IV
For anaphylaxis	0.3–0.5 mg of 1:10,000 IV 0.3–0.5 mg of 1:1000 IM
For airway obstruction	0.5 mL/kg of 1:1000 (max 5 mL) nebulised
Amiodarone (loading dose)	5 mg/kg IV over 1 h
Atropine	0.5 mg IV (max total dose 3 mg)
Benztropine	2 mg IV/IM/PO
Bupivacaine ± adrenaline For local anaesthesia	Maximum single dose 2 mg/kg SC Do not repeat at intervals less than 4 h Usual dose is 12.5–150 mg (= 5–60 mL of 0.25% = 2.5–30 mL of 0.5%)
Calcium	5–10 mL of 10% calcium chloride IV 10 mL of 10% calcium gluconate IV
Charcoal	50 g PO
Clonazepam	0.5–1 mg IV
Dexamethasone	4–8 mg IV/IM
Dextrose	25–50 mL (12.5–25 g) of 50% slow push
Diazepam	2.5–5 mg IV
Digoxin (loading dose)	Adults: 250–500 microg PO/IV q4-6h to a max of 1500 microg PO or 1000 microg IV Elderly: 250–500 microg PO/IV q4-6h to a max of 500 microg
Digoxin (maintenance dose)	Adults: 125–250 microg PO Elderly: 62.5–125 microg PO
Fentanyl	
For analgesia/sedation	25–50 microg IV or 50–100 microg SC/IM
Flumazenil	0.2–0.5 mg IV (max total dose 2 mg)
Glucagon	1 mg IV/IM
Haloperidol	2.5–5 mg IV or IM
Hydrocortisone	100–200 mg IV

Continues

3

Miscellaneous drugs used in ADULTS (continued)

Drug	Dose and route of administration	
Hyoscine butylbromide	10–20 mg PO qid 20–40 mg IV/IM up to 100 mg/d	
Ibuprofen	200–400 mg PO tds	
Ketamine		
For analgesia	0.3–1 mg/kg IV given slowly over 2 min *or* 4–5 mg/kg IM	
For anaesthesia	1–2 mg/kg IV *or* 10 mg/kg IM	
Lignocaine For local anaesthesia	Max single dose 3–4 mg/kg SC (up to 200 mg) Do not repeat max dose at intervals < 1.5 h	
Lignocaine + adrenaline For local anaesthesia	Maximum single dose 7 mg/kg SC (up to 500 mg)	
Loratadine	10 mg PO daily	
Magnesium	2 g IV over 5–10 min Eclampsia up to 4 g IV	
Mannitol	1 g/kg IV (= 5 mL/kg of 20% mannitol), max 50 g per dose	
Metoclopramide	10 mg PO/IV/IM q6h	
Midazolam	1–2.5 mg IV 0.07–0.1 mg/kg IM	
Morphine	2.5–5 mg IV 5–10 mg IM/SC	
Naloxone	200–400 microg IV/IM/SC; repeat every 2–3 min to a max 10 mg	
Olanzapine	5–10 mg PO/IM	
Ondansetron	4–8 mg PO/IV	
Oxycodone	2.5–5 mg PO qid	
Pamidronate	**Calcium level**	**Dose**
For hypercalcaemia—dose depends on calcium level (mmol/L)	< 3.0 3.0–3.5 3.5–4.0 > 4.0	30 mg 30–60 mg 60–90 mg 90 mg
Phenytoin (loading dose)	15–20 mg/kg IV infused at a rate < 50 mg/min	
Promethazine		
For allergy	10–25 mg PO tds 25 mg IM as a single dose	
For nausea, vomiting	25 mg PO or 12.5–25 mg IM q6h	

Drug	Dose and route of administration
Propofol	
For induction of anaesthesia	1 mg/kg IV
For maintenance of sedation during ventilation	1–3 mg/kg/h IV
Rocuronium	
For induction	0.6–1 mg/kg IV
For maintenance of paralysis	0.15 mg/kg IV (0.075 mg/kg IV in elderly)
Sugammadex	
For immediate reversal	16 mg/kg IV
For routine reversal	2–4 mg/kg IV
Suxamethonium	
For induction of general anaesthesia	0.5–1.2 mg/kg IV
Thiopentone	
For induction of general anaesthesia	3–5 mg/kg IV

Commonly used antibiotics in ADULTS

Antibiotic	Dose and route of administration
Amoxycillin	500 mg PO q8h
Amoxycillin/clavulanic acid	500/125 mg PO q8h (Augmentin Duo) 875/125 mg PO q12h (Augmentin Duo Forte)
Ampicillin	1 g IV q6h
Azithromycin	500 mg–1 g PO daily 500 mg IV daily
Ceftriaxone	1–2 g IV daily
Cefepime	1–2 g IV q8h
Cefotaxime	1 g IV q8h 2 g IV q6h (severe infections) up to 6 g/d
Ceftazidime	2 g IV q8h
Cephalexin	500 mg PO q6h
Cephazolin	1–2 g IV q8h
Ciprofloxacin	250–500 mg PO q12h 400 mg IV q12h
Clarithromycin	500 mg PO q12h
Clindamycin	150–450 mg PO q8h 200–900 mg IV q8h
Dicloxacillin	500 mg PO q6h 1 g IV q6h

Continues

Commonly used antibiotics in ADULTS (continued)

3

Antibiotic	Dose and route of administration
Doxycycline	100 mg PO q12h
Erythromycin	250 mg PO q6h
Flucloxacillin	500 mg PO q6h 1 g IV q6h
Gentamicin	3–5 mg/kg as initial dose only (dosing frequency depends on creatinine clearance and drug monitoring)
Imipenem	1 g IV q6h
Lincomycin	600 mg IV q8h
Meropenem	1 g IV q8h
Metronidazole	400 mg PO tds 500 mg IV bd
Moxifloxacin	400 mg PO/IV daily
Penicillin V (phenoxymethylpenicillin) Penicillin G (benzylpenicillin)	500 mg PO q6h 1.2–2.4 g IV q6h
Piperacillin + tazobactam	4 + 0.5 g IV q8h
Roxithromycin	300 mg PO daily
Ticarcillin + clavulanate	3 + 0.1 g IV q6h
Vancomycin	1–1.5 g IV as a stat dose 250 mg PO q6h (dosing frequency depends on creatinine clearance and drug monitoring)

4 Miscellaneous drugs—paediatrics

The following tables have been adapted from Shann F, *Drug Doses*, 15th edn, and the *Australian Medicines Handbook.*

Miscellaneous drugs used in PAEDIATRIC patients

Drug	Dose and route of administration
Adenosine	
For arrhythmia	
1st dose	0.1 mg/kg IV push (followed by a rapid saline flush)
Subsequent doses	Increase by 0.1 mg/kg IV every 2 min to a max of 0.5 mg/kg (max adult dose 18 mg) (followed by a rapid saline flush)
Adrenaline	
For anaphylaxis	0.05–0.1 mL/kg of 1:10,000 IV *or* 0.01 mL/kg (= 0.01 mg/kg) of 1:1000 IM (up to max 0.3 mg)
For croup	0.5 mL/kg of 1:1000 nebulised diluted to 6 mL (max 6 mL)
Calcium chloride 10%	0.2 mL/kg IV (max 10 mL)
Calcium gluconate 10%	0.5 mL/kg IV (max 20 mL)
Charcoal	1 g/kg PO/NG
Dexamethasone	0.1–1 mg/kg PO/IM/IV daily
For severe croup	0.6 mg/kg IV/IM (max 20 mg)
Diazepam	0.1–0.4 mg/kg IV/PR 0.04–0.2 mg/kg q8–12h PO
Fentanyl	1–2 microg/kg IM/IV
Glucagon (1 mg = 1 unit)	0.04 mg/kg IV/IM stat
Glucose	
For hypoglycaemia	0.5 mL/kg IV of 50% dextrose < 2 y, use 10% dextrose at 2.5 mL/kg
For hyperkalaemia	2 mL/kg of 50% dextrose IV + 0.1 unit/kg neutral insulin (Actrapid) IV
Hydrocortisone	2–4 mg/kg/dose IV/IM q6h
Ketamine	
For anaesthesia	1–2 mg/kg IV or 5–10 mg/kg IM
For analgesia/ sedation	0.3–1 mg IV or 2–4 mg/kg IM
Loratadine	> 30 kg: 10 mg PO 2–12 y < 30 kg: 5 mg PO 1–2 y: 2.5 mg PO

Continues

Miscellaneous drugs used in PAEDIATRIC patients (continued)

Drug	Dose and route of administration
Midazolam	0.1–0.2 mg/kg IV/IM (up to 0.5 mg/kg) 0.2 mg/kg nasally
Morphine	0.1 mg/kg IV 0.1 mg/kg IM (neonate) 0.2 mg/kg IM (child)
Naloxone	0.01 mg/kg IV/IM (max 0.4 mg) can be repeated every 2 min as necessary
Ondansetron	0.1–0.2 mg/kg PO (usual max 8 mg) 0.2 mg/kg IV over 5 min (max 8 mg)
Phenobarbitone (loading dose)	20 mg/kg IM/IV over 30 min
Phenobarbitone (maintenance dose)	5 mg/kg (max 300 mg) PO/IV/IM
Phenytoin (loading dose)	15–20 mg/kg IV (max 1.5 g) over 1 h
Phenytoin (maintenance dose)	2–3 mg/kg/dose (max 100 mg) PO/IV q8–12h, depending on the age of the child
Prednisolone (initial dose)	1 mg/kg PO stat
Rocuronium	0.6–1.2 mg/kg IV stat, then 0.1–0.2 mg/kg IV boluses
Salbutamol—acute asthma attack	< 6 y: 4–6 puffs via spacer > 6 y: 8–12 puffs via spacer < 2 y: 0.1 mg/kg up to 2.5 mg nebulised > 2 y: 2.5–5 mg nebulised **IV infusion:** — initially 5–10 microg/kg/min for 1 h; — then 1–2 microg/kg/min
Suxamethonium	3 mg/kg IV (neonate) 2 mg/kg IV (child) *Note*: double IV dose for IM
Thiopentone	2–5 mg/kg IV

Commonly used antibiotics in PAEDIATRIC patients

Antibiotic	Dose and route of administration
Amoxycillin	15–25 mg/kg/dose PO q8h
Amoxycillin + clavulanic acid	Dose as for amoxycillin
Ampicillin	15–25 mg/kg/dose IV q6h
Cefaclor	10–15 mg/kg/dose PO q8h
Cefotaxime	< 4-week-old: 25 mg/kg/dose IV q12h > 4-week-old: 25 mg/kg/dose IV q8h
For severe infections	1-week-old: 50 mg/kg/dose IV q8h > 2-week-old: 50 mg/kg/dose IV q6h
Ceftazidime	15–25 mg/kg/dose IV q8h
Ceftriaxone	25 mg/kg/dose IV/IM q12–24h
For severe infections	50 mg/kg/dose IV (max 2 g) q12–24h
For epiglottitis	100 mg/kg (max 2 g) IV (once only)
Cephalexin	7.5 mg/kg/dose PO q6h
Cefalotin	15–25 mg/kg/dose IV q6h
Cephazolin	10–15 mg/kg/dose IV q6h
Dicloxacillin	15–25 mg/kg/dose PO/IV q6h
For severe infections	1-week-old: 25–50 mg/kg/dose (max 2 g) IV q12h 2–4-week-old: 25–50 mg/kg/dose (max 2 g) IV q8h > 4-week-old: 25–50 mg/kg/dose (max 2 g) IV q6h
Flucloxacillin	12.5–25 mg/kg/dose PO q6h 25 mg/kg/dose IV q6h
For severe infections	1-week-old: 50 mg/kg/dose IV q12h 2–4-week-old: 50 mg/kg/dose IV q8h > 4-week-old: 50 mg/kg/dose IV q6h
Gentamicin (initial dose only)	Neonate: 5 mg/kg IV/IM stat 1 month–10 y: 8 mg/kg IV/IM stat > 10 y: 7 mg/kg IV/IM stat *Dose ↓ after initial stat injection*
Penicillin G (benzylpenicillin)	30 mg/kg/dose q6h IV
For serious infections	1-week-old: 50 mg/kg/dose (max 2 g) IV q12h 2–4-week-old: 50 mg/kg/dose (max 2 g) IV q6h > 4-week-old: 50 mg/kg/dose (max 2 g) IV q4h
Penicillin V (phenoxymethylpenicillin)	7.5–15 mg/kg/dose PO q6h
Roxithromycin	2.5–4 mg/kg PO q12h

5 Cardiology

5

Reversible causes of cardiac arrest ('4Hs and 4Ts')	
Hypoxia **H**ypovolaemia **H**ypo/**h**yperkalaemia and metabolic disturbances **H**ypo/**h**yperthermia	**T**ension pneumothorax **T**amponade (cardiac) **T**oxins **T**hromboembolism (pulmonary/ cardiac)

Post-resuscitation care

Aims:
- Maximise neurological outcome.
- Look for and treat the cause of the cardiac arrest.
- Treat complications (arrhythmias).

Re-evaluate A, B, C, D, E.
Perform ECG and CXR.
- Look for STE or new LBBB post arrest.
- Look for trauma related to CPR (e.g. rib fracture).
- Check placement of tubes (ETT, NGT, OGT)/lines.

Check adequacy of perfusion, oxygenation and ventilation (may require advanced airway if not already placed).
- Aim for systolic BP ≥ 100 mmHg.
- Aim for O_2 sats 94–98%

Induce hypothermia (32–34°C) for patients who are unresponsive to verbal command (continue for 12–24 h post arrest).
- Ice packs to neck, axillae, groin.
- Infuse cold fluids (30 mL/kg 0.9% saline).
- Cooling mattress.

Monitor BSLs
- Treat hyperglycaemia (> 10 mmol/L) with insulin but *avoid hypoglycaemia*.

Identify and treat underlying cause of cardiac arrest.
- See table above (4Hs and 4Ts)
- PCI may be indicated even in the absence of STE or new LBBB post arrest.

Adapted from Guideline 11.7, Post-resuscitation therapy in adult advanced life support, 2010, Australian Resuscitation Council. www.resus.org.au.

CARDIAC MARKERS

Cardiac markers—approximate time sequence from onset of symptoms

Cardiac marker	Earliest rise (h)	Peak rise (h)	Normalise (d)
CK-MB	4–6	24	2–3
Troponin I	4–6	12	3–10
Troponin T (includes high sensitivity test)	3–12	12	7–10

Causes of elevated troponins other than ACS

Cardiovascular	Arrhythmias HOCM Coronary vasospasm CCF Aortic valve disease Aortic dissection LVH
Respiratory	PE Severe pulmonary hypertension
CNS	Acute neurological disease Stroke SAH
Drug toxicity or toxins	Adriamycin Fluorouracil Snake venom
Infiltrative diseases	Amyloidosis Haemochromatosis Sarcoidosis Scleroderma
Inflammatory diseases	Myocarditis Kawasaki disease
Trauma	Cardiac contusion or other trauma/surgery Cardiac surgery Cardiac interventions Pacing Cardioversion Burns, especially if > 25% of BSA
Miscellaneous	Renal failure Critically ill patients Strenuous exercise Rhabdomyolysis with cardiac injury

MANAGEMENT OF STEMI (STEACS)

Thrombolysis/fibrinolysis versus percutaneous coronary intervention (PCI)

5

- Always consider PCI as the preferred primary reperfusion therapy.
- Primary PCI is superior to thrombolysis **IF** it occurs:
  within 1 hour if the onset of chest pain < 1 hour
  or
  within 90 minutes if a patient presents later.
- PCI or CAGS = preferred treatment options for cardiogenic shock secondary to STEMI.

Contraindications for thrombolysis for AMI

Absolute contraindications

- Any prior ICH
- CVA in the preceding 3 months
- Intracranial neoplasms or cerebral structural vascular lesions (e.g. AVM)
- Significant closed head or facial trauma (within 3 months)
- Active bleeding or known bleeding disorder (excluding menses)
- Suspected aortic dissection

Relative contraindications

- CVA > 3 months ago
- Dementia
- Current anticoagulant therapy
- Pregnancy
- Non-compressible vascular punctures
- Traumatic or prolonged (> 10 min) CPR
- Refractory hypertension (SBP > 180 mmHg or DBP > 110 mmHg)
- Recent major surgery (within 3 weeks)
- Recent internal bleeding (within 4 weeks)
- Active peptic ulcer

STEMI high-risk features

- Advanced age
- Hypotension
- Tachycardia
- Heart failure
- Anterior MI

A TIMI (thrombolysis in myocardial infarction) risk score for STEMI which predicts 30-day mortality after an MI is available at http://circ.ahajournals.org/content/102/17/2031.abstract.

MANAGEMENT OF UA AND NSTEMI (NSTEACS)

(Adapted from the Australian Resuscitation Council Guidelines and the National Heart Foundation.)

High-risk features

Presentation with clinical features consistent with ACS and any of:

History	Signs	Investigations
• Repetitive/ prolonged (> 10 min) chest pain • Syncope • LVEF < 40% • Prior PCI within 6 months • Prior CAGS • Diabetes or chronic kidney disease (EGFR < 60 mL/min) with classic chest pain	• Haemodynamic compromise • Sustained VT	• Elevated cardiac marker • ST depression ≥ 0.5 mm • New T wave inversion ≥ 2 mm • Transient ST elevation (≥ 0.5 mm) in more than two contiguous leads

5

Intermediate-risk features

Presentation with clinical features consistent with ACS and any of the following AND NOT meeting any criteria for high-risk NSTEACS:

History	Investigations
• Chest pain within past 48 h — at rest — repetitive — prolonged • Age > 65 y • Known IHD • ≥ 2 of the following risk factors: — hypertension — family history — smoking — hyperlipidaemia • Diabetes or chronic kidney disease with non-classical chest pain • Prior aspirin use	• No high risk ECG changes

5

Management of UA/NSTEMI patients

High-risk	Intermediate-risk
• Aggressive medical therapy — aspirin 300 mg — clopidogrel (600 mg if PCI planned; 300 mg if fibrinolysis) — heparin/enoxaparin — beta-blocker • Coronary angiography	• Require further investigation to reclassify as high- or low-risk • Options include: — exercise stress test — sestamibi — CT coronary angiogram

A TIMI (thrombolysis in myocardial infarction) risk score for UA/NSTEMI, indicating risk of death and ischaemic events, is available at stroke.ahajournals.org/content/41/12/2731.figures-only.

CHADS$_2$ SCORE FOR AF

CHADS$_2$ score: a clinical prediction rule to determine the risk of stroke in a patient with non-rheumatic atrial fibrillation

	Condition	Points
C	Congestive cardiac failure	1
H	Hypertension	1
A	Age ≥ 75 y	1
D	Diabetes	1
S$_2$	Prior stroke/TIA	2

CHADS$_2$ score	Stroke risk %	95% CI
0	1.9	1.2–3.0
1	2.8	2.0–3.8
2	4.0	3.1–5.1
3	5.9	4.6–7.3
4	8.5	6.3–11.1
5	12.5	8.2–17.5
6	18.2	10.5–27.4

Score	Risk	Anticoagulation therapy	Considerations
0	Low	None or aspirin	Aspirin daily
1	Moderate	Aspirin or warfarin	Aspirin daily or raise INR to 2–3
≥ 2	Moderate/high	Warfarin	Raise INR to 2–3, unless contraindicated

The CHA$_2$DS$_2$VASc score, a refinement incorporating additional stroke risk factors, can be found at: http://jama.jamanetwork.com/article.aspx?articleid=192996#tab3.

6 ECGs

ECG FEATURES

Speed and calibration of the ECG

	Measurement	Duration
Horizontally (width/duration)		
Speed	25 mm/sec	
1 small box	1 mm^2	0.04 s = 40 ms
1 large box	5 mm^2	0.2 s = 200 ms
5 large boxes	25 mm^2	1 s
300 large boxes		1 min
Vertically (amplitude/voltage)		
1 small box	1 mm	0.1 mV
2 large boxes	10 mm	1 mV

ECG TERMINOLOGY

Concordance: same polarity—i.e. deflections are occurring in the same direction.

Disconcordance: deflections are occurring in opposite directions.

R wave progression: normally see a relative increase in R wave size and decrease in S wave size when moving from V_1 to V_6.

Transition zone: the chest lead where the R wave approximately equals the S wave—usually V_3/V_4.

Time to onset of intrinsicoid deflection: the time from the beginning of QRS to the peak of the R wave.

Axis:

- Is the average direction of the spread of depolarisation through the ventricles when looking at the front of the patient.
- Leads aVR and II look at the heart from opposite directions.
- Looking at the front of a patient, depolarisation spreads from approx 11 o'clock to 5 o'clock (i.e., deflections are mainly negative in aVR and positive in II).
- Normal axis is a positive deflection in I, II, III as the depolarising wave is spreading towards these leads.

Normal waves, intervals and complexes in the ECG

	Represents	Duration: Width	Duration: Amplitude	Features	Special cases/ abnormalities
P wave	Atrial depolarisation	< 120 ms	< 1 mm	Positive in II, negative in aVR, biphasic in V_1	Bifid P waves > 120 ms = P mitrale (left atrial enlargement) Peaked P wave amplitude > 2.5 mm = P pulmonale (right atrial enlargement)
PR interval	Time taken for conduction from atria to ventricles	120–200 ms (3–5 small squares)	N/A		PR > 200 ms = 1st degree heart block
QRS complex	Ventricular depolarisation	< 120 ms (< 3 small squares)			
ST segment	Beginning of ventricular repolarisation	N/A	N/A	J point = beginning of the ST segment (i.e., junction of the QRS complex and ST segment)	
T wave	Ventricular repolarisation			Normally is asymmetrical in shape and concordant with QRS	Peaked and symmetrical = hyperacute AMI or hyperkalaemia
QT interval		Average QTc ≤ 440 ms		Bazett's formula QTc = QT (in ms) ÷ √RR —QTc = QT interval corrected for HR —RR = 60/HR	'Abnormal' QTc values > 450 ms (males) > 470 ms (females) Prolongation = increased risk of developing ventricular arrhythmias
U wave	Last phase of ventricular repolarisation		≤ 1 mm or < 25% the amplitude of T wave Looks bigger as the HR ↓	Small rounded deflection following T wave (usually of same polarity as T wave)	↑ amplitude = hypokalaemia, drugs (amiodarone, sotalol, quinidine, procainamide)

ECG AXIS

ECG axis features

Axis		ECG features
Normal	–30° to +90°	Positive in leads I, II and III
Left axis deviation	< –30°	Positive in lead I, negative in II, III
Right axis deviation	> +100°	Negative in lead I, positive in II, III
Extreme axis deviation	–100° to +180°	Negative in I and aVF

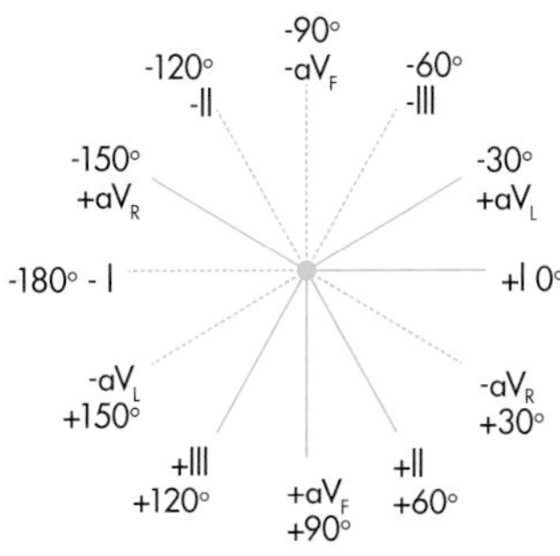

Figure 6.1 Hexaxial lead diagram

Causes of axis deviation

Deviation	Causes
Right axis	Right ventricular hypertrophy MI of lateral wall of LV Left posterior fascicular block Chronic lung disease Acute massive pulmonary embolism
Left axis	Left ventricular hypertrophy Left anterior fascicular block Inferior MI

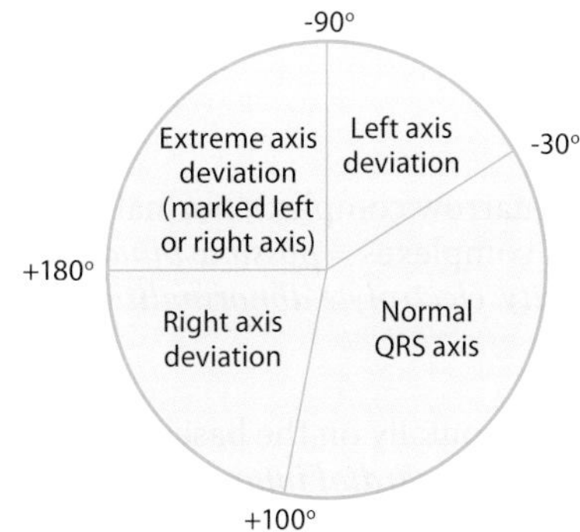

Figure 6.2 Normal QRS axis and axis deviation
Most ECGs show either a normal axis or left or right axis deviation. Occasionally, the QRS axis is between –90° and 180°. Such an extreme shift may be caused by marked left or right axis deviation.

Figures 6.1 and 6.2 adapted from Goldberger AL, Clinical electrocardiography: a simplified approach, 7th edn, Philadelphia: Mosby, 2006: Figs 5-2 and 5-13. Available: www.mdconsult.com/books/bbmapAsset?appID=MDC&isbn=0-323-04038-1&eid=4-u1.0-B0-323-04038-1..50006-8..gr13&assetType=full.

6

ECG INTERPRETATION

ECG parameters to check

Standardisation:

- Check the paper speed (25 mm/s) and voltage (1 mV = 10 mm).

Rate:

- Count the number of large boxes between successive QRS complexes (use the R–R interval).
- Divide 300 by the above number (e.g. if there are 5 large boxes between successive QRS complexes, then the heart rate is 300 ÷ 5 = 60/min).
- < 60/min = bradycardia.
- > 100/min = tachycardia.

Rhythm:

- Regular versus irregular.
- If irregular, is it regularly irregular (*2nd degree heart block, trigeminy*) or irregularly irregular (*atrial fibrillation*)?

P waves:

- Relationship of P waves to QRS complex: is each P wave followed by a QRS complex?
- Is the PR interval the same duration for all complexes?
- If all P waves and QRS complexes are completely unrelated = *AV dissociation.*

QRS complex:

Look at the:

- axis
- amplitude
- duration—short (narrow complex), normal or widened (broad complex)? Broad complexes = *possible bundle branch block (BBB), drug toxicity, electrolyte abnormalities.*

ST segment:

Is the ST segment:

- isoelectric (lies horizontally on the baseline)—*normal*?
- elevated = possible *myocardial infarction* or *pericarditis* (if widespread)?
- depressed = possible *ischaemia*, drug effect (*digoxin gives 'reverse tick' pattern*)?

T wave:

Look at polarity, *height* and shape:

- Inverted in aVR, upright in I, II
- May be normally inverted in III, V1
- Inversion in V_1–V_2 'persistent juvenile pattern'
- Examples of patterns:
  - Peaked = hyperkalaemia or hyperacute in early AMI
  - Flattened or inverted = ischaemia
  - Wellen's syndrome = symmetrical deep T wave inversion (usually > 2 mm) in praecordial leads; indicative of critical proximal LAD stenosis

6

Conduction abnormalities

Type	Pattern	Causes
LBBB 'WILLIAM'	QRS > 120 ms Broad, monophasic R waves in I, V_5, V_6 (usually notched/slurred) > 40 ms to peak of R wave in V_5, V_6 (delayed intrinsicoid deflection)	AMI Degenerative Cardiomyopathies Brugada syndrome
RBBB 'MARROW'	QRS > 120 ms rSR' ('M' shape) in V_1 or V_2 Late intrinsicoid deflection in V_1 S wave > 40 ms (or at least longer than R wave duration) in I and V_6 2nd R' is greater in amplitude than 1st r deflection May be associated T wave inversion	Can be normal PE Cor pulmonale Brugada syndrome AMI Myocarditis
Brugada syndrome	RBBB (may be incomplete) with ST ↑ in V_1–V_3 Abnormalities may be transient Normal QT	Channelopathy (Na)—mutation of the *SCN5A* gene in 10–30%
WPW syndrome	Normal P wave axis and morphology PR < 120 ms Delta wave (initial slurring of the QRS)	Alternative conduction pathway

6

Myocardial infarction localisation

Myocardial infarction	Leads involved
Inferior	II, III, aVF Reciprocal changes in aVL
Anterior	V_1–V_4 Reciprocal changes in III, aVF
Septal	V_1–V_2
Lateral	V_5–V_6, I, aVL
Posterior	ST depression, large R wave in V_1–V_3 ST elevation in posterior leads (V_7–V_9)
Right ventricular	ST elevation > 1 mm in V_4R Associated with 40% of inferior MI

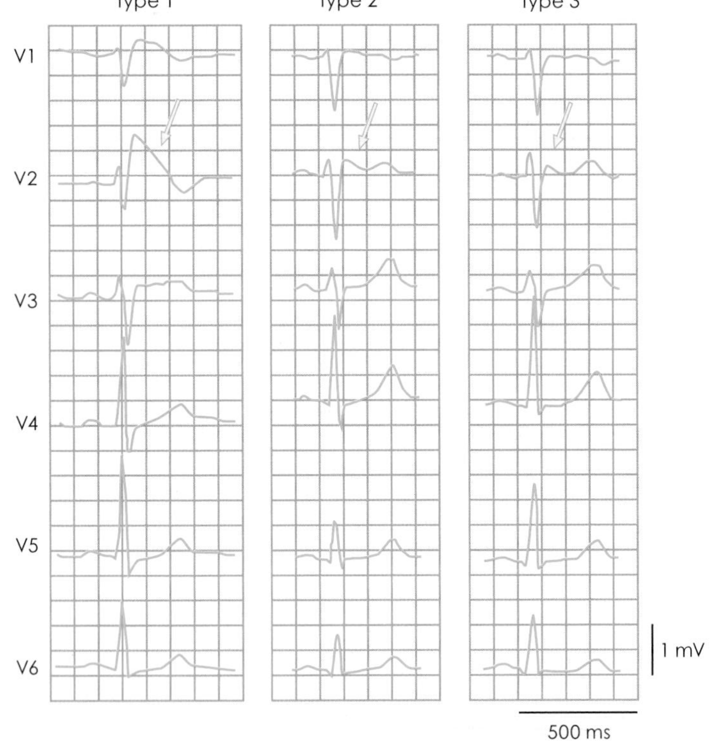

Figure 6.3 Brugada syndrome
(From Wilde AA, Strickberger SA et al: J Am Coll Cardio 47:473–484, 2006, Fig. 3.) In Ferri's Clinical Advisor 2013, 1st ed. Copyright © 2012 Mosby

BBB and AMI

Sgarbossa criteria

ECG criteria that increase specificity of AMI in patients that present with chest pain and new/old LBBB:

- A score ≥ 2 is > 85% specific for AMI.
- Remember, new LBBB or LBBB with a concordant segment → reperfusion recommended.

ECG changes	Points
Concordant ST elevation ≥ 1 mm in one lead	5
Concordant ST depression ≥ 1 mm in one of leads V_1–V_3	3
Disconcordant ST elevation ≥ 5 mm	2

6

RBBB

- Any ST elevation, even if disconcordant, is abnormal.
- In V_1–V_3, there is often up to 1 mm ST depression, so minimal ST elevation may be seen in an anterior AMI.

Differentiating VT versus SVT with aberrancy

Features making VT more likely	
Clinical features	**ECG features**
• Age > 35 y • IHD • CCF • History of AMI • Positive family history	• AV dissociation • Fusion beats • Capture beats • Extreme 'NW axis' • Concordance of QRS complexes in limb leads (all negative or all positive) • Brugada's sign – > 100 ms from onset of QRS to nadir of S wave • Absence of LBBB or RBBB morphology

7 Respiratory

OXYGEN SATURATION/INSPIRED OXYGEN

Oxygen dissociation curve (approximations)

% Oxygen saturation	Approximate pO_2 (mmHg)
60	30
70	40
80	50
90	60

Correlation between FiO_2 and expected pO_2: 'factor of 5' rule

7

Examples:
21% FiO_2 = pO_2 ~ 100 mmHg
90% FiO_2 = pO_2 ~ 450 mmHg
100% FiO_2 = pO_2 ~ 500 mmHg

Approximate FiO_2 related to flow rates of semi-rigid masks (i.e. Hudson, non-rebreathing masks)

O_2 flow rate (L/min)	Approximate FiO_2
4	0.35
6	0.50
8	0.55
10	0.60
12	0.65
15	0.70

ALVEOLAR OXYGEN AND A–a GRADIENT

Alveolar gas equation

$$P_AO_2 = PiO_2 - (P_ACO_2 \times 1.25)$$

where:

- P_AO_2 is the alveolar pO_2
- PiO_2 is the inspired $pO_2 = 713 \times FiO_2$
- P_ACO_2 is the alveolar pCO_2 (assumed to be equal to the measured arterial blood gas estimation of CO_2)

Example:

If at room air (21% FiO_2) P_ACO_2 = 40 mmHg, then

$$\begin{aligned} P_AO_2 &= (713 \times 0.21) - (40 \times 1.25)\ \text{mmHg} \\ &= 150 - 50\ \text{mmHg} \\ &= 100\ \text{mmHg} \end{aligned}$$

A–a gradient

$$\text{A–a gradient} = P_AO_2 - P_aO_2$$

where:

- P_AO_2 is the alveolar pO_2
- P_aO_2 is the arterial blood gas estimation of O_2

Normal value of A–a gradient:

$$\text{Calculating normal A–a gradient} = (\text{age} \div 4) + 4$$

Note: P_aO_2 decreases with age. As an approximate guide,

$$P_aO_2 \text{ at room air} = [100 - (\text{age} \div 3)] \text{ mmHg}.$$

CURB-65 SCORE

A severity scoring system for community-acquired pneumonia.

	Criterion	Score
C	Confusion	1
U	Urea > 7 mmol/L	1
R	Respiratory rate ≥ 30/min	1
B	BP (SBP ≤ 90 mmHg or DBP ≤ 60 mmHg)	1
65	≥ 65 years	1

Score	% 30-day mortality	Treatment considerations
1	2.7 (low risk)	Outpatient
2	6.8 (moderate risk)	Inpatient or close outpatient follow-up
3	14 (severe risk)	Inpatient ± intensive care admission
4 or 5	27.8 (highest risk)	Inpatient ± intensive care admission

7

SPIROMETRY PATTERNS OF OBSTRUCTIVE AND RESTRICTIVE RESPIRATORY DISEASES

Spirometric values

Definitions		
FVC	Forced vital capacity; the total volume of air that can be exhaled during a maximal forced expiration effort	
FEV_1	Forced expiratory volume in one second; the volume of air exhaled in the first second under force after a maximal inhalation	
FEV_1/FVC ratio	The percentage of the FVC expired in 1 second	
Patterns		
	Obstructive	**Restrictive**
FEV_1	↓	↓ or normal
FVC	Normal or ↓ if very severe	↓
FEV_1/FVC	< 0.70	> 0.70

CLASSIFICATION OF SEVERITY OF COPD

Stage	FEV_1 / FVC*	FEV_1	Clinical features
I (mild)	< 0.70	≥ 80% predicted	Chronic cough, sputum production
II (moderate)	< 0.70	50% ≤ FEV_1 < 80% predicted	Cough, sputum production, SOB
III (severe)	< 0.70	30% ≤ FEV_1 < 50% predicted	↑SOB, ↓exercise tolerance, fatigue, ↑frequency of exacerbations
IV (very severe)	< 0.70	FEV_1 < 30% or < 50% predicted plus chronic respiratory failure	Cor pulmonale, hypoxia, impaired quality of life, life-threatening exacerbations

* Post-bronchodilator measurements are recommended.
Adapted from the Global Initiative on Chronic Obstructive Lung Disease, Table 2. At-a-glance Outpatient Management Reference for Chronic Obstructive Pulmonary Disease (COPD).

NORMAL VALUES OF PEAK EXPIRATORY FLOW

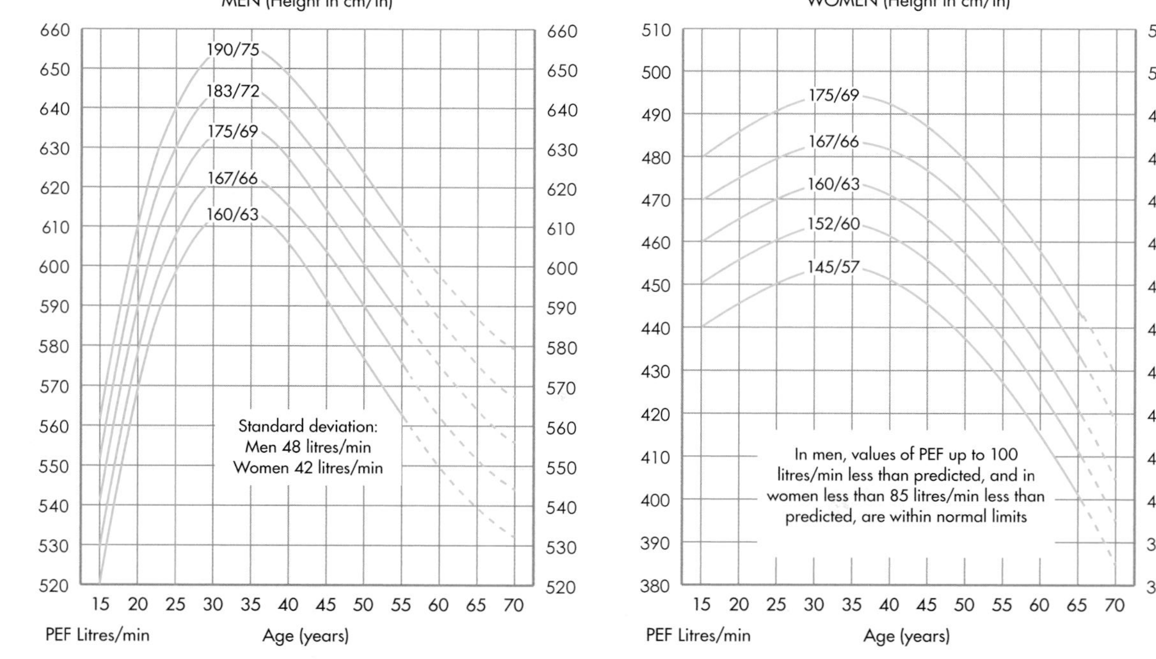

Figure 7.1 Normal values of peak expiratory flow for adult males

Figure 7.2 Normal values of peak expiratory flow for adult females

8 Trauma

TRANSFUSION

Massive transfusion in severe trauma

(Replacement of a patient's total blood volume over 24 hours or replacement of > 50% blood volume)

Practical points:

- After 6 units or as soon as the patient is recognised as potentially requiring a massive transfusion, **activate** the massive transfusion protocol.
- Use a blood warmer.
- Priority should be placed in early definitive haemostasis (e.g. surgery or interventional radiology).
- Identify patients who are on anticoagulants or antiplatelet therapy.
- Acidosis and hypothermia can impair coagulation.

Possible complications of massive transfusion:

- Transfusion of 10–12 units of PRBCs can cause:
  - dilutional thrombocytopenia (up to 50%)
  - dilutional effect on coagulation factors (approx 10% per 500 mL of red cells transfused).
- Hypothermia
- Hypocalcaemia (citrate binds ionised calcium)
- Hyperkalaemia

Other products to use:

- Aim for a ratio of 1 PRBCs:1 FFP.
- Be guided by bleeding visually stopped, haemodynamics.
- Role of factors and plasma probably greater than role of platelets.
- Aim for 4–6 units PRBCs:1 unit pooled platelets.
- Consider 6 units cryoprecipitate.

Monitoring

- Suggest:
  - arterial/venous gas sampling every 60–90 min
  - FBC, UEC, coagulation studies, fibrinogen every 3 h.
- Aim for:
  - platelets > 50×10^9/L
  - fibrinogen > 1 g/L
  - PT, APTT > 1.5 × mean control
  - Hb > 80 g/L

Adjunctive agents to consider:

- Tranexamic acid
  - Antifibrinolytic agent
  - 1 g IV bolus (over 10 min) **within 3 h** of injury
- Recombinant factor VIIa
  - Controversial
  - Use mainly in blunt trauma
- Prothrombinex
- Vitamin K

CANADIAN CT HEAD RULE

Role: to assist in determining who may need CT imaging to determine the presence of intracranial injury.

This rule **only applies** to those with GCS 13–15, witnessed LOC, amnesia to the head injury event or confusion.

8

GCS < 15 at 2 h after injury	Yes	High risk*
Suspected open or depressed skull #	Yes	High risk*
Any sign of base of skull #: —Haemotympanum, — 'Racoon eyes' —CSF otorrhoea/rhinorrhoea —Battle's sign	Yes	High risk*
Vomiting ≥ 2 episodes	Yes	High risk*
Age ≥ 65 years	Yes	High risk*
Amnesia before impact ≥ 30 min	Yes	Medium risk**
Dangerous mechanism: —Fall from height > 1 m (3 ft) or 5 stairs —Pedestrian struck by motor vehicle —Occupant ejected from motor vehicle	Yes	Medium risk**

* High risk of injury requiring neurosurgical intervention.
** Medium risk of brain injury on CT.

CANADIAN C-SPINE RULE

Canadian C-spine criteria (see Figure 8.1 also):

1 Perform imaging on the patient who has any of the following **high-risk criteria**:
   - Age ≥ 65 years
   - Dangerous mechanism of injury:
     - Fall from 1 m (3 ft) or 5 stairs
     - Axial load to the head, such as diving accident
     - MVA at high speed (> 100 km/h)

    - Motorised recreational vehicle accident
    - Ejection from a vehicle
    - Bicycle collision with an immovable object, such as a tree or parked car
  - Paraesthesiae in the extremities
2. If none of the above, assess for any **low-risk factor** that allows assessment of ROM of the neck:
   - Simple rear end MVA. This excludes:
     - Pushed into oncoming traffic
     - Hit by bus or large truck
     - Rollover
     - Hit by high speed (> 100 km/h) vehicle
   - Sitting position in the ED
   - Ambulatory at any time
   - Delayed onset of neck pain
   - Absence of midline cervical spine tenderness

   If the patient has none of the low-risk criteria, imaging must be done.

   If the patient has any of the low-risk criteria, assess ROM of the neck.
3. Test active ROM of the neck:
   - Can the patient rotate their neck actively 45° both left and right?
     - If YES → no imaging is required.
     - If NO → imaging is recommended.

NEXUS CRITERIA FOR C-SPINE IMAGING

C-spine imaging is indicated for all trauma patients UNLESS they have ALL the following criteria:

1. No posterior midline cervical tenderness
2. No evidence of intoxication
3. A normal level of alertness
4. No focal neurological deficit
5. No distracting painful injuries

(Based on Hoffman JR et al, Selective cervical spine radiography in blunt trauma: methodology of the National Emergency X-Radiography Utilization Study (NEXUS). Ann Emerg Med 1998;32(4):461–9.)

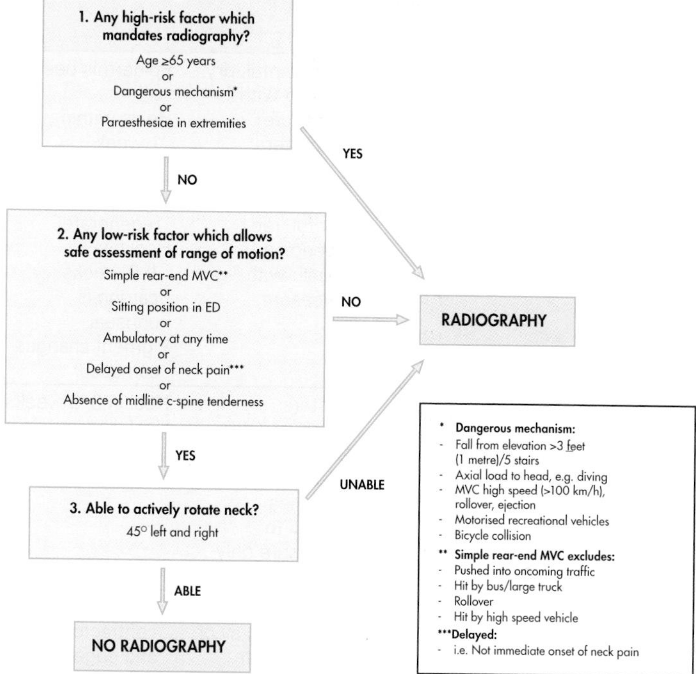

Figure 8.1 Canadian C-spine rule
Adapted from Stiell IG et al. The Canadian CT head rule for patients with minor head injury. Lancet 2001;357:1391–6.

8

BURNS

Classification of burns

Depth	Structures involved	Clinical features	Healing
Superficial	Epidermis only	Red, painful, dry, blanch with pressure No blisters	Epidermis peels off Heals within 1 week No scarring
Partial thickness—superficial	Epidermis and superficial dermis	Blisters Painful, red, weeping Blanch with pressure	Skin can regenerate Heal by 1–3 weeks Scarring is unusual Pigment changes can occur
Partial thickness—deep (can be difficult to differentiate from full thickness)	As above plus damage to hair follicles/glandular tissue	Blisters Wet/waxy dry Dark red or yellow-white patches Painful to pressure only Do not blanch	Heal in 3–8 weeks Heal by scarring
Full thickness	All layers of dermis plus often subcutaneous tissue	Charred or leathery gray or waxy white Insensate	Heal by wound contracture and edge epithelialisation Skin cannot regenerate

Eschar

- Dead and denatured dermis
- Can compromise viability of limb/torso if circumferential

Burn treatment tips

- Remove from source of burning
- Remove burnt clothing
- A, B, C assessment
- O_2 (ideally humidified)
- Water to cool the burn (only useful in 1st 3 h post injury)
- Cover burn
- Watch for hypothermia and no ice

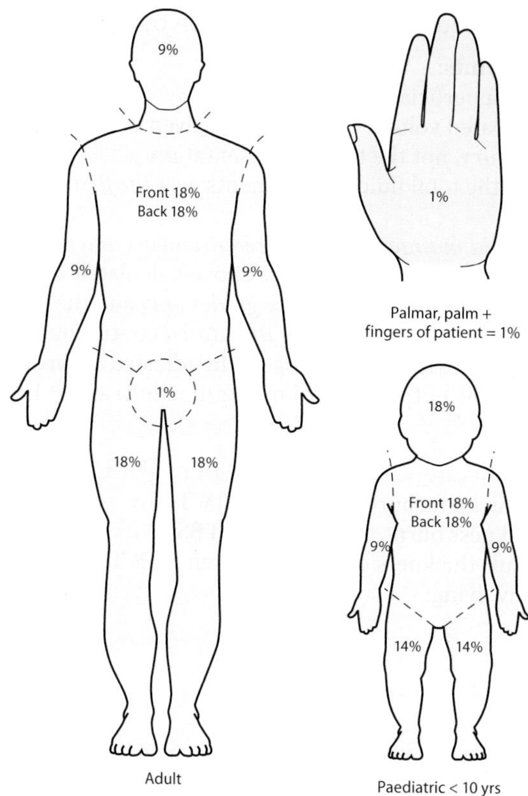

Figure 8.2 Rule of Nines: determining the percentage total body surface area (TBSA) involved; ignore simple erythema

- Assess % TBSA affected
- For burns > 15% TBSA:
  - IV access and begin fluid resuscitation
  - IV morphine
  - NBM
  - ± IDC
- Analgesia
- Check tetanus immunisation status

Parkland formula for fluid requirement

4 mL × bodyweight (kg) × % TBSA burned (adults)

Important points:

- Excludes superficial burns.
- The calculated volume above is to be given over 24 h from the *time of injury*, not the time of presentation.
- Give *half* the total fluid requirements *over the first 8 h*, the rest over 16 h.
- Need to *add maintenance fluid requirements and other losses* (e.g. traumatic blood loss) to the above-calculated volume.
- Fluid resuscitation formulas are *guides only* and the patient's *haemodynamic status must be monitored* continuously (HR, BP, urine output) with fluid management adjusted accordingly.
- Aim for urine output of > 0.5 mL/kg/h (adult) and ≥ 1 mL/kg/h (child).

Consultation/referral criteria to a specialist burns unit

- Partial-thickness burns in adults > 0% TBSA
- Full-thickness burns in adults > 5% TBSA
- Partial/full-thickness burns in children > 5% TBSA
- Burns involving:
  - Face
  - Eyes
  - Ears
  - Hands
  - Feet
  - Genitalia
  - Perineum
  - Major joints
- Chemical burns
- Electrical/lightning burns
- Burns associated with inhalational injury
- Circumferential burns to the limbs or chest
- Burns associated with other traumatic injuries
- Burns associated with comorbidities that could affect management and outcome
- Suspected child abuse

TETANUS PROPHYLAXIS

National Health and Medical Research Council (NHMRC) recommendations for tetanus prophylaxis (adapted from NHMRC, The Australian Immunisation Handbook, *9th edn, 2008. Online. Available: www.health.gov.au/internet/immunise/publishing.nsf/content/handbook-home).*

	Clean, minor wounds		All other wounds	
Tetanus immunisation history	**Tetanus booster**	**Tetanus Ig**	**Tetanus booster**	**Tetanus Ig**
Uncertain or < 3 doses	Yes	No	Yes	Yes
≥ 3 doses plus < 5 y since last dose	No	No	No	No
≥ 3 doses plus 5–10 y since last dose	No	No	Yes	No
≥ 3 doses plus > 10 y since last dose	Yes	No	Yes	No

Features of tetanus-prone wounds

Wounds contaminated with soil, dust or horse manure
Bite wounds
Deep penetrating wounds
Compound fractures
Wounds with foreign bodies (especially wood)
Wounds with extensive tissue damage (e.g. contusions, burns)
Reimplantation of an avulsed tooth
Wounds complicated by pyogenic infection

Tetanus booster options

For < 8 y:

(*Note*: DTPa = child formulations of diphtheria, tetanus, acellular pertussis-containing vaccines)

- DTPa-combinations
  - Infanrix Hexa DTPa (DTPa + hepB + inactivated polio, Hib)
  - Infanrix-IPV (DTPa + inactivated polio)
  - Infanrix Penta (DTPa + hepB + inactivated polio)

For > 8 y:

(*Note*: dTpa = adult and adolescent formulations of diphtheria, tetanus, acellular pertussis)

- ADT booster (adult formulation of diphtheria, tetanus): 0.5 mL
- Adacel (dTpa)
- Boostrix (dTpa)
- dTpa combinations:
  - Adacel Polio (dTpa + polio)
  - Boostrix-IPV (dTpa + polio)

Tetanus immunoglobulin (TIG):

- 250 IU IM
- If > 24 h have elapsed, use 500 IU
- Give a tetanus toxoid-containing vaccine concurrently in a different site

LOCAL ANAESTHETICS

Types of local anaesthetics

(*Note*: allergies = more common with esters than amides.)

Amides	Bupivacaine Levobupivacaine Lignocaine Prilocaine Ropivacaine
Esters	Amethocaine Cocaine

Local anaesthesia—buffering

When infiltrating lignocaine subcutaneously for local anaesthesia, buffering with sodium bicarbonate benefits in several ways:

- It reduces the pain of the injection.
- It decreases the time to onset of action.
- It maintains efficacy and duration of the local anaesthetic effect.

To buffer the lignocaine, use 1 part of sodium bicarbonate 8.4% injection (containing bicarbonate 1 mmol/mL) to 9 parts of lignocaine 1%.

Local anaesthetic concentration

Concentrations of local anaesthetics are expressed as a % or in mg/mL.

Multiply by 10 to convert from percentage to mg/mL (e.g. 0.5% = 5 mg/mL).

% Concentration	Concentration in g/100 mL	Dose per mL
0.25%	0.25 g/100 mL	2.5 mg/mL
0.5%	0.5 g/100 mL	5 mg/mL
1%	1 g/100 mL	10 mg/mL
2%	2 g/100 mL	20 mg/mL

Local anaesthetics combined with adrenaline

Do not use in:

- nose
- digits
- ears
- genitals.

9 Metabolic equations and electrolytes

ANION GAP (AG)

AG acidosis

$$AG = (Na^+) - (HCO_3^- + Cl^-)$$
$$\text{Normal AG} = 3\text{–}12$$

Causes of ↑ AG acidosis (mnemonic—'CATMUDPILES'):

C Cyanide
A Alcoholic ketoacidosis
T Toluene
M Methanol, Metformin
U Uraemia
D Diabetic ketoacidosis
P Paraldehyde, Propylene glycol
I Iron, Isoniazid
L Lactic acidosis
E Ethylene glycol
S Starvation ketoacidosis, Salicylates

Causes of normal AG acidosis (mnemonic—'USED CARP'):

U Ureteroenterostomy
S Small bowel fistula
E Extra chloride (hyperchloraemic acidosis)
D Diarrhoea, resolving DKA, Drugs (acetazolamide, cholestyramine)
C Carbonic anhydrase deficiency
A Adrenal insufficiency
R Renal tubular acidosis (type 1, 2, 4)
P Pancreatic fistula

ACID–BASE DISORDERS FORMULAS: COMPENSATORY MECHANISMS

These formulas are used to assess the appropriateness of the compensatory response. Deviations from these values indicate mixed metabolic/respiratory disorders.

Metabolic acidosis (Winter's formula)

$$\text{Expected } PCO_2 = (1.5 \times HCO_3^-) + 8 \text{ mmHg } (\pm 2)$$

If the actual PCO_2 > expected PCO_2, there is a concomitant respiratory acidosis.

9

Metabolic alkalosis

$$\text{Expected } PCO_2 = (0.7 \times HCO_3^-) + 20 \text{ mmHg } (\pm 5)$$

If the actual PCO_2 < expected PCO_2, there is a concomitant respiratory alkalosis.

Respiratory acidosis

Acute: ↑ 1 mmol HCO_3^- per 10 mmHg ↑ PCO_2 above 40 mmHg

$$\text{Expected } HCO_3^- = 24 + [(\text{actual } PCO_2 - 40) \div 10] \text{ mmol/L}$$

Chronic: ↑ 4 mmol HCO_3^- per 10 mmHg ↑ PCO_2 above 40 mmHg

$$\text{Expected } HCO_3^- = 24 + 4\,[(\text{actual } PCO_2 - 40) \div 10] \text{ mmol/L}$$

Respiratory alkalosis

Acute: ↓ 2 mmol HCO_3^- per 10 mmHg ↓ PCO_2 below 40 mmHg

9

$$\text{Expected } HCO_3^- = 24 - 2\,[(40 - \text{actual } PCO_2) \div 10] \text{ mmol/L}$$

Note: This rarely leads to a HCO_3^- < 8 mmol/L. If HCO_3^- < 18 mmol/L, a metabolic acidosis co-exists.

Chronic: ↓ 5 mmol HCO_3^- per 10 mmHg ↓ PCO_2 below 40 mmHg

$$\text{Expected } HCO_3^- = 24 - 5\,[(40 - \text{actual } PCO_2) \div 10] \text{ mmol/L } (\pm 2)$$

Note: Compensation is limited to HCO_3^- of about 12–15 mmol/L.

OSMOLAR GAP

Calculating the osmolar gap

Osmolar gap = Measured osmolarity – Calculated osmolarity
(Normal osmolar gap ≤ 10 mOsm/L.)

Calculated osmolarity = (2 × Na^+) + Glucose + Urea
(where all parameters are in mmol/L).

Exogenous agents causing ↑ osmolar gap

- Ethanol
- Methanol
- Ethylene glycol
- Isopropyl alcohol
- Propylene glycol
- Mannitol
- Sorbitol
- Glycine
- Glycerol

Non-toxicological conditions associated with ↑ osmolar gap

- DKA
- Alcoholic ketoacidosis
- Severe lactic acidosis
- Chronic renal failure
- Trauma and burns
- Hyperlipidaemia
- Hyperproteinaemia
- Massive hypermagnesaemia

HYPERKALAEMIA

- Severe > 7 mmol/L
- Signs and symptoms:
  - Often asymptomatic
  - Neuromuscular (weakness → paralysis)
  - Arrhythmias (including palpitations, syncope, chest pain)

Causes of true hyperkalaemia

↑ cellular release of K^+	Massive blood transfusion Massive haemolysis Rhabdomyolysis Burns Trauma Tumour lysis syndrome
Shift of K^+ out of cells	Metabolic acidosis Insulin deficiency Beta blockers Digoxin overdose Suxamethonium
↓ renal excretion of K^+	Renal failure Mineralocorticoid deficiency: — Hypoaldosteronism — Addison's disease Medications: — ACEIs — Angiotensin receptor blockers — Cyclosporin — Tacrolimus — Spironolactone (K^+ sparing)

ECG changes of hyperkalaemia

- Tall peaked T waves (> 5 mm)
- PR prolongation
- Small amplitude P waves/loss of P wave
- ↑ QRS width
- Intraventricular blocks, BBB
- Fusion of QRS complex with T wave (→ sine wave)
- Bradycardias, AV dissociation, VT, VF, PEA

Treatment options for true hyperkalaemia

Note: Patients with hyperkalaemia and normal ECGs can suddenly go into cardiac arrest. The ECG is not an indicator of how serious the hyperkalaemia is in that particular patient.

Treatment	Dose	Time to onset of effect	Duration of effect
Temporary			
Calcium gluconate 10% (if patient awake)	10 mL IV; can be repeated at 10-min intervals	Should improve ECG within 3 min	30 min
Calcium chloride 10% (if patient in cardiac arrest)	10 mL IV		
Glucose and short-acting insulin (Actrapid)	50 mL 50% dextrose IV, 10 U of Actrapid IV (if BSL > 15 mmol/L dextrose is not required)	Within 15 min (K ↓ by 0.5–1 mmol/L)	4–6 h
Salbutamol	10–20 mg nebulised	Within 30 min (K ↓ by 0.5–1 mmol/L)	2 h
Sodium bicarbonate 8.4% (IF patient is acidotic)	50–100 mmol IV	Within 30 min	2 h
Permanent (removes potassium)			
Resonium	30–60 g PO/PR	Within 1 h (K ↓ by 0.5–1 mmol/L)	6 h
Dialysis		Immediate	3 h

Note: Avoid calcium in hyperkalaemia caused by digoxin toxicity.

HYPOKALAEMIA

- Severe < 2.5 mmol/L
- Signs and symptoms of hypokalaemia
  - Weakness (begins in lower extremities, moves cephalad)
  - Muscle cramps and tenderness
  - Flaccid paralysis
  - Hyporeflexia
  - Ischaemic rhabdomyolysis
  - Paraesthesiae
  - Constipation, ileus
  - Ventricular/atrial ectopic beats
  - Arrhythmias

Causes of hypokalaemia

↑ gastrointestinal loss	Diarrhoea (including laxative abuse) Vomiting Intestinal/pancreatic fistulae Ileostomy
Shift of K^+ into cells	During treatment of DKA Alkalosis Treatment of asthma (frequent beta-agonists)
↑ renal loss	Diuretics (loop, thiazides, carbonic anhydrase inhibitors) Hypomagnesaemia Hyperaldosteronism: — 1° (adrenal hyperplasia, adenoma, ca) — 2° (renal artery stenosis, CCF, liver cirrhosis) Alkalosis Congenital syndromes (Bartter and Gitelman) Renal tubular damage: — RTA type I, II — Interstitial nephritis — Analgesic nephropathy — Drug toxicity (amphotericin, gentamicin, toluene)

ECG changes of hypokalaemia

- Low amplitude, flattened or inverted T waves
- U waves
- ST depression
- Wide PR interval
- Illusion of prolonged QT (T wave disappears, U wave = prominent)
- Ectopic beats and arrhythmias

9

Useful lab investigations in hypokalaemia

Test	Result	Possible underlying cause
HCO_3^-	High	Vomiting Diuretic abuse Mineralocorticoid excess Bartter, Gitelman
	Low	Renal tubular disease Diarrhoea
Na^+	High	1° hyperaldosteronism
	Low	Diuretic use Hypovolaemia (GI loss)
Urine K^+	< 20 mmol/L	GI loss Intracellular shift of K^+ Poor oral intake
	> 40 mmol/L	Renal loss
Urine Na^+	< 20 mmol/L (with ↑ urine K^+)	2° hyperaldosteronism

Treatment of hypokalaemia

- Replace with IV/PO potassium chloride depending on symptoms, severity and cause of hypokalaemia.
- PO is the safer route.
- IV if:
  - — neuromuscular dysfunction
  - — arrhythmias
  - — ongoing GI losses
  - — severe.
- KCl IV at 10 mmol/h is the safest rate. (Higher rates → pain, phlebitis, ventricular arrhythmias)

HYPERNATRAEMIA

- Severe > 155 mmol/L
- High mortality rate (~50%)

Causes of hypernatraemia

Hypovolaemic (most common)	Loss/deficiency of water *or* Loss of Na^+ and water with Na^+ losses > water losses	Inability to drink/obtain water Impaired thirst mechanism Osmotic diuresis: — Glycosuria — Mannitol Extreme sweating Severe watery diarrhoea Vomiting Burns
Euvolaemic	Water loss without Na^+ loss	Diabetes insipidus: — Hypothalamic — Nephrogenic
Hypervolaemic	Gain of Na^+ and water with Na^+ gain > water gain	Iatrogenic (NaCl tablets, hypertonic saline, administration of $NaHCO_3$, hypertonic dialysis) Hypertonic medicines (ticarcillin) Cushing disease Adrenal hyperplasia Primary aldosteronism Sea water drownings

Treatment of hypernatraemia

Volume resuscitation if hypovolaemic	0.9% NS IV bolus
Calculate water deficit	Free water deficit (in L) = bodyweight (kg) × %TBW* × (actual Na^+ ÷ desired Na^+] – 1)
Correct slowly (rapid correction precipitates seizures)	↓ by < 1 mmol/L/h

***%TBW = percentage total body water**

%TBW	Population group
0.6	Young men
0.5	Young women Elderly men
0.4	Elderly women

9

HYPONATRAEMIA

- Concerning level: < 130 mmol/L
- Symptoms occur when the fall in sodium occurs rapidly or when adaptive responses fail to develop.

Useful investigations

- Serum
  - Osmolality
  - Uric acid
  - TSH, cortisol
- Urinalysis
  - Electrolytes
  - Uric acid
  - Urea
  - Creatinine
  - Osmolality

Treatment of hyponatraemia

- **Hypertonic saline** (3%) IV for CNS dysfunction (altered mental state, coma, seizures):
  - 100 mL IV (can go through peripheral IV access) over 10–20 min (for seizure)
  - Can repeat once (10 min between doses)
  - Send repeat Na^+
  - Each bolus will raise Na^+ 2 mmol

  Note: Risk of osmotic demyelination with treatment.
- **Fluid restrict** unless hypotensive
- **Monitor urine output**
- **'Rule of 6s':**
  - For those with CNS dysfunction, no more than 6 mmol correction in 6 h
  - Then no more than 6 mmol correction over 24 h

HYPERCALCAEMIA

Serum calcium:

- 45% ionised = physiologically active form of Ca^{2+}
- 40% bound to albumin
- 15% bound to other ions (citrate, phosphate, carbonate)

Causes of hypercalcaemia

- Primary hyperparathyroidism
- Malignancy
- Vitamin D excess
- Granulomatous disease (sarcoidosis)
- Renal failure
- Milk–alkali syndrome
- High bone turnover rates
  - Paget's
  - Prolonged immobilisation
  - Multiple myeloma

Symptoms of hypercalcaemia

Stones	Renal Biliary
Bones	Bone pain
Abdominal groans	Abdominal pain Nausea Vomiting Anorexia Pancreatitis
Psychiatric overtones	Confusion Depression Anxiety Coma

Useful lab investigations

- UEC
- Ionised calcium, phosphate
- BSL
- LFTs (albumin)
- PTH level

ECG changes of hypercalcaemia

- Prolongation of PR interval
- Shortening of QT interval
- QRS widening
- Sinus bradycardia
- BBB, AV block
- Cardiac arrest

Treatment of hypercalcaemia

Treatment option	Dose
Hydration (0.9% saline)	Titrate
Diuretics—e.g. frusemide	10–40 mg IV
Bisphosphonates—e.g. pamidronate	60–90 mg IV
Calcitonin	4U/kg IM/SC q12h

HYPOCALCAEMIA

- Severe: total Ca^{2+} < 2.175 mmol/L (8.7 mg/dL)
- If ionised Ca^{2+} normal, then asymptomatic
- Symptoms when ionised Ca^{2+} < 0.8 mmol/L
- ↑ 0.1 unit of pH → ↓ ionised Ca^{2+} by 3–8%

Causes of hypocalcaemia

9

Factitious	Hypoalbuminaemia
↓ PTH	Hypoparathyroidism Pseudohypoparathyroidism Parathyroid/thyroid surgery Radical neck dissection Radiation therapy for head/neck ca
↓ Vitamin D	Nutritional malabsorption ↓ Intake Renal disease Pronounced hypophosphataemia
↑ Calcitonin	Medullary thyroid ca
↑ Phosphate	Tumour lysis syndrome Rhabdomyolysis CRF
↑ Citrate in serum	Massive blood transfusion Plasmapheresis
↑ Bone formation/	Malignancy (prostate, breast, lung, chondrosarcoma) Osteomalacia
Medications	Phenytoin Phenobarbitone Colchicine Cisplatin
Others	Sepsis Severe burns Pancreatitis (calcium complex formation)

Symptoms and signs of hypocalcaemia

Symptoms dependent on the absolute value and rate of fall in Ca^{2+}.

Neuromuscular	Paraesthesiae Hyperreflexia Muscle spasm Tetany Chvostek's sign (facial N tap) Trousseau sign (BP cuff pumped up) Laryngeal stridor Seizures Choreoathetosis
Cardiovascular	Arrhythmias Hypotension Impaired contractility (heart failure)
Psychiatric	Anxiety, irritability Psychosis Depression Confusion Delusions

9

Chvostek's sign:

- Tap 0.5–1 cm below zygomatic process, 2 cm anterior to ear lobe.
- Positive if see twitching of circumoral Ms and orbicularis oculi.

Trousseau's sign:

- Inflate BP cuff to above systolic BP for several minutes.
- Positive if see carpopedal spasm.

ECG changes of hypocalcaemia

- Bradycardia
- Prolongation of QT interval
- Heart block
- T wave inversion
- Torsades de pointes

DIFFERENCES BETWEEN Ca CHLORIDE AND Ca GLUCONATE

Ca chloride	Ca gluconate
3 times more potent	⅓ potency of Ca chloride
Ca^{2+} ions immediately available post injection	Requires liver to metabolism gluconate component and release Ca
Can be given as a slow push	Given over 10 min due to sugar load (gluconate) which can cause hypotension
Highly irritant to veins	Less irritant
10% solution → 0.70 mmol/mL	10% solution → 0.22 mmol/mL

ION CORRECTION FORMULAS

Sodium corrected for hyperglycaemia

9

$$\text{corrected Na}^{+} = \text{measured Na}^{+} + [\text{glucose (mmol/L)} \div 4]$$

Calcium corrected for hypoalbuminaemia

$$\text{corrected Ca}^{2+}\text{ (mmol/L)} = \text{measured Ca}^{2+}\text{ (mmol/L)} + [40 - \text{measured albumin (g/L)}] \times 0.02$$

10 Thromboembolism and coagulopathy

Pulmonary embolism rule-out criteria (PERC)

- Age < 50 years
- HR < 100/min
- O_2 sats on room air ≥ 95%
- No prior history of DVT/PE
- No trauma or surgery requiring hospitalisation within 4 weeks
- No haemoptysis
- No exogenous oestrogen
- No unilateral leg swelling

Note: Low clinical suspicion for PE + ALL the above criteria = < 2% probability of PE and no further work-up is required.

WELLS' CRITERIA FOR PE

Determines the pre-test probability of PE. This can then be used in conjunction with a D-dimer assay to determine the need for imaging.

Clinical feature		Points
Clinical symptoms of DVT		3
Other diagnosis less likely than PE		3
Heart rate > 100/min		1.5
Immobilisation or surgery in past 4 weeks		1.5
Previous DVT/PE		1.5
Haemoptysis		1
Malignancy		1
Risk score (probability of PE)		
Points	**Risk of PE at 3 months**	
> 6	High (40.6% chance of PE in the ED population)	
2–6	Moderate (16.2% chance of PE in the ED population)	
< 2	Low (1.3% chance of PE in the ED population)	

Based on Wells PS et al. Excluding pulmonary embolism at the bedside without diagnostic imaging: management of patients with suspected pulmonary embolism presenting to the emergency department by using a simple clinical model and D-dimer. Ann Intern Med 2001;135(2):98–107.

WELLS' CRITERIA FOR DVT

Clinical feature	Points
Active cancer (treatment within past 6 months, palliation)	1
Paralysis, paresis or immobilisation of lower extremity	1
Bedridden for more than 3 days and/or surgery within 4 weeks	1
Localised tenderness along distribution of deep veins	1
Entire leg swollen	1
Unilateral calf swelling > 3 cm (measured below tibial tuberosity)	1
Unilateral pitting oedema	1
Collateral superficial veins	1
Alternative diagnosis as likely or more likely than DVT	–2
Risk score (probability of DVT)	
Points	**Risk of DVT**
≥ 3	High
1–2	Moderate
< 1	Low

THROMBOPHILIA (PROTHROMBOTIC) SCREEN

Clotting-based assays	Protein C Protein S Antithrombin III Activated protein C resistance Lupus anticoagulant Shortened 'APTT'
Immunological	Anti-cardiolipin antibody Anti-beta-2-glycoprotein antibodies
DNA-based testing	Factor V Leiden Prothrombin *G20210A* mutation MTHFR *C677T* mutation
Others	Homocysteine levels

MTHFR = methylene tetra-hydrofolate reductase.

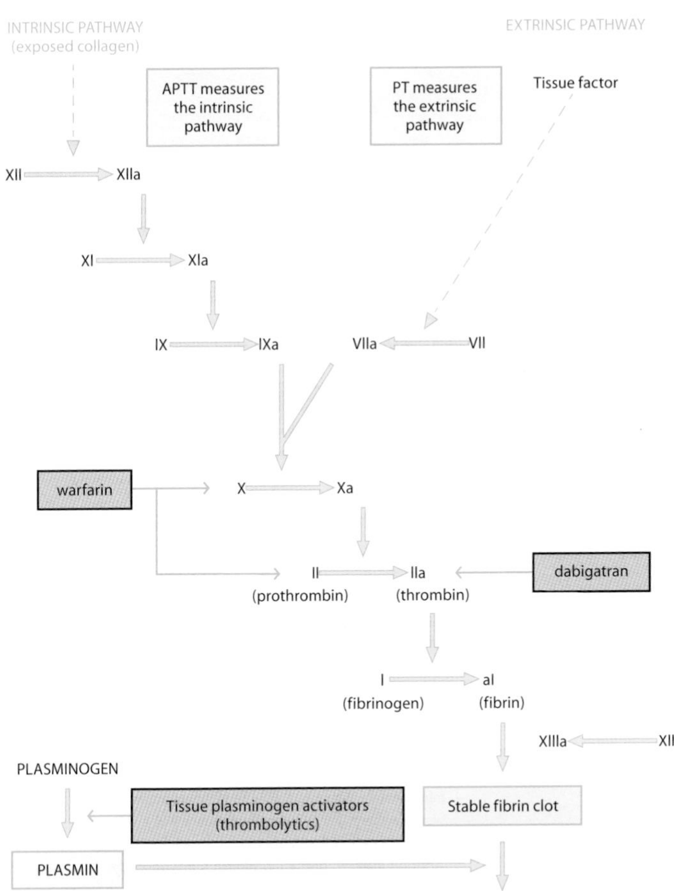

Figure 10.1 Coagulation cascade flow chart

St Vincent's Hospital
GUIDELINES FOR THE MANAGEMENT OF AN ELEVATED INTERNATIONAL NORMALISED RATIO (INR) IN ADULT PATIENTS WITH OR WITHOUT BLEEDING

Note:

- ***Prothrombinex-HT* can only be prescribed after consultation with a haematologist.**
- The anticoagulant effect of warfarin may be difficult to re-establish for some time after vitamin K is used. Use the lowest dose possible and, if possible, consult the treating specialist prior to using vitamin K.
- Small oral doses of vitamin K are obtained by measuring the dose from the injectable formulation and administering orally. Vitamin K effect on INR can be expected within 6–12 hours; however, the full effect of vitamin K in reducing the INR can take up to 24 hours.

Table 1 Guidelines for the management of an elevated international normalised ratio (INR) in adult patients with or without bleeding

Clinical setting	Action
INR higher than the therapeutic range but < 5; bleeding absent	Lower the dose or omit the next dose of warfarin. Resume therapy at a lower dose when the INR approaches therapeutic range. If the INR is only minimally above therapeutic range (up to 10%), dose reduction may not be necessary.
INR 5–9; bleeding absent	Cease warfarin therapy; consider reasons for elevated INR and patient-specific factors. Bleeding risk increases exponentially from INR 5 to 9; INR ≥ 6 should be monitored closely. If bleeding risk is high (see Table 2), give vitamin K (1–2 mg orally or 0.5–1 mg intravenously). See the notes above for further information about vitamin K. Measure INR within 24 hours and resume warfarin at a reduced dose once INR is in therapeutic range.
INR > 9; bleeding absent	Where there is a low risk of bleeding, cease warfarin therapy, give 2.5–5 mg vitamin K orally or 1 mg intravenously. Measure INR in 6–12 hours, resume warfarin therapy at a reduced dose once INR < 5.0. Where there is high risk of bleeding (see Table 2), cease warfarin therapy, give 1 mg vitamin K intravenously. Consider Prothrombinex-HT (25–50 IU/kg) and fresh frozen plasma (150–300 mL), measure INR in 6–12 hours, resume warfarin therapy at a reduced dose once INR < 5. ***Prothrombinex-HT* can only be prescribed after consultation with a haematologist.** See the notes above for further information about vitamin K.

Figure 43.1 St Vincent's Hospital guidelines for the management of an elevated INR in adult patients with or without bleeding (continues)
FFP, fresh frozen plasma; INR, international normalised ratio; PTX, Prothrombinex
Based on Tran HA, Chunilal SD, Harper PL et al, on behalf of the Australasian Society of Thrombosis and Haemostasis. An update of consensus guidelines for warfarin reversal. Med J Aust 2013;198(4):198–9

Clinical setting	Action
Any clinically significant bleeding where warfarin-induced coagulopathy is considered a contributing factor	Cease warfarin therapy, give 5–10 mg vitamin K intravenously, as well as Prothrombinex-HT (25–50 IU/kg) and fresh frozen plasma (150–300 mL), assess patient continuously until INR < 5, and bleeding stops. OR If fresh frozen plasma is unavailable, cease warfarin therapy, give 5–10 mg vitamin K intravenously, and Prothrombinex-HT (25–50 IU/kg), assess patient continuously until INR < 5, and bleeding stops. OR If Prothrombinex-HT is unavailable, cease warfarin therapy, give 5–10 mg vitamin K intravenously, and 10–15 mL/kg of fresh frozen plasma, assess patient continuously until INR < 5, and bleeding stops. Prothrombinex-HT can only be prescribed after consultation with a haematologist. In all situations carefully reassess the need for ongoing warfarin therapy.

Table 2 Risk factors for bleeding complications of anticoagulation therapy

Risk factor category	Specific risk factors
Age	> 65 years
Cardiac	Uncontrolled hypertension
Gastrointestinal	History of gastrointestinal haemorrhage, active peptic ulcer, hepatic insufficiency
Haematological/oncological	Thrombocytopenia (platelet count $< 50 \times 10^9$/L), platelet dysfunction, coagulation defect, underlying malignancy
Neurological	History of stroke, cognitive or psychological impairment
Renal	Renal insufficiency
Trauma	Recent trauma, history of falls (> 3 within previous treatment year, or recurrent, injurious falls)
Alcohol	Excessive alcohol intake
Medications	Aspirin, non-specific non-steroidal anti-inflammatory drugs (COX-II inhibitors do not impair platelet function, but can influence warfarin effect), 'natural remedies' that interfere with haemostasis. Careful monitoring of warfarin effect is critical to minimise risk in patients taking multiple medications.

Figure 43.1 Continued

MANAGEMENT OF THROMBOLYTIC-INDUCED MAJOR BLEEDING

1 Ensure large bore IV access.
2 Draw bloods for FBC, platelet count, PT/INR, APTT, bleeding time, G&H.
3 Volume resuscitation—including packed RBCs.
4 Stop heparin/LMWH: consider protamine.
5 6–12 U cryoprecipitate.

6 Stop antiplatelet therapy.
7 If the patient is still bleeding, check fibrinogen level:
 —if fibrinogen > 1 g/L → FFP 2 U
 —if fibrinogen < 1 g/L → cryoprecipitate 8–12 U.
8 If patient is still bleeding, consider aminocaproic acid.
9 Recheck PT/INR, APTT, fibrinogen, bleeding time.
10 Haematology consult.

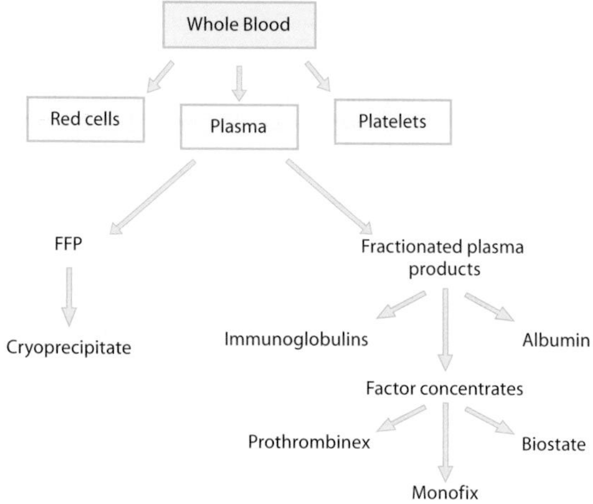

Figure 10.2 Blood components flow chart

REVERSING ANTICOAGULATION: PROTAMINE

- SLOW IV infusion (if rapid → hypotension, anaphylactoid reaction)

Protamine vs enoxaparin:

- 1 mg protamine will approximately neutralise 1 mg enoxaparin.
- Time since last dose of LMWH also determines protamine dose.

Time elapsed since last enoxaparin dose	Dose
< 8 h	1 mg protamine per 1 mg enoxaparin
> 8 h	0.5 mg protamine per 1 mg enoxaparin
> 12 h	Protamine may not be required

Protamine vs heparin:

- 10 mg protamine over 10 min followed by 10–20 mg protamine over 10–20 min.
- This will neutralise 2000–3000 U of heparin.

INHIBITING FIBRINOLYSIS: AMINOCAPROIC ACID

- Initially 5 g in 250 mL 5% dextrose or NS over 1 h.
- Followed by 5 g in 250 mL 5% dextrose or NS over 5 h.
- Cease infusion if bleeding stops.

BLOOD COMPONENTS – SPECIFICS

Product	Contents (per unit)	Volume
Red cells	Hb (> 40 g) Haematocrit (0.50–0.70)	200 mL
Platelets	200–240 × 10^9	> 160 mL
FFP	Coagulation factors (200 IU of factor VIII) Other proteins	250 mL
Cryoprecipitate	Factor VIII (≥ 70 IU) Fibrinogen (≥ 140 mg) Fibronectin Factor XIII vWF (≥ 100 IU)	30–40 mL
Prothrombin complex concentrate (Prothrombinex)	Factors II, IX, X (500 IU of each) Low levels of VII	Vials of powder reconstituted to 20 mL
Biostate	Factor VIII vWF	Variety of preparations
MonoFIX	Factor IX concentrate	Variety of preparations

Adapted from the Australian Red Cross.

BLEEDING DISORDERS

Disorder	Defect	Treatment options
Haemophilia A *Mild* *Moderate* *Severe*	Absence/low factor VIII *6–25% factor VIII* *1–5%* *< 1%*	Desmopressin for mild (> 15%) Recombinant factor VIII Biostate
Haemophilia B	Absence/low factor IX	Recombinant factor IX MonoFIX
Von Willebrand	Quantitative ± qualitative defect in vWF	Desmopressin Biostate
Coagulopathy 2° liver disease		Vit K FFP Platelets Cryoprecipitate
Thrombolytic drugs	Systemic fibrinolysis	Cryoprecipitate FFP

Note: Treatment should be guided by a specialist haematologist.

10

11 Neurology
ADULT CEREBROSPINAL FLUID (CSF) STUDIES

CSF studies in adults in normal and infected fluid

CSF studies	Normal	Bacterial	Viral	TB/fungi
Pressure (cmH_2O)	7–25	↑↑↑	Normal / ↑	Variable
WCC (per mm_3)	< 5	> 200–20,000	< 100	< 1000 ?variable
Predominant cell type	Lymphocytes, no polymorphs	Polymorphs (10% lymphocytes)	Lymphocytes	Lymphocytes
Glucose	≥ 0.6 × serum	↓ / normal	↑ / normal	↓ / normal
Protein (mg/L)	< 400 mg/L	↑ / normal	↑ / normal	↑
Organisms	0	+ve gram stain in 80%		+ve India ink stain with cryptococcal

Causes of increased protein in CSF

- Inflammation
- Tumour
- Demyelinating disorders
- Subarachnoid haemorrhage
- Traumatic tap

TRAUMATIC LUMBAR PUNCTURE (TAP)

Differences between traumatic lumbar puncture (tap) and pathological bleeding

Traumatic tap	Pathological bleeding
Decreasing blood in subsequent tubes	Same amount of blood in all tubes
Clear supernatant	Xanthochromia
Clots	No clots

Calculation to correct for falsely elevated WBC count due to a traumatic tap

$$\text{WBC artificially introduced} = \text{WBC in blood} \times [\text{RBC in CSF} \div \text{RBC in blood}]$$

Therefore:

$$\text{WBC in CSF (predicted)} = \text{WBC in CSF (measured)} - \text{WBC artificially introduced}$$

COMMON UPPER LIMB NERVE PALSIES

Inspection and signs

Nerve	Inspection	Motor signs	Sensory signs	Pearls
Median	Thenar atrophy 'Ape-hand' deformity (thumb lies in the same plane as the palm)	Weak pronation of forearm Weak flexion of wrist and fingers (especially index and middle)Unable to make a fist or close hand around a bottle Unable to flex or oppose thumb	Numbness of radial 3½ digits and corresponding portions of the palm	Superficial branch of median supplies thenar eminence—distinguishes low from high lesion
Ulnar	'Claw-hand' deformity (ring and little fingers curl up)	Froment's sign—testing thumb adduction causes thumb to flex instead of remaining straight	Numbness of entire little finger and ulnar half of ring finger	Less clawing in a high lesion Low lesion at level of wrist will have normal sensation Check intrinsic function by crossing middle finger over index finger
Radial	Wrist drop	Weak elbow extension Weak extension at wrist/digits Weak forearm supination	Dorsum of the hand	If weak elbow extension present then high lesion

11

11

Autogenous zones for median, ulnar and radial nerves

Nerve	Zone
Median	Volar aspect of the index finger
Ulnar	Volar aspect of the little finger
Radial	Dorsal aspect of 1st web space

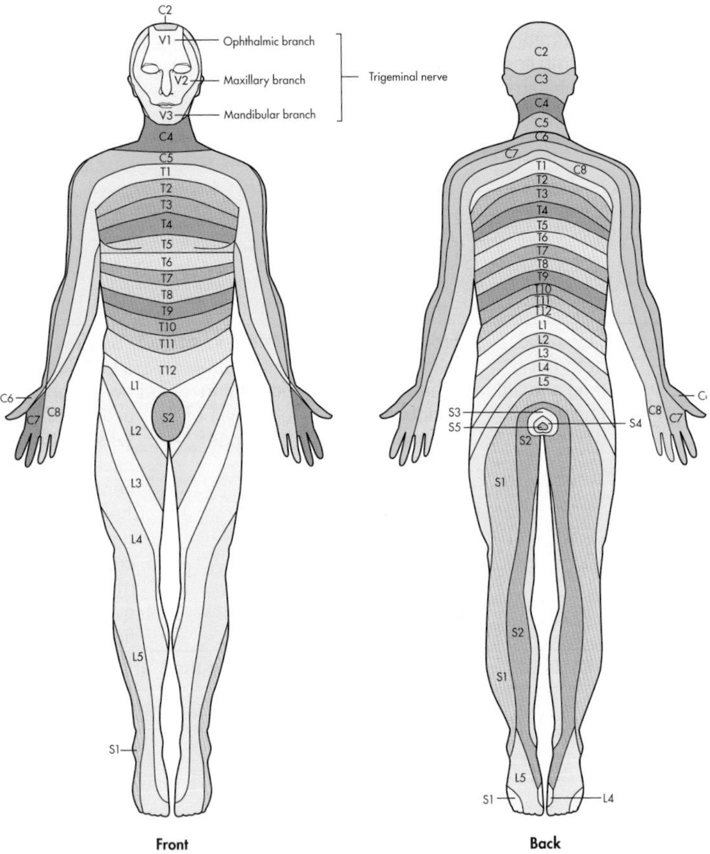

Figure 11.1 Dermatome maps

Reproduced with permission from Standring S, Gray's anatomy, 40th edn. Philadelphia: Churchill Livingstone, 2008: Fig 15.2A.

12 Important procedures

INTRAOSSEOUS PUNCTURE

Positioning of patient and insertion sites

- Supine.
- For proximal tibial placement:
  - Sufficient padding under the knee of the uninjured lower limb with approximately 30° flexion of the knee.
  - Anteromedial surface of the proximal tibia, approximately 2 cm below patella and 2 cm medial to tibial tuberosity.
- For distal tibial placement:
  - 3 cm proximal to most prominent part of medial malleolus.
  - Check the anterior and posterior borders and ensure insertion occurs on the flat part of the bone.
- For humeral placement:
  - Ensure patient's hand on abdomen with elbow adducted.
  - Slide your thumb up the anterior shaft of humerus until greater tuberosity is felt (this is the surgical neck).
  - Insert approximately 1 cm above the surgical neck.

Method of insertion into the proximal tibia

Sterile technique.

1. Initially at 90°, insert the intraosseous needle through skin and periosteum.
2. After gaining access into bone, direct the needle 45–60° away from the epiphyseal plate (i.e. towards the foot).
3. Use a gentle twisting motion to advance the needle through the bone cortex and into the marrow.
4. Remove stylet, attach syringe and withdraw, aspirating bone marrow.
5. Flush with saline and check for no evidence of swelling/ subcutaneous infiltration.

Note: There are now intraosseous insertion devices (drills) that are easier to use.

Other sites of insertion for adults

- Distal tibia
- Proximal humerus

CHEST TUBE INSERTION

Positioning of patient

- Semi-upright 30–60°, head up
- Ipsilateral arm abducted and hand placed behind patient's head (for lateral approach)

Insertion sites

- 5th intercostal space just anterior to mid-axillary line on the affected side
  or
- 2nd intercostal space in mid-clavicular line on the affected side

Size

- Use large bore (28–32 Fr) for trauma

Method of insertion

Sterile technique—including sterile field.

1. Clamp the proximal end of the chest tube with Kelly forceps and place aside.
2. Locally anaesthetise the skin, subcutaneous tissues, periosteum and parietal pleura.
3. Make a 2–3-cm horizontal incision in the insertion site and bluntly dissect with curved Kelly forceps through the subcutaneous tissues, just over the top of the rib.
4. Puncture the parietal pleura with the tip of the artery forceps and put a gloved finger into the dissected tract to avoid other tissue damage and to clear clots, adhesions etc with a circumferential sweep.
5. Keep your finger in the tract.
6. Advance chest tube (using forceps clamped to its tip) into the pleural cavity, alongside your finger, to the desired length (ensure fenestrations are within the thoracic cavity).
7. Try to direct the tube posteriorly along the inside of the chest wall.
8. Look for fogging of the tube and connect to an underwater seal drain and suction.
9. Suture and secure the chest tube in place and apply sterile dressings.
10. Tape all connections to ensure secure.
11. Check position of the tube ± re-expansion of the lung (CXR) and continue close cardiorespiratory monitoring.

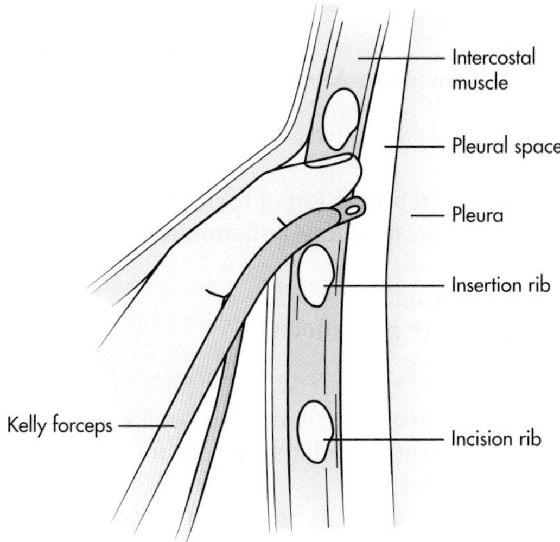

Figure 12.1 Tip placement in the pleural cavity, using the finger as a guide
Reproduced with permission from Pfenninger JL, Fowler GC, eds. Pfenninger and Fowler's procedures for primary care, 3rd edn. Philadelphia: Mosby, 2010: Fig 212.7.

12

13 Toxicology

POISONS INFORMATION

Call 131126 (nationwide in Australia).

PRINCIPLES OF MANAGEMENT OF POISONINGS

1 Resuscitation
2 Risk assessment and prediction of toxic effects
3 Supportive care, investigations and monitoring
4 Decontamination
5 Enhanced elimination
6 Specific treatment (e.g. antidotes)

PRINCIPLES OF GI DECONTAMINATION

- Always perform a risk–benefit analysis—risks from the decontamination process vs likely benefit for that particular toxicity and patient.
- Not routinely used—depends on time of presentation following ingestion and risk of toxicity.
- Not recommended for non-toxic or sub-toxic ingestions.
- Not recommended for toxins that may → seizures or ↓ LOC.
- Not recommended for hydrocarbon ingestions.
- Not recommended for corrosive ingestions.
- Single-dose charcoal is the preferred modality. Best used within 1 h post-toxic ingestion.

Decontamination methods

Modality	Agent/method	Dose	Contraindications
Activated charcoal (AC)	Place in cup Mix with ice cream for kids Can give via OGT/NGT once tube placement confirmed	1 g/kg (kids) 50 g (adults)	As text above plus: — ↓ LOC — Toxin does not bind to AC*
Gastric lavage	Patient position left lateral, head down 36–40 G lavage tube inserted into oesophagus Aspirate gastric contents Instil 200 mL warm water into stomach Drain fluid into dependent bucket Continue instilling/draining until effluent is clear Finish with administering AC		As text above plus: — Unprotected airway — Small kids

Continues

Decontamination methods (continued)

Modality	Agent/method	Dose	Contraindications
Whole-bowel irrigation**	Polyethylene glycol electrolyte solution (PEG) Place NGT and administer PEG at rate of 2 L/h (adults) or 25 mL/kg/h (kids) Give metoclopramide (minimise vomiting and ↑ gastric emptying) Easy access to toilet/commode Continue until effluent is clear or packages/drug preparations apparent Monitor for abdominal distension or ↓ bowel sounds		

* See table below: Drugs not well adsorbed by activated charcoal
** See box below: Poisonings where whole-bowel irrigation MAY be useful

Drugs not well adsorbed by activated charcoal

Drug group	Examples
Alcohols	Ethanol, methanol, isopropyl alcohol, ethylene glycol
Metals	Lithium, iron, mercury, potassium, lead, arsenic
Acids and alkalis	
Hydrocarbons	Turpentine, kerosene, eucalyptus oil, benzene

Poisonings where whole bowel irrigation MAY be useful

- Life-threatening ingestions of sustained-release preparations (e.g. verapamil, diltiazem, potassium)
- Life-threatening ingestions of enteric-coated preparations
- Agents that do not bind to charcoal (e.g. lead, arsenic)
- 'Body packers/stuffers' (illicit drug 'mules')
- Iron overdose

13

Complications associated with GI decontamination

- GI trauma or perforation
- Bowel obstruction
- Nausea, vomiting
- Aspiration pneumonitis
- Laryngospasm
- Hypoxia

Measurable (serum) toxin levels useful in assessing toxicity

- Alcohol
- Carbamazepine
- Carboxyhaemoglobin
- Digoxin
- Iron
- Lithium
- Methaemoglobin
- Paracetamol
- Phenytoin
- Salicylate
- Sodium valproate
- Theophylline

Enhanced elimination techniques

	Multiple-dose activated charcoal	Urinary alkalinisation	Haemodialysis
Toxins technique may be used in	Carbamazepine Dapsone Phenobarbitone Quinine Theophylline	Phenobarbitone Salicylates	Alcohols Lithium Metformin Potassium Salicylate Theophylline Valproate

RISK-ASSESSMENT CHART FOR COMMON OVERDOSES

This table highlights *approximate* doses associated with significant toxicity requiring observation, treatment and discussion with a toxicologist or Poisons Centre.

Drug	Adult	Children
Aspirin	150 mg/kg > 300 mg/kg = severe intoxication	
Carbamazepine	20–50 mg/kg	
Carbon monoxide	> 10%	
Chlorpromazine	> 5 g	1 tablet
Cocaine	> 1 g = potentially lethal	
Colchicine	> 0.2 mg/kg Any intentional OD = potentially lethal	
Digoxin—acute ingestion	> 10 mg = potentially lethal	> 75 microg/kg > 4 mg = potentially lethal
Ibuprofen	> 100 mg/kg	> 300 mg/kg
Iron	20–60 mg/kg	> 60 mg/kg
Lithium—acute ingestion	> 25 g	
Metformin	> 10 g	> 1700 mg
Olanzapine	40–100 mg	> 0.5 mg/kg
Opioids		> 2 mg/kg codeine PO
Paracetamol—acute single ingestion	> 150 mg/kg *or* > 10 g	> 200 mg/kg
Phenelzine	> 2 mg/kg 4–6 mg/kg potentially lethal	1–2 tablets
Phenytoin	> 20 mg/kg	> 200 mg

Drug	Adult	Children
Quetiapine	> 3 g	> 100 mg
Quinine	> 1 g	600 mg = potentially lethal
Risperidone		> 1 mg
Salicylates	150–300 mg/kg	> 5 mL of methyl salicylate (oil of wintergreen)
Sulfonylureas	1 tablet (especially if non-diabetic)	1 tablet
Tramadol	> 1.5 g	> 10 mg/kg
Tricyclic antidepressants (TCAs)	> 10 mg/kg	> 5 mg/kg
Valproate	> 400 mg/kg	> 200 mg/kg

RATIO OF ACUTE EQUIPOTENCY OF OPIOID ANALGESICS

When changing opioid start at 50%, the equipotent dose, then titrate according to response.

Drug	Oral dose	Parenteral dose	Approximate duration of action
Buprenorphine	0.8 mg sublingual	0.4 mg IM	6–8 h
Codeine	200 mg	120–130 mg IM/SC	3–4 h
Fentanyl	–	100–150 microg IV/SC	0.5–1 h
Methadone	Complex	–	8–24 h
Morphine	30 mg	10 mg IM/SC	2–3 h 12–24 h (controlled release
Oxycodone	15–20 mg	–	3–4 h 12–24 h (controlled release)
Pethidine	–	75–100 mg IM	2–3 h
Tramadol	150 mg	100–120 mg IM/IV	

Based on the *Australian Medicines Handbook*, 2011. Online. Available: www.amh.hcn.com.au

ANTIDOTES

Drug	'Antidote'
Benzodiazepines	Flumazenil
Beta-blockers	High-dose insulin therapy
Calcium channel blockers	Calcium chloride Calcium gluconate High-dose insulin therapy
Carbon monoxide	Oxygen (enhances elimination)
Cyanide	Hydroxocobalamin (Cyanokit) = 1st line Sodium thiosulfate = 2nd line
Digoxin	Digoxin immune Fab (antibody fragments)
Heparin	Protamine
Hydrofluoric acid (skin exposure)	Calcium gel 2.5% Calcium gluconate 1 g/10 mL DO NOT USE CALCIUM CHLORIDE (it causes tissue damage)
Insulin	Glucose
Iron	Desferrioxamine
Isoniazid	Pyridoxine
Lead	Dimercaptosuccinic acid (DMSA) Sodium calcium edetate (for lead encephalopathy/severe poisoning)
Lignocaine	Intralipid 20%
Methanol, ethylene glycol	Ethanol
Methaemoglobinaemia	Methylene Blue
Opiates	Naloxone
Organophosphates	Atropine Pralidoxime
Paracetamol	N-acetylcysteine
Sulfonylureas	Octreotide + glucose
Tricyclic antidepressants	Bicarbonate
Warfarin	Vitamin K Prothrombin complex concentrates (e.g. Prothrombinex, FFP)

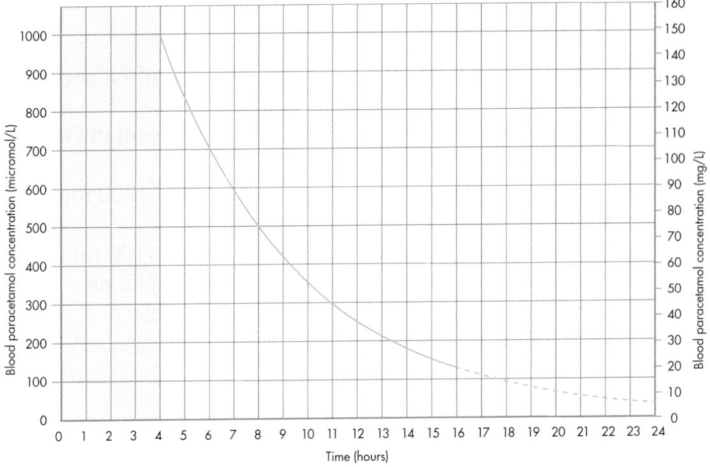

Figure 13.1 Paracetamol treatment nomogram

Important pitfalls

- Serum paracetamol is reported in different units from different laboratories. Ensure the correct units are being used before interpreting results with the nomogram.
- To convert paracetamol results in micromol/L to mg/L, multiply the result by 0.151.

From Daly FFS, Fountain JS, Murray L et al. Guidelines for the management of paracetamol poisoning in Australia and New Zealand—explanation and elaboration. MJA 2008; 188(5)296–302.

14 Drug infusions

AMIODARONE

Loading dose: 5 mg/kg over 20 min to 1 h (over < 3 min if cardiac arrest)

Concentration: 900 mg in 500 mL 5% glucose (dextrose) in GLASS bottle (1.8 mg/mL)

Dose required: 15 mg/kg over 24 h to a maximum of 1200 mg intravenously.

Note: For fluid restricted patients only use 900 mg/100 mL. Prepare this by removing 18 mL from 100 mL 5% glucose GLASS bottle then add 900 mg (9 mg/mL); see table 'Amiodarone infusion' below.

Cautions:

- Cardiac monitoring
- Glass must be used due to adsorption of amiodarone to plastic bags
- Central line is preferable for infusion

Side effects:

- Rapid injection can cause hypotension/circulatory collapse
- Bradycardia plus other arrhythmias
- Hot flushes, sweating, nausea, vomiting
- Acute pulmonary toxicities, bronchospasm

Amiodarone infusion

Weight (kg)	15 mg/kg over 24 h	900 mg/500 mL	*900 mg/100 mL
		Rate mL/h	
60	900 mg	21	4.2
65	975 mg	23	4.5
70	1050 mg	24	4.9
75	1125 mg	26	5.2
> 80	1200 mg	28	5.5

GLYCERYL TRINITRATE (GTN)

Concentration: See table 'GTN infusion'; use 5% glucose

Intravenous infusion rate:

- Starting dose usually 5 microg/min
- Increments of 5 microg can be made every 3–5 minutes according to clinical response (pain and BP)

Side effects:

- Hypotension
- Headache, nausea, vomiting

Cautions:

- — Glass bottle used to minimise GTN adsorption to plastic bag
- — BP monitoring

GTN infusion

Loaded concentration	50 mg in 500 mL = 100 microg/mL	100 mg in 500 mL = 200 microg/mL	200 mg in 500 mL = 400 microg/mL
		Flow rate mL/h	
3	5 microg/min	10 microg/min	20 microg/min
6	10 microg/min	20 microg /min	40 microg /min
9	15 microg/min	30 microg/min	60 microg/min
12	20 microg/min	40 microg/min	80 microg/min
15	25 microg/min	50 microg/min	100 microg/min
18	30 microg/min	60 microg/min	120 microg/min
21	35 microg/min	70 microg/min	140 microg/min
24	40 microg/min	80 microg/min	160 microg/min
48	80 microg/min	160 microg/min	320 microg/min
72	120 microg/min	240 microg/min	480 microg/min
96	160 microg/min	320 microg/min	640 microg/min

HEPARIN

Concentration: 15,000 units in 100 mL 5% glucose

Intravenous infusion rate

Weight (kg)	Rate (mL/h)
< 54	5
55–64	6
65–74	7
75–84	8
85–94	9
> 95	10

INOTROPE INFUSIONS

'Rule of 6s'

For adrenaline, noradrenaline and isoprenaline

- 6 mg in 100 mL of 5% glucose = 60 microg/mL
- ∴ 1 mL/h = 1 microg/min
- Run infusion at 1–20 microg/min = 1–20 mL/h

14

For dopamine and dobutamine

- 6 mg/kg in 1000 mL 5% glucose = 6 microg/kg/mL
- ∴ 10 mL/h = 1 microg/kg/min

For dopamine

- 3–5 microg/kg/min (renal dose) = 30–50 mL/h
- > 5 microg/kg/min (inotropic dose) = > 50 mL/h

For dobutamine

- 1–20 microg/kg/min = 10–200 mL/h

LIGNOCAINE

Loading dose: 1 mg/kg over 2–3 min
Concentration: 4 g in 500 mL 5% glucose (= 8 mg/mL)
Intravenous infusion rate:
8 mg/min (60 mL/h) for 20 min (total volume infused = 20 mL)
THEN 2 mg/min (15 mL/h) as maintenance infusion
Side effects:
- — GI
  - Nausea, vomiting
- — CNS
  - Paraesthesiae
  - Drowsiness
  - Blurred vision
  - Tinnitus
  - Confusion
  - Tremors
  - Seizures
- — CVS
  - Bradycardia
  - Arrest

ACETYLCYSTEINE INFUSION: 3-STEP IV INFUSION PROTOCOL

The 3 infusions take approximately 20 h to complete. If the infusion needs to be continued after 20 h, do so at the dose and rate indicated in step 3.

1. 150 mg/kg IV in 200 mL 5% glucose over 15–60 min
2. 50 mg/kg IV in 500 mL 5% glucose over 4 h
3. 100 mg/kg IV in 1 L of 5% glucose over 16 h

Acetylcysteine (Parvolex) infusion dosage guide in adults
(According to Parvolex product information)

Bodyweight (kg)	1st infusion (mL)	2nd infusion (mL)	3rd infusion (mL)	Total (mL)
50	37.5	12.5	25	75
60	45.0	15.0	30	90
70	52.5	17.5	35	105
80	60.0	20.0	40	120
90	67.5	22.5	45	135
x	$0.75x$	$0.25x$	$0.5x$	$1.5x$

Acetylcysteine infusion dosage guide in children
The volume of 5% glucose should be appropriate for the patient's weight.

Bodyweight	1st infusion	2nd infusion	3rd infusion	4th infusion
Children < 20 kg	150 mg/kg in 3 mL/kg of 5% glucose over 15 min	50 mg/kg in 7 mL/kg of 5% glucose over 4 h	50 mg/kg in 7 mL/kg of 5% glucose over 8 h	50 mg/kg in 7 mL/kg of 5% glucose over 8 h
Children > 20 kg	150 mg/kg in 100 mL of 5% glucose over 15 min	50 mg/kg in 250 mL of 5% glucose over 4 h	50 mg/kg in 250 mL of 5% glucose over 8 h	50 mg/kg in 250 mL of 5% glucose over 8 h

NALOXONE

Concentration: 2 mg per 100 mL 5% glucose or 0.9% saline
Intravenous infusion rate:

—5–135 mL/h (0.1–2.7 mg/h); titrate to GCS and RR
—Set rate to ½ to ⅓ of total bolus dose required for initial clinical response

Naloxone infusion

Initial dose required (mg)	Hourly naloxone required (mg)	Infusion rate (mL/h)
0.2	0.1	5
0.4	0.2	10
0.8	0.5	25
1.2	0.8	40
1.6	1	50
2	1.3	65
4	2.7	135

14

OCTREOTIDE

Bolus: 25 microg IV
Concentration: 100 microg in 100 mL 5% glucose
Intravenous infusion rate: 25 microg/h (25 mL/h)
Side effects:

— Pain, redness and swelling at site of injection
— Impaired glucose tolerance
— Liver dysfunction
— Bradycardia
— Abdominal pain, diarrhoea, bloating

Cautions: Monitor blood sugar levels (may increase)

15 Paediatrics
EQUIPMENT

Defibrillation paddle size

Weight of child	Size
< 10 kg	4.5 cm
> 10 kg	4.5 cm or adult size

Self-inflating bags

Bag volume	Age group
250 mL	Very small babies only
500 mL	Up to 8 y
1500 mL	> 8 y to adults

PAEDIATRIC FORMULAS
Formulas for approximate weight (kg) based on age

Age	Approximate calculated weight
Age < 9 y	(2 × age) + 9
Age > 9 y	3 × age
Age < 12 mo	(Age in months ÷ 2) + 4

BP

Approximate systolic BP (mmHg) = 80 + (age in years × 2)

Formulas for ETT size

Age > 1 year	
ETT size (mm)	(age ÷ 4) + 4
ETT length (cm) at lips	(age ÷ 2) + 12
ETT length (cm) at nose	(age ÷ 2) + 15
For the newborn	
Weight	**ETT size (mm)**
< 1 kg	2.5
1–3.5 kg	3.0
> 3.5 kg	3.5

(Adapted from Shann F, *Drug Doses*, 15th edn. Melbourne: The Royal Children's Hospital; 2010.)

15

PAEDIATRIC VITAL SIGNS: NORMAL RANGES

Age (years)	Heart rate (beats/min)	Systolic BP (mmHg)	Respiratory rate (breaths/min)
< 1	110–160	70–90	30–40
1–2	100–150	80–95	25–35
2–5	95–140	80–100	25–30
5–12	80–120	90–110	20–25
> 12	60–100	100–120	15–20

PAEDIATRIC MODIFIED GLASGOW COMA SCALE

Eyes open	
Any age	**Score**
Spontaneously	4
To speech	3
To pain	2
No response	1

Best verbal response			
> 5 y	**2–5 y**	**0–23 mo**	**Score**
Orientated and converses	Appropriate words and phrases	Smiles, coos, cries appropriately	5
Confused	Inappropriate words	Cries but consolable	4
Inappropriate words	Cries and/or screams	Persistent cries and/ or screams	3
Incomprehensible sounds	Grunts	Grunts	2
No response	No response	No response	1

Best motor response		
> 1 y	**< 1 y**	**Score**
Obeys command	Spontaneously moves	6
Localises pain	Localises pain	5
Flexion–withdrawal	Flexion–withdrawal	4
Flexion–abnormal (decorticate rigidity)	Flexion–abnormal (decorticate rigidity)	3
Extension (decerebrate)	Extension (decerebrate)	2
No response	No response	1

PAEDIATRIC PEAK EXPIRATORY FLOW

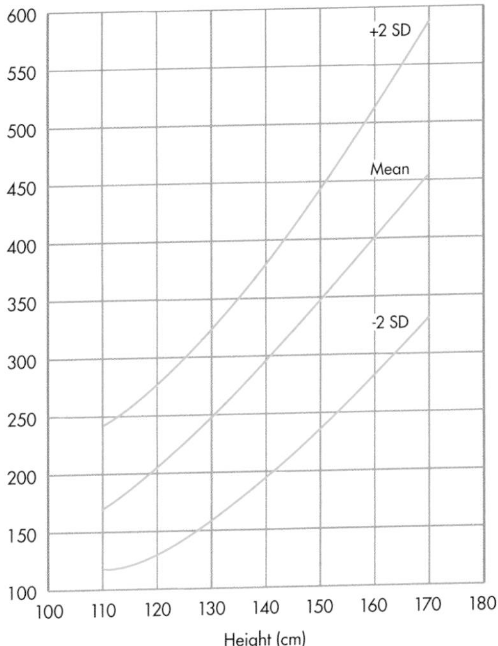

Figure 15.1 Peak expiratory flow chart for children 5–18 y (male and female)

PAEDIATRIC FLUID THERAPY

Bolus for resuscitation: 20 mL/kg IV with usually 0.9% saline

Maintenance fluids:

— < 10 kg child: 10% glucose + 0.45% saline

— > 10 kg child: 5% glucose + 0.45% saline)

Weight in kg	mL/kg/day	mL/kg/h
0–10	100	4
11–20	50	2
> 20	20	1

Example 1: 3-kg child

Maintenance fluids = (3 × 100) mL/day
= 300 mL/day

Example 2: 13-kg child

$$\begin{aligned}\text{Maintenance fluids} &= (10 \times 100) + (3 \times 50) \text{ mL/day}\\ &= 1000 + 150 \text{ mL/day}\\ &= 1150 \text{ mL/day}\end{aligned}$$

Example 3: 25-kg child

$$\begin{aligned}\text{Maintenance fluids} &= (10 \times 100) + (10 \times 50) + (5 \times 20) \text{ mL/day}\\ &= 1000 + 500 + 100 \text{ mL/day}\\ &= 1600 \text{ mL/day}\end{aligned}$$

Note: This formula does not include any losses or additional fluid requirements. Add any deficits and ongoing losses to the above.

Example 4: 11-kg child with 5% dehydration

$$\begin{aligned}\text{Maintenance fluids} &= (10 \times 100) + (1 \times 50) \text{ mL/day}\\ &= 1000 + 50 \text{ mL/day}\\ &= 1050 \text{ mL/day}\end{aligned}$$

$$\begin{aligned}\text{Deficit} &= 5\% \times 11 \text{ kg}\\ &= 0.05 \times 11{,}000 \text{ mL}\\ &= 550 \text{ mL}\end{aligned}$$

$$\begin{aligned}\text{Total fluids required} &= 1050 + 550 \text{ mL/day}\\ &= 1600 \text{ mL/day}\end{aligned}$$

16 Pathology

Haematology

Anaemia type	Laboratory findings	More common causes
Iron deficiency	Hb = N/ ↓ MCV = N/ ↓ (microcytic) MCH = N/ ↓ (hypochromic) Fe ↓ ferritin ↓ TIBC ↑ Transferrin ↑	Blood loss, diet low in iron, poor absorption of iron
Pernicious and vitamin B deficiency	Hb ↓ MCV ↑ (macrocytic) Reticulocyte count ↓ B_{12} or folate level ↓ if deficient	Intrinsic factor antibodies Diet low in vitamin B_{12}, folate
Haemolytic	Hb ↓ MCH ↑ Reticulocyte count ↑ Abnormal forms of RBC in peripheral smear (spherocytes, elliptocytes, spur cells, tear drops, inclusions) Unconjugated (indirect) bilirubin ↑ LDH ↑ Haptoglobin ↓	Sickle cell anaemia, thalassaemia, autoimmune diseases, transfusion reaction, drugs
Aplastic	Hb ↓ RBC and WBC counts ↓ Platelet count ↓ MCV, MCH usually N WBC differential usually shows ↓ all white cell types except lymphocytes Reticulocyte count ↓	Cancer therapy, toxins, autoimmune, viral infections

Fe = iron; Hb = haemoglobin; LDH = lactate dehydrogenase; MCH = mean corpuscular haemoglobin (average amount of Hb in RBCs); MCV = mean corpuscular volume (average size of RBCs); N = normal; RBC = red blood cell; TIBC = total iron-binding capacity; WBC = white blood cell.

PLEURAL FLUID

What tests to order:

- Differential cell count
- Protein
- LDH

(*pto*)

- Glucose
- Culture (also put fluid into blood culture bottles—this improves yield of anaerobic organisms)
- Cytology

Note: There must be simultaneous measurement of the equivalent serum values of protein, LDH and glucose in order to do the calculations below.

Normal pleural fluid

Colour	Clear
pH	7.60–7.64
Protein content	< 2% (1–2 g/dL)
Cell count	< 1000 WBC per mm^3
Glucose	Similar to that of plasma
LDH	< 50% that of plasma

Exudate if:

Pleural fluid protein:serum protein > 0.5 Pleural fluid LDH:serum LDH > 0.6 Pleural LDH > ⅔ the upper limit of the normal serum value	Light's criteria
Pleural fluid LDH > 0.45 the upper limit of the normal serum value Pleural fluid cholesterol level > 45 mg/dL Pleural fluid protein level > 2.9 g/dL	Additional criteria

Transudates Low protein and LDH	Exudates Relatively high protein or LDH, pH < 7.2
• CCF • Cirrhosis, ascites • Hypoalbuminaemia • Nephrotic syndrome • Peritoneal dialysis • Myxoedema • Constrictive pericarditis	• Parapneumonic causes • Malignancy • PE • Infection • Pancreatitis • Sarcoidosis • Autoimmune (RA, SLE) • Chylothorax • Haemothorax • Intra-abdominal abscess

Laboratory result on pleural fluid	Possible cause
LDH > 1000 IU/L	Empyema Malignancy RA
Low glucose (30–50 mg/dL)	Malignancy TB Oesophageal rupture SLE
Very low glucose (< 30 mg/dL)	RA Empyema
pH < 7.30 with a normal serum pH	Malignancy TB Oesophageal rupture SLE
> 85% lymphocytes	Lymphoma TB Sarcoidosis Chronic rheumatoid pleurisy Yellow nail syndrome Chylothorax
50–70% lymphocytes	Malignancy
Eosinophilia (> 10%)	Air/blood in pleural space PE/pulmonary infarction Benign asbestos disease Parasitic disease Fungal infection Drugs

SYNOVIAL FLUID ANALYSIS

	Appearance	WBCs/mm^3	PMN%	Crystals
Normal	Clear	< 200	< 25%	None
Non-inflammatory	Clear	< 400	< 25%	None
Acute gout	Cloudy	2000–5000	> 75%	Negative birefringence
Pseudogout	Cloudy	5000–50,000	> 75%	Positive birefringence
Septic arthritis	Purulent	15,000–> 50,000	> 75% (> 90% = very suggestive)	None
Inflammatory (e.g. RA)	Cloudy	5000–50,000	50–75%	None

16

17 Orthopaedics

SYSTEMATIC APPROACH TO DESCRIBING A FRACTURE

1. **Age** and **sex** and **occupation** of patient
2. Name the **bone(s) involved**
3. **Open versus closed** injury—if open, describe the wound (e.g. abrasion, full thickness laceration) and its relationship to the fracture site
4. **Location** of the fracture
   a. Is it in the proximal, middle or distal part of the bone?
   b. Is it at a junction?
      Examples:
      - Junction of the proximal ⅔ and distal ⅓
      - Junction of the proximal ¼ and distal ¾
      - Junction of the lateral ⅓ and medial ⅔
   c. Is it involving the head, neck, shaft or base of the bone?
      Examples:
      - Head of the 5th metacarpal
      - Middle part of the shaft of the humerus
   d. Is it involving an anatomical part of the bone?
      Examples:
      - Greater trochanter of the femur
      - Greater tuberosity of the head of the humerus
5. **Pattern/direction** of the fracture (horizontal, spiral, oblique, comminuted [more than 2 pieces], segmental [several large fragments in one bone], T-shaped, Y-shaped etc)
6. **Alignment**
   a. Is it displaced or undisplaced?
   b. Is it straight or angulated (estimate degree of and anatomical direction)?
7. **Special features**
   a. Number of malleoli in ankle (unimalleolar/bimalleolar/trimalleolar)
   b. Medial and lateral plateau of tibia
   c. Colles number (distal radius)
   d. Neck of femur—subcapital, transcervical, pertrochanteric, intertrochanteric

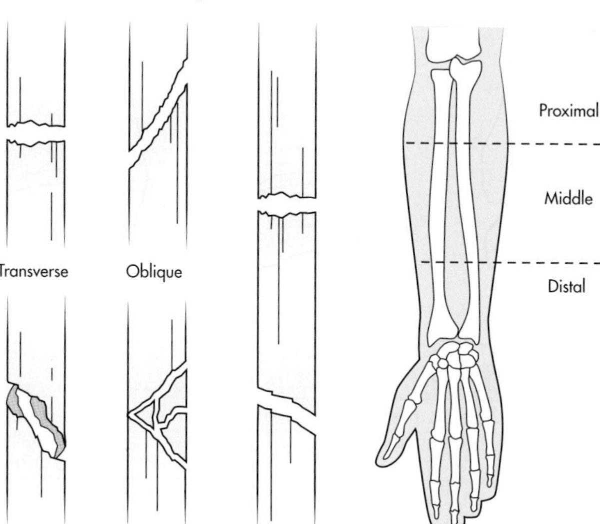

Figure 17.1 Common types of fractures

OTTAWA ANKLE RULES

An ankle X-ray is required if:

There is any pain in the malleolar region and one of the following:

- bone tenderness at the posterior edge of the distal 6 cm of the fibula or the tip of the lateral malleolus *or*
- bone tenderness at the posterior edge of the distal 6 cm of the tibia or the tip of the medial malleolus *or*
- inability to weight bear both immediately and in emergency department.

A foot X-ray is required if:

There is any pain in the midfoot region and one of the following:

- bone tenderness over the base of the 5th metatarsal *or*
- bone tenderness over the navicular *or*
- inability to weight bear both immediately and in emergency department (not applicable to < 18 y).

Clinical judgment is required for those intoxicated, uncooperative, ↓ sensation in leg or with distracting injuries.

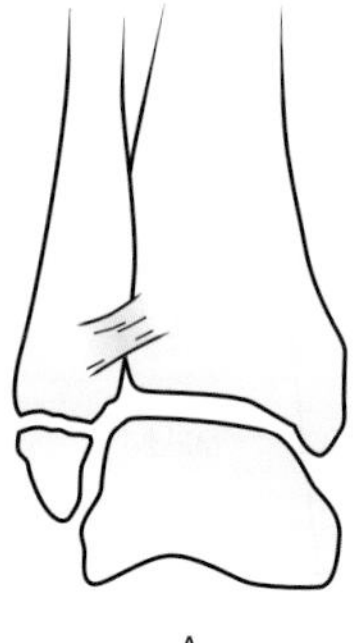

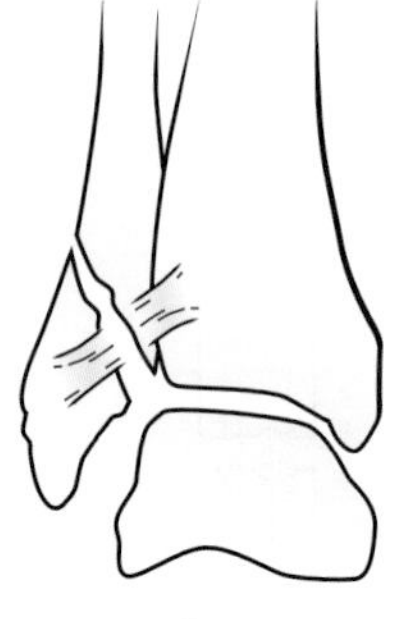

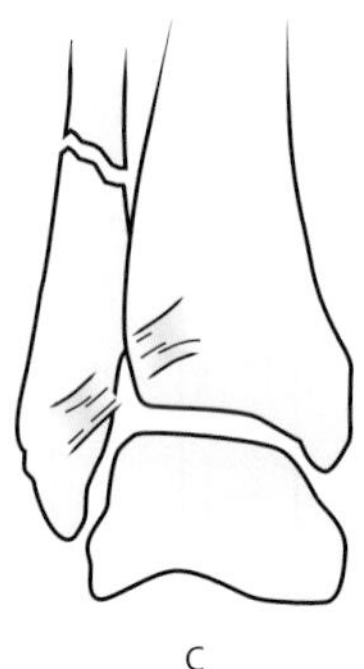

Classification	Location of fracture line	Integrity of syndesmosis	Stability
A	Below the level of the ankle joint	Intact	Usually stable; occasionally needs ORIF
B	At the level of the ankle joint	Disruption in 50%	Variable
C	Above the level of the ankle joint	Always disrupted	Unstable ORIF

Syndesmosis is made up of anterior–inferior tibiofibular ligament, interosseous ligament and posterior–inferior fibular ligaments, inferior transverse tibiofibular ligament and interosseous ligament.
ORIF = open reduction internal fixation.

Figure 17.2 Weber classification of ankle (fibular) fractures

OTTAWA KNEE RULES

A knee X-ray is required if:

- Age > 55 y
- Unable to transfer weight for 4 steps both immediately after injury and in emergency department
- Unable to flex to 90°
- Tenderness over fibular head
- Isolated tenderness of patella

17

INTERPRETATION OF ELBOW FRACTURES IN CHILDREN

Is there a joint effusion?

- Fat pad sign—present with effusion
- Look for upward displacement of anterior fat pad
  or
- a visible posterior fat pad (not normally seen).

Is there normal alignment of the bones?

- Radiocapitellar line—line drawn through the centre of the proximal radius should pass through the centre of the capitellum on all views. If not, the radial head is subluxed or dislocated.
- Anterior humeral line—line drawn on a lateral view along the anterior border of the humerus should pass through the medial ⅓ of the capitellum—in supracondylar fractures, it often intersects with anterior ⅓ or beyond.

Are there normal ossification centres?

These appear at highly variable times but, as a general guide, the following can be used. The significance is the order in which they appear to help you decide whether a small piece of bone is a fracture fragment or an ossification centre.

Elbow ossification order—CRITOE

	Ossification centre	Age of appearance
C	Capitellum	1 y
R	Radial head	3 y
I	Internal (medial) epicondyle	5 y
T	Trochlea	7 y
O	Olecranon	9 y
E	External (lateral) epicondyle	11 y

X-ray changes to look for

Features to look for	What it means	Likely cause
Elevation of anterior fat pad	Joint effusion	Fracture or dislocation of radial head in elbow joint
Presence of a posterior fat pad (not normally visible at all)	Joint effusion	Fracture or dislocation of radial head in elbow joint
Radiocapitellar line (evident on all views)	Displacement of radial head	Subluxation or dislocation of the radial head
Anterior humeral line (use a TRUE lateral view)	Displacement of the distal part of the humerus	Supracondylar fracture

17

Supracondylar fractures

- Represent 60% of paediatric elbow fractures
- Commonly distal fragment angulates and displaces posteriorly
- Pay close attention to neurovascular status of the limb—10% incidence of nerve injury—radial most commonly then median and finally ulnar

SALTER-HARRIS CLASSIFICATION OF PHYSEAL (GROWTH PLATE) FRACTURES IN CHILDREN

- Grades I–V (see also Figure 17.3)
- Significance: higher grades have greater risk of growth abnormalities

Grade	Description	Pearls and pitfalls
I	# within the growth plate	May not be visible on X-ray or may see widening or displacement of the growth plate on X-ray
II	Involves metaphysis and growth plate	Most common Rarely cause future functional limitations
III	Involves epiphysis and growth plate	Intra-articular therefore can cause chronic disability but rarely significant deformity
IV	Intra-articular # which involves the metaphysis, growth plate and epiphysis	Can cause deformity due to premature fusion of bones
V	Compression injury	Difficult to see on X-ray Cause functional limitations due to growth disturbance History of axial load injury might be only clue to diagnosis

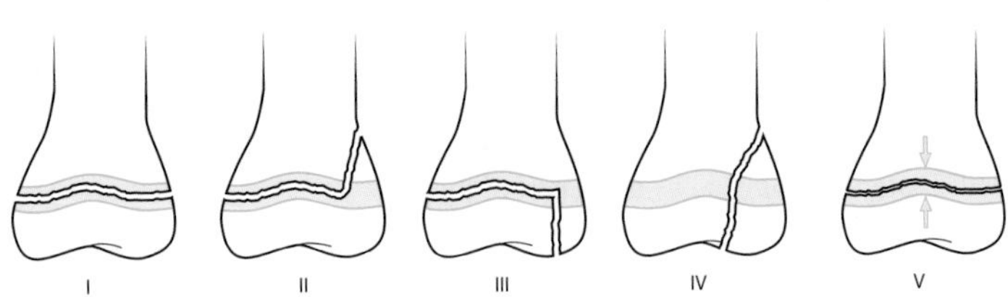

Figure 17.3 Salter-Harris classification of physeal (growth plate) fractures in children

18 Obstetrics and gynaecology

BETA-HUMAN CHORIONIC GONADOTROPHIN (beta-hCG)

- In normal pregnancy, levels double every 2 days.
- Transvaginal ultrasound (TVUS) will detect:
  - gestational sac at ~4.5–5 weeks gestation
  - yolk sac at 5–6 weeks (until 10 weeks)
  - fetal pole with cardiac activity (5.5–6 weeks).
- Discriminatory zone:
  - This is the serum beta-hCG level at which a gestational sac should be visualised by ultrasound if the pregnancy is intrauterine.
  - For TVUS, this is 1500–2000 IU/L.
  - For transabdominal ultrasound (TAUS), this is 6500 IU/L.
  - These may vary according to individuals/multiple gestation.

Rh D IMMUNOGLOBULIN (ANTI-D) ADMINISTRATION

Dose:

- If < 12 weeks gestation → 250 IU IM
- If > 12 weeks gestation → 625 IU IM

Indications:

- Possible fetomaternal haemorrhage (see box below)

Indications for Anti-D administration

- Antenatal haemorrhage
- Induced abortion
- Miscarriage
- Ectopic pregnancy
- Maternal abdominal trauma
- Delivery
- Partial molar pregnancy
- Chorionic villus sampling, amniocentesis
- Cordocentesis
- Percutaneous fetal procedures (e.g. fetoscopy)
- External cephalic version
- Abruptio placenta
- Manual removal of the placenta

PRETERM LABOUR SUPPRESSION

- Between 24 and 34 weeks.
- Accounts for only 10% of births but is associated with 75% of neonatal morbidity and mortality.

- To prevent respiratory distress syndrome, administer betamethasone 11.4 mg IM. Repeat the dose 24 h later, unless delivery has occurred.
- Tocolytic agent (see table) = *nifedipine is preferred*; salbutamol may also be used

Tocolytic agent	Nifedipine	Salbutamol infusion
Initial dose	20 mg PO (onset of tocolysis = 30–60 mins)	6 mL/h of 10 mg in 100 mL 0.9% saline*
Subsequent dosing	20 mg PO at 30-minute intervals for 2 more doses (if required)	↑ rate by 3 mL/h every 10 min until response
Maintenance dose	20–40 mg PO q6h depending on uterine activity and side effects (max 160 mg/24 h)	If contractions cease, maintain infusion rate for 6 h and then ↓ by 3 mL/h each hour until maintenance level reached
Side effects	Hypotension Tachycardia Palpitations Flushing Headache Nausea	Tremor Anxiety Nausea Palpitations
Tips	Do not use if hypotensive, established cardiac disease BP reduction may be potentiated by other antihypertensives Caution using magnesium concurrently	Cease if maternal chest pain, SOB, vomiting Slow rate if maternal HR > 140/min or FHR > 180/min

* To make up infusion, withdraw 10 mL from a 100-mL bag of 0.9% saline and replace with 10 mL (10 mg) of obstetric salbutamol. This results in 100 microg/mL.
FHR = fetal heart rate.

19 Dental

Dental trauma

Trauma	Definition	Treatment
Concussion	Tooth is immobile and undisplaced, normal X-ray; sensitive to percussion	Rest (no biting)
Subluxation	Loosening of tooth but no displacement; sensitive to percussion	Use local anaesthetic Return tooth to correct anatomical position without further damage to tissues and bone and secure to adjacent teeth with a periodontal splint Analgesia Antibiotic cover Early dental follow-up
Avulsion	Complete extraction of tooth	
Intrusive luxation	Forcing of tooth into its socket (in apical direction)	
Extrusive luxation	Tooth forced in axial direction out of socket	
Lateral luxation	Tooth is forced into a sideways direction	
Dental fracture	Ellis class I: enamel only; non-tender, no colour change, rough edges	File rough edges if necessary
	Ellis class II: enamel and dentin involved; tender to touch and air exposure; may see yellow layer of dentin	Cover exposed site with calcium hydroxide composition Analgesia Antibiotic cover
	Ellis class III: pulp involved; tender as with class II and pink/red or blood seen in centre of tooth	Cover exposed site with calcium hydroxide composition Analgesia Antibiotic cover

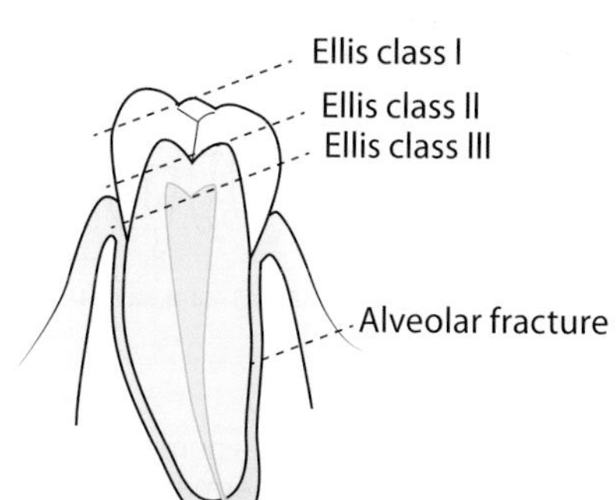

Figure 19.1 Ellis fracture classification

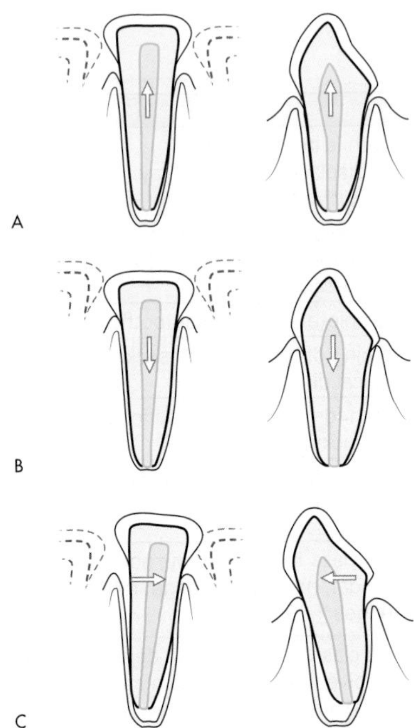

Figure 19.2 Patterns of luxation
A, Extrusive luxation. **B**, Intrusive luxation. **C**, Lateral luxation.

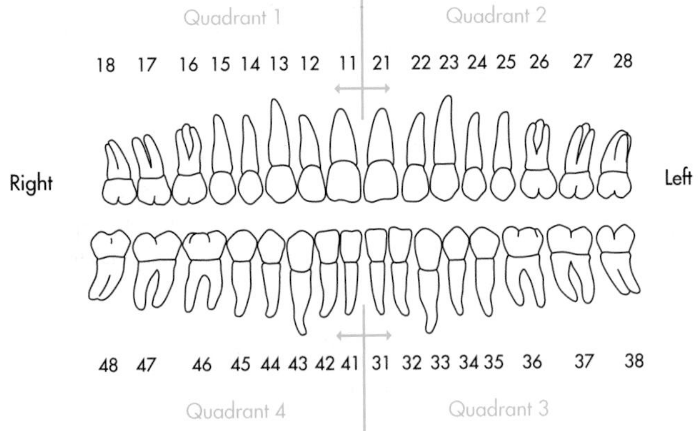

Figure 19.3 Dental chart—nomenclature and universal numbering system for permanent (adult) dentition

LOCAL ANAESTHESIA – SUPRAPERIOSTEAL INFILTRATION

This technique is useful for a single tooth or closely clustered group of teeth.

- Place the needle in the mucobuccal fold with the bevel facing the bone.
- Direct the needle tip toward the apex of the desired tooth (usually several millimetres deep).
- If bone is contacted, withdraw slightly to avoid periosteal infiltration.
- Inject anaesthetic once satisfied the needle is in the correct place (i.e., not intravascular).
- Generally 1–2 mL of local anaesthetic is sufficient.
- It may take up to 10 min to achieve complete anaesthesia.

REIMPLANTATION OF AVULSED TOOTH

- Gently clean tooth in either normal saline or sterile auxiliary solution (e.g. Hank's balanced salt solution).
- Avoid scrubbing the tooth or any unnecessary delay before reimplantation.
- Return tooth to its original position by applying firm finger pressure.
- Handle the tooth by the crown, and avoid trauma to the tooth root.
- Stabilise the tooth with a temporary periodontal splint.
- Ensure early dental follow-up.
- Give antibiotics to cover intraoral flora (e.g. penicillin, clindamycin).

20 Common conversions

Conversion table/calculator

	To convert from	To	Multiply by	To convert from	To	Multiply by
Albumin	g/L	g/dL	0.1	g/dL	g/L	10
Bicarbonate	mEq/L	mmol/L	1.0	mmol/L	mEq/L	1.0
Bilirubin	micromol/L	mg/dL	0.0584	mg/dL	micromol/L	17.1
Calcium	mmol/L	mg/dL	4	mg/dL	mmol/L	0.25
	mEq/L	mmol/L	0.5	mmol/L	mEq/L	2
Carbamazepine	micromol/L	mg/L	0.236	mg/L	micromol/L	4.2372
Cholesterol	mmol/L	mg/dL	38.61	mg/dL	mmol/L	0.0259
Creatinine	micromol/L	mg/dL	0.01131	mg/dL	micromol/L	88.4
Digoxin	nmol/L	ng/L	0.78064	ng/L	nmol/L	1.281
Ethanol	mg/dL	mmol/L	0.2174	mmol/L	mg/dL	4.6
	%	mg/dL	1000	mg/dL	%	0.001
Glucose	mmol/L	mg/dL	18.0182	mg/dL	mmol/L	0.0555
Iron	micromol /L	microg/dL	5.5866	microg/dL	micromol/L	0.179
Lead	microg/dL	micromol/L	0.0483	micromol/L	microg/dL	20.704
Lithium	mEq/L	mmol/L	1.0	mmol/L	mEq/L	1.0
Magnesium	mmol/L	mg/dL	2.43	mg/dL	mmol/L	0.4115
	mEq/L	mmol/L	0.5	mmol/L	mEq/L	2
Oxygen	mmHg	kPa	0.133	kPa	mmHg	7.5188
Paracetamol	microg/mL	micromol /L	6.62	micromol /L	microg/mL	0.151

	To convert from	To	Multiply by	To convert from	To	Multiply by
Phenobarbitone	mg/L	micromol/L	4.31	micromol/L	mg/L	0.232
Phenytoin	microg/mL	micromol/L	3.96	micromol/L	microg/mL	0.2525
Protein	g/L	g/dL	0.1	g/dL	g/L	10
Salicylate	mg/dL	mmol/L	0.0724	mmol/L	mg/dL	13.8
Urea	mmol/L	mg/dL	2.8011	mg/dL	mmol/L	0.357
Valproate	micromol/L	mg/L	0.144	mg/L	micromol/L	6.94
Temperature	°C	°F	(9/5 × °C) + 32	°F	°C	5/9 × (°F – 32)

21 Antibiotic prescribing

TREATMENT OF COMMON INFECTIONS

Drug choice may be influenced by local factors, susceptibilities. For children, check the dose of the antimicrobials.

Condition		Antimicrobial options (paediatric dose in mg/kg up to a max of adult dose)	Options if penicillin allergy* (paediatric dose in mg/kg up to a max of adult dose)	Options if penicillin anaphylaxis** (paediatric dose in mg/kg up to a max of adult dose)	Special cases
Febrile neutropenia		Cefepime 2 g IV q8h OR Ceftazidime 2 g IV q8h OR Piperacillin + tazobactam 4 + 0.5 g IV q8h			Add vancomycin 1.5 g IV q12h if not resolving after 48 h Consider antifungals if ongoing fever
Osteomyelitis & septic arthritis		Di/flucloxacillin 2 g (50 mg/kg up to 2 g) IV q6h	Cephazolin 2 g (50 mg/kg) IV q8h	Vancomycin 1.5 g (< 12 y: 30 mg/kg) IV q12h	Adjust therapy to known culture results
Compound fractures	Simple	Dicloxacillin 2 g (50 mg/kg) IV q6h	Cephazolin 2 g (50 mg/kg) IV q8h	Clindamycin 450 mg (10 mg/kg) IV or PO q8h OR Lincomycin 600 mg (15 mg/kg) IV q8h	
	Contaminated or soiled wound	Piperacillin + tazobactam 4 + 0.5 g (100 + 12.5 mg/kg) IV q8h OR Ticarcillin + clavulanate 3 + 0.1 g (50 + 1.7 mg/kg) IV q6h	Cephazolin 2 g (50 mg/kg) IV q8h PLUS Metronidazole 500 mg (12.5 mg/kg) IV q12h	Ciprofloxacin 400 mg (10 mg/kg) IV q12h PLUS EITHER Clindamycin 450 mg (15 mg/kg) IV or PO q8h OR Lincomycin 600 mg (15 mg/kg) IV q8h	

Endocarditis	Empirical treatment	Benzylpenicillin 1.8 g (45 mg/kg) IV q4h PLUS Di/flucloxacillin 2 g (50 mg/kg) IV q4h PLUS Gentamicin 4–6 mg/kg (< 10 y: 7.5 mg/kg, > 10 y 6 mg/kg) IV for 1 dose	Seek expert advice. Consider rapid desensitisation	Vancomycin 1.5 g (< 12 y: 30 mg/kg) IV q12h PLUS Gentamicin 4–6 mg/kg (< 10 y: 7.5 mg/kg, > 10 y 6 mg/kg) IV for 1 dose	All pts should have 3 sets of blood cultures taken. If any of: prosthetic heart valve PPM or intracardiac device in situ healthcare-associated infection immediate penicillin hypersensitivity then use vancomycin regimen instead
Meningitis	Empirical treatment Adults and children > 3 mo	Dexamethasone 10 mg (0.15 mg/kg) IV Before or with 1st dose of: Ceftriaxone 4 g (100 mg/kg) IV daily OR Cefotaxime 2 g (50 mg/kg) IV q6h		Vancomycin 1.5 g (< 12 y: 30 mg/kg) IV q12h PLUS EITHER Ciprofloxacin 400 mg (10 mg/kg) IV q12h OR Moxifloxacin 400 mg (10 mg/kg) IV daily	Consider adding in: Penicillin g 2.4 g IV q4h for immunocompromised, age > 50 y or hx of alcohol abuse to cover listeria Add vancomycin if Gram +ve diplococci seen or pneumococcal antigen assay in CSF +ve
Encephalitis—herpes simplex		Acyclovir 10 mg/kg IV q8h for at least 14/7			For full-term neonates use 20 mg/kg IV q8h for 21/7

* Hypersensitivity excluding immediate hypersensitivity.

** Immediate hypersensitivity characterised by development of urticaria, angio-oedema, bronchospasm or cardiovascular collapse within an hour or two of antibiotic administration.

Continues

Condition		Antimicrobial options	Options if penicillin allergy*	Options if penicillin anaphylaxis**	Special cases
		(paediatric dose in mg/kg up to a max of adult dose)			
Epididymo-orchitis	UTI source Mild	Trimethoprim 300 mg (6 mg/kg) PO for 14/7 OR Cephalexin 500 mg (12.5 mg/kg) PO q12h for 14/7 OR Amoxycillin + clavulanate 500 + 125 mg (12.5 + 3.1 mg/kg) q12h for 14/7			If resistance to drugs at left, use norfloxacin 400 mg IV q12h
	Severe	Ampicillin 2 g (50 mg/kg) IV q6h PLUS Gentamicin 4–6 mg/kg (< 10 y 7.5 mg/kg, > 10 y 6 mg/kg) IV for 1 dose	Gentamicin 4–6 mg/kg (< 10 y 7.5 mg/kg, > 10 y 6 mg/kg) IV for 1 dose	Gentamicin 4–6 mg/kg (< 10 y 7.5 mg/kg, > 10 y 6 mg/kg) IV for 1 dose	If gentamicin contraindicated: ceftriaxone 1 g (25 mg/kg) IV daily
	Sexually acquired source	Ceftriaxone 500 mg in 2 mL of 1% lignocaine IMI or 500 mg IV daily for 3 days PLUS EITHER Doxycycline 100 mg PO q12h for 14/7 OR Azithromycin 1 g orally as a single dose 1 week later		Seek expert advice	

Pelvic inflammatory disease	**Mild**	Ceftriaxone 500 mg in 2 mL 1% lignocaine IMI or 500 mg IV as a single dose PLUS Metronidazole 400 mg PO q12h for 14/7 PLUS Azithromycin 1 g PO as single dose PLUS EITHER Azithromycin 1 g PO 1/52 later OR Doxycycline 100 mg q12h for 14/7		Metronidazole 400 mg PO q12h for 14/7
	Severe	Ceftriaxone 1 g daily PLUS Azithromycin 500 mg IV daily PLUS Metronidazole 500 mg IV q12h		Gentamicin 4–6 mg/kg IV for 1 dose PLUS EITHER Clindamycin 450 mg IV q8h OR Lincomycin 600 mg IV q8h
Cholecystitis, ascending cholangitis		Ampicillin 1 g (25 mg/kg) IV q6h PLUS Gentamicin 4–6 mg/kg (< 10 y, 7.5 mg/kg, > 10 y 6 mg/kg) IV daily PLUS IF BILIARY OBSTRUCTION Metronidazole 500 mg (12.5 mg/kg) IV q12h	Ceftriaxone 1 g (25 mg/kg) IV daily OR Cefotaxime 1 g (25 mg/kg) IV q8h	Seek expert advice

* Hypersensitivity excluding immediate hypersensitivity.

** Immediate hypersensitivity characterised by development of urticaria, angio-oedema, bronchospasm or cardiovascular collapse within an hour or two of antibiotic administration.

Continues

Condition	Antimicrobial options (paediatric dose in mg/kg up to a max of adult dose)	Options if penicillin allergy*	Options if penicillin anaphylaxis**	Special cases
Peritonitis due to perforated viscus	Ampicillin 1 g (50 mg/kg) IV q6h PLUS Metronidazole 500 mg (12.5 mg/kg) IV q12h PLUS Gentamicin 4–6 mg/kg (< 10 y 7.5 mg/kg, > 10 y 6 mg/kg) for 1 dose	Metronidazole 500 mg (12.5 mg/kg) IV q12h PLUS EITHER Ceftriaxone 1 g (25 mg/kg) IV daily OR Cefotaxime 1 g (25 mg/kg) IV q8h	Seek expert advice	
Spontaneous bacterial peritonitis	Ceftriaxone 1 g (25 mg/kg) IV daily OR Cefotaxime 1 g IV q8h OR Piperacillin + tazobactam 4 + 0.5 g (100 + 12.5 mg/kg) IV q8h OR Ticarcillin + clavulanate 3 + 0.1 g (50 + 1.7 mg/kg) IV q6h			If already on prophylaxis add ampicillin 1 g IV q6h to regimen

Diverticulitis	Mild	Amoxycillin + clavulanate 875 + 125 mg PO q12h for 5/7 OR Cephalexin 500 mg PO q6h for 5/7 PLUS Metronidazole 400 mg PO q12h for 5/7		Metronidazole 400 mg PO q12h for 5/7 PLUS Trimethoprim + sulfamethoxazole 160 + 800 mg PO q12h for 5/7	
	Severe	Ampicillin 1 g IV q6h PLUS Gentamicin 4–6 mg/kg IV PLUS Metronidazole 500 mg IV q12h	Metronidazole 500 mg IV q12h PLUS EITHER Ceftriaxone 1 g IV daily OR Cefotaxime 1 g IV q8h	Seek expert advice	
Acute pyelonephritis	Mild	Amoxycillin + clavulanate 875 + 125 mg PO q12h for 10/7 OR Cephalexin 500 mg PO q6h for 10/7 OR Trimethoprim 300 mg PO daily for 10/7			If resistant use: Norfloxacin 400 mg PO q12h for 10/7 OR Ciprofloxacin 500 mg PO q12h for 10/7
	Severe	Gentamicin 4–6 mg/kg IV PLUS Ampicillin 2 g IV q6h			If gentamicin contraindicated use: Ceftriaxone 1 g IV daily OR Cefotaxime 1 g IV q8h

* Hypersensitivity excluding immediate hypersensitivity.

** Immediate hypersensitivity characterised by development of urticaria, angio-oedema, bronchospasm or cardiovascular collapse within an hour or two of antibiotic administration.

Continues

21

Condition		Antimicrobial options	Options if penicillin allergy*	Options if penicillin anaphylaxis**	Special cases
		(paediatric dose in mg/kg up to a max of adult dose)			
Acute cystitis	Non-pregnant women	Trimethoprim 300 mg PO for 3/7 OR Cephalexin 500 mg PO q12h for 5/7 OR Amoxycillin + clavulanate 500 + 125 mg PO q12h for 5/7 OR Nitrofurantoin 100 mg PO q12h for 5/7			If resistant to drugs at left use: Norfloxacin 400 mg PO q12h for 3/7
	Pregnant	Cephalexin 500 mg PO q12h for 5/7 OR Nitrofurantoin 100 mg PO for 5/7 OR Amoxycillin + clavulanate 500 + 125 mg PO q12h for 5/7			
	Men	Trimethoprim 300 mg PO daily for 14/7 OR Cephalexin 500 mg PO q12h for 14/7 OR Amoxycillin + clavulanate 500 + 125 mg PO q12h for 14/7			

Community acquired pneumonia	**Mild**	Amoxycillin 1 g PO q8h for 5–7/7	Doxycycline 200 mg PO for the first dose, then 100 mg daily for 5/7		If *M. pneumoniae* suspected use: Doxycycline 200 mg then 100 mg daily for 5/7
	Moderate	Benzylpenicillin 1.2 g IV q6h OR Ceftriaxone 1 g IV daily PLUS EITHER Doxycycline 100 mg q12h OR Clarithromycin 500 mg q12h	Substitute benzylpenicillin with: Ceftriaxone 1 g IV daily OR Cefotaxime 1 g IV q8h	Moxifloxacin 400 mg PO daily for 7/7	In tropical regions, if risk of melioidosis then use: Ceftriaxone 2 g IV daily PLUS Gentamicin 4–6 mg/kg IV daily
	Severe	Benzylpenicillin 1.2 g IV q4h PLUS Gentamicin 4–6 mg/kg OR Ceftriaxone 1 g IV daily OR Cefotaxime 1 g IV q8h PLUS WITH EACH OF ABOVE Azithromycin 500 mg IV daily		Moxifloxacin 400 mg IV daily PLUS Azithromycin 500 mg IV daily	In tropical regions use as first-line: Meropenem 1 g IV q8h OR Imipenem 1 g IV q6h PLUS WITH EACH OF ABOVE REGIMENS Azithromycin 500 mg IV daily
Aspiration pneumonia		Benzylpenicillin 1.2 g IV q6h PLUS Metronidazole 500 mg IV q12h	Clindamycin 450 mg (10 mg/kg) IV or PO q8h OR Lincomycin 600 mg (15 mg/kg) IV q8h	Clindamycin 450 mg (10 mg/kg) IV or PO q8h OR Lincomycin 600 mg (15 mg/kg) IV q8h	

* Hypersensitivity excluding immediate hypersensitivity.

** Immediate hypersensitivity characterised by development of urticaria, angio-oedema, bronchospasm or cardiovascular collapse within an hour or two of antibiotic administration.

Continues

Condition	Antimicrobial options	Options if penicillin allergy*	Options if penicillin anaphylaxis**	Special cases
	(paediatric dose in mg/kg up to a max of adult dose)			
Bacterial tonsillitis	Phenoxymethylpenicillin 500 mg PO q12h for 10 days	Roxithromycin 300 mg daily (4 mg/kg q12h) PO for 10/7	Roxithromycin 300 mg daily (4 mg/kg q12h) PO for 10/7	Dexamethasone 10 mg IV/PO or prednisolone 60 mg helps with severe difficulty swallowing Quinsy—drainage, IV penicillin/clindamycin plus metronidazole
Acute epiglottitis	Ceftriaxone 1 g (25 mg/kg) IV daily OR Cefotaxime 1 g (25 mg/kg) IV q8h			Dexamethasone 10 mg IV (child 0.15 mg/kg)
Otitis media	Amoxycillin 15 mg/kg PO q8h for 5/7	Cefuroxime (3 mo–2 y: 10 mg/kg, > 2 y 15 mg/kg) PO q12h for 5/7 OR Cefaclor 10 mg/kg up to 250 mg PO q8h for 5/7	Cefuroxime (3 mo–2 y: 10 mg/kg, > 2 y 15 mg/kg) PO q12h for 5/7 OR Cefaclor 10 mg/kg up to 250 mg PO q8h for 5/7	If poor response, try amoxycillin + clavulanate 22.5 + 3.2 mg/kg PO q8h

Human and animal bites	Infection not established	Amoxycillin + clavulanate 875 + 125 mg (22.5 + 3.2 mg/kg) PO q12h for 5/7			Ensure tetanus status up to date
	Infection established	Piperacillin + tazobactam 4 + 0.5 g (100 + 12.5 mg/kg) IV q8h OR Ticarcillin + clavulanate 3 + 0.1 g (50 + 1.7 mg/kg) IV q6h OR COMBINATION OF Metronidazole 400 mg (10 mg/kg) PO q 12h PLUS EITHER Ceftriaxone 1 g (child 25 mg/kg) IV daily OR Cefotaxime 1 g (25 mg/kg) IV q8h	Moxifloxacin 400 mg (10 mg/kg) PO daily OR COMBINATION OF Metronidazole 400 mg (10 mg/kg) PO q12h PLUS EITHER Doxycycline 200 mg (> 8 y: 5 mg/kg) PO for the first dose then 100 mg (> 8 y: 2.5 mg/kg) PO daily OR Trimethoprim + sulfamethoxazole 160 + 800 mg (> 2 mo: 4 + 20 mg/kg) PO q12h	Moxifloxacin 400 mg (10 mg/kg) PO daily OR COMBINATION OF Metronidazole 400 mg (10 mg/kg) PO q12h PLUS EITHER Doxycycline 200 mg (> 8 y: 5 mg/kg) PO for the first dose then 100 mg (> 8 y: 2.5 mg/kg) PO daily OR Trimethoprim + sulfamethoxazole 160 + 800 mg (> 2 mo: 4 + 20 mg/kg) PO q12h	

* Hypersensitivity excluding immediate hypersensitivity.

** Immediate hypersensitivity characterised by development of urticaria, angio-oedema, bronchospasm or cardiovascular collapse within an hour or two of antibiotic administration.

Continues

Condition		Antimicrobial options	Options if penicillin allergy*	Options if penicillin anaphylaxis**	Special cases
		(paediatric dose in mg/kg up to a max of adult dose)			
Cellulitis	Mild	Di/flucloxacillin 500 mg	Cephalexin 500 mg PO q6h	Clindamycin 450 mg PO q8h	NORSA—use clindamycin/ doxycycline/ trimethoprim + sulfamethoxazole MRSA—use vancomycin
	Severe	Di/flucloxacillin 2 g IV q6h	Cephazolin 2 g (25 mg/kg) IV q8h	Clindamycin 450 mg (10 mg/kg) PO or IV q8h OR Lincomycin 600 mg (15 mg/kg) IV q8h OR Vancomycin 1.5 g (< 12 y: 30 mg/kg) IV q12h	
	Home IV therapy indicated	Cephazolin 2 g IV daily PLUS Probenecid 1 g PO daily			
Diabetic foot infections	Mild to moderate	Amoxycillin + clavulanate 875 + 125 mg PO q12h OR Cephalexin 500 mg PO q6h PLUS Metronidazole 400 mg PO q12h	Ciprofloxacin 500 mg PO q12h PLUS Clindamycin 600 mg PO q8h	Ciprofloxacin 500 mg PO q12h PLUS Clindamycin 600 mg PO q8h	
	Severe	Piperacillin + tazobactam 4 + 0.5 g IV q8h OR Ticarcillin + clavulanate 3 + 0.1 g IV q6h	Ciprofloxacin 400 mg IV q12h or 750 mg PO q12h PLUS EITHER Clindamycin 900 mg IV q8h OR Lincomycin 900 mg IV q8h	Ciprofloxacin 400 mg IV q12h or 750 mg PO q12h PLUS EITHER Clindamycin 900 mg IV q8h OR Lincomycin 900 mg IV q8h	
Necrotising fasciitis		Meropenem 1 g (25 mg/kg) IV q8h PLUS EITHER Clindamycin 600 mg (15 mg/kg) IV q8h OR Lincomycin 600 mg (15 mg/[illegible]			Early surgical debridement Hyperbaric O_2 if available

Severe sepsis (unclear source)	**Adults**	Di/flucloxacillin 2 g IV q6h PLUS Gentamicin 7 mg/kg IV for 1 dose	Substitute for di/flucoxacillin: Cephazolin 2 g IV q8h	Substitute for di/flucoxacillin: Vancomycin 1.5 g IV q12h	If meningococcal infection suspected, add benzylpenicillin If MRSA suspected, add vancomycin
	Children, meningitis not excluded	Age < 6 mo: Ampicillin 50 mg/kg IV q6h PLUS Cefotaxime 50 mg/kg q6h Age > 6 mo: Cefotaxime 50 mg/kg q6h			If pneumococcal meningitis likely add: Vancomycin 30 mg/kg IV q12h
	Children, meningitis excluded	Age < 4 mo: Ampicillin 50 mg/kg IV q6h PLUS Gentamicin 7.5 mg/kg IV for 1 dose Age > 4 mo: Cefotaxime 25 mg/kg IV q6h OR COMBINATION OF Ceftriaxone 25 mg/kg IV daily PLUS di/flucloxacillin 50 mg/kg IV q6h			

* Hypersensitivity excluding immediate hypersensitivity.

** Immediate hypersensitivity characterised by development of urticaria, angio-oedema, bronchospasm or cardiovascular collapse within an hour or two of antibiotic administration.

22 Normal values

(Approximate reference ranges)

Blood chemistry

Sodium	137–146 mmol/L
Potassium	3.5 –5.0 mmol/L
Chloride	95–110 mmol/L
Bicarbonate	24–31 mmol/L
Urea	3.0–8.5 mmol/L
Creatinine	Male: 60–120 micromol/L Female: 40–90 micromol/L
Glucose	3.0–7.8 mmol/L
Phosphate	0.70–1.40 mmol/L
Magnesium	0.70–1.05 mmol/L
Calcium	2.10–2.60 mmol/L
Albumin	36–52 g/L
Total protein	66–82 g/L
Total bilirubin	0–18 micromol/L
ALT	0–30 U/L
AST	0–30 U/L
ALP	30–100 U/L
GGT	0–35 U/L
Lipase	< 60 U/L
Troponin T (hs)	0–14 ng/L

Full blood count

Haemoglobin	130–180 g/L (men) 115–165 g/L (women)
MCV	76–96 fL
Platelets	150–400 × 10^9/L
WCC	4.0–11.0 × 10^9/L
APTT	25–35 s
PT	11–15 s

Abbreviations

1°, 2° primary, secondary
3D three-dimensional
AAA abdominal aortic aneurysm
AAI acute arterial insufficiency
ABC airway, breathing, or ABCs circulation (the ABCs of resuscitation)
ABCDE (in medical retrieval) airway, breathing, circulation, disability, exposure/expectations
ABG arterial blood gas
AC acromioclavicular; alternating current
ACE angiotensin-converting enzyme
ACEM Australasian College for Emergency Medicine
ACI acute cardiac ischaemia
ACL anterior cruciate ligament
ACLS advanced cardiac life support
ACS acute coronary syndrome
ACTH adrenocorticotrophic hormone
AD Addison's disease, atopic dermatitis
ADC AIDS dementia complex
ADH antidiuretic hormone
ADHF acute decompensated (chronic) heart failure
ADL or ADLs activities of daily living
ADT adult diphtheria tetanus
AED automatic external defibrillator
AF atrial fibrillation
AG anion gap
AGE arterial gas embolism
AGEP acute generalised exanthematic pustulosis
AGVHD acute graft-versus-host disease
AHF acute heart failure
AIDS acquired immune deficiency syndrome
AIR assessment, intervention, reassessment
ALS (adult) advanced life support
ALT alanine aminotransferase
AMC area medical coordinator
AMI acute myocardial infarction
AML acute myelocytic leukaemia
ANUG acute necrotising ulcerative gingivitis
AP anteroposterior
APLS advanced paediatric life support
APO acute pulmonary oedema
APTT activated partial thromboplastin time
ARDS acute respiratory distress syndrome
ARF acute renal failure
ARS adjective rating scale (for pain)
ART antiretroviral therapy
ASCOT a severity characteristic of trauma
ASD atrial septal defect
ASET aged service emergency team
AST aspartate aminotransferase
ATLS advanced trauma life support
ATMS Abbreviated Mental Test Score
ATN acute tubular necrosis
ATP adenosine triphosphate
ATS Australasian Triage Scale
AV arteriovenous; atrioventricular
AVM arteriovenous malformation
AVN avascular necrosis
AVNRT AV nodal re-entry tachycardia
AVRT AV re-entry tachycardia
AWS Alcohol Withdrawal Scale
AXIS electrical pathway mapping
BAC blood alcohol concentration
BD, bd, bid twice daily
BBB bundle branch block
β-hCG beta human chorionic gonadotrophin
BiPAP bi-level positive airway pressure

BLS basic life support
BNP B-type natriuretic protein
BP blood pressure
bpm beats per minute
BPV benign positional vertigo
BPPV benign paroxysmal positional vertigo
BSA body surface area
BSL blood sugar level
BURP backward, upward, rightward pressure
BVM bag–valve–mask
Ca calcium
CABG coronary artery bypass graft
CAL (acute-on)-chronic airflow limitation, chronic airway limitation
CA-MRSA community-acquired methicillin-resistant *Staphylococcus aureus*
CAM Confusion Assessment Method
CAPD continuous ambulatory peritoneal dialysis
CAS coloured analogue scale (for pain)
CBR chemical, biological, radiological
CCF congestive cardiac failure; chronic cardiac failure
CCO casualty collecting (ambulance) officer
CCR5 chemokine (C–C motif) receptor 5 (blockers)
CCU coronary care unit
CHB complete heart block
CIN clinical initiatives nurse
CO cardiac output
COPD chronic obstructive pulmonary disease
CHB complete heart block
CIAP Clinical Information Access Program
CIN clinical initiatives nurse
CJD Creutzfeldt–Jakob disease
CK creatine kinase
CLL chronic lymphocytic leukaemia
CMC central medical coordinator
CML chromic myeloid leukaemia
CMO career medical officer
CMV cytomegalovirus
CNS central nervous system
CO carbon monoxide
CO_2 carbon dioxide
COAD chronic obstructive airways disease
COLD chronic obstructive lung disease
COPD chronic obstructive pulmonary disease
CPAP continuous positive airway pressure
CPK creatine phosphokinase
CPP cerebral perfusion pressure
CPR cardiopulmonary resuscitation
CRAG cryptococcal antigen
CRF chronic renal failure
CRP C-reactive protein
CSF cerebrospinal fluid
C-spine cervical spine
CSL Commonwealth Serum Laboratories
CT computed tomography
CTCA CT coronary angiography
CTG cardiotocography
CTPA computed tomography pulmonary angiogram
CTR cardiothoracic ratio
CVA cerebrovascular accident
CVC central venous catheter
CVP central venous pressure
CVS cardiovascular system
CXR chest X-ray
D&C dilation and curettage
DBP diastolic blood pressure
DC direct current
DD differential diagnosis/diagnoses
DFA direct fluorescent antibody
DI diabetes insipidus
DIC disseminated intravascular coagulation

DIP distal interphalangeal
DISPLAN medical response plan
DKA diabetic ketoacidosis
DM diabetes mellitus
DNA deoxyribonucleic acid
DPL diagnostic peritoneal lavage
DRESS drug reaction/rash with eosinophilia and systemic symptoms
DRS disability rating scale
DSA digital subtraction angiography
DTP diphtheria, tetanus, pertussis (vaccine)
DTaP, DTPa diphtheria, tetanus, acellular pertussis (vaccine)
DTs delirium tremens
DUB dysfunctional uterine bleeding
DVT deep vein thrombosis, deep venous thrombosis
EB epidermolysis bullosa
EBV Epstein–Barr virus
ECC emergency control centre
ECF extracellular fluid
ECG electrocardiogram, electrocardiography
ECMO extracorporeal membrane oxygenation
ED emergency department
EDH extradural haematoma
EDIS Emergency Department Information System
EER external emergency response
EEG electroencephalogram, electroencephalography
EF ejection fraction
eFAST extended FAST (focused assessment with sonography in trauma)
eGFR estimated glomerular filtration rate
EGFRI epidermal growth factor receptor inhibitor
EIA enzyme immunoassay
ELISA enzyme-linked immunosorbent assay
ELS emergency life support
EM erythema multiforme
EMA Emergency Medicine Australia
EMD electromechanical dissociation
EMR Electronic Medical Record
EMLA trade name for topical anaesthetic
EMST early management of severe trauma (guidelines)
EOC emergency operation centre
ENT ear, nose, throat
EOC emergency operation centre
EPAP expiratory positive airway pressure
EPS electrophysiological study
ERCP endoscopic retrograde cholangiopancreatography
ESR erythrocyte sedimentation rate
ESWL extracorporeal shock-wave lithotripsy
EtCO$_2$ end-tidal carbon dioxide
ETT endotracheal tube
EUC electrolytes, urea and creatinine (also UEC)
EVD external ventricular drain
FAS facial affective scale (for pain)
FAST focused assessment with sonography in trauma
FBC full blood count
FBE full blood examination
FDP fibrin degradation products; flexor digitorum profundus (deep digital flexor)
FDS flexor digitorum superficialis (superficial digital flexor)
FEV$_1$ forced expiratory volume in the first second
FFP fresh frozen plasma
FIM functional independence measure
FiO$_2$ fraction of inspired oxygen
Fr French gauge
FRC functional residual capacity

FSH follicle-stimulating hormone
FVC forced vital capacity
G&H group and hold (blood)
GABA gamma-aminobutyric acid
GBHS group B beta-haemolytic *Streptococcus*
GCS Glasgow Coma Scale
GDR Geriatric Depression Scale
GFR glomerular filtration rate
GHB gamma-hydroxybutyrate
GI gastrointestinal
GIT gastrointestinal tract
GM-CSF granulocyte–macrophage colony-stimulating factor
GNR Gram-negative rods
GORD gastro-oesophageal reflux disease
GP general practitioner
GTN glyceryl trinitrate
GVHD graft-versus-host disease
HAART highly active antiretroviral treatment
HADS Hospital Anxiety and Depression Scale
HAPE high-altitude pulmonary (o)edema
HAV hepatitis A virus
HA-MRSA hospital-acquired methicillin-resistant *Staphylococcus aureus*
Hb haemoglobin
HBC hepatitis B core antibody
HBO hyperbaric oxygen therapy
HBS hepatitis B surface antibody
HBV hepatitis B virus
hCG human chorionic gonadotrophin
HCM hypertrophic cardiomyopathy
Hct haematocrit
HCV hepatitis C virus
HDL high-density lipoprotein
HDV hepatitis delta agent
HEV hepatitis E virus
HF hydrofluoric acid
HFMD hand, foot and mouth disease
HGV hepatitis G virus
HHNS hyperosmolar hyperglycaemic non-ketotic state
HHS hyper-osmolar hyperglycaemic syndrome
HIDA hepatobiliary iminodiacetic acid (scan)
Hib *Haemophilus influenzae* type b
HIDA hepatobiliary iminodiacetic acid scan
HITH hospital in the home
HITTS heparin-induced thrombotic thrombocytopenia syndrome
HIV human immunodeficiency syndrome
HLA human leucocyte antigen
HOCM hypertrophic cardiomyopathy
HONK hyperosmolar non-ketosis
HPI history of present illness
HPV human papillomavirus
HR heart rate
HRT hormone replacement therapy
HSV herpes simplex virus
HTLV-1 human T-lymphotropic virus type 1
HZ herpes zoster
IABC intra-aortic balloon counterpulsation
IBS irritable bowel syndrome
ICC intercostal catheter
ICD implantable cardiac defibrillator
ICF intracellular fluid
ICH intracerebral haemorrhage
ICP intracranial pressure
ICRP International Commission on Radiological Protection
ICS intercellular space
ICU intensive care unit
IDC indwelling (urinary) catheter
IDU injecting drug user
IIOC immediate initiation of care

Ig immunoglobulin
IHD ischaemic heart disease
ILCOR International Liaison Committee on Resuscitation
IM intramuscular(ly)
IMI intramuscular injection
IMV intermittent mandatory ventilation
IN intranasal, nasally
INH isoniazid
INR international normalised ratio (for prothrombin time)
IO intraosseous(ly)
IOP intraocular pressure
IP intraperitoneal
IPAP inspiratory positive airway pressure
iPEEP intrinsic PEEP (positive end-expiratory pressure)
IPPV intermittent positive-pressure ventilation
IRIS immune reconstitution inflammatory syndrome
IRT incident response team
ISS Injury Severity Score
IT information technology
ITN ischaemic tissue necrosis
ITP idiopathic thrombocytopenia, idiopathic thrombocytopenic purpura
IUD, IUCD intrauterine (contraceptive) device
IV intravenous(ly)
IVC inferior vena cava
IVDU intravenous drug use/user
IVI intravenous injection
IVP intravenous pyelogram
IVS intravascular space
IVT intravenous therapy
JRA juvenile rheumatoid arthritis
JVP jugular venous pressure
JVT jugular venous distension
K potassium
KPI key performance indicator
KS Kaposi's sarcoma
KUB kidneys–ureters–bladder (X-ray or CT)
LAD left-axis deviation (in ECG); left anterior descending
LAFB left anterior fascicular block (anterior hemiblock)
LAP left atrial pressure
LBBB left bundle branch block
LBFB left posterior fascicular block (posterior hemiblock)
LCA left coronary artery
LCL lateral collateral ligament; lateral cruciate ligament
LDH lactate dehydrogenase
LDL low-density lipoprotein
LFT liver function test
LH luteinising hormone
LIF left iliac fossa
LMA laryngeal mask airway
LMO local medical officer
LMP last (normal) menstrual period
LMWH low-molecular-weight heparin
LOC level of consciousness; loss of consciousness
LP lumbar puncture
LPFB left posterior fascicular block
LR likelihood ratio
LSD lysergic acid diethylamide
LTBI latent tuberculosis infection
LV left ventricular
LVEF left ventricular ejection fraction
LVF left ventricular failure
LVH left ventricular hypertrophy
m, mo, mths months
M/C/S or M&S microculture and sensitivity (both used)
MAC *Mycobacterium avium–intracellulare* complex
MAOI monoamine oxidase inhibitor
MAP mean arterial (blood) pressure
MAST military antishock trousers

MCH mean corpuscular haemoglobin
MCI mass-casualty incident
MCL medial collateral ligament
MCP metacarpophalangeal
MCU micturating cystourethrogram
MCV mean corpuscular volume
MDI metered-dose inhaler
MDMA 3,4-methylene dioxymethylamphetamine (ecstasy)
MET mobile emergency team
Mg magnesium
MILS manual in-line stabilisation/ immobilisation
MIMMS major incident medical management and support
MMR measles, mumps, rubella
MMSE Mini Mental State Examination
MODS multi-organ dysfunction syndrome
MR magnetic resonance
MRA magnetic resonance angiography
MRI magnetic resonance imaging
MRSA multi-resistant *Staphylococcus aureus*; methicillin-resistant *Staphylococcus aureus*
MS mitral stenosis
MSM men who have sex with men
MSU midstream urine
MVP mitral valve prolapse
N/2 half normal
N/4 quarter normal
N_2O nitrous oxide
Na sodium
NAAT nucleic acid amplification testing
NAC *N*-acetylcysteine
NAD nothing abnormal detected
NAPA *N*-acetylprocainamide
NAPQI *N*-acetyl-*p*-quinoneimine
NAT nucleic acid testing
NBM nil by mouth
NFR not for resuscitation
NG nasogastric
NGO non-government organisation
NGT nasogastric tube
NHL non-Hodgkin's lymphoma
NIBP non-invasive blood pressure (monitoring)
NIPPV non-invasive positive-pressure ventilation
NIV non-invasive ventilation
NMDA *N*-methyl-D-aspartate
NMR nuclear magnetic resonance
NMS neuroleptic malignant syndrome
NNRTI non-nucleoside reverse transcriptase inhibitor
NO nitric oxide
NOF neck of femur
NORSA non-multiresistant oxacillin-resistant *Staphylococcus aureus*
NP nurse practitioner
NRS numeric rating scale (for pain)
NRTI nucleoside reversion transcriptase inhibitor
NSA normal serum albumin
NSAID non-steroidal anti-inflammatory drug
NSTEACS non-ST-segment elevation acute coronary syndrome
NSTEMI non-ST-elevation myocardial infarction
NT *N*-terminal
NTT nasotracheal tube
O&G obstetrics and gynaecology
O_2 oxygen
OCP oral contraceptive pill
od once daily
OI opportunistic infection
OM occipitomental
OPG orthopantomogram
ORIF open reduction internal fixation
OT occupational therapy; operating theatre
PA posteroanterior

$PACO_2$ partial pressure (tension) of alveolar carbon dioxide
$PaCO_2$ partial pressure of arterial carbon dioxide
PACS Patient Archiving and Communication System
PAN polyarteritis nodosa
Pap smear Papanicolaou smear test
PAWP pulmonary artery wedge pressure
PBL problem-based learning
PC platelet count
PCA patient-controlled analgesia; percutaneous coronary angioplasty
PCI percutaneous coronary intervention
PCL posterior cruciate ligament
PCO_2 partial pressure of carbon dioxide (may be arterial or venous)
PCP *Pneumocystis jiroveci (carinii)* pneumonia
PCR polymerase chain reaction
PCV packed cell volume
PDN paroxysmal nocturnal dyspnoea
PE pulmonary embolism
PEA pulseless electrical activity
PEEP positive end-expiratory pressure
PEFR peak expiratory flow rate
PEP post-exposure prophylaxis
PERC PE Rule-out Criteria
PET positron emission
PG prostaglandin
PGL persistent generalised lymphadenopathy
PI product information (drugs); protease inhibitor
PID pelvic inflammatory disease
PiO_2 partial pressure of inspired oxygen
PIOPED prospective investigation of pulmonary embolism diagnosis
PIP peak inspiratory pressure; proximal interphalangeal
PML progressive multifocal leucoencephalopathy
PND paroxysmal nocturnal dypnoea
PNS peripheral nervous system
PO per orem, by mouth
POP plaster of Paris
POSI position of safe immobilisation
P_{osm} plasma osmolarity
PPE personal protective equipment
PPI proton-pump inhibitor
PPNG penicillinase-producing *Neisseria gonorrhoeae*
PPV patency, protection, ventilation
PR per rectum, rectally
PRN, prn as required
PRVC pressure-regulated volume control
PSA prostate-specific antigen
PSI Pneumonia Severity Index
PSVT paroxysmal supraventricular tachycardia
PT prothrombin time
PTCA percutaneous transluminal coronary angioplasty
PTH parathyroid hormone
PTHrp parathyroid hormone related protein
PTSD post-traumatic stress disorder
PTT partial thromboplastin time
PUD peptic ulcer disease
PUO pyrexia of unknown origin
PUVA psoralen ultraviolet A (therapy)
PV per vaginam, vaginally
q4h every 4 hours (etc)
QID, qid 4 times daily
R respiratory quotient; right
RA radiofrequency ablation; rheumatoid arthritis
RAA renin–angiotensin–aldosterone (system)
RAD right-axis deviation (in ECG)
RAP right atrial pressure
RAT rapid assessment team

RBBB right bundle branch block
RBC red blood cell
RCA right coronary artery
RF radiofrequency
RICE rest, ice, compression and elevation
RMO resident medical officer
RNA ribonucleic acid
ROM range of movement
ROSC return of spontaneous circulation
RPFB right posterior fascicular block
RPR rapid plasma reagin (test)
RR relative risk
RSI rapid-sequence induction, rapid-sequence intubation
RSV respiratory syncytial virus
RTA road traffic accident
rTPA tissue plasminogen activator
RTS Revised Trauma Score
RUQ right upper quadrant
RV right ventricle
RVH right ventricular hypertrophy
SA sinoatrial
SAED semi-automated external defibrillator
SAH subarachnoid haemorrhage
SaO_2 peripheral oxygen saturation
SARS severe acute respiratory syndrome
SBP systolic blood pressure
SBT skin bleeding time
SC subcutaneous(ly)
SCA sickle-cell anaemia
SCAR serous cutaneous adverse reaction
SCD sickle-cell disease
SCID severe combined immune deficiency
SCIWORA spinal cord injury without radiological abnormality
SDH subdural haematoma/ haemorrhage
SF-36 a 36-item health survey (Medical Outcomes Study)
SFFS sitting fetal feet supported
SGOT serum glutamic oxaloacetic transaminase
SIADH syndrome of inappropriate antidiuretic hormone
SIDS sudden infant death syndrome
SIMV synchronised intermittent mandatory ventilation
SIRS systemic inflammatory response syndrome
SJS Stevens–Johnson syndrome
SK streptokinase
SLE systemic lupus erythematosus
SLS sodium lauryl sulfate
SMA superior mesanteric artery
SNRI selective serotonin and noradrenaline re-uptake inhibitor
SOB shortness of breath
SOL space-occupying lesion
SPC suprapubic catheter
SpO_2 peripheral oxygen saturation
SR sinus rhythm
SSD silver sulfadiazine
SSLR serum-sickness-like reaction
SSNRI selective serotonin norepinephine release inhibitor
SSRI selective serotonin re-uptake inhibitor
SSSS staphylococcal scalded skin syndrome
stat at once
STD sexually transmitted disease
STEMI ST-elevation myocardial infarction
SV stroke volume
SVC superior vena cava
SvO_2 central venous oxygen saturation
SVT supraventricular tachycardia
TAC tetracaine, adrenaline and cocaine in a gel preparation
TASER Thomas A Swift Electric Rifle
TB tuberculosis

TBI traumatic brain injury
TBSA total body surface area
TED thromboembolism
TCA tricyclic antidepressant
TDS 3 times daily
TEN toxic epidermal necrolysis
TENS transcutaneous electrical nerve stimulation
TFT thyroid function test
TGA Therapeutic Goods and Administration
THC tetrahydrocannabinol
TIA transient ischaemic attack
TIG tetanus immunoglobulin
TIMI thrombolysis in myocardial infarction (score)
TIPS transjugular intrahepatic portosystemic shunt
TLS tumour lysis syndrome
TMJ temporomandibular joint
TNF tumour necrosis factor
TPHA *Treponema pallidum* haemagglutination assay
TOE transoesophageal echocardiogram/echocardiography
TORCH toxoplasmosis, rubella, cytomegalovirus, herpes simplex and HIV
TOV trial of void
TPA tissue plasminogen activator
TPHA Treponema pallidum haemagglutination assay (syphilis test)
TPN total parenteral nutrition
TPR total peripheral resistance
TRALI transfusion-related acute lung injury
TRISS Revised Trauma Score and Injury Severity Score combined
TRTS Triage Revised Trauma Score
TSH thyroid-stimulating hormone
TSST toxic shock syndrome toxin
TT thrombin time
U/A urinalysis
UA urinalysis; unstable angina
U&E urea and electrolytes
UEC urea, electrolytes and creatinine (also EUC)
UNH unfractionated heparin
URTI upper respiratory tract infection
US ultrasound
UTI urinary tract infection
VAS visual analogue scale (for pain)
VBG venous blood gas
vCJD variant Creutzfeldt–Jakob disease
VDK venom detection kit
VDRL venereal disease reference laboratory (test)
VEB ventricular ectopic beat
VF ventricular fibrillation
VP ventriculoperitoneal
V/Q ventilation–perfusion
VSD ventricular septal defect
VT ventricular tachycardia
VTE venous thromboembolism
vWF Von Willebrand's factor
VZIG varicella zoster immune globulin
VZV varicella zoster virus
WBC white blood cell
WCC white (blood) cell count
WHO World Health Organization
WPW Wolfe-Parkinson-White (syndrome)
y, yrs years

emergency medicine

the principles of practice

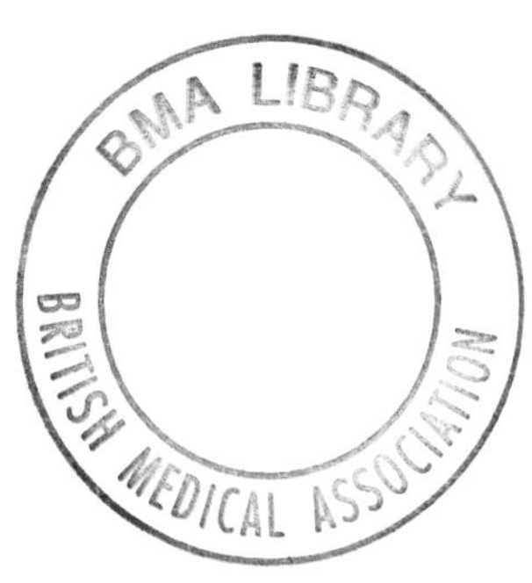

emergency medicine

the principles of practice

SIXTH EDITION

Edited by

Gordian W O Fulde

MBBS, FRACS, FRCS (Edin),
FRCS/RCP (A&E) (Edin), FACEM

Director, Emergency Department
St Vincent's Hospital, Sydney

and

Sascha Fulde

MBBS, BSc
Registrar in Emergency Medicine,
St Vincent's Hospital, Sydney

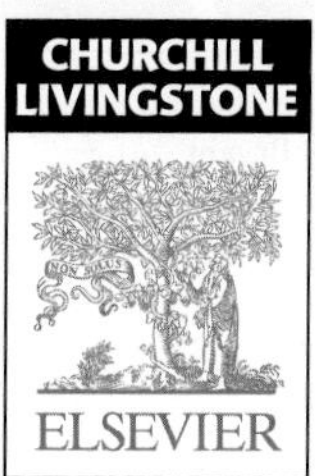

Sydney Edinburgh London New York
Philadelphia St Louis Toronto

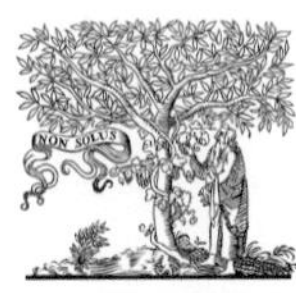

Churchill Livingstone
is an imprint of Elsevier

Elsevier Australia. ACN 001 002 357
(a division of Reed International Books Australia Pty Ltd)
Tower 1, 475 Victoria Avenue, Chatswood, NSW 2067

eISBN: 9780729581462

5th edn 2009; 4th edn 2004; 3rd edn 1998; 2nd edn 1992; 1st edn 1988

National Library of Australia Cataloguing-in-Publication Data

---

Fulde, Gordian W. O., author.

Emergency medicine : the principles of practice / Gordian W O Fulde; Sascha Fulde.

6th edition.
9780729541466 (paperback)
Includes index.

Emergency medicine–Handbooks, manuals, etc.

Fulde, Sascha, author.

616.025

Content Strategist: Larissa Norrie
Content Development Specialist: Neli Bryant
Senior Project Manager: Natalie Hamad
Edited by Teresa McIntyre
Proofread by Tim Learner
Technical editing by Jerry Perkins and Lynne MacKinnon
Cover and internal design by Shaun Jury
Index by Robert Swanson
Typeset by Midland Typesetters
Printed in China by China Translation & Printing Services Limited

Preface

Since the first edition of this book in 1988 and following editions in 1992, 1998, 2004 and 2009, emergency medicine has — fortunately — continued to advance. In this edition much new information, many new approaches and extensive refinements of existing clinical management have been incorporated. Again, current and respected practising clinicians have been chosen as authors for their clinical expertise and experience, so that they can compact their knowledge into the pocket-sized format. As healthcare resources continue to be stretched, the first hours of a patient's illness or initial contact with healthcare providers, outside and inside a hospital, are even more critical to the outcome. It is also very pertinent given the challenge of re-engineering patient flow, e.g. the '4-hour rule', which is coupled to funding. The aim of this book is to help with this initial contact.

Any suggestions for improving this will be very much appreciated: please send them to gfulde@stvincents.com.au.

Acknowledgements

Once again I am very grateful to the busy clinician authors for their excellent contributions. Also, the support and stimulation from many doctors, nurses, students and other professionals who use this book and have helped with ideas are greatly appreciated.

How do I adequately thank my wife, Lesley, for her unfailing encouragement and support?

Brigette Veen and Rory Banwell typed, collated, chased up details and much more; I most sincerely thank them.

Also, to all the fabulous staff of the emergency department who are so great to work with — not only are the patients lucky to have such people care for them, but also the way they support and care for each other is wonderful.

Contents

Contributors

Judy E Alford, MBBS, FACEM
Staff Specialist, Emergency Medicine, St Vincent's Hospital, Sydney, NSW; Conjoint Lecturer, University of New South Wales

Glenn Arendts, MBBS, MMed, FACEM
Consultant Emergency Physician, Royal Perth Hospital, WA; Associate Professor, School of Primary, Aboriginal and Rural Health, University of Western Australia; Member, Scientific Committee, Australasian College for Emergency Medicine

Shalini Arunanthy, MBBS, FACEM
Senior Staff Specialist, Emergency Department, Westmead Hospital, Westmead, NSW; VMO, Emergency Department, Bankstown Hospital, Bankstown, NSW; Clinical Senior Lecturer, University of Sydney, Sydney, NSW; Australasian College for Emergency Medicine Censor for NSW; Member, Court of Examiners, ACEM; Member, SCE Subcommittee, Fellowship Examination Committee; Chair, Pathology Subcommittee, Primary Examination Committee; Member, Credentials Committee, ACEM

Neil Ballard, MBBS, FACEM
Senior Staff Specialist, Ambulance Service of NSW Aeromedical and Retrieval Services; Senior Staff Specialist, Prince of Wales Hospital Emergency Department, Randwick, NSW; Medical Coordinator, Careflight Medical Services, Queensland

Melinda J Berry, MBBS, FACEM
Staff Specialist, Emergency Medicine, St Vincent's Hospital, Sydney, NSW; Medical Coordinator, Don Harrison Patient Safety Simulation Centre, St Vincent's Hospital, Sydney; Conjoint Senior Lecturer, Faculty of Medicine, University of New South Wales

Nick Brennan, MBBS (Hons), FRACP
Senior Specialist, Department of Geriatric Medicine, St Vincent's Hospital, Sydney, NSW

Phillip Brenner, MBBS, FRACS
Urologist, St Vincent's Clinic, Sydney, NSW; Senior Conjoint Lecturer, University of New South Wales, Sydney

Anthony F T Brown, MB ChB, FRCP, FRCS(Ed), FACEM, FCEM
Senior Staff Specialist, Department of Emergency Medicine, Royal Brisbane and Women's Hospital, Brisbane, Queensland; Professor of Emergency Medicine, Discipline of Anaesthesiology and Critical Care, School of Medicine, University of Queensland; Editor-in-Chief, *Emergency Medicine Australasia*; Senior Court of Examiners, Australasian College for Emergency Medicine

Gary Browne, MBBS, MSpMed, FRACP, FACEM
Professor of Medicine, University of Sydney, Sydney, NSW; Head, Discipline of Emergency Medicine; Senior Staff Specialist, Children's Hospital at Westmead; Member, Court of Examiners, Australasian College for Emergency Medicine

Adam Chiu Fat Chan, MBBS, FACEM, Grad Dip Couns
Senior Consultant, Department of Emergency Medicine, St George Hospital, NSW, Australia; Conjoint Senior Lecturer in Emergency Medicine, Faculty of Medicine, University of New South Wales; Senior Court of Examiners, Australasian College for Emergency Medicine

Nicholas Cheng, MBBS, BSc (Med), DCH, FRACP
Paediatric Emergency Physician, Children's Hospital at Westmead; Chair, Kidsafe NSW; Conjoint Senior Lecturer, University of New South Wales; Conjoint Senior Lecturer, University of Western Sydney

Fiona Chow, MBBS, FACEM
Staff Specialist, Emergency Medicine, St Vincent's Hospital, Sydney, NSW; Conjoint Lecturer, University of New South Wales, Sydney

Carmel Crock, MBBS, FACEM, BLitt
Director, Emergency Department, Royal Victorian Eye and Ear Hospital, Melbourne, Victoria; Chair, Quality Management Subcommittee, Australasian College for Emergency Medicine

Bill Croker, MBBS, BMedSc, FACEM, MMedEd
Emergency Physician, Nepean Hospital, Penrith, NSW; Emergency Physician, The Sanitarium Hospital, Wahroonga, NSW; Member, Court of Examiners, Australasian College for Emergency Medicine

Shane Curran, MBBS, BMedSc, FACEM
Director Emergency Medicine, Wagga Wagga Base Hospital, Wagga Wagga, NSW; Associate Professor, Rural Clinical School, University of New South Wales, Wagga Wagga; Associate Professor, Wagga Wagga Clinical School, University of Notre Dame; Associate Professor, School of Biomedical Sciences, Charles Sturt University, Wagga Wagga

Barbara Daly, RN, BHA, MHA
Senior Nurse Manager, Department of Emergency Medicine, Prince of Wales Hospital, Randwick, NSW; Co-Chair of Critical Care Priority Health Taskforce; Member, Health Care Advisory Council; Member, Emergency Department Ministerial Taskforce

Linda Dann, MBBS, FANZCA, FACEM
Director, Emergency Medicine, Bankstown-Lidcombe Hospital, Bankstown, NSW; Conjoint Lecturer, University of New South Wales, Sydney; Former Member, Court of Examiners, Australasian College for Emergency Medicine

Michael R Delaney, MBBS, FRACO, FRACS
Visiting Ophthalmic Surgeon, St Vincent's Hospital, Sydney, NSW; Clinical Lecturer in Ophthalmology, University of New South Wales, Sydney

Anthony Dodds, MBBS (Hons), FRACP, FRCPA
Director of Haematology and Bone Marrow Transplantation, St Vincent's Hospital, Sydney, NSW; Former Head, Division of Haematology, SydPath; Associate Professor of Medicine (conjoint), University of New South Wales, Sydney; Former Co-Chair Bone Marrow Transplant Network NSW; Former Vice President, Bone Marrow Transplant Society of Australia and New Zealand

Martin Duffy, MBBS, MMed (Clin Epi), FACEM
Senior Staff Specialist, Emergency Medicine, St Vincent's Hospital, Sydney, NSW; Senior Instructor, Early Management of Severe Trauma, Royal College of Surgeons; Lecturer/Examiner, Ambulance Service of New South Wales; Conjoint Senior Lecturer, Emergency Medicine, University of New South Wales, Sydney

Stephen John Dunjey, MBBS, FACEM, DDU
Senior Consultant Emergency Medicine, Royal Perth Hospital, King Edward Memorial Hospital for Women, WA; Senior Lecturer, Emergency Medicine, University of Western Australia; Senior Member of the Court of Examiners, Australasian College for Emergency Medicine

Rob Edwards, MBBS, FACEM
Senior Staff Specialist in Emergency Medicine & Department of Trauma, Westmead Hospital, Sydney, NSW; Clinical Senior Lecturer, Western Clinical School, The University of Sydney

Bruce Fasher, MBBS, DRCOG, DCH, FRCP(L), FRACP
Paediatric Physician, Emergency Department, Royal Alexandra Hospital for Children, Westmead, NSW

Andrew Finckh, BA, MBBS, FACEM
Senior Staff Specialist, Department of Emergency Medicine, St Vincent's Hospital, Sydney, NSW; Conjoint Senior Lecturer, University of New South Wales

Peter Foltyn, BDS(Syd)
Consultant Dentist, Dental Department, St Vincent's Hospital, Sydney, NSW

S Lesley Forster, MBBS, MHP, FRACMA, DipIndRel&LabLaw(Syd), FAFPHM
Associate Dean; Head, Sydney Campus, Rural Clinical School, University of New South Wales, Sydney

Jeremy Fry, MBBS, FACEM
Co-Director of Emergency Medical Training, Wagga Wagga Base Hospital, Wagga Wagga, NSW; VMO Emergency Specialist, Gosford Hospital, Gosford, NSW; VMO Emergency Specialist, Sutherland Hospital, Sydney, NSW

Gordian W O Fulde, MBBS, FRACS, FRCS(Ed), FRACS/RCP (A&E) Ed, FACEM
Director, Emergency Medicine, St Vincent's Hospital, Sydney, NSW; Director, Emergency Department, Sydney Hospital; Director Emergency Services, South East Sydney Illawarra Area Health Service; Member, Senior Court of Examiners, Australasian College for Emergency Medicine; Professor, Emergency Medicine, The University of Notre Dame, Sydney; Associate Professor, Emergency Medicine, University of New South Wales, Sydney

Sascha Fulde, MBBS, BSc
Registrar in Emergency Medicine, St Vincent's Hospital, Sydney, NSW

Tiffany Fulde, MBBS (Hons)
Resident, St Vincent's Hospital, Sydney, NSW

Paul Gaudry, MBBS, FACEM
Emergency Physician, Blacktown and Mt Druitt Hospitals, NSW

Mark Gillett, MBBS, Dip RACOG, FRACGP, FACEM, MClinEd (UNSW), Grad Cert U/S (USyd)
Director of Education and Research and Senior Staff Specialist, Emergency Department, Royal North Shore Hospital, Sydney, NSW; Senior Clinical Lecturer, Northern Clinical School, University of Sydney; Senior Examiner, Australasian College for Emergency Medicine Court of Examiners; Former ACEM State Censor (NSW) and Chair, ACEM Fellowship Examination Committee; Medical Director, Immediate Assistants, Sydney

Anthony J Grabs, MBBS, FRACS (Gen&Vasc)
Director, Trauma Service, St Vincent's Hospital, Sydney, NSW; Conjoint Associate Professor in Surgery, St Vincent's Hospital, Sydney, University of New South Wales

Robert Ian Graham, MBBS, FAChAM
Staff Specialist, Addiction Medicine; St Vincent's, Blacktown, Mt Druitt and Nepean Hospitals, NSW; Conjoint Lecturer, University of New South Wales

Tim Green, MBBS, FACEM
Director, Emergency Department, Royal Prince Alfred Hospital, Sydney, NSW; Clinical Senior Lecturer, Sydney Medical School, University of Sydney; Senior Member, Court of Adjudicators, Australasian College for Emergency Medicine

Michael J Golding, BMed, Dip Ped, Grad Cert Tox, Adv Dip Gov, MPHTM, MHM, FRACMA, FACRRM, FACEM
Director of Emergency Department, Prince of Wales Hospital, Sydney, NSW

Anna Holdgate, MBBS, FACEM, MMed
Emergency Medicine Research Unit, Liverpool Hospital, Sydney, NSW

Craig Hore, MBBS, FACEM, FCICM, MHPol
Senior Staff Specialist, Sydney Helicopter Emergency Medical Service, Ambulance Service of NSW; Staff Specialist, Intensive Care Unit, Liverpool Hospital, Sydney, NSW; Senior Lecturer, Faculty of Medicine, University of New South Wales; Member, Court of Examiners, Australasian College for Emergency Medicine

Beaver Hudson, RMN, RN, MN, MRCNA
Clinical Nurse Consultant, Emergency Psychiatry, St Vincent's Hospital, Sydney, NSW; Clinical Coordinator Emergency Psychiatry, Emergency Department, St Vincent's Hospital, Sydney; Lecturer, Institute of Psychiatry, NSW

Sarah Hoy, BN, Grad Dip VocLrn, MEd (Adult Ed)
Nurse Educator, Department of Emergency Medicine, Prince of Wales Hospital, Randwick, NSW; Committee Member, College of Emergency Nursing Australasia (CENA), NSW Branch; Education Chair and Trauma Nursing Program (TNP) Coordinator, CENA NSW

Anthony Kelleher, PhD, MBBS, FRACP, FRCPA
Head, Immunovirology and Pathogenesis Program, National Centre in HIV Epidemiology and Clinical Research; Associate Professor, Faculty of Medicine, University of New South Wales; Consultant Immunologist and Immunopathologist, St Vincent's Hospital, Sydney, NSW

Diane King, MBBS, FACEM
Director, Emergency Medicine, Flinders Medical Centre, Adelaide, SA; Regional Director, Southern Adelaide Area Health Service, SA; Divisional Director, Emergency and Perioperative Medicine, Flinders Medical Centre, Adelaide; Senior Lecturer, Emergency Medicine, Flinders University, Adelaide; Member, Court of Examiners, Australasian College for Emergency Medicine

Julie Leung, MBBS, FACEM, Grad Cert Tox
Senior Staff Specialist, Department of Emergency Medicine, St Vincent's Hospital, Sydney, NSW; Conjoint Lecturer, University of New South Wales

David J Lewis-Driver, MBBS (Hons), FACEM, FRACGP, MRACMA
Senior Staff Specialist, Department of Emergency Medicine, Sunshine Coast Health Service, Queensland; Senior Lecturer, Department of Anaesthesiology and Critical Care, University of Queensland, Brisbane; Member, Senior Court of Examiners, Australasian College for Emergency Medicine

Peter Locke, VMO-MNCLHD (Mid North Coast Local Health District)
ACRRM (Australian College of Rural and Remote Medicine), Brisbane, Queensland

Derek Louey, MBBS (Adel), FACEM
Senior Staff Specialist, Emergency Department, Flinders Medical Centre, Adelaide, SA; Senior Clinical Lecturer, Graduate Entry Medical Program, Flinders University, Adelaide

Kevin Maruno, MBBS, FACEM, BMedSc (Hons)
Staff Specialist, Emergency Medicine, St Vincent's Hospital, Sydney, NSW; Academic Coordinator, Senior Conjoint Lecturer, The University of Notre Dame, Sydney; Conjoint Lecturer, Faculty of Medicine, University of New South Wales

Sally McCarthy, MBBS, FACEM, MBA
Director, Emergency Medicine, Prince of Wales Hospital, Randwick, NSW; Senior Lecturer, Emergency Medicine, University of New South Wales; President, Australasian College for Emergency Medicine, University of New South Wales

Thomas McDonagh, MBBS, FACEM
Staff Specialist, Emergency Department, Northwest Regional Hospital, Burnie, Tasmania; Senior Lecturer in Emergency Medicine, University of Tasmania

Greg McDonald, MBBS, FACEM
Director of Emergency Care, Sydney Adventist Hospital, NSW; Member, Senior Court of Examiners, Australasian College for Emergency Medicine; Chair, Private Practice Committee, ACEM; Member, Management Committee, Emergency Life Support Course

Karon McDonnell, RN, Dip Hlth Sc, Grad Cert Em Nsg
Trauma Service Manager, St Vincent's Hospital, Sydney, NSW

Kirsty McLeod, RN, PCB HA
Nurse Manager, Emergency Department, St Vincent's Hospital, Sydney, NSW

Paul M Middleton, RGN, MBBS, Dip IMCRCS (Ed), MMed (Clin Epi), MD FRCS (Eng), FACAP, FCEM, FACEM
Clinical Associate Professor, Discipline of Emergency Medicine, University of Sydney, NSW; Director, Australian Institute for Clinical Education; Chair, Australian Resuscitation Council, NSW Branch

Christopher J Mobbs, MBBS, FACEM
Staff Specialist, Emergency Department, The Geelong Hospital, Geelong, Victoria; Conjoint Lecturer, Deakin University, Victoria; Advanced Paediatric Life Support Instructor

Edmond Park, MBBS, FACEM
Emergency Physician, Liverpool and Campbelltown Emergency Departments, Sydney, NSW

Veronica A Preda, BSc (Med), MBBS (Hons), MPH
Research Fellow, Oxford, England; Conjoint Associate Lecturer, University of New South Wales

Paul Preisz, MBBS, FACEM
Deputy Director, Emergency Department, St Vincent's Hospital, Sydney, NSW; Senior Staff Specialist, Emergency Department, Sydney Hospital; Associate Professor, Emergency Medicine, The University of Notre Dame, Sydney; Senior

Lecturer, Emergency Medicine, University of New South Wales, Sydney; Former Member, Senior Court of Examiners, Australasian College for Emergency Medicine

Donald S Pryor, MBBS, MD, FRACP
VMO Neurologist, St George Hospital, Sydney, NSW; Conjoint Senior Lecturer University of NSW, Sydney

John Raftos, MBBS (Hons), FACEM
Senior Staff Specialist Emergency Medicine, St Vincent's Hospital and Sutherland Hospital, Sydney, NSW; Conjoint Associate Professor, Faculty of Medicine, University of New South Wales, Sydney; Early Management of Severe Trauma Instructor; Medico-Legal Consultant

Drew Richardson, MBBS (Hons), FACEM, Grad Cert HE
Senior Staff Specialist, Emergency Department, The Canberra Hospital, Canberra, ACT; NRMA-ACT Road Safety Trust Chair of Road Trauma and Emergency Medicine, Australian National University Medical School, Canberra, ACT; Member, Court of Examiners, Australasian College for Emergency Medicine

John Roberts, MBBS, FACEM
Director of ICU, Manning Rural Referral Hospital, Taree, NSW; VMO Critical Care, Port Macquarie Base Hospital, NSW; Senior Lecturer, School of Rural Health, University of New South Wales

Patricia A Saccasan-Whelan, MBBS, FACEM
Director, Emergency Department, Goulburn Base Hospital, Goulburn, NSW; Director of Critical Care and Deputy Health Services Functional Area; Coordinator for Disasters, Murrumbidgee and Southern NSW Local Health Districts; Rural Medical Adviser, NSW Ambulance Service; Medical Co-Chair NSW Rural Critical Care Taskforce

Iromi Samarasinghe, MBBS, FACEM
Emergency Physician, Sydney Hospital and St Vincent's Hospital, Sydney, NSW; Conjoint Lecturer, University of New South Wales

E S Seelan, MBBS, FRANZCR
Managing Radiologist, Healthcare Imaging, Miranda, NSW; Former Director of Radiology, Sutherland Hospital, Caringbah, NSW

Emma Spencer, MBBS BSc (Med) NSW, FRACP
Infectious Diseases and General Physician, Royal Darwin Hospital, NT

John R Sullivan, MBBS, FACD
Consultant Dermatologist, Skin and Cancer Foundation Darlinghurst, St Vincent's Hospital, Sydney, NSW; Senior Lecturer, University of New South Wales, Sydney

Richard Sullivan, MBBS (Hons)
Resident, Prince of Wales Hospital, Sydney, NSW

Wayne Varndell, BSc (Hons) Nsg, PGDip (AP), PGCert (Ed)
Acting Clinical Nurse Consultant, Prince of Wales Hospital Emergency Department, Sydney, NSW; Associate Clinical Lecturer, Faculty of Nursing, Midwifery and Health, University of Technology, Sydney

John Vinen, MBBS, MHP, FACEM, FIFEM, FACBS
Senior Staff Specialist, Deputy Director Emergency Department, Calvary Hospital, Canberra; Medico-Legal Consultant

Rebecca Walsh, BSc (Hons), BMed, BSurg (Hons)
Senior Haematology Registrar, St Vincent's Hospital, Sydney, NSW

Jeff Wassertheil, CS&J, MBBS, FACEM, MClinEd, MRACMA, MACLM
Formerly Head, Emergency Medicine Academic Stream, Southern Clinical School, Monash University, Faculty of Medicine, Nursing and Health Sciences; Associate Professor/Director, Emergency Medicine, Peninsula Health, Frankston, Victoria; Deputy Chief Medical Coordinator, Medical DISPLAN, Victoria.

Anthony J Whelan, MBBS, Grad Cert Ed, FRACP
Physician, Goulburn Base Hospital, Goulburn, NSW; Senior Lecturer, Rural Clinical School, Australian National University, ACT

Margot J Whitfield, MBBS, FACD
Consultant Dermatologist, Director, Dermatology Department, St Vincent's Hospital, Sydney, NSW; Skin and Cancer Foundation, St Vincent's Hospital, Sydney; Senior Lecturer, University of New South Wales, Sydney

F X Luis Winoto, BA, BSc (Med), MBBS
Registrar, Emergency Department, St Vincent's Public Hospital, Sydney, NSW; Conjoint Lecturer, University of New South Wales

Alex Wodak, MBBS, FRACP, FAFPHM, FAChAM
Emeritus Senior Specialist, Alcohol and Drug Service, St Vincent's Hospital, Sydney, NSW; Senior Lecturer, School of Public Health and Community Medicine, School of Medicine, National Drug and Alcohol Research Centre, Centre for HIV Epidemiology and Clinical Research, University of New South Wales, Sydney

Christopher Ern-Yoong Wong, MBBS (Singapore), FRCSEd (A&E), FAMS (Emerg)
Fellow, Emergency Care, Sydney Adventist Hospital, NSW; Fellow, Royal College of Surgeons, Edinburgh (Accident and Emergency); Fellow, Academy of Medicine, Singapore (Emergency Medicine); Visiting Specialist, Jurong General Hospital, Singapore

Nikki Woods, MBBS, FACEM
Staff Specialist, Emergency Department, St Vincent's Hospital, Sydney, NSW

Allen Yuen, MBBS (Hons), FRACGP, FACEM
Honorary Clinical Associate Professor, Monash University, Melbourne, Victoria; Examiner, Australian Medical Council

Reviewers

Deepak Doshi, FACEM, FCEM, DCH, MRCS A&E (Edin), MRCS (Glasgow), MS, MBBS
Emergency Medicine Consultant, Logan Hospital, Meadowbrook, Queensland

Melissa Gan, BSc (UQ), MBBS (Hon 1), BSc (Med) (UNSW), FACEM
Emergency Medicine Consultant, Gold Coast Hospital, Gold Coast, Queensland

Sarah Mahoney, MBBS
Senior Lecturer, Flinders University, Adelaide, SA

Larry McGuire, MBChB, MRCP (UK), FFAEM, FACEM
Senior Emergency Medicine Consultant, Logan Hospital, Meadowbrook, Queensland

Shashidhar Venkatesh Murthy, BSc, MBBS, MD (Pathology), GCTT, PG Cert in HSM, MBA (Educational Leadership)
Associate Professor, Head of Pathology, School of Medicine and Dentistry, Adjunct Professor of Pathology and Medical Education, Manipal University, India

Jim Reid, MB ChB, DipObs (Otago), FRNZCGP, FCCP, MPS (NZ)
Acting Dean and Head of Section of Rural Health, Dunedin School of Medicine, University of Otago, Dunedin, New Zealand

Chapter 1
Cardiopulmonary resuscitation

Gordian W O Fulde, Paul Preisz and Melinda J Berry

A patient in cardiac arrest is not an uncommon situation in the emergency department. Medical and nursing staff should all be familiar with the delivery of basic and advanced life support.

Time to defibrillation remains the most important feature of cardiac arrest management. Rapid defibrillation makes the biggest impact on patient outcome of any intervention. Uninterrupted, effective chest compressions have now also been shown to improve outcomes, but this should not delay defibrillation.

Cardiac arrest is a stressful situation for everyone involved. The basic life support (BLS) and adult advanced life support (ALS) algorithms are kept clear and simple so that people can follow them under duress. The algorithms should be clearly displayed so that they can be referred to during the course of an arrest.

Effective management of a patient in cardiac arrest also involves communication and teamwork skills in the context of a highly pressured situation. Simulation of arrest scenarios allows learning and rehearsal of these skills in addition to practising the steps of the algorithm.

Basic life support (BLS)

The principles of BLS are the same in children and adults, and the Australian Resuscitation Council recommends the same BLS algorithm for all ages. This allows for ease of learning and retention for lay people in the community (as well as many healthcare workers!)

There are obviously differences in anatomy, physiology and pathology between children and adults, and this is reflected in the recommendations for healthcare workers providing more-advanced life support for these different groups (see following sections).

BLS commences with looking for danger, quickly assessing the response of the patient and calling for help. If there is life-threatening

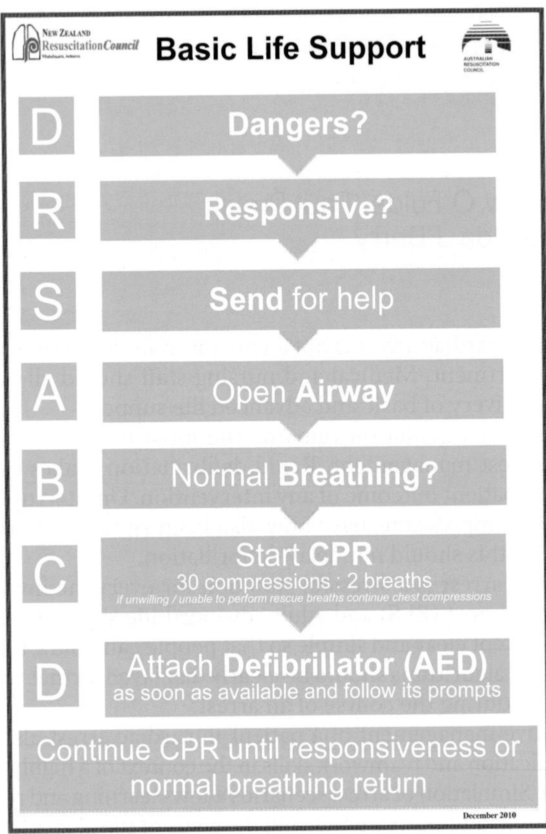

Figure 1.1 Basic life support

AED, automatic external defibrillator; CPR, cardiopulmonary resuscitation

From Australian Resuscitation Council; reproduced with permission

external bleeding, it must be stopped by applying direct pressure and elevating the wound above the level of the heart.

Open the airway with a head tilt, chin lift and/or jaw thrust. Any visible obstructing material can be removed, but a routine finger sweep is not recommended. Look, listen and feel for normal breathing.

Commence chest compressions if the patient is unresponsive and not breathing normally. Healthcare workers may feel for a pulse, but this has been found to be alarmingly unreliable and can cause delays in commencing chest compressions. No more than 10 seconds should be spent feeling for a pulse before moving on to start chest compressions. Chest compressions are commenced prior to delivering ventilations.

Chest compressions are delivered at a rate of 100/min to the lower half of the sternum and to a depth of at least one-third of the depth of the chest. After 30 compressions, pause briefly to deliver 2 ventilations. Early, effective and uninterrupted chest compressions have been shown to improve survival outcomes from cardiac arrest.

Chest compressions to an adult are delivered with a two-handed technique. For infants and small children, only one hand may be needed; and for babies, two fingers or the thumb/hand encircling technique. In late pregnancy, position the arrested patient supine but with something under the right buttock to provide sideways pelvic tilt to lift the gravid uterus off the inferior vena cava.

Performing chest compressions is tiring, even in a paediatric patient, and effectiveness declines over time with the same compressor. Change compressors every 2 minutes wherever possible, but with minimal interruption to the compressions.

Ventilations can be delivered by mouth-to-mouth expired air (mouth-to-nose in babies and infants), mouth-to-mask or by bag-and-mask. The volume delivered just needs to be enough to see the chest wall rise. Overventilation causes hyperinflation of the chest which impairs venous return to the heart, limiting cardiac output. Overventilation can also cause gastric distension, predisposing to regurgitation of stomach contents and aspiration of this into the lungs.

Early defibrillation improves outcome. Automatic external defibrillators (AEDs) allow early defibrillation in community areas and low-acuity hospital areas where advanced life support is not immediately available. If an AED is available, it should be used as soon as possible.

Adult advanced life support (ALS)

ALS involves defibrillation, oxygenation of the vital organs and reversing any causes of the arrest. Minimal interruptions to effective chest compressions and prompt defibrillation remain the priority.

Defibrillation of a shockable rhythm (ventricular fibrillation VF or pulseless ventricular tachycardia VT) must occur as soon as possible. The praecordial thump is no longer recommended. Maximum joules (200 J for biphasic defibrillator) are used for the first and all subsequent shocks. Stacked shocks are no longer recommended.

Defibrillation electrode pads are now widely available. Place one pad at the right parasternal area over the 2nd intercostal space, and

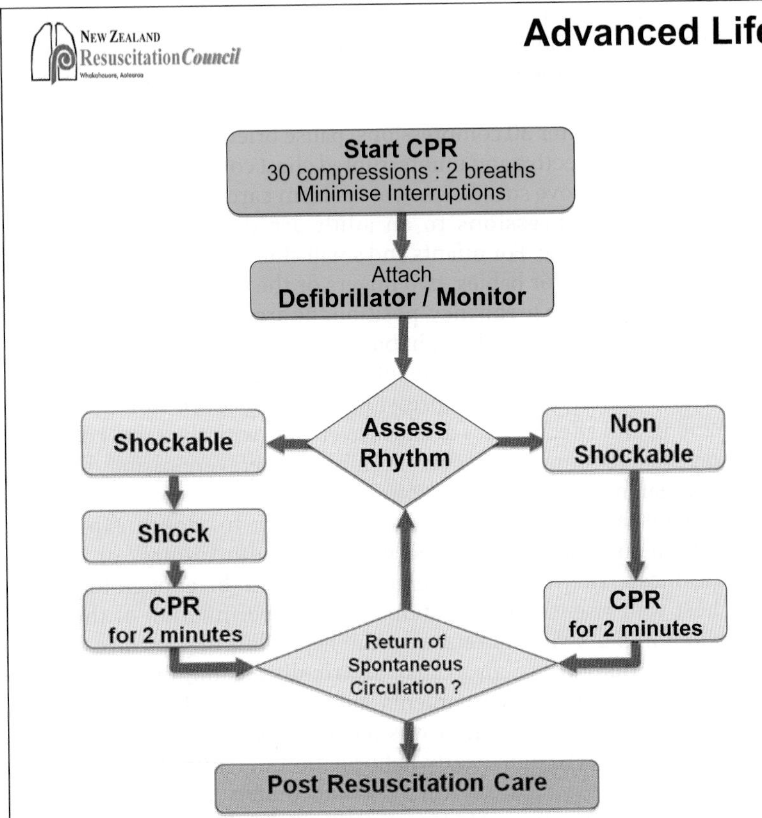

Figure 1.2 Advanced life support for adults

ABCDE, airway, breathing, circulation, disability, exposure algorithm; CPR, cardiopulmonary resuscitation; ETT, endotracheal tube; IO, intraosseus; IV, intravenous; LMA, laryngeal mask airway

the other pad in the left mid-axillary line over the 6th intercostal space. Antero-posterior (left parasternal area and just below the left scapula) is an alternative, but involves rolling the patient to apply the posterior pad and hence interrupting chest compressions. Avoid ECG electrodes, medication patches and pacemaker boxes.

Rhythm analysis occurs every 2 minutes. The defibrillator can be charged up while compressions are continuing. A pause in compressions allows for rhythm analysis and shock delivery if VT or VF is present. This sequence minimises interruptions to compressions.

Support for Adults

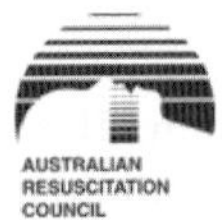

During CPR
Airway adjuncts (LMA / ETT)
Oxygen
Waveform capnography
IV / IO access
Plan actions before interrupting compressions
(e.g. charge manual defibrillator)
Drugs
Shockable
* Adrenaline 1 mg after 2nd shock
(then every 2nd loop)
* Amiodarone 300 mg after 3rd shock
Non Shockable
* Adrenaline 1 mg immediately
(then every 2nd loop)

Consider and Correct
Hypoxia
Hypovolaemia
Hyper / hypokalaemia / metabolic disorders
Hypothermia / hyperthermia
Tension pneumothorax
Tamponade
Toxins
Thrombosis (pulmonary / coronary)

Post Resuscitation Care
Re-evaluate ABCDE
12 lead ECG
Treat precipitating causes
Re-evaluate oxygenation and ventilation
Temperature control (cool)

From Australian Resuscitation Council; reproduced with permission

Every 2 minutes, the manual defibrillator can be charged up ready for shock delivery at the same pause in chest compressions as for rhythm analysis. The charge can be dumped if the rhythm is non-shockable (pulseless electrical activity PEA or asystole).

Chest compressions are resumed immediately after every shock, regardless of a change in rhythm. The theory behind this is that the heart is 'stunned' after defibrillation and cardiac output may still be very poor, even if an organised rhythm has been achieved. Unless the patient has obvious signs of a good cardiac output (moving or talking!), chest compressions continue until the next 2-minute mark when the rhythm is analysed and the patient is examined for a pulse. If a pulse is not detected after 10 seconds, chest compressions are resumed.

Adrenaline is administered in an attempt to direct more blood flow to the heart and brain. The recommended dose is adrenaline 1 mg (10 mL of 1:10,000 solution) intravenous IV (or intraosseous IO) every 4 minutes (every 2nd cycle). If the patient is not in a shockable rhythm, adrenaline is administered immediately. If the rhythm is shockable, adrenaline is administered after the 2nd unsuccessful shock as chest compressions are recommenced.

Amiodarone is recommended for refractory VF or VT. Amiodarone 300 mg is administered (IV or IO) after the 3rd unsuccessful shock with the recommencement of chest compressions.

Where IV access is not attainable, the IO route is recommended. Endotracheal administration of medications is no longer recommended. IO access devices for adults (drills) are becoming more widely available.

Two-person bag-and-mask ventilation with simple airway manoeuvres and adjuncts is the first-line technique to deliver oxygen to the lungs. Endotracheal intubation has advantages, such as a secure and protected airway, but does not take priority over chest compressions and defibrillation. If intubation is performed, chest compressions should not be interrupted for more than 20 seconds. A traumatised airway or an oesophageal intubation *worsens* the outcome for the patient, so this needs to be taken into consideration. Once the patient is intubated, chest compressions can be continuous at 100/min with ventilations at a rate of 6–8/min.

Reversible causes need to be considered in all arrests. These can be recalled by using the 'four Hs and four Ts' mnemonic:

H Hypoxia
H Hypovolaemia
H Hyper/hypo K, Mg, Ca, glucose
H Hypothermia (temperature below 30°C)
T Tension pneumothorax
T Tamponade
T Toxins (including anaphylaxis)
T Thromboembolus

Once cardiac output is re-established, post-resuscitation care is an opportunity to lessen morbidity and mortality for these patients. This includes appropriate airway management, achieving normal oxygen levels while avoiding hyperoxia and maintaining a blood pressure that provides adequate perfusion to the vital organs and a normal blood glucose level. The underlying cause of the arrest needs to be addressed, including consideration of cardiac angiography in many adult cases.

Patients who remain unconscious post arrest may have a greater chance of a good neurological outcome if they are cooled in the first few hours to 32–34°C for 12–24 hours. Cooling can start right from the beginning of the resuscitation.

It is impossible to predict accurately the degree of neurological recovery during or immediately after cardiac arrest. Relying on the neurological examination during or immediately after cardiac arrest to predict outcome is not recommended and should not be used.

In cases where there is no return of spontaneous circulation, senior medical staff may decide to stop resuscitation efforts and declare the person deceased. This decision is made in the context of the duration and nature of the arrest, the premorbid state of the patient and the likelihood of significant neurological recovery.

Advanced life support in children

The basic life support (BLS) algorithm given above is the same for children as adults, but for healthcare workers providing *advanced* life support, 2 ventilations should be given after every 15 compressions.

Bradycardia and asystole are common initial rhythms in paediatric cardiac arrest and hypoxia or hypovolaemia are more commonly the cause than primary cardiac disease. However, VF and VT do still occur in children and so rhythm analysis and defibrillation of shockable rhythms must occur as soon as possible. Defibrillation dose is 4 J/kg for the first and all subsequent shocks.

Effective uninterrupted chest compressions are just as important in children as in adults. Again, two-person bag-and-mask ventilation with simple airway manoeuvres and adjuncts is the first-line technique to deliver oxygen to the lungs.

Adrenaline 10 microg/kg IV (or IO) is administered immediately in cases of asystole or PEA and after the 2nd unsuccessful defibrillation in VF or VT with the recommencement of chest compressions. Amiodarone 5 mg/kg is recommended for refractory VF or VT after the 3rd unsuccessful defibrillation attempt.

IV access is the first-line route of drug administration. No more than 90 seconds should be spent attempting IV access before resorting to IO access.

The reversible causes need to be considered and this can be remembered with the four Hs and four Ts (see opposite). Hypovolaemia is prominent in paediatric arrest, so a fluid bolus of 20 mL/kg (normal

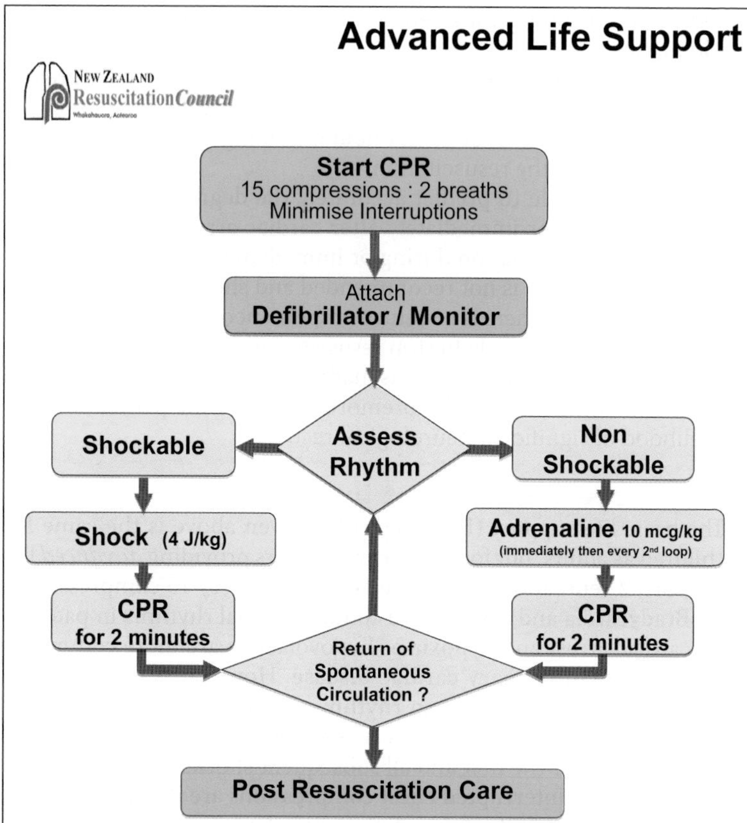

Figure 1.3 Advanced life support in children

saline) is routinely administered. Blood sugar level should be tested early on, with administration of dextrose 10% 5 mL/kg if hypoglycaemic.

Parents or primary caregivers may wish to be present during the resuscitation process. This should be encouraged, with the provision that there is a senior nursing or medical staff member allocated solely to explaining events and answering questions.

Resuscitation of the newborn

A small percentage of newborn babies require some resuscitation at birth, usually initial breathing assistance. Deliveries in the ED are unexpected or precipitous and so carry a higher risk of neonatal

for Infants and Children

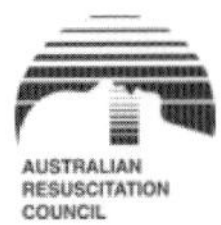

During CPR

Airway adjuncts (LMA / ETT)
Oxygen
Waveform capnography
IV / IO access
Plan actions before interrupting compressions
(e.g. charge manual defibrillator to 4 J/kg)
Drugs
Shockable
* Adrenaline 10 mcg/kg after 2nd shock (then every 2nd loop)
* Amiodarone 5mg/kg after 3rd shock
Non Shockable
* Adrenaline 10 mcg/kg immediately (then every 2nd loop)

Consider and Correct

Hypoxia
Hypovolaemia
Hyper / hypokalaemia / metabolic disorders
Hypothermia / hyperthermia
Tension pneumothorax
Tamponade
Toxins
Thrombosis (pulmonary / coronary)

Post Resuscitation Care

Re-evaluate ABCDE
12 lead ECG
Treat precipitating causes
Re-evaluate oxygenation and ventilation
Temperature control (cool)

From Australian Resuscitation Council; reproduced with permission

complications. All deliveries in the ED warrant preparations for full neonatal resuscitation with a team that is separate from the staff assisting the mother.

Initial assessment occurs while the newborn is being dried, the cord clamped and the baby placed on dry bedding under a radiant heater, or placed on the mother's chest and covered with a dry blanket if it is obvious that no resuscitation is required.

Assess response to stimulation, colour, tone, respiratory rate/effort and heart rate (which should be 110–160 bpm). If the baby is not moving or breathing, place on the neonatal resuscitation bed under a radiant heater and provide stimulation by drying with a soft towel.

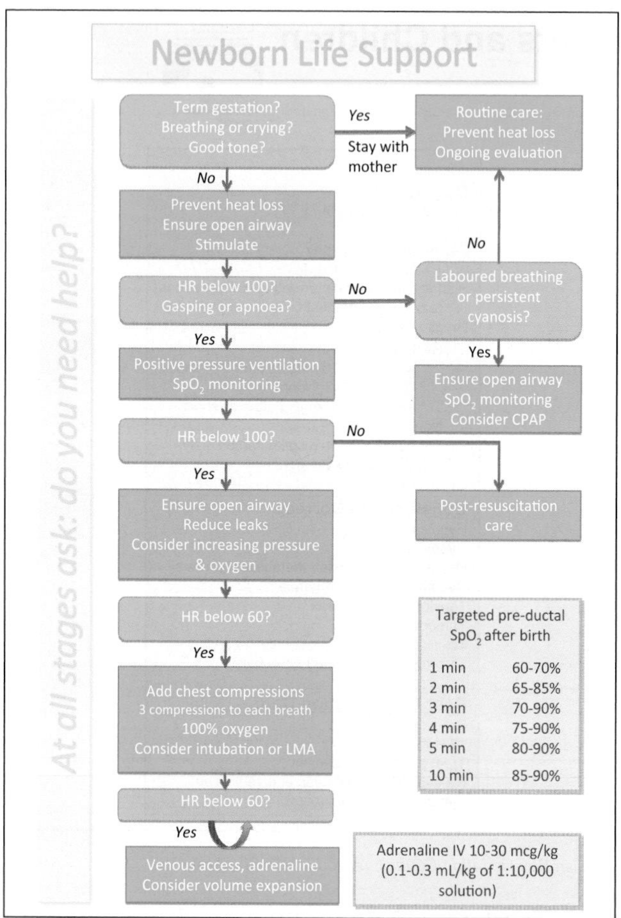

Figure 1.4 Newborn life support

CPAP, continuous positive airway pressure; HR, heart rate; LMA, laryngeal mask airway; SpO_2, peripheral oxygen saturation

From Australian Resuscitation Council; reproduced with permission

Ensure the airway is open. Routine suctioning is not recommended, but if there are secretions causing obstruction, these can be very gently and briefly suctioned.

If the baby has not started breathing or the heart rate is < 100 bpm, provide positive-pressure ventilation with air via a self-inflating 500 mL paediatric resuscitation bag (240 mL bag is used for pre-term babies under 2.5 kg). Use a soft-rimmed mask that covers the mouth and nose, but not the eyes. Keep the head in a neutral position as extension or flexion can kink and obstruct the airway.

Deliver breaths at a rate of 40–60/min with just enough volume to see the chest wall rise. The heart rate should rise above 100 bpm. Ongoing bradycardia is usually due to hypoxia and inadequate ventilation. Oxygen can be added if there is no improvement in heart rate after the first few minutes.

If the heart rate is < 60 bpm after 30 seconds of positive-pressure ventilation with oxygen, commence chest compressions. Use two fingers on the lower half of the sternum, or both hands encircling the chest with both thumbs on the lower half of the sternum. Compress the chest to one-third of its depth at a rate of 100/min. Perform 3 compressions before pausing to deliver ventilation. Intubation can then be performed if there is an experienced operator available.

Drugs and IV fluids are rarely required. If the heart rate remains below 60 bpm despite adequate ventilation, oxygenation and chest compressions, adrenaline 10–30 microg/kg IV may be administered but must not detract from the above measures. IV access is usually readily available through the umbilical vein.

Foreign body airway obstruction

Sudden onset of noisy breathing, stridor and coughing can be signs of partial airway obstruction by a foreign body. The patient's own coughing can be the most effective way of relieving the obstruction, but if coughing is inadequate, call an ambulance or cardiac arrest team and move on to the manoeuvres outlined below.

The conscious patient who is unable to cough and clear their own airway needs assistance. Deliver up to 5 back blows with the heel of the hand to the middle of the back between the shoulder blades, checking after each to see if it has been successful in clearing the airway. If this is unsuccessful, up to 5 chest thrusts can be performed. This is a sharp blow with the heel of the hand delivered to the same area of the chest as chest compressions. Continue 5 back blows and 5 chest thrusts until the obstruction is relieved.

If it is a baby or infant, they can be placed prone and head down across your lap. Firm blows are delivered with the heel of your hand to the baby's back between the shoulder blades. Deliver up to 5 blows, checking in between to see if the airway has been cleared. If not successful, turn the infant over and perform up to 5 chest thrusts. Again, these are sharp blows delivered to the same location as for

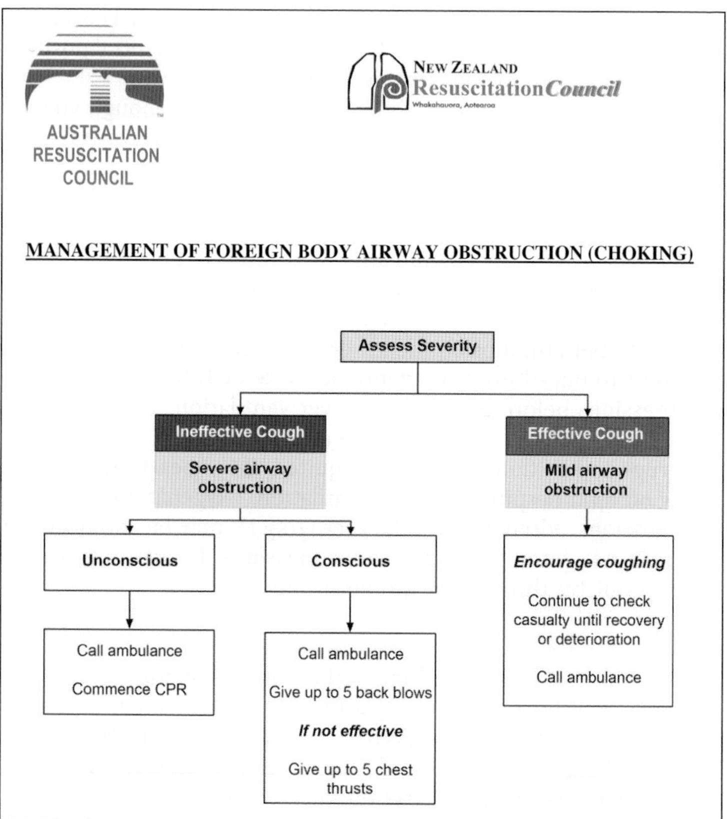

Figure 1.5 Management of foreign body airway obstruction (choking)
From Australian Resuscitation Council; reproduced with permission

chest compressions. Continue 5 back blows and 5 chest thrusts until the obstruction is relieved.

If the patient becomes unconscious, commence basic life support while waiting for the ambulance or arrest team to arrive.

Online resources

Australian Resuscitation Council (ARC)
www.resus.org.au

International Liaison Committee on Resuscitation (ILCOR)
www.ilcor.org

Chapter 2

Securing the airway, ventilation and procedural sedation

Judy Alford, Melinda Berry, Paul Gaudry and Andrew Finckh

Securing the airway

(Paul Gaudry and Melinda Berry)

Assessment and stabilisation of the airway have priority over other aspects of resuscitation in patients with life-threatening illness or injury.

Editorial Comment

Lack of an adequate airway is still the most common cause of preventable death outside and inside a hospital.

DIFFERENCES BETWEEN THE AIRWAY ANATOMIES OF CHILDREN AND ADULTS

The anatomy of the airways of infants and young children differs significantly from that of older children and adults in ways that are relevant to airway management:

1 larger and more mobile head, which tends to flex the neck in the supine position
2 larger tongue, more prominent oropharyngeal tonsils and larger epiglottis
3 higher and more anterior larynx in an infant (cervical vertebrae 3–4) than in a child or an adult (cervical vertebrae 5–6)
4 narrowest at cricoid cartilage rather than at vocal cords
5 smaller diameter and shorter length of trachea
6 small amounts of mucosal swelling producing large effects on airway resistance.

CAUSES OF AIRWAY OBSTRUCTION AND RESPIRATORY FAILURE

1. Decreased level of consciousness (cerebrovascular accident, seizure, infection, poisoning, head injury, near-drowning)
2. Trauma (maxillofacial fractures, blunt and penetrating neck injuries, laryngotracheal and bronchial rupture, chest injury, spinal cord injury)
3. Burns (face and neck burns, inhalational burns)
4. Foreign bodies (supraglottic, trachea, bronchus, oesophagus)
5. Infection (peritonsillar abscess, retropharyngeal abscess, epiglottitis, croup, pneumonia)
6. Inflammation (angioneurotic oedema, caustic ingestion, asthma, aspiration pneumonitis, parenchymal lung disease)
7. Shock (haemorrhagic, septic, anaphylactic, spinal)
8. Tumours (pharynx, larynx, trachea, bronchus)
9. Generalised weakness (neuropathies, myopathies)
10. Congenital anomalies in children (vascular ring)

ASSESSMENT AND ANTICIPATION OF AIRWAY OBSTRUCTION

Establish whether the airway is patent and protected, threatened, or partially or completely obstructed. A patent airway is an absolute first priority. Protection from aspiration is only a relative priority and does not take priority over initial assessment and treatment of the patient's breathing and circulation.

1. Observe and listen for air movement and the rate and depth of respirations (at the mouth and nose, movement of the chest wall, presence of tracheal tug).
2. Listen for noisy or abnormal sounds (gurgling, snoring, choking, coughing, stridor, wheeze).
3. Assess the sound and quality of the voice (weak, painful, hoarse).
4. Determine the level of consciousness (Glasgow Coma Scale score).
5. Inspect the mouth for foreign body.
6. Test the tone of the jaw, mouth and oropharyngeal muscles.
7. Test the gag reflex.
8. Feel the maxillofacial and neck regions (swelling, deformity, subcutaneous emphysema).

Upper airway obstruction. Initially the airway may only be threatened, but the pathological process may be progressive, as with burns and infection or movement of a foreign body. Priority must be given to securing the airway, as delay may itself precipitate complete obstruction. Intravenous sedation may also precipitate complete obstruction and should be avoided. If anaesthesia is required, inhalational induction may be preferred and relaxants avoided until bag–valve–mask ventilation is confirmed.

AIRWAY EXAMINATION FINDINGS

Several examination findings correlate with difficult mask ventilation or laryngoscopy. They should be taken into account. Positive findings tend to overestimate the chance of difficulty, but it is preferable to be over-prepared than under-prepared. Multiple abnormalities are more highly suggestive of difficulty. Negative findings do not exclude difficulty, and so problems may still arise unexpectedly. Difficult airway management algorithms help to work through problems when they occur.

Difficult mask ventilation

A poor seal between face and mask impedes bag–valve–mask ventilation. Six risk factors for difficult mask ventilation have been defined: beard, age > 57, snoring, BMI > 26, Mallampati III/IV, limited mandibular protrusion.

A commonly used mnemonic for a quick assessment of ventilation difficulty is BONES:

B Beard
O Obesity
N No teeth
E Elderly
S Stiffness

Difficult intubation

The following section reviews the commonly used clinical tests and examination to predict difficult laryngoscopy.

The LEMON mnemonic can be used as a reminder:

L Look externally: gestalt view—trauma, trismus, obesity
E Evaluate 3:3:2 rule (below)
M Mallampati score (below)
O Obstruction
N Neck immobility: cervical collar, rheumatoid arthritis, surgery

3:3:2 rule

- **Inter-incisor distance (3 fingers)**
  - Measure with the mouth fully open and head extended.

    - Less than 3 fingerbreadths imply more difficulty with intubation.
    - Average adult values are 3.5–4.5 cm.
- **Hyo-mental distance (3 fingers)**
    - Measure accurately from mental process to the hyoid bone with the head extended.
    - As a general rule a thyro-mental distance (mental process to thyroid cartilage) < 6.5 cm predicts a difficult intubation.
- **Thyro-hyoid distance (2 fingers)**
    - Measure from the thyroid cartilage to hyoid bone (or base of mouth) with neck extended.

Mallampati examination

This examination is performed with the patient sitting upright, head neutral, mouth fully opened, tongue extended and not talking (i.e. we can rarely ascertain a true Mallampati score in an ED patient requiring intubation but it can often be done prior to procedural sedation).

It was originally described with three classes and later modified by Samsoon and Young into four classes:

- Class I: soft palate, fauces, uvula, anterior and posterior pillars
- Class II: soft palate, fauces, uvula
- Class III: soft palate, base of uvula
- Class IV: hard palate

Difficult surgical airway

Look for factors which may obscure surgical landmarks. These can be remembered using the mnemonic SHORT:

S Surgery/Scar
H Haematoma
O Obesity
R Radiation
T Trauma/Tumour

FACTORS CONFOUNDING AIRWAY MANAGEMENT

Cervical spine injury. Head and neck immobilisation must be maintained in the victim of blunt trauma until injury to the cervical spine is definitely excluded. If endotracheal intubation is indicated, it must be achieved without flexion, extension or distraction of the neck. Intubation should be performed while an assistant maintains in-line immobilisation, without traction, of the head and neck.

Full stomach. All seriously ill or injured patients requiring intubation must be presumed to have a full stomach. Apply cricoid pressure during intubation to prevent regurgitation and aspiration.

Limited haemodynamic reserves. A patient with any form of shock is subject to haemodynamic deterioration during intubation, from the drugs used to facilitate intubation or from hypoxaemia before or during intubation. Pre-intubation oxygenation volume resuscitation and sometimes inotrope support are needed. The drugs used, and especially the drug dosage, must be individualised.

MANOEUVRES TO OPEN OR MAINTAIN THE AIRWAY

Head tilt, chin lift and jaw thrust help to open the airway by pulling the tongue off the back of the oropharynx. In patients with suspected cervical spine injury, this is limited to jaw thrust.

MANOEUVRES TO RELIEVE FOREIGN BODY OBSTRUCTION

If the patient is capable of air movement, spontaneous coughing and breathing should be encouraged. The patient with poor or no air movement requires immediate help.

Back blows. Deliver four forcible blows between the scapulae with the heel of the hand. This may relieve partial or complete obstruction.

Chest thrust. Deliver four chest compressions with the hands over the sternum with the patient lying or sitting.

Finger sweep. To relieve obstruction in the oropharynx. Not recommended in infants.

Repeated sequence. Back blows, chest thrust, finger sweep, Heimlich manoeuvre and mouth-to-mouth ventilation is recommended.

Suction or Magill forceps can then remove obstructing material.

Infants under 1 year of age. The recommended sequence is back blows, chest thrust and mouth-to-mouth ventilation.

OROPHARYNGEAL AND NASOPHARYNGEAL AIRWAYS

Oropharyngeal airway (Guedel airway). Must be placed over the tongue, so that the tongue is lifted off the hypopharynx. Insert using a tongue depressor or insert concave side up and then rotate 180°. Only tolerated if gag reflex is impaired. Can be used as a bite block in the intubated patient.

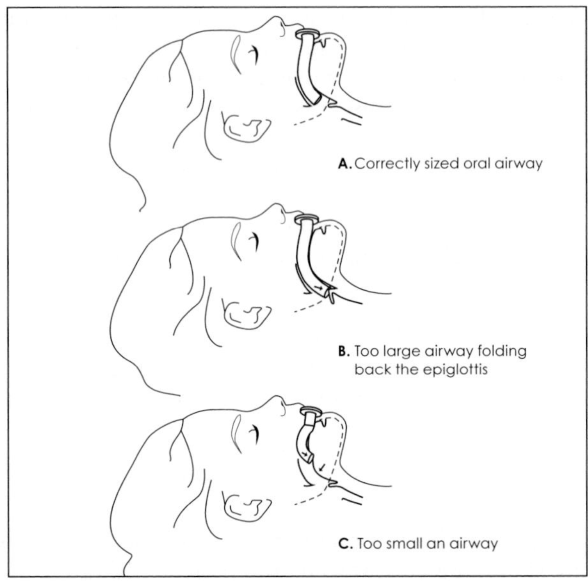

Figure 2.1 Correct placement and sizing of an oropharyngeal airway
From St Vincent's and Mater Health Campus Emergency Airways Handbook, produced and published by the Don Harrison Patient Safety Simulation Centre and Emergency Department St Vincent's Hospital, Sydney.

Nasopharyngeal airway. Lubricate well and insert through medial and inferior aspect of nasal cavity. Can be inserted in patients with tightly clenched teeth. Tolerated even if the patient has an active gag reflex. Tip needs to lie behind the tongue and low in the hypopharynx but above the larynx.

Editorial Comment

LMAs (laryngeal mask airways) are now increasingly used in the field as formal ETT (endotracheal tube) insertion may not be effective. Evidence is accumulating that even in the ED an LMA first-line can provide oxygenation and protect the airway as a step in a crashed patient before formal, difficult intubation.

TYPES OF VENTILATION

Mouth-to-mask ventilation

Mask should incorporate a one-way valve. It is preferable to mouth-to-mouth ventilation. Patients can be adequately ventilated until definitive assisted ventilation techniques are obtained.

Bag–valve–mask ventilation

Use 2 L bag for adults and children over 5 years of age, 500 mL bag for younger children and infants, 250 mL bag for premature infants.

Mask-to-face seal is maintained with even pressure using thumb and index finger on the mask and the other fingers applying chin lift or jaw thrust, depending on the size of the patient. A second resuscitator may be needed to assist with jaw thrust.

Endotracheal intubation

Endotracheal intubation is the most effective and reliable means of securing an airway. It provides airway patency, prevents aspiration, assures oxygenation and permits high ventilatory pressures and the use of positive end-expiratory pressure. It readily allows suctioning and can be used for administration of drugs if there is no intravenous access.

1. Approximate tube size (internal diameter) in adults is 7.5–8.0 mm in females and 8.0–8.5 mm in males.
   In pre-term infants use 2.5 mm, in term infants 3.0 mm, in 3- to 9-month-olds 3.5 mm, and in 9- to 24-month-olds 4.0 mm.
   Tube size for patients over the age of 2 years is calculated from the formula:

   $$\text{Diameter (mm)} = [\text{Age (in years)} + 4] \div 4$$

2. Uncuffed tubes are used in patients under the age of 8–10 years, allowing for an audible leak to prevent excessive pressure on the subglottis.
   Large-volume, low-pressure cuffs are used in older children and adults.
3. Orotracheal intubation is faster and easier than nasotracheal intubation.

Technique of orotracheal intubation

1. Precheck equipment (airways, tubes, introducers, forceps, bag–valve–mask, laryngoscopes).
2. Oxygen, suction and monitoring equipment must be available.
3. Skilled assistance is invaluable (with knowledge of the equipment used, to provide in-line manual immobilisation of the head and neck, and to apply cricoid pressure).
4. The 'sniffing' position allows optimal visualisation of the vocal cords. Positioning obese patients by placing the head on a pillow may not achieve adequate neck flexion or head extension. A ramp effect may be needed, achieved by placing a pillow under the shoulders and two pillows under the head.

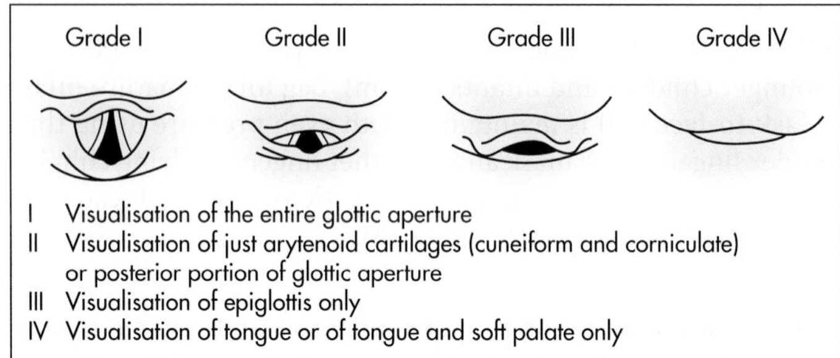

Grade I
Grade II
Grade III
Grade IV
I Visualisation of the entire glottic aperture
II Visualisation of just arytenoid cartilages (cuneiform and corniculate) or posterior portion of glottic aperture
III Visualisation of epiglottis only
IV Visualisation of tongue or of tongue and soft palate only

Figure 2.2 Cormack-Lehane laryngoscopic grading system

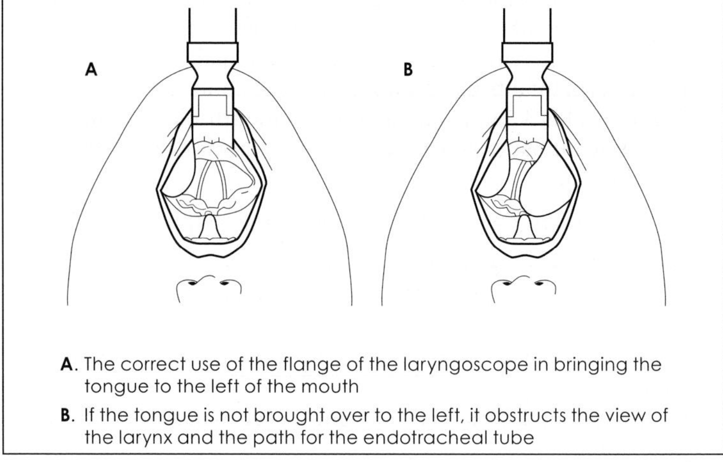

A
B
A. The correct use of the flange of the laryngoscope in bringing the tongue to the left of the mouth
B. If the tongue is not brought over to the left, it obstructs the view of the larynx and the path for the endotracheal tube

Figure 2.3 Correct placement of the laryngoscope blade
From St Vincent's and Mater Health Campus Emergency Airways Handbook, produced and published by the Don Harrison Patient Safety Simulation Centre and Emergency Department St Vincent's Hospital, Sydney.

5 Be calm and orderly.
6 Monitor oxygen saturation, ECG and BP during the procedure.
7 ‘Stiffen’ the tube to aid manipulation of the tube tip, by placing a lubricated ‘introducer’ inside the tube.
8 Aid visualisation of the larynx by the application of backward, upward, rightward pressure (BURP) to the thyroid cartilage.
9 Maintain visualisation of the tube passing through the vocal cords until the proximal end of the cuff is 2 cm beyond the cords.

10 Observation and auscultation should be performed to verify bilateral lung expansion.
11 Secure the tube in position, then insert an intragastric tube.
12 Capnography is required to confirm tube placement in the trachea.
13 Chest X-ray will ascertain the position of the tube tip in relation to the carina.

RAPID-SEQUENCE INDUCTION (RSI)

This is employed to induce unconsciousness and muscular paralysis to provide optimal intubating conditions, to avoid aspiration from a probable full stomach and to protect against reflex bradycardia and raised intracranial pressure due to manipulation of the airway. It is contraindicated if 'difficult' intubation is predicted and successful bag–valve–mask ventilation is considered unlikely. This will depend on the patient, the equipment and assistance available and the skill of the operator.

1 **Preoxygenation.** Administration of 100% oxygen, using a well-fitting bag–mask for 2 minutes, will result in 95–98% nitrogen washout. This will protect against hypoxia during apnoea for up to 8 minutes. Manual ventilation is preferably avoided until intubation is accomplished. Preoxygenation in a semi-sitting or head-up position may be more effective in the obese patient.
2 **Simultaneous in-line manual immobilisation of the head and neck.** Used in the blunt trauma victim when cervical spine injury is a possibility.
3 **Cricoid pressure.** As soon as consciousness is lost, cricoid pressure is applied with the thumb and index finger to compress the oesophagus between the cricoid cartilage and the cervical spine. Compression is maintained until the tube cuff is inflated. This technique helps to prevent regurgitation and aspiration, but is contraindicated if the patient vomits. It should not be confused with BURP (backward, upward, rightward pressure) to bring the vocal cords into view.
   - **Note:** At this time, the routine application of cricoid pressure is considered a standard of care. There is, however, no evidence absolutely supporting its routine use in RSI.
   - When properly applied by a *trained* individual, cricoid pressure tends to improve laryngoscopy. It can also be used to assist in the BURP manoeuvre, which can improve laryngoscopic view by one grade.
   - It should be remembered that improperly applied cricoid pressure can render laryngoscopy more difficult.

Table 2.1 Drugs in airway management

Drug	Dose	Important effects
Induction agents		
Thiopentone	3–5 mg/kg Less (0.5–1 mg/kg) in elderly or unstable	Hypotension, especially in hypovolaemia Respiratory depression Reduces cerebral metabolism, ICP Increases laryngeal sensitivity
Propofol	1–2.5 mg/kg	Decreases BP, especially in hypovolaemia Respiratory depression Reduces cerebral metabolism
Ketamine	1–2 mg/kg IV 3–5 mg/kg IM	Raises BP Raises HR Airway reflexes maintained Respiration not depressed Bronchodilation Raises ICP and IOP Hallucinations more common in adults
Fentanyl	2–3 microg/kg	Dose-related respiratory depression Analgesia Large doses may cause chest wall rigidity Relative cardiovascular stability
Midazolam	0.1–0.4 mg/kg	Some decrease in BP Respiratory depression
Muscle relaxants		
Suxamethonium	1 mg/kg	Drug of choice for RSI Raises K by 0.5 mEq/L, more in burns (>48 h old), paralysis and denervation (>3 days old), crush injury Raises IOP (avoid in open eye injury) Triggers malignant hyperthermia Prolonged apnoea (rare, inherited)
Rocuronium	1 mg/kg for RSI 0.6 mg/kg for non-RSI 0.15 mg/kg PRN	Use for RSI when suxamethonium contraindicated Use for maintaining paralysis
Vecuronium	0.1 mg/kg	Use for maintaining paralysis Not suitable for RSI

BP, blood pressure; HR, heart rate; K, potassium; ICP, intracranial pressure; IOP, intraocular pressure; PRN, as needed; RSI, rapid-sequence induction

Editorial Comment

There is some controversy about how effective BURP is.
At intubation be prepared to be flexible—nothing works in all cases.

4 **Secure intravenous infusion site,** for fluid and drug administration.
5 **Atropine** (10–20 microg/kg) is given as pretreatment to prevent bradycardia, which is more likely in children under 8 years of age and after repeated doses of suxamethonium.
6 **Induction.** Thiopentone 2.5% (3–5 mg/kg) induces unconsciousness within seconds of a single IV dose; its duration is a few minutes. Use a smaller dose (1–2 mg/kg) if depressed level of consciousness is already present. Its main side effects are cardiovascular and respiratory depression. Hypotension is managed with intravenous fluids. The dose must be reduced if there is already hypovolaemia or hypoxaemia. Propofol (2.0–2.5 mg/kg) also induces unconsciousness; a single induction dose lasts 5–10 minutes; avoid in children under 3 years. Alternatives are midazolam (0.1–0.2 mg/kg) combined with morphine (0.1–0.2 mg/kg) or fentanyl (2–4 microg/kg). Preinduction treatment of depressed cardiac output (from hypovolaemia, hypoxaemia, septic or cardiogenic shock) and titrating the drug dose against response are important, regardless of the agent. Lignocaine 1.5 mg/kg may be used as pretreatment in patients at risk of elevation of intracranial pressure.
7 **Suxamethonium** (1–2 mg/kg, 2–3 mg/kg in infants) induces neuromuscular depolarisation (fasciculations) followed by relaxation. Relaxation occurs within 60 seconds and generally lasts 3–10 minutes. Hypertension and tachycardia may occur due to stimulation of autonomic ganglia, or there may be bradycardia and salivation due to muscarinic effects. Other side effects include potassium flux from muscle cells, myoglobinaemia, muscle pain, a rise in intragastric, intraocular and intracranial pressure and triggering of malignant hyperthermia. Prolonged relaxation occurs if there is pseudocholinesterase deficiency. An alternative is an 'intubating dose' of vecuronium (0.2–0.3 mg/kg), which produces relaxation by non-depolarising neuromuscular block. Onset is within 90 seconds and duration is 90–120 minutes.
8 **Propofol infusion** (1.0–3.0 mg/kg/h) is used to provide sedation to facilitate control of oxygenation and ventilation in adults. Alternatives are sedation and analgesia (midazolam and morphine). Add muscle relaxant if absolute control of ventilation is required. Under no circumstances give relaxants without sedation and analgesia. Usually vecuronium

(0.1–0.15 mg/kg) or pancuronium (0.1–0.15 mg/kg) are used for maintenance relaxation. Vecuronium has a shorter duration of action, does not cause histamine release and produces less tachycardia and hypertension than pancuronium.

9 **Monitoring** is essential during and following the procedure—ECG, BP, oxygen saturation, capnography.

SUCTIONING

Suctioning is an adjunct to manoeuvres to open or maintain the airway. It is used to remove tracheobronchial secretions via an endotracheal tube.

- Yankauer sucker is used to remove secretions, blood, vomitus or foreign body from mouth and pharynx. In the unintubated patient, turn the patient on the side during suctioning.
- Y-suction catheter with a soft tip is used for nasopharyngeal and tracheobronchial secretions. Catheter diameter should not be more than half the diameter of the endotracheal tube.
- Preoxygenate and bag–valve–tube ventilate the patient before and after suctioning to prevent hypoxaemia and pulmonary collapse.

OXYGENATION AND VENTILATION

Ventilator settings require decisions about minute ventilation, respiratory rate, inspired oxygen concentration, peak airway pressure and the use of positive end-expiratory pressure. (See the section 'Choosing initial settings for ventilation' in this chapter.)

Monitor peak airway pressure as well as oxygen saturation, capnography and blood gases. Aim for oxygen saturation above 95% and mild hypocapnia.

A disconnection alarm must be used during mechanical ventilation.

COMPLICATIONS OF INTUBATION

- **During intubation:** trauma to any structure from lips to the trachea; inability to oxygenate, ventilate or intubate; exacerbation of spinal cord injury; aspiration; haemodynamic collapse.
- **While tube is in place:** misplacement; blockage; problems related to the ventilator.
- **After extubation:** laryngospasm; aspiration; complications of trauma.

EXTUBATION

1 The patient must be fully awake and have a gag reflex before extubation.
2 Non-depolarising neuromuscular blockade can be reversed with neostigmine (an anticholinesterase) and atropine (prophylactic antimuscarinic). Antagonists to midazolam and morphine are only rarely required.
3 Preoxygenation, suctioning of pharynx and trachea and intragastric tube should precede extubation, which is performed at the peak of inspiration.
4 Ensure oxygenation after extubation with a bag–valve–mask or a non-rebreathing mask.

ALTERNATIVE AIRWAY TECHNIQUES

Nasotracheal intubation. Can be performed without direct laryngoscopy in the non-apnoeic patient (the 'blind' technique). It is an appropriate alternative to orotracheal intubation in confirmed unstable cervical spine injury or spinal cord injury, in severely dyspnoeic awake patients who can be intubated in the sitting position, and in patients unable to fully open their mouth. It is contraindicated in patients with maxillofacial and anterior cranial fractures, and with conditions such as nasal polyps, upper airway foreign bodies and retropharyngeal abscesses.

Airway bougie. An extension of the use of an 'introducer', this is used for a 'difficult' intubation. A long semi-rigid bougie is inserted between the vocal cords and the endotracheal tube is then passed over the bougie into the trachea. The bougie is then removed.

Video-laryngoscope. Video-assisted laryngoscopy can provide an improvement in glottis visualisation and may be of particular use in anticipated difficult airways and cases with limited neck motion.

Laryngeal mask airway (LMA). Consists of airway with elliptical cuffed 'mask' on distal end which rests over the larynx when inserted. Low-pressure ventilation may be performed, but it does not reliably prevent aspiration. Is quicker and an easier technique to learn than endotracheal intubation. Has an established role to provide an airway in the fasted patient during anaesthesia. Is a useful temporising technique if intubation skills are not available. When direct laryngoscopy and intubation fails, it may serve to provide a functional airway until definitive intubation by cannulation of the trachea through the mask is performed.

Fibre-optic intubating laryngoscope. Alternative to intubation guided by transillumination (Trachlight) if RSI is contraindicated. Intubation is performed under local anaesthesia, preferably via the nasotracheal route. The laryngoscope is directed into the larynx and then acts like a guidewire for the tube. Requires a significant amount of training and is not in widespread use. Devices aiding view and intubation via a visual monitor are increasingly available as back-up.

Editorial Comment

There are an increasing number of video-visualisation devices. While they can be quicker, all need training—never to be used first time in an emergency airway crisis. Routine intubation by direct laryngoscopy remains the essential core skill that must be mastered.

Oesophageal–tracheal airway ('Combitube'). Consists of twin-lumen tube with one lumen inserted into the oesophagus and the other lying above the trachea. A pharyngeal balloon provides a seal to enable ventilation. A distal balloon seals against gastric inflation and aspiration. Is an alternative to LMA if intubation skills are not available.

Translaryngeal oxygenation. Indicated when non-surgical airway management has failed, is contraindicated or is not available (total upper airway obstruction). Preferred to cricothyroidotomy in children under 8 years of age. Temporising oxygenating procedure does not prevent aspiration, may lead to hypercarbia and is not effective if a foreign body is present below the cricoid cartilage.

Cricothyroidotomy. Alternative to translaryngeal oxygenation. May be used after temporising with translaryngeal oxygenation. Preferred to tracheostomy, which should be reserved for the operating room. Percutaneous approach (Seldinger technique) is easiest and fastest. Using a surgical approach, insert a small endotracheal tube or tracheostomy tube. When the patient is stable, convert to tracheostomy or orotracheal tube.

GUIDELINES FOR 'DIFFICULT' INTUBATION

1 If 'difficult' intubation is predicted but is not urgent, seek assistance from an experienced operator.
2 Assemble the available 'difficult' airway equipment. In many institutions it is thought that direct visualisation of the larynx with a standard laryngoscope handle and blade in the

management of the anticipated difficult airway is no longer acceptable. Consideration of tools such as the GlideScope or fibre-optic bronchoscope is strongly recommended in such situations. Use of these devices in routine securing of the airway results in proficient use in the emergency situation.

3. Assess whether successful bag–valve–mask ventilation is likely.
4. Use an airway bougie (or intubation guided by transillumination if available) if 'difficult' intubation is predicted.
5. Nasotracheal intubation, awake intubation or use of the fibre-optic intubating laryngoscope are options if successful bag–valve–mask ventilation is considered unlikely.
6. Avoid use of muscle relaxants if successful bag–mask–valve ventilation is considered unlikely.
7. If the initial attempt at orotracheal intubation fails and the patient has been paralysed, institute bag–valve–mask oxygenation and ventilation, then use BURP or an airway bougie and re-attempt intubation.
8. A 'difficult' intubation occurs if orotracheal intubation cannot be achieved after 2 attempts under direct laryngoscopy. Resume bag–valve–mask oxygenation and ventilation. Then re-attempt intubation using BURP or an airway bougie, or consider using a laryngeal mask airway, an oesophageal–tracheal airway or fibre-optic intubation.
9. If attempts at bag–valve–mask oxygenation and ventilation fail, escalate the use of an LMA or oesophageal–tracheal airway to reoxygenate. Consider passing airway bougie or endotracheal tube though the laryngeal mask.
10. Translaryngeal oxygenation or cricothyroidotomy are indicated when non-surgical airway management fails.

FAILED INTUBATION

(Andrew Finckh)

Following failed intubation, a reassessment of the situation and an analysis of possible reasons for the failure should be made.

1. Patient factors
   - Can the patient positioning be improved?
   - Can laryngeal positioning be improved (e.g. BURP manoeuvre)?
2. Equipment
   - Is the choice of blade (type/size) correct?
   - Consider use of other airway tools, such as a fibre-optic laryngoscope, e.g. GlideScope.

3 Drugs
— Has adequate patient relaxation been achieved?

THE DIFFICULT AIRWAY TROLLEY

It is essential that all emergency departments have a difficult airway trolley. It should be well organised and have clearly labelled contents. The exact contents of a difficult airway trolley may vary, but should include a limited selection of tools to assist in securing the airway. The field of airway management is changing rapidly with new and, sometimes, improved devices becoming available. The trolley should reflect this. Its contents should be revised regularly and, if necessary, updated.

Suggested contents of a difficult airway trolley include:

- laryngeal mask airways
- supraglottic devices, such as Combitube
- lighted stylet, such as Trachlight
- flexible fibre-optic laryngoscope
- surgical airway, including commercial devices to perform cricothyroidotomy with a modified Seldinger technique.

SECURING THE AIRWAY ALGORITHMS

An algorithmic approach to securing the airway can assist in a systematic and reliable management of the airway.

1 **Management of the difficult airway**

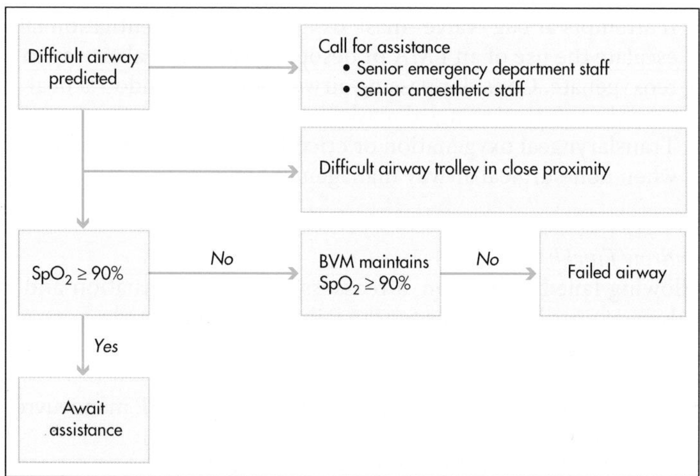

Figure 2.4 Difficult airway algorithm
BVM, bag–valve–mask; SpO_2, oxygen saturation via pulse oximetry

2 Management of the failed airway

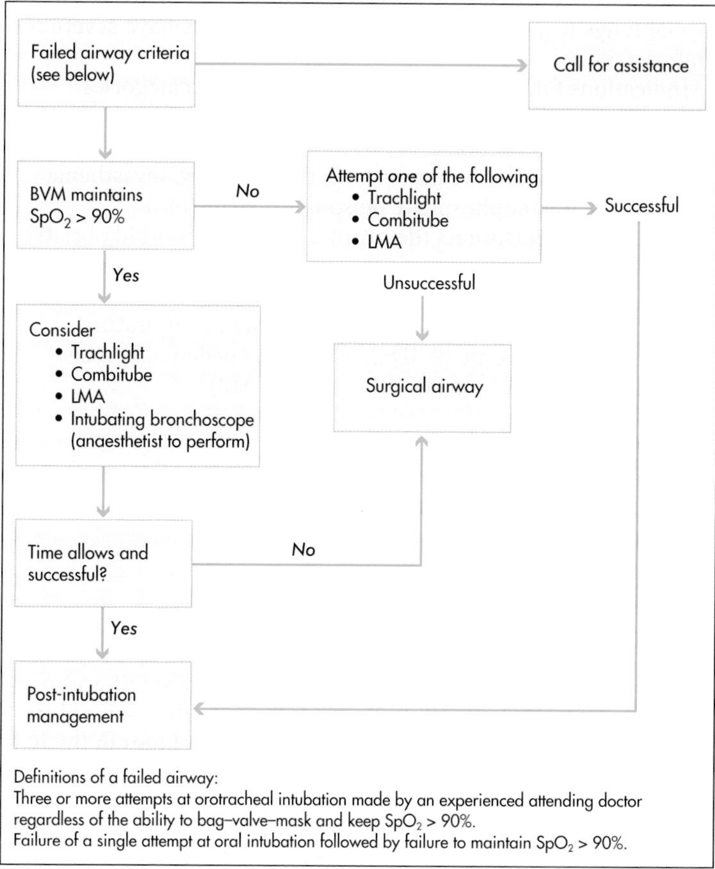

Figure 2.5 Failed airway algorithm
LMA, laryngeal mask airway

Surgical airway

Refer to Chapter 3, 'Resuscitation and emergency procedures'.

Ventilators

(Judy Alford)

Ventilators are used in the ED to assist or control the respiration of patients. Patients needing invasive ventilation need an artificial airway, most commonly an endotracheal tube. The level of ventilatory support needed by a patient varies widely. Some have essentially normal lungs (e.g. sedative overdose), while others have severe respiratory failure.

Indications for ventilation fall into three broad categories:

1 **Respiratory failure**
- Airway obstruction
- Neuromuscular weakness (spinal cord injury, myasthenia gravis, organophosphate poisoning, exhaustion)
- Chest wall disorders (deformity, flail chest, morbid obesity)
- Pleural disease (massive effusions, pneumothorax or haemothorax)
- Parenchymal lung disease (infection, adult respiratory distress syndrome (ARDS), pulmonary oedema, fibrosis, asthma, chronic airflow limitation (CAL))

2 **CNS disease**
- Poisoning
- Trauma
- Cerebrovascular accident (CVA)
- Infections

3 **Circulatory failure**
- Hypovolaemia
- Sepsis
- Cardiogenic shock

The type of ventilator used in the ED is usually small and portable. The range of ventilatory modes available varies, but is usually less than is available on more complex machines in the ICU. Nonetheless most patients can be managed in the short term.

CHOOSING INITIAL SETTINGS FOR VENTILATION

Initially, ventilator settings are estimated; adjustments should be made according to the patient's clinical progress and serial blood gas measurements.

Is the patient breathing spontaneously?

Spontaneously breathing patients are ventilated using a mode that assists each inspiratory effort by providing extra pressure or volume. Examples are continuous positive airway pressure (CPAP) and pressure support. Some ventilators and their circuits increase the work of breathing significantly and spontaneous breathing may not be tolerated. In these cases, the patient may need to be sedated and fully ventilated.

The patient who is not breathing adequately needs a mode that does all the work for them. Intermittent positive-pressure ventilation (IPPV) or intermittent mandatory ventilation (IMV) provides a breath at a preset rate regardless of the patient's respiratory effort. Some ventilators can deliver a breath synchronised to an inspiratory effort; this is known as synchronised intermittent mandatory ventilation (SIMV).

How much oxygen does the patient need?

In most cases, start ventilation with 100% oxygen and titrate downwards as soon as possible according to the patient's arterial blood gases (ABG) results. Prolonged ventilation with high levels of inspired oxygen may be associated with complications such as absorption atelectasis and oxidative injury.

Some ventilators have limited options in selecting an inspired oxygen level. In patients who are inadequately oxygenated, positive end-expiratory pressure (PEEP) can increase the arterial oxygen tension for a given level of inspired oxygen.

How much gas should the patient receive?

The **minute volume** is the amount of gas moved every minute:

$$\text{Minute volume} = \text{Respiratory rate} \times \text{Tidal volume}$$

The arterial tension of carbon dioxide is sensitive to changes in minute volume. Increasing the minute volume reduces the partial pressure of arterial CO_2 ($PaCO_2$), and decreasing the minute volume raises $PaCO_2$. In patients with raised intracranial pressure, it may be necessary to deliberately hyperventilate to maintain a modest decrease in $PaCO_2$. In some patients with lung injury, trying to deliver a 'normal' minute volume may pose a risk of barotrauma. In these cases, the $PaCO_2$ may be allowed to rise quite significantly, an approach called permissive hypercapnia.

The ventilators in common use apply positive pressure to the lungs to enable gas movement. The amount of gas moved per breath depends on the ventilator settings and the lung compliance.

Ventilators can be set to deliver a given tidal volume at each breath. This mode is called **volume control** and is available on even the most basic machines. It may be possible to limit the delivery of the set volume if the airway pressures exceed a limit chosen by the operator (pressure-regulated volume control (PRVC) mode).

Pressure control is a mode commonly used in the ICU but not always available on smaller ventilators. A constant airway pressure is provided during inspiration, with the tidal volume varying. This approach is often used where barotrauma is a concern.

Lung compliance is the change in lung volume for a given change in transpulmonary pressure. Diseased lungs often have abnormal compliance (e.g. in pulmonary oedema the lung is less compliant or 'stiffer'). Trying to deliver a 'normal' tidal volume to a poorly compliant lung can cause high airway pressures, increasing the risk of pneumothorax. Overdistension can worsen lung damage. The approach to ventilating is usually one of providing limited tidal volumes (6–8 mL/kg, sometimes less) with PEEP. This can be done using either volume or pressure control.

The choice of **initial tidal volume** depends on the clinical situation. In patients with respiratory failure or shock, a volume of 6–8 mL/kg is safest, as this will minimise barotrauma and volutrauma. Inspiratory pressures should not exceed 30 cmH_2O.

POSITIVE END-EXPIRATORY PRESSURE (PEEP)

PEEP leaves a constant pressure on the lungs at the end of expiration, preventing the collapse of alveoli. Constant opening and closing of alveoli can damage them. Using PEEP may prevent further lung injury as well as maintaining functional residual capacity. As noted earlier, PEEP has a positive effect on oxygenation. However, PEEP has a negative effect on cardiac output because high intrathoracic pressures impede venous return. High levels of PEEP may not be tolerated in haemodynamically unstable patients. Another factor to be considered is 'auto-PEEP'. This is the pressure difference between the alveoli and the proximal airway at end-expiration, which can be raised in conditions with air-trapping, such as severe asthma. 'Auto-PEEP' can contribute to haemodynamic instability in some patients. Prolonging expiration may help to reduce air-trapping in affected patients.

Choosing a level of PEEP

PEEP of 5 cmH_2O is tolerated by most patients. In patients with severe lung disease, increases in PEEP up to about 12 cmH_2O may be needed. PEEP may not be tolerated in patients with haemodynamic instability. Another group of patients who may not tolerate PEEP have raised intracranial pressure. In some cases the reduction in cerebral venous return may be enough to exacerbate the increase in intracranial pressure.

Special situations

Asthma

Use low respiratory rates with a prolonged expiratory phase to limit air-trapping. Auto-PEEP may be significant, so additional PEEP may lead to hypotension. Avoid large tidal volumes. Permissive hypercapnia may be needed.

Raised intracranial pressure

Avoid hypercapnia. Maintain $PaCO_2$ between 30 and 35 mmHg, using end-tidal monitoring and ABG. High levels of PEEP should be avoided.

Adult respiratory distress syndrome (ARDS)

ARDS is a difficult problem. The ideal ventilatory strategy is controversial. In the ED the key points are: (1) to avoid barotrauma by using small tidal volumes and avoiding high airway pressures; and (2) to use PEEP as tolerated and tolerate a high $PaCO_2$. Paralysis may be necessary. Frequent adjustments to tidal volume and respiratory rate may be needed, along with recruitment manoeuvres to reopen collapsed alveoli. Specialised techniques such as prone ventilation and high-frequency oscillatory ventilation may be undertaken in the ICU. In the rapidly deteriorating patient with refractory hypoxaemia, early referral for consideration of ECMO (extracorporeal membrane oxygenation) may be life-saving.

Troubleshooting

- Ask for advice early.
- Never assume the monitor is at fault.
- If there is difficulty ventilating the patient:
  - Immediately remove the patient from the circuit and commence bag ventilation with 100% oxygen.
  - Check the endotracheal tube for kinking, displacement (in or out), obstruction and leaking.
  - Examine the patient for equal and adequate breath sounds. Check the trachea is midline.
  - If breath sounds are diminished, suction for mucous plugs and consider treating for a pneumothorax. Treat bronchospasm or pulmonary oedema if present.
  - Get a chest X-ray.
  - Consider bronchoscopy.

(pto)

- If all of the above are normal, the problem may be with the machine.
  - The ventilator may have become disconnected (from the circuit, the gas supply or the power supply).
  - There may be leaks in the tubing or valves, or tubing may be obstructed.
  - Consider changing the circuit.

NON-INVASIVE VENTILATION (NIV)

Non-invasive ventilation using positive pressure via a face or nasal mask has become widely used in EDs. Most commonly, a bi-level positive airway pressure (BiPAP) machine is used, although conventional pressure-cycled ventilators can also be used.

The machine delivers a constant low level of positive pressure, which is increased upon sensing the patient's inspiratory effort. This increased inspiratory pressure is equivalent to pressure-support ventilation but, when setting the machine, the inspiratory positive airway pressure (IPAP) should be set at a level equal to the sum of PEEP and pressure support (e.g. an IPAP of 15 and an expiratory positive airway pressure (EPAP) of 5 is equivalent to pressure support of 10 and PEEP of 5).

Indications

- Acute respiratory failure due to pulmonary oedema, CAL, asthma, pneumonia
- Chronic respiratory failure due to neuromuscular conditions
- Obstructive sleep apnoea

Contraindications

- Apnoea or impending cardiorespiratory arrest
- Haemodynamic instability
- Risk of aspiration
- Decreased level of consciousness
- Inability to cooperate with mask

Problems with BiPAP

The mask may not be tolerated for the following reasons:

1. Skin irritation and pressure necrosis
2. Conjunctival irritation or injury
3. Aspiration
4. Gastric over-distension
5. Hypotension due to raised intrathoracic pressure

6 Progressive respiratory failure despite BiPAP, which is an indication for intubation

Procedural sedation

Procedural sedation (also known as conscious sedation) refers to administration of sedative drugs to facilitate performance of a distressing or painful procedure. The level of sedation required varies with the procedure and the individual patient. The level of sedation falls short of general anaesthesia. The patient should retain the ability to respond to stimulus, and airway reflexes should be maintained.

INDICATIONS

Procedures involving significant pain and/or anxiety are tolerated to varying degrees by individual patients. For example, a child may require sedation for wound suturing where an adult may not.

Procedures requiring sedation in nearly all patients

- Reduction of dislocations of large joints
- Reduction and splinting of long-bone fractures
- Cardioversion

Procedures requiring sedation in some patients

- Lumbar puncture
- Central line insertion
- Wound suturing
- Foreign body removal
- Burn dressing
- Chest drain insertion

REQUIREMENTS

Procedural sedation should be undertaken in an area with working suction and oxygen. Pulse oximetry should be used. Continuous ECG and BP monitoring may be used in selected patients (e.g. older or with cardiac history). Ready access to resuscitation equipment and emergency drugs is essential. At least one person should be present who has the skills to manage any complications, including airway obstruction and cardiac arrest. All patients should have details recorded on a standard form. See Figure 2.6.

Fasting status does not necessarily preclude the use of sedation, but does influence the depth of sedation induced.

St Vincent's Hospital
EMERGENCY DEPARTMENT

Anaesthetic/Procedural
Sedation Assessment Form

MRN		SURNAME	
OTHER NAMES			
DOB	SEX	AMO	WARD/CLINIC

(Please enter information or affix patient information label)

Reason for intubation/procedural sedation: ______

Emergency procedure (unable to complete form) (tick if applicable)

Reason ______

HISTORY

Allergies: ______

Medications: ______

Past health Comorbidities (tick if present) Diabetes COPD
Asthma IHD

Other significant history: ______

Anaesthetic history: ______

Tobacco: ______ Alcohol: ______ Other: ______

Fasting time (in hours): ______

EXAMINATION

BP: ______ PR: ______ SpO_2: ______

Mallampati: Class I Class II Class III Class IV

Teeth: ______

Neck mobility: ______

Other relevant physical findings: ______

INVESTIGATIONS

Consent obtained: Yes ☐ No ☐ If no, reason ______

MEDICAL OFFICER

Name: ______ Signature: ______

Designation: ______ Date: ______

Name of supervising medical officer (if applicable): ______

ANAESTHETIC/PROCEDURAL SEDATION ASSESSMENT FORM

Figure 2.6 Anaesthetic procedural sedation assessment

Table 2.2 Drugs used in procedural sedation

Drug	Dose	Duration
Midazolam	0.02–0.1 mg/kg IV 0.5 mg/kg PO (onset about 20 minutes)	30 minutes IV 45–60 minutes PO
Fentanyl	2–3 microg/kg IV	20–30 minutes
Propofol	0.5–1 mg/kg IV	10 minutes
Ketamine	1–2 mg/kg IV 3–5 mg/kg IM	15 minutes IV 30 minutes IM
Nitrous oxide	Given as 30–50% mix in oxygen Causes expansion of gas-filled structures (e.g. pneumothorax)	5 minutes

DRUGS

The ideal drug for procedural sedation has rapid onset and offset, has no significant side effects, preserves airway reflexes and is easily titrated. Some commonly used agents are found in Table 2.2.

AFTERCARE

The patient should be monitored until they have emerged from sedation. It is not uncommon for patients to become more deeply sedated once painful stimulus has ceased.

Patients should not be discharged from the ED until they have returned to their baseline mental state, are ambulant and have safe transport and supervision. Patients with poor social circumstances may require a longer period of observation.

Editorial Comment

In the management of an urgent airway problem, always have a prepared back-up plan in case the current manoeuvre is unsuccessful.

Chapter 3
Resuscitation and emergency procedures

Drew Richardson

This chapter gives a brief overview of major procedures which may be carried out in the emergency department. It is meant to be used as a reminder for a doctor who has already been trained in these techniques, and not as a training manual. The common procedures should be practised under supervision, and the uncommon procedures should be formally taught before they are attempted solo. Some procedures require both training and experience, and some institutions require formal accreditation for operators (e.g. for focused assessment with sonography in trauma (FAST) scanning). Many procedures and their integration into complex, team-based resuscitation are best learnt in a simulator laboratory rather than in an ED.

For all procedures, the following steps are essential:

1. Use the appropriate sterile technique and standard precautions. Minimally invasive procedures such as peripheral intravenous access require only gloves and a clean technique, but more-invasive procedures mandate formal sterile technique with a sterile field, appropriate drapes, gown, gloves, mask and eye protection. Less-formal technique may be acceptable only when the procedure is required within seconds (e.g. cricothyroidotomy or ED thoracotomy), and full protection for the staff must still be observed.
2. Obtain the patient's informed consent whenever possible. The level of explanation obviously varies with the invasiveness of the procedure and the urgency of the patient's condition, but all conscious patients should give their consent (even if only implied).
3. Ensure patient comfort and the safety of all parties by using appropriate analgesia and, if necessary, sedation. Do not attempt difficult procedures on patients who are unable or unwilling to lie still.

4 Utilise a 'time-out routine'. Stop and reflect at least for a moment to ensure that the right procedure is being undertaken on the right patient at the right site—look again at any relevant imaging to confirm it is the right way around.
5 Ensure continuing care and resuscitation of the patient, particularly during long procedures, utilising other staff and patient monitoring throughout.
6 Document the time, operator and result of the procedure appropriately, in line with local practice. Even minor procedures such as insertion of an intravenous cannula normally require a standardised form of documentation such as a date written on the dressing.

Editorial Comment

Ask: can I do this procedure more safely with ultrasound guidance?

Intravenous access techniques

There are four basic IV access techniques:

1 Indwelling metal needle is now used only rarely and in peripheral sites, e.g. 'a butterfly'.
2 Catheter over needle technique includes common IV cannula.
3 Catheter through needle technique is used infrequently. A large-bore needle is inserted into the relevant vessel, and a smaller catheter advanced up the needle, usually into a central vein. The metal needle is then withdrawn and rendered safe in a plastic guard. This technique carries the disadvantage of a small-bore catheter and the risks of catheter-tip embolisation with poor technique and ongoing ooze due to the diameter difference.
4 Seldinger technique is widely accepted for all large or long IV lines. The vessel is punctured with a long needle on a syringe, and a flexible guidewire passed down the needle (sometimes through the syringe). The syringe and needle are removed, and appropriate dilators passed over the wire, and then removed. The catheter is passed over the wire into the vessel, and the wire is then removed. With this technique it is important to:
   a check and understand the equipment before starting (various sets are available)
   b have cardiac monitoring in place if the wire is to be near the heart
   c secure the catheter properly (usually by stitching)
   d above all, never let go of the wire.

Ultrasound guidance

All of the following techniques benefit from appropriate ultrasound guidance. If small veins cannot be seen or palpated, then ultrasound assists in location. Large deep veins are beyond visualisation, so skin marking using ultrasound before the procedure and/or direct visualisation using ultrasound (with sterile technique) during the procedure increases success and decreases complications. In settings where large deep vessels are regularly cannulated, availability of ultrasound is now considered to represent 'standard of care'.

Editorial Comment

Ultrasound guidance is increasingly being used for all access and is considered very desirable for any central access procedures.

INTRAVENOUS LINES—PERIPHERAL

Indications

- Administration of fluid—resuscitative and/or maintenance
- Administration of drugs
- Obtaining blood (rare)

Contraindications

- Overlying skin damage (e.g. burns) or infection
- Venous damage proximal to site insertion
- Arteriovenous (AV) fistula in the limb

Technique

1. Apply a venous tourniquet.
2. Identify a suitable vessel, ideally as peripheral as possible. Start looking on the back of the hands. Use cubital fossa veins only when large-volume resuscitation is required or other sites have proven unsuitable.
3. Prepare the area with a disinfectant-soaked swab, swabbing in a distal direction.
4. Stretch the skin slightly over the vein.
5. Insert the needle, bevel upwards, until a flushback is obtained.
6. Advance the catheter over the needle.
7. Remove the needle, attach the IV line or bung and secure the catheter.
8. Check position and patency by infusion or injection to clear blood from the catheter.

Complications

- Haematoma
- Subcutaneous extravasation of fluid
- Damage to nearby structures
- Inter-arterial cannulation

INTRAVENOUS LINES—PAEDIATRIC

The selection of a site for IV infusion in the neonate or young child should include consideration of the femoral vein in the groin and the scalp veins.

Of these, the femoral vein is probably the best to use in the critically ill child. Although no tourniquet can be applied, the vein is reliably located medial to the femoral artery pulse just below the inguinal ligament.

The scalp veins can be rendered more visible by use of a rubber band tourniquet around the head, and entered in the usual fashion. Always inject saline and check for blanching to exclude arterial puncture. Careful strapping and use of a protector (e.g. plastic cup) are essential to avoid displacement of the scalp vein catheter.

INTRAOSSEOUS (IO) INFUSION—PAEDIATRIC OR ADULT

This is a rapid technique for reliably obtaining vascular access in sick, small children. It can be used in patients of all ages, but the thicker bones of older children and adults mandate the use of a specially designed drill rather than manual insertion, and such a drill should be available for all patients in a setting where this is likely. Blood can usefully be drawn for biochemistry (not haematology) and large volumes of fluid or drug infused. It is highly recommended that this technique be practised on animal bones before it is attempted on a patient.

Indications

- Critically ill patient (especially small child) in urgent need of drug or fluid administration
- No other vascular access readily available

Editorial Comment

IOs are becoming standard use in some acute resuscitations and problematic access. Practise with a kit available to you on a simulation trainer/bone to get the feel. Also ensure you know laboratory limitations for any blood tests, care of the IO site and safe length of use.

Contraindications

- Infection at puncture site
- Fracture of the bone
- Osteogenesis imperfecta
- Recent nearby IO puncture (relative contraindication that is likely to lead to extravasation)

Technique

1. Identify infusion site: preferably upper medial surface of the tibia, 1–2 cm distal to the tibial tuberosity, but the lower tibia (at the junction of the medial malleolus and the shaft) may be suitable.
2. Prepare the area with an iodine swab.
3. Insert IO needle (16- to 18-gauge special needle with stylet) into the bone at 45°, aiming distally. If performed manually, this requires a rotary 'grinding' motion until a 'crunch' is felt as the cortex is penetrated. Using a drill, go at 90° and expect progress to be faster, but the definite penetration will still be felt.
4. Remove stylet and attempt to aspirate marrow contents. Success clearly indicates correct placement, but failure sometimes occurs despite placement.
5. Begin infusion or injection of fluids and drugs. Flow should be relatively free.
6. Secure and protect the infusion site.

Complications

- Extravasation of fluid
- Needle blockage
- Infection (rare, reduced by good technique and removal as soon as practicable)

INTRAVENOUS LINES—CENTRAL

Indications

- Central venous pressure monitoring
- Infusion of concentrated/irritant solutions (e.g. inotropes, parenteral nutrition)
- Insertion of specialised equipment (e.g. plasma exchange catheter, Swan-Ganz catheter, transvenous pacemaker)
- Emergency venous access when peripheral access is impossible

Contraindications

- Distorted local anatomy
- Known or suspected vessel damage (current trauma, previous radiation therapy, previous surgery)

- Coagulopathy or vasculitis
- Inability to provide cardiac monitoring
- Pneumothorax in central venous access on the opposite side (risk of bilateral pneumothoraces)

Technique—general

All of the techniques below carry different risks and benefits. All require ongoing cardiac monitoring, but the choice of technique should depend on the experience of the operator and the technique favoured in the particular hospital.

Remember: The ICU may have to care for 'your' catheter for days or weeks so, if a choice is available, use the method preferred by the inpatient team.

1. Use local anaesthesia liberally, following down the intended track.
2. Have cardiac monitoring in place, and always withdraw the catheter/wire slightly when arrhythmias (usually ventricular ectopics) occur.
3. After catheter placement, always aspirate each part then inject adequate saline to clear the line.
4. Secure the catheter by stitching, and apply dressing.

Complications

Arterial puncture. When detected, remove the needle or catheter and apply pressure over the site for a full 10 minutes, followed by arterial observation of the limb.

Pneumothorax. Always obtain chest X-ray (CXR).

Malposition of catheter tip. Always check X-ray.

- Wrong vein—passing into jugular vein from subclavian vein instead of superior vena cava (SVC). This is difficult to reposition without an image intensifier and may require repuncture.
- Excessive length—in right atrium or ventricle rather than SVC. The CXR should show that the tip is not below the carina. If it is too low, the catheter can be easily withdrawn.

Damage to mediastinal contents. Haemothorax, hydrothorax, arteriovenous fistula and perforation of any structure in the chest (even an endotracheal cuff has been reported) may occur.

Infection.

Embolism of air, wire or catheter parts.

Knotting/kinking of catheter.

SUBCLAVIAN CANNULATION

Infraclavicular technique

1. Position the patient supine in 15° Trendelenburg with the arm adducted.
2. Enter at the junction of the middle and medial thirds of the clavicle.
3. Aim along the inferior surface of the clavicle towards the suprasternal notch, with a needle bevel facing inferomedially.
4. Advance 1–2 mm after first flush of blood to obtain reliable flow back into the syringe.

Complications

- Pneumothorax
- Arterial puncture
- Others as described above

Supraclavicular technique

1. Position the patient supine in 15° Trendelenburg.
2. Enter the neck just lateral to the lateral border of the clavicular head of the sternocleidomastoid and just above the clavicle.
3. Aim approximately at the contralateral nipple with the bevel of the needle towards the patient's toes.
4. Advance 1–2 mm after first flush of blood to obtain reliable flow back into the syringe.

Complications

Although the full range of complications as above is described, they occur significantly less frequently with the supraclavicular approach.

INTERNAL JUGULAR VEIN CATHETERISATION

Technique

1. Position the patient's head down 10° and turned slightly away from side of entry.
2. Enter just above the point of the triangle formed by the two heads of the sternocleidomastoid and 1 cm lateral to the internal carotid pulsation.
3. Aim parallel to the carotid artery ('straight down the neck').

Complications

- Arterial puncture
- More easily displaced by movement than subclavian lines
- Others as above (rare)

Arterial access techniques

The same basic types of cannula used for venous access are available for arterial access, often again in specialised kits. Note that arterial puncture is painful, and for a single-sample puncture the smallest practical needle should be used—usually 25-gauge (radial) or 23-gauge (femoral). Indications for arterial blood gas (ABG) measures are very limited in the emergency setting: the venous pH and PCO_2 are normally close enough to the arterial values for diagnostic purposes, and the peripheral oxygen saturation (SaO_2) is usually a good measure of gas exchange.

Editorial Comment

Even in the critically ill we should be doing fewer arterial punctures.

INDICATIONS

- ABG measurement (see above)
- Need for recurrent (e.g. hourly) blood sampling—normally patients going to ICU
- Ongoing monitoring of arterial blood pressure—also ICU and theatre patients

CONTRAINDICATIONS

- Overlying skin damage (e.g. burns) or infection
- Arteriovenous fistula in the limb
- Clotting diathesis (relative)

RADIAL ARTERY CANNULATION

1. With the wrist in mild extension, palpate the radial arterial pulse over the distal radius.
2. Insert the catheter or needle into the centre of the pulsation, parallel to the long axis of the forearm with the bevel forward.
3. Pulsatile flushback into the syringe or cannula indicates successful puncture. If inserting a cannula, proceed another 1–2 mm to ensure that the tip of the needle is entirely within the artery.
4. If puncture fails, apply pressure to the site to reduce haematoma formation.

FEMORAL ARTERY CANNULATION

1. Palpate the femoral pulse at the midpoint of the inguinal ligament.
2. Insert the catheter or needle into the centre of the pulsation parallel to the thigh.

3 Pulsatile flushback into the syringe or cannula indicates successful puncture. If inserting a cannula, proceed another 1–2 mm to ensure the tip of the needle is entirely within the artery.
4 If puncture fails, apply pressure to the site to reduce haematoma formation.

COMPLICATIONS

- Haematoma or haemorrhage (apply pressure)
- Venous cannulation (check for pulsation, pressure wave)
- Thrombosis or embolism (rare and usually late)
- Infection

Chest drainage procedures

NEEDLE THORACOSTOMY

Needle thoracostomy is performed with either a soft flexible catheter 'over a needle', such as an IV cannula, or a specialised drainage set which may utilise a catheter through needle or the Seldinger technique. The location depends on setting and urgency. For a tension pneumothorax, the procedure is performed rapidly and without anaesthetic over the anterior chest wall. For therapeutic drainage of an effusion, it is performed posteriorly; and for aspiration of a simple pneumothorax, laterally or posteriorly. Note that many readily available IV cannulae are too short for emergency drainage in an obese population, and that ultrasound may be useful in localising intrapleural fluid.

Indications

- Tension pneumothorax—drain direct to air
- Simple pneumothorax (spontaneous) up to 75% collapse
- Pleural effusion—drainage or sampling

Contraindications

- Traumatic pneumothorax (unless tension is present), since tube thoracostomy indicated
- Haemothorax
- Bleeding dyscrasias (relative)

Technique

1 Check equipment. For drainage of fluid or simple pneumothorax, a large syringe and three-way tap are required in addition to the soft catheter. A syringe is normally attached if an IV cannula is being used.

2 Position the patient:
   a lying flat for anterior puncture of tension pneumothorax—2nd interspace, midclavicular line
   b head of bed elevated for lateral puncture of simple pneumothorax—4th to 5th interspace, just anterior to midaxillary line
   c leaning forwards over a pillow for posterior puncture of pleural effusion—8th to 10th interspace, midscapular line.
3 Inject local anaesthetic if needed.
4 Insert the needle just over the lower rib of the interspace (in order to avoid the neurovascular bundle that lies beneath the rib above).
5 Aspiration of air/fluid through a cannula or a 'pop' into the pleural space indicates correct placement—advance the catheter and remove the needle, or follow the technique appropriate to the individual kit.
6 For a tension pneumothorax, leave open and undertake subsequent tube thoracostomy.
7 For other drainage, connect a three-way tap and syringe to the catheter.
8 Aspirate air or fluid, emptying the syringe and sealing the catheter by means of the tap.
9 Remove catheter when aspiration is finished or when the tube thoracostomy is in place.
10 Always obtain repeat chest X-ray.

Complications

- Damage to local structures—neurovascular bundle, internal thoracic artery (anterior approach)
- Inadequate drainage due to small size of catheter, adhesions or blockage
- Underlying lung damage—a pneumothorax will be created if one is not already present
- Infection at the site

INTERCOSTAL CATHETER (ICC)—TUBE THORACOSTOMY

Indications

- Tension pneumothorax—only after needle thoracostomy
- Traumatic pneumothorax
- Simple pneumothorax that has not responded to needle drainage or is causing significant respiratory compromise

- Haemothorax
- Haemopneumothorax
- 'Prophylactic' use in the chest trauma patient who is to receive positive-pressure ventilation or aeromedical transport—depends on available skills and circumstance

Contraindications (all relative)

- Multiple adhesions
- Need for immediate thoracotomy
- Bleeding dyscrasias

Technique

1 Provide appropriate sedation/analgesia. The majority of conscious patients will tolerate narcotics well and should receive them.
2 Position the patient by:
   a elevating the head of the bed 45° if possible
   b raising the arm on the relevant side over the head and placing the fingers behind the head
   c tilting the patient slightly away.
3 Select and mark the site, the 4th or 5th interspace and just in front of the midaxillary line, i.e. at the level of the nipple just behind the muscle bulk of the anterior chest wall muscles.
4 Select appropriate tube size—in general the largest reasonable tube (32 Fr to 36 Fr) should be used in adults with haemothorax, but much smaller tubes are appropriate if only air is to be drained.
5 Prepare drainage system—normally disposable plastic sets with an in-built water trap, but bag drainage with some form of flutter valve is often used in the field.
6 Prepare the area and inject local anaesthetic down to the pleura over the line of the rib below.
7 Incise skin 3–4 cm along the line of the rib below.
8 Bluntly dissect through the subcutaneous tissue and muscle layers to the pleura, passing just above the rib to avoid the neuromuscular bundle. A hiss will normally be heard when the pleural space is entered.
9 Enlarge the tract with a finger and insert the finger into the chest cavity to ensure full penetration and check for adhesions.
10 Insert tube without stylet in one of three ways:
   a hold tube and advance through hole manually
   b grasp tip of tube in curved forceps and advance through hole

   c use specially designed forceps (Pollard forceps) to open a path through which the tube is passed.

   Advance the tube to at least 3 cm beyond the last lateral hole.

11 Immediately connect the tube to the drainage system. If there is to be any delay, the tube should be clamped for a spontaneously breathing patient, but must not be clamped for a patient who is ventilated. 'Fogging' of the tube normally confirms its location inside the chest cavity.
12 Check that the underwater drain is bubbling or swinging; ask the patient to cough to confirm position. If it is not swinging, rotate the tube or remove and re-insert.
13 Close the skin wound with sutures and stitch the tube in place. Dress the wound and anchor the dressing to the tube.
14 X-ray to check position of tube and re-expansion of pneumothorax or drainage of haemothorax.

Complications

- Blockage or failure to drain due to blood clots, position against chest wall, multiple adhesions or kinks
- Puncture of solid organs—should not occur if stylet is not used and technique is followed, even in the presence of diaphragmatic hernia
- Reverse flow—keep drainage bottle below patient
- Re-expansion pulmonary oedema
- Local injury or infection
- Persistent bubbling or failure of re-expansion due to leakage in circuit, ICC hole outside pleural cavity or (rare) oesophageal rupture/broncopleural fistula

PERICARDIOCENTESIS

Pericardiocentesis is an emergency procedure for the diagnosis of pericardial tamponade—a diagnosis made clinically, on the basis of high central venous pressure, hypotension, tachycardia and muffled heart sounds, or via ultrasonography (either FAST or formal echocardiography). It is relatively common after penetrating chest trauma, relatively uncommon after blunt chest trauma, and is seen in left ventricular free-wall rupture after myocardial infarction. In any setting where pericardiocentesis is expected to occur, it should be done with ultrasound guidance, but lack of ultrasound is not a contraindication to a potentially life-saving intervention. Survival is poor unless the patient is reasonably fit and there is access to cardiothoracic surgery facilities.

Indications

- Diagnostic—if the patient is stable, not indicated in the ED
- Pericardial tamponade or suspicion in deteriorating patient
- Electromechanical dissociation in cardiac arrest when other causes are excluded—low success rate as tamponade is a rare cause of cardiac arrest unless there is a sizeable hole in the ventricular wall

Contraindications

- Immediate need for thoracotomy, particularly in cases of trauma
- Stable patient—seek echocardiographic evidence before proceeding
- Prolonged cardiac arrest when good outcome is not possible

Technique

1. Position the patient with head up at 45°.
2. Pass a nasogastric tube if abdominal distension present.
3. Prepare equipment—syringe, three-way tap and large needle. Ideally an insulated 10 cm needle, purpose-designed for such taps, or a pericardial catheter ('catheter over a needle') should be used. However, when the diagnosis is clear or when the patient is in cardiac arrest, then a large needle or large-bore IV catheter may be used. The metal hub of the needle should be attached to a V lead of the ECG monitor, and monitoring must be ongoing throughout the procedure.
4. Approach—insert needle between xiphoid process and left costal margin at 30–45°, advancing towards the left shoulder.
5. The pericardium is normally entered 6–8 cm below the skin, and any fluid will be aspirated. If the needle touches the epicardium, an injury current with high ST segment should be seen on the ECG. In this case, withdraw the needle a few millimetres.
6. Aspirate with a syringe, using the three-way tap to disperse the contents if necessary. If a catheter has been inserted, withdraw the needle and re-connect the catheter to the tap.
7. Withdraw whatever fluid can be obtained, but if blood continues to flow freely, suspect ventricular penetration. Pericardial fluid may have a lower haematocrit than blood and may not clot, but neither of these tests is absolutely reliable nor helpful within the first few minutes of aspiration.
8. If a response is obtained, leave the catheter in place and be prepared to re-aspirate prior to a thoracotomy.

9 Perform chest X-ray after the procedure to check for a pneumothorax.

Complications

- Myocardial damage—ventricular puncture or coronary artery laceration
- Arrhythmias—ventricular ectopics, ventricular fibrillation (VF), cardiac arrest
- Pneumothorax or lung laceration
- Air embolism if accidental injection of air occurs
- Local infection

Urinary catheterisation

INDICATIONS

- Urinary retention
- Monitoring of urinary output
- Drainage of neurogenic bladder
- Diagnostic urinary specimen
- Preoperative procedure for pelvic surgery
- Management of the unconscious patient

CONTRAINDICATIONS

- Clinical suspicion of urethral injury—if there is a perineal haematoma and blood at the meatus, then an ascending urethrogram should be performed to identify urethral damage and/or a suprapubic catheter used as an alternative
- Urinary tract infection (UTI)—relative contraindication, as introducing a foreign body to an infected area is undesirable

TECHNIQUE—MALES

1. Position is supine.
2. Prepare penis using no-touch technique, retracting the foreskin and swabbing the glans and surrounding areas. Drape with a fenestrated sheet and repeat swab.
3. Instil lignocaine gel into urethral opening while holding the penis in the 'dirty' hand. From this point on, the hand holding the penis should be considered 'dirty' and only the other hand should touch the tray and catheter equipment.
4. After a delay for the gel to take effect, hold the catheter in forceps and insert into the bladder to a distance of 20–25 cm.
5. Inflate the catheter balloon using 5–10 mL sterile saline.

6 Check for free flow of urine and collect a specimen if necessary.
7 Connect an appropriate drainage bag.

Editorial Comment

Ensure the foreskin is fully replaced after every catheterisation.

TECHNIQUE—FEMALES

1 Position is supine with heels drawn up and thighs abducted.
2 Prepare external genitalia by swabbing and drape with a fenestrated sheet. Separate labia with gauze squares and identify urinary meatus and re-swab.
3 Apply sterile lubricant liberally to the catheter.
4 Insert catheter into bladder using forceps, to a distance of 10–12 cm.
5 If catheter is to be left indwelling, inflate balloon with 5–10 mL sterile saline.
6 Collect any specimens necessary and connect appropriate drainage bag.

COMPLICATIONS—BOTH SEXES

- Failure to catheterise:
  - Inability to identify urethra (females). The urinary orifice is frequently displaced by gynaecological surgery or obscured by oedematous tissue. A more thorough examination, repositioning and better light are appropriate.
  - Strictures of the urethra. Excessive force should not be used, but a smaller catheter may be tried.
  - Prostatic obstruction. This is commonly the indication for catheterisation. Once again, a smaller catheter, and possibly an introducer, should be tried.
- Trauma—creation of false passage, partial or complete urethral tear, long-term risk of stricture
- Infection—urethritis, epididymitis, pyelonephritis
- Haemorrhagic cystitis—rare complication of rapid decompression of a chronically distended bladder
- Paraphimosis in males—always replace a retracted foreskin

Removal of trapped urinary catheter

Emergency medicine doctors may be called upon to remove a urinary catheter which is either blocked and unable to be removed or simply 'stuck' at a time of routine removal. The usual cause is a 'flap valve' in the balloon tubing which prevents balloon deflation.

Various techniques are described. Cutting the catheter is rarely effective, since the blockage is usually proximal. If the patient's bladder is not excessively distended and the catheter balloon definitely lies within the bladder, then the balloon may be overinflated with sterile water or saline until it bursts. If there is doubt about the position of the balloon, then ultrasound should be used to identify it, since it must not be overinflated in the urinary tract. The balloon within the bladder can also be punctured using a suprapubic needle.

Suprapubic cystostomy

Ultrasound localisation of the bladder should be considered mandatory before this procedure unless it is being performed 'in the field' or for replacement of a pre-existing catheter.

INDICATIONS

- As for urinary catheter, but catheter cannot be passed due to a suspected or definite urethral trauma
- Failed catheterisation, usually strictures or prosthetic disease
- Other reasons, such as blockage of an existing catheter

CONTRAINDICATIONS

- Previous lower abdominal surgery/scarring/radiation
- Inability to palpate the bladder (or visualise on ultrasound)
- Bleeding diathesis
- Urinary tract infection

TECHNIQUE

1. Check equipment—a number of suprapubic catheter sets are available, mostly relying on a variant of the 'catheter over the needle' technique.
2. Position patient supine.
3. Inject local anaesthetic starting 2–3 cm above the pubic symphysis and heading down the expected track at approximately 20° towards the pelvis. When urine is drawn back into the anaesthetic syringe, the bladder has been reached.
4. Incise the skin with an appropriate scalpel blade.
5. Puncture the bladder down the same track used for the anaesthetic.
6. Follow appropriate technique to secure the catheter in the bladder. This varies between suprapubic catheter sets.

7 Collect any necessary specimens and connect the catheter to an appropriate drainage bag.
8 Apply adhesive and/or sutures as appropriate to maintain the catheter in place.

COMPLICATIONS

- Failure to catheterise the bladder
- Bowel perforation
- Extravasation of urine—intraperitoneal or extraperitoneal
- Local bleeding—intraperitoneal, extraperitoneal or into bladder
- Infection
- Obstruction

Cricothyroidotomy

INDICATIONS

- Supralaryngeal airway obstruction when tracheal intubation not possible (e.g. epiglottitis, burns, facial trauma)
- Ventilatory support required (e.g. apnoea) and tracheal intubation failed

TECHNIQUE

1. Position the patient supine with the neck extended if possible.
2. Identify the cricothyroid membrane as a horizontal depression in the midline anteriorly between the notch of the thyroid cartilage and the cricoid cartilage. Prepare the area.
3. Make a 1.5 cm incision across the lower half of the cricothyroid membrane, then incise the membrane. This is best done with a guarded scalpel blade, usually supplied in cricothyroidotomy kits. However, it can be accomplished with any scalpel.
4. Open the cricothyroidotomy by dilating with artery forceps or gently twisting the scalpel blade.
5. Insert the tube (either a 6 mm cuffed endotracheal tube for an adult, or a 4.5 mm uncuffed cricothyroidotomy tube) in a downward direction.
6. Remove trocar, secure tube and ventilate the patient.
7. Check ventilation in the same way as for endotracheal intubation.

COMPLICATIONS

- Local bleeding—external or into the airway
- Creation of a false passage

- Damage to larynx, trachea, oesophagus
- Local infection

Lumbar puncture (LP)

INDICATIONS

- Clinical suspicion of CNS infection, particularly meningitis
- Sample of cerebrospinal fluid (CSF) required for non-emergent evaluation (e.g. Guillain-Barré syndrome)
- Therapeutic—drainage of CSF or installation of chemotherapy

CONTRAINDICATIONS

- Clinical or CT evidence of raised intracranial pressure or localising signs
- Infected site of puncture
- Bleeding diathesis

Editorial Comment

Always explain, and obtain consent (preferably written) as complaints and complications frequently follow.

TECHNIQUE

1. Position the patient: if measurement of CSF pressure is indicated, in the lateral recumbent position with knees drawn up; otherwise sitting up leaning forwards with the feet over the side of the bed on a chair (sitting fetal feet supported, 'SFFS'). Mark the L4 spinous process which is palpable in a line connecting the posterior and superior iliac crests.
2. Prepare and drape the area.
3. Infiltrate local anaesthetic in L3/L4 or L4/L5. Gently insert a spinal needle in the midline. A non-cutting needle with side port is preferred, in which case the skin may need to be punctured first with a sheath. If a cutting needle is used, position the bevel horizontal. After penetrating the skin, aim approximately for the patient's umbilicus.
4. Advance, feeling for the loss of resistance as the needle penetrates the ligamentum flavum.
5. Remove the stylet to check for CSF flow. If the subarachnoid space has not been reached, carefully re-insert the stylet and continue.

6 When CSF is obtained, connect a manometer to measure CSF pressure if needed and then collect a sample, normally into 3 sterile bottles.
7 Remove the needle and dress the site.

COMPLICATIONS

- CSF infection—rare but potentially fatal
- Spinal cord or corda equina damage—should not occur if performed at the correct level
- Uncal herniation—described after LP in cases with raised intracranial pressure
- Post-LP headache

Emergency department thoracotomy

ED thoracotomy should be considered only if the operator is experienced, there is some hope of meaningful survival based on the patient's presentation, and facilities exist for rapid removal of the patient to a thoracic operating facility.

INDICATIONS

- Penetrating chest trauma with all of the following:
  - signs of life present during pre-hospital phase
  - any pneumothorax drained
  - pericardiocentesis undertaken
  - fluid load given
  - continued poor response—in cardiac arrest or cardiac arrest clinically eminent.
- Blunt trauma—only when signs of life have been present in the ED, no other lethal injuries (e.g. severe head injury) present, no response to standard resuscitation and electrical cardiac activity still present.

Note: Even in these circumstances, the response rate to ED thoracotomy in blunt form is exceedingly low. The aim of ED thoracotomy is to drain pericardial tamponade, repair cardiac lacerations or cross-clamp the aorta. Internal cardiac massage or internal defibrillation may be performed, but does not constitute an indication for thoracotomy alone.

CONTRAINDICATIONS

- Inadequately skilled personnel
- Thoracic operating theatre not available
- 'Medical' cardiac arrest

TECHNIQUE

1. Patient is normally supine, intubated, undergoing CPR.
2. Prepare the left side of the chest.
3. Incise along the top of the left 5th rib down to the chest wall muscles. Begin 2 cm lateral to the sternum and extend beyond the posterior axillary line.
4. Dissect through the intercostal muscles into the pleura with Mayo scissors, stopping ventilation so that the lung collapses momentarily. Divide the intercostal muscles with a sweep of the Mayo scissors along the top of the 5th rib.
5. Insert rib spreaders with a handle and ratchet bar downwards and retract the ribs.
6. If pericardotomy is required (history consistent with pericardial tamponade, pericardium swollen and tense), perform it with scissors starting at the diaphragm and moving upwards, 1 cm anterior to the phrenic nerve. Use fingers to gently sweep clots of blood from the pericardium.
7. If direct cardiac compression is required use two hands, anterior and posterior to the heart, to gently compress.
8. If aortic cross-clamping is required, this is difficult to perform with a vascular clamp since the aorta must be separated from the oesophagus. It is easier to apply pressure through the pleura to compress the aorta against the thoracic spine.
9. Repair of lacerations in the myocardium is particularly difficult in the emergency setting, but may be attempted if necessary.
10. Proceed immediately to the operating theatre for further definitive treatment.

Editorial Comment

Most problems arise when procedures are ill-prepared, ill-explained and performed with inadequate analgesia and in haste.

Chapter 4
Diagnostic imaging in emergency patients

E S Seelan

The aim of this chapter is to explain briefly the need and usefulness of diagnostic imaging services in emergency situations. Many of these emergencies arise 'after hours', and staff in most emergency departments have no immediate access to radiologists. The chapter also outlines the various diagnostic imaging modalities available, the basic principles involved in each modality and some clues to interpreting some of the most obvious lesions.

Editorial Comment

Although long, this chapter contains a wealth of practical information. Very few emergency patients escape diagnostic tests. Always, if there is any doubt, talk to the radiographers/radiologists about any study. Always arrange for follow-up of the formal report, as emergency doctors are not radiologists. Even if the images and reconstructions look easy—you are not an expert and are simply giving the patients an impression.

Imaging modalities

PLAIN X-RAYS

Plain X-rays are a commonly used modality. An X-ray beam is passed through the body.

Different tissues of the body absorb different amounts of X-rays. Unabsorbed X-rays are recorded on a film placed on the opposite side. Bone absorbs the most, hence it looks white on film. Air absorbs almost none, hence it looks black on film. Other tissues are demonstrated in shades between black and white.

Plain X-rays are performed as the first line of emergency investigations in many instances, as in fractures and abdominal or chest pain.

ULTRASOUND

Transducers used in this examination pass ultrasound into the body and also receive the echoes. The intensity of the echoes depends on the degree of absorption of sound waves by various tissues. On the image, echogenic areas appear white and sonolucent areas (that transmit sound, e.g. fluid) appear black.

Immediate and instant demonstration of organs by real-time ultrasound imaging and the fact that it is non-invasive and harmless (no radiation) have made this tool very popular. It is used in the following:

- To find out whether a lesion or lump is solid or cystic.
- Abdominal and pelvic organs—liver, gall bladder, bile ducts, pancreas, spleen, kidneys, aorta, inferior vena cava (IVC), bladder, prostate, uterus and ovaries, renal stones, gall stones, aortic aneurysm, traumatic and other haematomas—abscess and abnormal fluid collections can be demonstrated.
- To examine small parts (thyroid, testes and breast) and neonatal heads for ventricular size, etc.
- For obstetrical work-up, including study of fetus for early detection of abnormalities, and for emergencies like ectopic pregnancy, vaginal ultrasound is extremely useful.
- Ultrasound-guided biopsy and interventional procedures.
- Musculoskeletal investigations, e.g. shoulder, knee, muscle and tendon injuries and acute tenosynovitis.
- Duplex and colour Doppler ultrasound:
  - With the advent of duplex and colour-flow Doppler it is now easy to identify arteries and veins non-invasively. This modality should be the first line of imaging for the detection of deep vein thrombosis (DVT) in the limbs. (This study can be difficult in extremely swollen, oedematous lower legs.) In difficult cases venography can be performed. It should be remembered that ultrasound is non-invasive and can be performed repeatedly even in pregnant patients with suspected DVT.
  - Duplex ultrasound is useful in identifying superficial thrombophlebitis.
  - While excluding thrombosis, ultrasound study can also diagnose other causes of a swollen, tender calf such as ruptured Baker's cyst, haematoma in calf muscle, e.g. a gastrocnemius tear, mass in groin, axilla.
  - Doppler ultrasound is useful in detecting and localising acute arterial occlusion in the limbs and in the investigation of peripheral vascular disease and carotid arterial disease.
  - It is also useful in assessing renal artery stenosis and renal parenchymal vascular disease in the investigation of hypertension.

COMPUTED TOMOGRAPHY (CT)

The same principles are applied in CT as in plain X-rays, but there are two main modifications:

1. The X-ray tube is rotated around the body in an axial plane.
2. Instead of an X-ray film, detectors are used on the opposite side. Multiple fixed detectors are placed around the body to pick up the signals as the X-ray tube rotates around the body. Signals from the detectors are digitalised and the computer builds up an image which can be seen on a TV monitor or recorded on a film.

The resulting images are transverse sections of the part examined. Using the stored information of consecutive thin transverse sections, the images can be reconstructed in sagittal, coronal and oblique planes. CT is now a proven diagnostic tool which delivers valuable information to help in the early diagnosis of many lesions and disease. Its use is greatly appreciated in many emergencies such as head injuries and some chest and abdominal emergencies. It is also useful in demonstrating fractures that are not shown by plain X-rays.

Helical CT scanning

Helical or spiral CT scanning is an improvement that allows very quick scanning of a patient (shorter scanning time than conventional CT) with increased accuracy of lesion detection resulting from volumetric data acquisition. In conventional CT, X-ray exposure and patient movement through the gantry alternate; whereas in helical CT, X-ray exposure and patient movement take place simultaneously giving a 'spiral impression'.

Advantages

- Greater length of patient's body can be scanned with one 'breath-hold' thus producing contiguous images without interruption, e.g. a 30-second scan can cover most of the chest.
- Eliminates respiratory artefacts and reduces partial volume effect, peristaltic and other movement artefacts.
- Produces overlapping images without extra radiation exposures.
- Using a window workstation the acquired images can be reconstructed in multiplanar and three-dimensional images with excellent clarity.

Multi-slice CT scans

This is a further advancement whereby the speed of scanning and resolutions are considerably improved by using more-efficient detectors and obtaining thinner slices per rotation of the X-ray tube as the patient passes through the gantry.

Scanners are available to obtain 4, 8, 16, 32 or 64 slices (per rotation) of up to 0.5 mm thickness. A few 300-slice scanners are also available in Australia. These are faster than a heartbeat.

Advantages and uses

- Speed—some scanners can complete a body scan in 20 seconds; useful in the ICU and in paediatric, elderly, trauma and postoperative patients, where a shorter breath-hold and quick scanning are required.
- High resolution and fewer artefacts.
- Less IV contrast usage by allowing the scanning to start when the contrast reaches the area of interest (contrast detection system).
- Multi-plane reconstruction without loss of resolution.
- 3D reconstruction useful for surgical planning.
- CT angiography (including pulmonary angiography to detect pulmonary embolism) and cholangiography.
- CT fluoroscopy—useful in interventional work, e.g. placement of needle for biopsy, facet joint injection, etc.
- Virtual endoscopy—enables a bronchoscopic view or colonoscopic view to be obtained.
- Coronary angiography—introduction of 300-slice CT will be useful for cardiac and coronary assessment without the need for catheterisation.

MAGNETIC RESONANCE IMAGING (MRI)

In the past 20 years MRI has gradually become the technique of first choice in the investigation of many diseases. The physics involved in MRI is more complex than for any other radiological technique. However, the basic principles are indicated by the original terminology, nuclear magnetic resonance (NMR).

Nuclear

Unlike X-ray images, which are produced by attenuation of X-ray photons by the outer orbital electrons in the atoms of the elements in the body tissue, the MRI signal arises from the centre of the atom—the nucleus. The nuclei used in MRI are those of hydrogen atoms.

Hydrogen is selected because:

- it makes up about 80% of the human body
- its nucleus has only 1 proton, which has magnetic properties
- the solitary proton gives it a larger magnetic field (or moment).

Magnetic

The hydrogen ion, or proton, is a small, positively charged particle with associated angular momentum or spin. This situation represents a current loop and results in the formation of a magnetic field with north and south poles (dipoles). In other words, the protons behave as tiny magnets within the tissues. All nuclei used in MRI must have this property.

In the absence of influence from any external magnetic fields, the protons tend to orientate randomly in all directions. However, when a strong static external magnetic field is applied, these dipolar protons tend to align parallel to the direction of the external magnetic field (longitudinal plane).

The strong external magnetic field must be homogeneous over a volume large enough to contain the human body. This explains why the magnet tunnel is much longer than the CT gantry.

Resonance

This is a phenomenon whereby an object is exposed to an external oscillating disturbance that has a frequency similar to its own frequency of oscillation. Therefore, when a hydrogen proton is exposed to an external disturbance with a similar frequency to its own, the proton gains energy from the external disturbance. This is called resonance. This can happen only if the external disturbance is applied at 90° to the magnetic field of the proton. The oscillation frequency of the hydrogen proton in a static magnetic field of the strength used in clinical MRI corresponds to the radiofrequency band (RF) in the electromagnetic spectrum.

Therefore, for resonance of hydrogen to take place, an RF pulse at the same frequency as the oscillation of the hydrogen proton must be applied at 90° to the magnetic field of the proton. The application of the RF pulse that causes resonance is called excitation, as it results in the nuclei gaining energy. This energy causes the magnetic field of the protons to change direction. Enough RF pulse energy is given to the proton to change the direction from the longitudinal to the transverse plane (flip angle of 90°). Now the protons are rotating in the transverse plane. According to the laws of electromagnetism, if a receiver coil is placed in the transverse plane, the transverse magnetisation will produce a voltage in the coil. This voltage constitutes the MR signal.

When the RF pulse is turned off, the hydrogen protons return to their original orientations in the longitudinal plane. This is called relaxation.

There are two main types of relaxation (T1 and T2). T1 is the return of net magnetisation to the longitudinal plane. T2 is the decay of magnetisation in the transverse plane. These two relaxations and their time variances are used to create imaging sequences. All relaxation times are based on fat and water. This is where most of the body's hydrogen protons are.

- T1 images are known for their anatomical details. In T1 images, fluid appears black and fat appears white.
- T2 images are known for their contrast. In these images, fluid appears white and fat appears grey.
- Proton density images are a combination of T1 and T2. These images specifically look at the concentration of hydrogen protons.

The above is a simple explanation of the basics, but more complex physics is involved in the formation of MR images which is beyond the scope of this chapter.

Summary

MRI involves the use of:

- large magnet to produce a static magnetic field
- RF generator to produce RF pulses
- hydrogen nuclei—different tissues have characteristic differences in hydrogen proton concentrations, therefore the MR signal and hence the image obtained basically represent the different distributions of hydrogen protons in the body
- computer to convert the signals into images in various anatomical planes.

Advantages of MRI

- No ionising radiation.
- Free of artefacts from adjacent bones and gas. Therefore it is excellent to demonstrate soft tissues adjacent to bones, e.g. base of brain and spinal cord.
- Excellent resolution—even without contrast enhancement, MR is much more sensitive than CD in detecting contrast differences between various tissues. This is due to the intrinsic differences in hydrogen proton density as well as T1 and T2 relaxation, magnetic susceptibility and motion in various tissues.

Uses of MRI

Brain

- Stroke—MRI can diagnose acute infarction within hours of onset when the CT scan is still normal. This is done by using diffusion imaging, which tracks the motion of water that becomes acutely restricted in the area of infarction. Once infarction has been diagnosed, an intravenous MR angiogram can be performed at the same time to assess the calibre of the neck arteries.

- Haematoma—subdural and parenchymal haematoma and dural sinus thrombosis.
- Aneurysm and other vascular malformations—MR angiography is very sensitive in finding small aneurysms up to about 2 mm and can also give some idea of the degree of any associated vasospasm.
- Intracranial mass—MRI can accurately stage both primary and metastatic tumours. It is more sensitive than CT for metastases. Some masses like abscess and epidermoid can be differentiated from other tumours with certainty, as they have restricted water diffusion. In certain cases spectroscopy can also help in the differential diagnosis. MRI is also superior to CT in detecting lesions closer to the skull base, such as acoustic neuroma and pituitary tumour.
- Other uses—demyelination, congenital abnormality, meningeal disease and investigation of epilepsy.

Spine

MRI is the modality of choice for assessing cord contusion and haematoma in the acute stage, especially when there is an associated spinal fracture and neurological signs. It is also excellent in demonstrating cord compression, infarction, tumour, neuromas, metastases, myelopathy, radiculopathy and brachial plexus avulsion. It is also useful in post-laminectomy complications such as haematoma or infection as well as investigation of infective spondylodiscitis where early changes, such as fluid in the disc, paraspinal collections and end-plate erosions, are seen.

Musculoskeletal

MRI has the ability to simultaneously characterise soft tissues (muscles, ligaments, tendons and cartilage) as well as bone marrow. It is very useful in the investigation of musculotendinous injury and pathology, joint injury and pathology (e.g. rotator cuff injury in shoulder, meniscal and ligamentous injury in knee) and fractures not detected by X-ray (e.g. fracture in the neck of femur) as well as bone infection, avascular necrosis, marrow disorders and bone and soft-tissue tumours.

Chest

Constrictive pericarditis, aortic and great vessel dissection, congenital cardiac and great vessel abnormality, lung cancers closer to the chest wall and apex (e.g. Pancoast's tumour).

Abdomen

Adrenal mass using chemical shift imaging, cholangiography, etc.

Pelvis

Uterine and cervical tumours and abnormalities, differentiation of adenomyosis from fibroids, endometriosis assessment, bladder tumour, etc.

Contrast-enhanced MRI

In spite of the excellent tissue contrast definition without use of intravenous contrast, contrast-enhanced MRI (gadolinium) provides even better imaging sensitivity and specificity.

The enhanced contrast shows subtle parenchymal lesions as well as leptomengingeal lesions not otherwise visible, e.g. very small metastatic lesions, acoustic neuromas of 2–3 mm, pituitary microadenomas, differentiation of the actual size of tumour from the surrounding oedema and differentiation of more-malignant areas from less-malignant areas. These are helpful for the purpose of treatment and to select the exact site for biopsy.

Ongoing research into the development of new contrast agents targeted at specific organs, disease processes, cells or gene type is likely to result in considerable expansion of the use of MRI.

MR angiography (MRA)

Protons in flowing blood (moving protons) produce a high signal against the background of little or no signal from the surrounding stationary tissues—hence the development of the MR angiogram with no display of the background soft tissue.

Contraindications to MRI

Cardiac pacemakers, ferromagnetic intracranial aneurysm clips (except where MR-compatible clips have been used), cochlear implants, intravascular stainless steel stents inserted less than 6 weeks previously, surgical clips in chest and abdomen inserted less than 1 week previously, metal-workers with metallic foreign body in the eye.

Disadvantages of MRI

Because of the length of the magnet (tunnel), some patients may experience claustrophobia. This can mostly be overcome by sedation.

Scanners are now available with open gantry which will alleviate claustrophobia, but these scanners are dedicated and are used mainly for musculoskeletal and spinal work-up.

CONTRAST STUDY

The main limitation in the use of plain X-rays is the superimposition of the shadows of various organs. In many instances this can be overcome by introducing contrast:

- Barium to demonstrate the gastrointestinal (GI) tract.
- Intravenous pyelogram (IVP)—IV contrast demonstrates kidneys, collecting system and bladder. Helpful to assess function (excretion) and to detect stones, obstruction, space-occupying lesion, deformities of renal tract, etc.
- Micturating cystourethrogram (MCU)—to demonstrate urethra, bladder and vesicoureteral reflux.
- Arthrography—e.g. shoulder, to detect rotator cuff tears. Sometimes this is combined with a CT scan, which helps to identify glenoid labral injury, etc. (Arthrograms may not be required if there is access to high-resolution ultrasound and MRI scan.)
- Herniography—contrast injected into the peritoneal cavity to detect clinically undetectable inguinal or femoral hernia that is producing symptoms.
- Myelography—contrast injected via lumbar puncture demonstrates the subarachnoid space around the spinal cord and nerve roots. With the advent of CT and MRI, the need for this examination is almost nil.
- Cholangiography—in the past, oral cholangiograms were performed, but this is now replaced by CT cholangiography. This examination requires slow infusion of contrast (which is excreted by bile) followed by helical CT scan and 3D reconstruction of the biliary tree.
- Sialography—contrast injected into the salivary ducts (parotid or submandibular) to identify stones, strictures, sialectasis and lesions in the glands.
- Hysterosalpingogram—contrast injected into the uterine cavity to demonstrate the uterine cavity, fallopian tubes and to detect patency of the tube in the investigation of infertility.
- Sinogram and fistulogram—contrast injection shows the cavities and communications.
- Venography—could detect clots, incompetent perforators and varicose veins (current trend is to do Doppler and colour Doppler ultrasound examination).

- Arteriography—contrast injected into various arteries using catheters demonstrates the arteries in various organs. It is used to demonstrate occlusions, narrowing of arteries, aneurysms, bleeding points, AV malformation and tumours. Digital subtraction angiography (DSA) has replaced the conventional angiograms. In this technique, the X-ray images are digitalised and stored and manipulated by computer. The image signal of an area or organ obtained before the injection of contrast is subtracted, by the computer, from the image signal obtained after injection of contrast into the vessels.

Advantages

The resulting image will demonstrate the vessels and branches without superimposition of bones and other soft-tissue shadows.

Owing to the fact that the image signals can be intensified by the computer, contrast media of low concentration and volume can be used with thinner catheters.

INTERVENTIONAL RADIOLOGY

Radiologists are able to perform certain therapeutic and interventional diagnostic procedures using various types of imaging equipment (fluoroscopy, ultrasound, CT and MRI), needles, catheters and guide wires.

- Dilation of narrowed arteries—transluminal angioplasty, insertion of vascular stents.
- Embolisation—of bleeding vessels, preoperative tumour embolisation to assist surgery by reducing blood loss and reducing the duration of surgery, palliative embolisation of tumours, embolisation of some vascular abnormalities.
- Thrombolysis—using local low-dose intra-arterial injection of thrombolytic agents to relieve thromboembolism in certain vessels such as coronary artery and peripheral arteries.
- IVC filter insertion to prevent pulmonary embolism caused by clots arising from pelvis and lower limbs.
- Percutaneous insertion of stents to relieve biliary or ureteric obstruction.
- Percutaneous drainage of cysts, abscesses, pleural effusion, etc.
- Percutaneous removal of renal or biliary stones when other methods are contraindicated.
- Biopsy of deep and superficial lesions—lesions in liver, pancreas, kidneys, other abdominal masses, chest lesions, breast, thyroid, lymph node and other superficial and deep lesions.

Intravenous contrast reaction

Even though the incidence of fatality is much lower than in street accidents, reaction to IV contrast is a great worry to doctors. Some statistics show that about 1 in 80,000 patients developed severe or fatal reaction when ionic contrast was used. Incidence of mild reaction is probably about 5–15%, moderate reaction about 1–2% and severe reaction is probably about 0.2%. However, with the use of non-ionic contrast and taking good precautions, the incidence of reaction is said to have reduced to about one-third to one-quarter of the frequency.

Usually patients who develop severe reaction have some other aggravating disease as well.

The exact pathogenesis of the reaction is not very clear. However, the following are possible mechanisms:

- chemotoxic effect
- hyperosmolar reactions causing erythrocyte or endothelial damage, blood–brain barrier damage and vasodilation
- vasomotor reactions with release of vasoactive substances such as histamine, serotonin and bradykinin
- vasovagal reaction with inhibition of enzymes such as cholinesterase.

SYMPTOMS AND SIGNS

Most reactions occur within minutes of injection. However, delayed reactions have also been reported.

Mild reactions—hot flush, burning sensation, arm pain, dizziness, nausea, vomiting, headache and urticaria—are thought to be due to systemic effects as a result of histamine liberation. Usually reassurance and restoration of the patient's confidence is all that is required, but sometimes oral antihistamine for urticaria, mild analgesics and sometimes tranquillisers for anxiety (5 mg diazepam) may also be helpful.

Moderate reactions involve a slightly more serious manifestation of the above symptoms, with or without a moderate degree of hypotension and bronchospasm. They usually respond to reassurance and antihistamine (IM or IV), diazepam 5 mg, salbutamol inhalation for bronchospasm, hydrocortisone (100–500 mg IM or IV) and occasionally adrenaline 0.3–1 mL of 1/1000 IM. Oxygen by mask is administered.

Severe reaction can be life-threatening and involve a severe form of the above reactions plus convulsion, unconsciousness, laryngeal oedema, bronchospasm, pulmonary oedema, arrhythmia, hypotension, cardiac arrest, anaphylactic shock. Severe reactions require urgent treatment (see treatment of anaphylaxis in Chapter 40, 'Dermatological presentations to emergency').

Predisposing factors—in the presence of these, the incidence of reaction can be about 2–10 times as severe:

- Previous adverse reaction to contrast.
- Significant allergic history including iodides.
- Asthma.
- Cardiac disease.
- Dehydration—all patients should be adequately hydrated as dehydration is dangerous, especially in patients with diabetes, renal impairment and multiple myeloma.
- Haematological and metabolic conditions such as sickle-cell anaemia, patients with known phaeochromocytoma.
- Renal disease—patients with pre-existing renal disease, especially patients with diabetes, have an increased risk of reaction as well as of renal failure. Metformin, an oral antidiabetic drug, is excreted by the kidneys and in patients with renal impairment this has been known to cause lactic acidosis and lead to acute alteration of renal function. In view of this, all diabetic patients treated with metformin drugs must have serum urea and creatinine levels reviewed before the IV contrast injection (serum urea must be less than 6.7 mmol/L and serum creatinine must be less than 0.10 mmol/L). The metformin drugs should be discontinued from 48 hours before until 48 hours after the injection, and should be recommenced only after checking the serum urea and creatinine. If required, another hypoglycaemic agent may be used during this period.

PREVENTION AND PRECAUTIONS

1. Always try to use non-ionic contrast.
2. Like other drugs, contrast agents should be used only if indicated and should be used in the smallest possible dose and concentration that will result in adequate imaging.
3. Weigh the possible advantages of using contrast against the possible risk. In patients with a strong family history of reaction, contrast should be avoided. In many cases the contrast study may be replaced by another examination such as ultrasound, CT or MRI.
4. A test dose may not help. However, some authors advise a small test dose of about 1 mL IV in high-risk patients who definitely require contrast for diagnosis.

(*pto*)

5 In some patients (e.g. asthmatic and allergic patients), premedication with oral corticosteroid and possibly antihistamines could be given during the 24 hours preceding the test. The patient should also be adequately hydrated.

Imaging of the head

Common emergencies are: trauma, severe headaches, collapse, syncope, seizures and stroke.

TRAUMA

Plain X-rays of skull

Indications

(Uncommon as CT is investigation of choice.)

- History of unconsciousness
- Palpable or visible depression on skull
- Laceration or penetrating wound
- Cerebrospinal fluid (CSF) or blood discharge from ear or nose
- Fits
- Presence of neurological signs

Views

- Include anteroposterior, lateral, Towne's and basal views.
- 'Shoot through' lateral (patient in supine position and X-ray beam horizontal) is useful to demonstrate air–fluid levels, especially in sinuses.

Interpretation

Every doctor working in the accident and emergency department should try to be familiar with the appearance of normal skull X-rays. The best way to detect abnormality is to know the normal. (This applies to every modality of imaging.)

- One should be familiar with the skull sutures, vascular markings, venous lakes along the inner table of the skull vault, appearance of normal sinuses and normal intracranial calcifications (e.g. pineal body, choroid plexus).
- Fracture of the skull can be an undepressed crack fracture or a depressed fracture.
- Do not misinterpret sutures and vascular markings as fractures. You can avoid this by knowing the normal positions of sutures and vascular markings. Sutures are usually serrated. Fracture lines are usually 'blacker' than the vascular markings.
- Beware of metopic sutures—in some patients such a suture may persist throughout life and may look like a fracture.

- In depressed fractures, one or more fragments may be depressed. In some cases, oblique or tangential views may be needed to demonstrate depression.
- If pineal calcification is present, look for shift. This indicates a space-occupying lesion such as a haematoma. (Towne's view is ideal for this.)
- Look for air–fluid level in sinuses or air in ventricles in the horizontal beam lateral view.

Plain X-rays of the face

Most facial injuries can be evaluated clinically. However, X-rays are performed for:

- confirmation
- assessment of the degree of displacement or depression of fragments
- detecting fractures in the presence of extreme facial swelling which makes palpation difficult.

In some cases facial fractures are associated with other serious emergencies, such as intracranial, neck or chest injuries, which may require emergency management such as maintenance of airway. In these patients, X-rays of the face can be postponed to the latter part of the management and may even be deferred for a few days.

Views

- Routine facial views—posteroanterior (PA), occipitomental (OM) and lateral
- Special views—nose (anteroposterior (AP), lateral and axial), zygoma (Towne's or modified basal view for the arch), orbital, mandible (PA, lateral, oblique and sometimes orthopantomogram (OPG) and occlusal view for symphysis menti)

Classification

For convenience, facial fractures can be divided into three types: upper third, middle third and lower third.

1. **Upper third.** The upper third, which is above the superior orbital margin, includes the superior orbital margin, the frontal sinuses and the adjacent frontal bone:
   - Fracture of superior orbital margin appears as interrupted cortical margin with or without depression, either craniocaudally or posteriorly.
   - Fracture of the frontal sinuses may involve anterior wall or both anterior and posterior walls.

- — Fracture may be linear or comminuted, depressed or undisplaced.
- — Fracture of sinus may extend into orbit—therefore look for orbital emphysema.
- — Fractures causing laceration of mucosa in sinus or fractures communicating with skin laceration are compound fractures.

2 **Middle third.** This includes the nose, zygoma, orbit (floor, lateral and medial walls) and maxillae (mid-facial bones):

- — *Nose.* Nasal fracture and deviations are easily detectable clinically, but X-rays are needed in patients with severe swelling or for confirmation of the degree of damage. Fractures of nasal bones are better seen in lateral view (soft-tissue exposure). Deviation is seen in axial view. PA view may demonstrate fracture of frontal process of maxilla and also deviation of fracture of the bony part of the nasal septum. Associated fractures in severe cases are: bony nasal septum, cribriform plate, frontal process of maxilla, anterior nasal spine of maxilla.
- — *Zygoma.* Fracture of the arch usually involves three sites causing depression of the arch. A commonly seen severe form of fracture is of the zygomaticomaxillary complex. One fracture line extends from the zygomaticofrontal suture across the orbital process of the zygoma (lateral wall of orbit) up to the lateral aspect of the inferior orbital fissure. Another fracture extends from the lateral wall of the maxilla to the inferior orbital margin (near the inferior orbital foramen) and extends along the floor of the orbit to the lateral aspect of the inferior orbital fissure, thus completing a circle. This fracture can cause separation of the zygomatic bone from the maxilla and orbit. (This fracture can be well understood if the reader takes a dry skull and follows the line of the fracture described above).
- — *Orbit*—blowout fracture. The orbital margin is stronger than the floor and medial wall of the orbit. The posterior half of the orbital floor is formed by the thin orbital plate of the maxilla. The medial wall is formed by the orbital plate of the ethmoid. These two orbital plates are very weak. Sometimes the orbital margin can be intact and the force of injury can be transmitted to the floor and medial walls of the orbit, causing blowout fractures into the adjacent sinuses. Therefore, in the presence of orbital emphysema, a blowout fracture should be suspected.

- *Maxilla*—fractures of mid-facial bones. These fractures tend to follow a certain pattern. There are three common patterns, which are named after the person who described them—Le Fort I, II and III fractures.
  a Le Fort I is the lowest and almost horizontal fracture through the maxilla, causing separation of the lower part of the maxilla. The fracture line extends from the inferolateral aspect of the nasal aperture horizontally across the lower part of the anterolateral and posterolateral walls of the maxilla. It then passes almost horizontally across the lower part of the medial and lateral pterygoid plates, reaches the medial wall of the maxillary antrum and extends to the inferolateral aspect of the nasal aperture, thus completing a circle.
  b Le Fort II fracture separates the midfacial bones from the cranium and the lateral aspect of the face. The medial part of the fracture line is across the nasal bone, nasal septum, frontal process of the maxilla and lacrimal bone, and runs posteriorly along the ethmoidal bone. Laterally the fracture runs obliquely downwards from the inferior orbital margin (near the zygomaticomaxillary suture) along the anterolateral wall of the maxilla and then slightly ascends up the posterolateral wall of the maxilla to the inferior orbital fissure.
  c Le Fort III is the highest of the fractures and is bilateral, causing complete separation of the midfacial bone from the base of the skull. The fracture line passes across the nasofrontal region to the ethmoid and runs posteriorly to the inferior orbital fissure. It also involves the pterygoid plates. Laterally the fracture involves the lateral wall of the orbit and the zygomatic arch.

  The Le Fort fractures may occur in combination. The above description is useful for surgical planning.

3 **Lower third.** This includes the mandible. Common sites of fractures are the alveolar process (weakest part), condyles, angle of the mandible, body (usually the fracture is around the canine tooth because of maximum convexity). Bilateral fractures are common. Fractures of the body on one side and the angle on the other side are also common.

CT findings in head injury

If CT is available, it is the quickest way of detecting intracranial trauma. It has been reported that about 10–15% of patients with head injury with no neurological signs were found to have abnormal CT findings. In contrast, about 75% of patients with neurological signs demonstrated abnormal CT findings.

The lesions described in the following sections may be seen in CT.

Haematomas and contusions (acute and delayed)

Haematomas appear as high-density areas (white) on CT without contrast. Haematomas are fairly homogeneous, but contusion shows patchy dense and low-density areas. Low-density areas are due to oedema. Fresh blood appears as dense areas due to haemoglobin. (In anaemic patients it may be isodense with the rest of the brain or even hypodense if the haemoglobin level is low.)

Most haematomas become isodense in 1–3 weeks and in some cases get even smaller and hypodense. The isodense haematomas may be missed unless other signs of mass effect are looked for.

Delayed haematomas may appear from 2–7 days after trauma. Haematomas and associated oedema usually cause space-occupying effects—midline shift, compression on ventricles, cisterns etc.

Subdural haematomas

These usually appear as dense areas and follow the brain surface with a concave inner border and convex outer border. They tend to be diffuse and extend along the subdural space. Thin haematomas (e.g. less than 5 mm) and haematomas near the vertex may be difficult to identify. However, indirect evidence such as midline shift may help. Beware of bilateral subdural haematomas, which may not cause any shift.

- Acute haematomas (occurring 0–1 week after trauma) are usually dense.
- Subacute haematomas (occurring 1–3 weeks after trauma) may be isodense.
- Chronic haematomas (more than 3 weeks after trauma) are usually hypodense.
- Acute-on-chronic haematomas show mixed density.

Epidural haematomas

These are caused by traumatic separation of the dura from the inner table, causing damage to the middle meningeal arterial branches, venous branches or diploic veins. An epidural haematoma is usually seen as a biconvex density under the inner table of the skull. The biconvex appearance is due to firm adhesion of the dura to the inner table. For this reason the epidural haematomas are demarcated by sutures.

Oedema

Oedematous areas appear as low-density areas in the CT. They may be focal, patchy or diffuse. Due to the oedema there may be space-occupying effects, such as compression on the adjacent ventricles and midline shift.

Note: Oedema may have other causes such as infarction. Therefore it should be differentiated. A history of trauma and the site of involvement may be helpful.

Intraventricular and subarachnoid haemorrhage

These may occur with some head injuries and appear as dense areas within the ventricles, basal cistern, sylvian fissures, interhemispheric fissure or cerebral sulci. Resolution of the haemorrhage within the ventricular system and subarachnoid space is fairly quick and may disappear within a week.

Fractures and displaced or depressed bony fragments

These can be seen in CT when viewed with bone windows. The CT is useful to identify soft-tissue contusion and foreign bodies in the scalp or in the intracranial region. It is also useful to identify any traumatic pneumocephalus.

Post-traumatic changes

- Acute or delayed hydrocephalus is caused by blood in the subarachnoid space causing some obstruction to the CSF pathways.
- Ischaemic infarction appears as low-density areas.
- Post-traumatic atrophy is seen in almost one-third of patients with severe head injury. Due to the atrophy there may be compensatory dilation of the ventricles usually adjacent to the site of atrophy.
- Post-traumatic abscess may be seen in penetrating injury or fracture, or as a complication following surgery. It appears as a low-density area with ring enhancement after contrast injection. This ring enhancement is usually surrounded by a large area of oedema. The lesion will also produce a space-occupying effect.

The use of CT in facial trauma

In some cases plain tomography is performed to demonstrate facial fractures. However, CT of facial bones in coronal, axial and sagittal planes is very useful, not only to demonstrate the fractures but also to show the extent and degree of depression of fragments and associated haematomas, especially in the adjacent sinuses, orbits, etc.

Angiography in cerebral trauma

This has been almost eliminated by CT scanners. However, it is indicated if there is suspicion of vascular damage such as occlusion of an artery or injury to an AV malformation.

MRI in head injury

Even though MRI is superior to CT in detecting small haematomas, especially near the bones, CT is preferable as the initial investigation not only because the examination time is shorter but also because sometimes haematomas that are less than 1–2 days old may not be shown by MRI. CT shows acute haemorrhages well.

Head injury in children—CT appearance

Appearance of haematoma is almost the same as in adults. However, haemorrhagic contusions are less common than in adults due to greater pliability of the skull.

The paediatric brain may demonstrate acute generalised oedema causing narrowing of ventricles and subarachnoid space. Oedema is less marked in adults.

ACUTE SEVERE HEADACHE AND COLLAPSE

Sudden onset of severe headache or sudden collapse may be caused by intracranial haemorrhage.

- The haemorrhage could be from: aneurysm, AV malformation, capillary bleed in hypertension, bleeding disorders or bleeding from a tumour.
- The haemorrhage may be intracerebral, subarachnoid or intraventricular.

In these cases CT is rewarding. Blood appears as dense areas. Valuable clues as to the site of bleeding and the cause may be shown by CT. However, in most cases angiograms (CT or DSA) will be required to show the exact site and cause of bleeding. Multiple vessel studies are necessary as there may be multiple aneurysms. An angiogram will also show the site of the lesion and, in cases of AV malformation, the feeding vessels to the malformation. Angiograms are not necessary in cerebral parenchymal haemorrhage.

In suspected **subarachnoid haemorrhage**, CT scan is performed before lumbar puncture. If haemorrhage is marked, or hydrocephalus or space-occupying effect is detected, lumbar puncture is avoided. However, in cases where no haemorrhage is detected, lumbar puncture could be performed. This is because very small haemorrhages may not be shown by CT. Small amounts of blood are not enough to change the CSF density, or in some (anaemic) patients the haemoglobin content may not be enough to change the CSF density.

SYNCOPE AND SEIZURES

Of the many causes of syncope only a few need radiological assistance for diagnosis or confirmation:

- Syncope caused by reduced cardiac output may need echocardiography, cardiac catheterisation and angiography.
- Syncope is rarely caused by cerebrovascular disease, e.g. transient ischaemic attacks, subclavian steal, vertebrobasilar insufficiency. In these cases Doppler ultrasound or angiography will be useful.
- In cases of seizures, CT of the head may be required to exclude any underlying pathology.

STROKE

Transient ischaemic attacks (TIAs) may represent an early warning sign of impending stroke. Therefore arteriography (DSA) of the neck vessels and cerebral arteries is performed in cases of TIA.

Even though arteriography gives a more definite answer, ultrasound examination of the neck vessels (Duplex and colour Doppler studies) could be performed initially.

In all patients with stroke, CT should be the initial radiological examination. However, if MRI is available, it is preferred to CT as MRI is better at detecting early infarction (within a few hours of vascular occlusion). CT sometimes gives negative results within the first 24–48 hours.

Emergencies in the neck

Major emergencies are trauma, foreign bodies, and croup and laryngeal inflammation in children.

TRAUMA

Cervical spine injuries are common and can be life-threatening. They range from nerve root compression and paralysis to death. Therefore, X-ray or CT evaluation of the cervical spine is important in trauma.

Plain X-ray views

1. The first film to obtain is a 'brow up—shoot through' lateral view. (Patient in supine position; movement of neck should be avoided.) Film should be well penetrated. All the cervical vertebrae and possibly the upper thoracic vertebrae should be demonstrated. Demonstration of the lower cervical and upper thoracic spine may be difficult in most patients. Swimmer's lateral projection or a lateral film with shoulder traction could be useful. Sometimes the patient's condition may not permit this. Alternative ways to demonstrate this area are tomography in lateral projection or CT scan if available.
2. If no abnormality is seen in the first film, do an open-mouth AP view of the odontoid process to exclude fracture of odontoid process. In suspicious cases the rest of the views are done only after expert examination of the film: a radiologist should be consulted if available.
3. If no abnormality is seen in the above two views, do the rest of the views, i.e. AP and two obliques. Patients must move the neck themselves.
4. Lastly, if there are no neurological signs, a flexion and extension view (functional view) could be done. Do not force the neck—the patient must move the neck. In suspicious cases the oblique and functional views should be done under the supervision of the attending doctor.
5. If no abnormality is seen in the above and the symptoms are still suspicious of fracture, tomography of selected areas could be done. If CT is available, it will be useful to show the vertebrae in transverse plane and to detect haematomas. If a helical or multiple-slice scanner is available, high-resolution images could be obtained in the sagittal and coronal planes as well as 3D images.

Clues for interpretation of X-rays

1. For proper interpretation one should be familiar with the normal appearance of the vertebrae, facetal joints, disc spaces and the soft tissues around the spine.
2. Lateral and odontoid process views should be inspected first.
3. Look for fracture lines or deformities in each vertebral body, neural arch and the facets. Look for dislocation or subluxation of facetal joints and any malalignment of vertebrae.
4. Loss of lordosis and scoliosis may indicate bony injury or soft-tissue injury.

5 If the disc is damaged the space may be narrow.
6 Soft tissues anterior to the spine (prevertebral soft tissue) should be inspected for swelling (haematomas). Normal AP distance of the prevertebral soft tissue in the retropharyngeal region (at the anteroinferior angle of C2) is about 6–7 mm in adults and children. Retrotracheal soft tissue at the level of the anteroinferior angle of C6 is about 14–15 mm in children and about 15–20 mm in adults (these measurements are upper limit of normal). Haematoma may be due to fracture or rupture of the anterior spinal ligament.
7 To identify upper cervical subluxation in the lateral view, draw a line along the anterior cortical margin of the spinous processes from C1 to C3 (posterior cervical line). If there is more than 2 mm displacement, it is diagnostic. This is usually seen in odontoid fracture or Hangman's fracture.
Note: In children slight anterior subluxation of the body of C2 on C3, especially in the flexion view, is normal. In these cases note the posterior cervical line, which will be normal.
8 Look for common fractures. Fractures are common at the C1–C2 articulation, odontoid process and from C5 to C7.
9 *Pitfalls:* In the AP view of the odontoid process, watch for superimposed shadow of an incisor tooth which will look like a fracture. Also look for a separate ossification centre of the odontoid process. (In some cases tomography of the odontoid process may be needed to identify the fracture.)
10 CT can be performed to determine the state of soft-tissue structures around the spine.
11 CT is also useful in cases of suspected instability at the fracture and also to identify suspected bony fragments within the vertebral canal.
12 CT (in bone windows) will demonstrate the neural arches and facetal joints. This will be useful to identify fractures or dislocation at the joints. Modern CT scanners can image the spine in various anatomical planes.
13 MRI is more sensitive than CT in demonstrating the spinal cord.

Classification of cervical spine injury

Cervical spine injuries can be classified according to the type of injury—flexion injury or extension injury. However, in many instances the patient is unconscious or cannot describe the injury. As far as treatment is concerned, it is important to decide whether the fracture is stable or unstable. The X-ray findings are useful in making this decision.

Flexion injury

The various kinds of flexion injury are described below in order of severity.

Hyperflexion sprain. Partial damage to posterior ligaments including interspinous ligaments. Flexion lateral view may demonstrate widening or fanning of the space between adjacent spinous processes.

Unilateral or bilateral facetal dislocation.

- In lateral view, look for anterior displacement of one vertebral body on the other by less than 50%.
- In AP view look for malalignment of spinous processes (especially in unilateral dislocation). Facets may be locked, i.e. inferior articular facet of the vertebra above is locked in front of the superior facet of the vertebra below.

Anterior wedging of vertebral bodies or compression fractures. If the neural arches are not fractured this may be a stable fracture.

Comminuted fracture of vertebral body ('teardrop' fractures). In these fractures look for any fragments in the vertebral canal. These fragments could cause damage to the spinal cord. CT scan would be useful in these cases to identify any fragments in the canal.

Extension injury

The various kinds of extension injury are described below in order of severity.

Hyperextension sprain. This causes damage to the anterior longitudinal ligament. Due to hyperextension there may be protrusion or bulging of the disc posteriorly. There may also be some haematoma and swelling from the ligamentum flavum. The disc bulging and the swelling from the ligamentum flavum can cause compression on the spinal cord. In these cases the X-ray may be normal. CT scan or MRI would be useful in these patients.

- Sometimes lateral plain X-ray may show soft-tissue swelling (haematoma) within prevertebral tissue.
- Extension injuries may be associated with fractures of the anterior angles of the vertebral bodies.
- Extension injuries may not be stable in extended positions of the neck but are stable in flexion.

Hangman's fracture. Fracture of both pedicles of axis with displacement of the body of C2 anteriorly and posterior displacement of neural arch of C2. This is well seen in the lateral view.

Jefferson bursting fracture. This fracture is unusual and is caused mainly by vertical compression injury causing bilateral fractures of anterior and posterior arches of C1. In the open-mouth AP view there will be lateral displacement—both lateral masses of C1.

Fracture of odontoid process. Look for fracture line (not to be confused with superimposed shadows and separate ossification centres). Also look for alignment in lateral view—posterior cervical line.

Stable fractures

- Unilateral fracture of lamina pedicle or lateral mass
- Unilateral facetal fracture or dislocation
- Wedge fracture
- Burst fracture—disc forced into fractured end plates of body
- Fracture of spinous process

Unstable fractures

- Bilateral fracture of lamina
- Bilateral dislocation of facets
- Comminuted fracture body (any fracture dislocation)
- Hangman's fracture
- Fracture of odontoid process

FOREIGN BODY IN NECK—PHARYNX AND UPPER OESOPHAGUS

Most swallowed foreign bodies lodge at the level of cricopharyngeal muscle or in the upper oesophagus. Commonest foreign bodies are fish bone, meat or chicken bone, large pieces of meat and coins.

Lateral film of the neck is the most useful view. Film of soft-tissue exposure may be necessary to identify faintly calcified bones. Radio-opaque materials are fairly easy to detect. Superimposition of calcified hyoid, thyroid, cricoid and laryngeal cartilages will be a problem. However, an understanding of their normal expected anatomical position will help to distinguish a foreign body. Pattern of calcification of cartilages (irregular) will also help. Swallowed bone may have a linear cortex. In difficult cases a barium swallow may help to identify the foreign body. Swallowing cottonwool soaked in barium (usually under fluoroscopic control) will occasionally help. This may get caught on the foreign body.

CT is also useful to locate smaller FBs not shown by X-ray.

EPIGLOTTITIS AND CROUP

Young children may develop severe acute inflammation of the epiglottis and larynx. In most cases where the condition is severe, radiological examination is postponed until the patient's condition is stable.

A lateral view of the neck (soft-tissue exposure) is the best view. Rarely, a single midline tomogram in lateral projection may be necessary.

- A swollen epiglottis will look like a thumb—the swollen aryepiglottis may also be seen.
- In croup usually the subglottic region from the vocal cord to the level of the inferior border of the thyroid cartilage shows mucosal swelling which causes narrowing of the airway. Vocal cords will also be affected. The need for radiology is debatable. However, if the patient's condition permits, it will be useful to perform an AP and lateral view of the neck. Swollen vocal cords, obliteration of laryngeal ventricles and narrowing of the subglottic airway by swelling can be easily seen.

Helical CT scan of larynx and trachea with sagittal and coronal reconstruction would be useful if clinically reasonable.

Emergencies in thoracic and lumbar spine

INJURY AND ACUTE DISC PROLAPSE OR RUPTURE

Views

- If the patient is immobilised, a 'shoot through' lateral view is initially performed.
- Lateral film of the thoracic spine is obtained while the patient is breathing. This is to 'blur' the superimposed ribs.
- Swimmer's lateral or lateral tomography may be required for demonstration of upper 3/4 thoracic vertebrae.
- AP view is fairly easy to obtain.
- In cases of suspected ligamentous rupture, flexion and extension views in lateral projection are obtained.
- In lumbar spine, if the condition of the patient permits, oblique views are also performed. These demonstrate the laminae and facetal joints well.
- CT scan is useful to demonstrate the integrity of disc and bony elements. They are also useful to detect facetal dislocation, subluxation and any posterior dislodgment of bony fragments into the vertebral canal. It is also useful to demonstrate the soft tissues around the spine.

Interpretation of X-rays

1 Look for:
   - reduction in the height of vertebral body and disc spaces (compression or wedge fractures)
   - fracture lines or displaced fragments in the vertebrae, including transverse process and spinous process (also look for posterior rib fracture in thoracic region)
   - paravertebral haematoma (loss of psoas shadow in lumbar region, displacement of pleural lining in thoracic region, etc)
   - subluxation, kyphosis, gibbus and scoliosis.

2 Look for any underlying causes of fracture such as secondary deposits, Paget's disease, osteoporosis, etc.

3 Beware of limbus vertebra non-united secondary ossification centres, butterfly vertebra and narrowing of vertebral bodies caused by long-standing scoliosis and kyphosis.

Unstable injury

- Transverse fractures through vertebral bodies and neural arches
- Fracture dislocation
- Rupture of ligaments (in the lateral view, the interspinous distance is wide, especially in flexion view)

Disc prolapse

- Plain X-ray may show disc narrowing—this is not always seen. Therefore, if symptoms persist, CT scan of the disc would be useful to show disc prolapse.
- High-resolution scanners can differentiate disc material, nerve roots, etc.
- MRI scan is superior in demonstrating spinal cord, nerve roots, discs, ligaments and bone oedema from trauma.

Chest emergencies

ROUTINE VIEWS

- PA and lateral—obtained in erect position, both in full inspiration.
- If patient cannot stand, erect PA or AP and lateral in sitting position (in full inspiration) are obtained.
- If patient cannot sit or stand, supine AP is obtained. This is unsatisfactory because the patient may not be able to take a full inspiration and the diaphragm appears elevated. It also causes magnification, especially of the mediastinum. Mobile views are AP.

ADDITIONAL VIEWS

- Oblique views for ribs.
- Apical lordotic view to demonstrate lung apices (to get the superimposed clavicle out of the way).
- Inspiration and expiration films to demonstrate pneumothorax.
- Penetrated film to see mediastinum or lung bases.
- Lateral decubitus (patient lying down on one side—right or left—and film obtained with horizontal beam). This demonstrates mobility of pleural fluid on the dependent side.

INTERPRETATION

There are two ways to interpret:

1 An experienced person will use a problem-oriented approach, depending on the clinical information.

2 An inexperienced person should look at a chest film in a routine, systematic manner.

   a Start looking at the mediastinal shadows. Cast your eyes along the:
      - anterior mediastinal structures—thymus (enlargement in infants; tumour in adults), thyroid (retrosternal), lymph nodes (if enlarged)
      - middle mediastinum—heart, aortic arch and branches, pulmonary artery, superior and inferior venae cavae.
      - posterior mediastinal structures—trachea, bronchi, oesophagus, descending thoracic aorta, lymph nodes, (abnormal) neural tissues, look for hiatus hernia, spine.

   b Look at the hilar shadows.

   c Look at the lung parenchyma and other lung markings (pulmonary vasculature and bronchi).

   d Look at the pleura.

   e Look at the chest wall (including ribs).

   f Cast your eyes along the periphery of the film, e.g. the shoulder, under the diaphragm.

TRAUMA

Rib fractures

First, second and third rib fractures are seen only in severe trauma. Commonest are from 4th to 9th ribs. Flail chest is seen when 3 or more ribs are fractured at 2 points. These are usually seen from the 4th to 8th ribs. A common site of fracture is usually the lateral angle. Because of this, oblique views are essential. Rib fractures can cause pneumothorax and haemothorax. Fracture of 10th, 11th and 12th ribs can cause damage to the liver, spleen and kidneys.

Lung contusion

Appears as an area of consolidation. It is not always associated with rib fracture. It may not appear immediately (sometimes a day later) and begins to resolve 2–3 days after injury. It usually resolves completely in about 10–15 days.

Rupture of thoracic aorta

Seen in motor vehicle accidents—usually seen near the ligamentum arteriosum. In this region the aorta is relatively fixed. Sudden deceleration and compression injury causes laceration at this relatively fixed portion of the aorta.

In chest X-rays there will be evidence of superior mediastinal widening, shift of the trachea to the right with obscuring of the aortic arch, and there may be haemothorax on the left. CT scan and aortography are the other radiological investigations in these patients.

Rupture of trachea or bronchus

Common findings in chest X-rays are pneumomediastinum, pneumothorax and surgical emphysema. Occlusion of fractured bronchus can cause collapse of the corresponding lung, lobe or segment.

Rupture of diaphragm

Seen in direct blunt trauma and penetrating injury. Sometimes not diagnosed immediately. In an X-ray the outline of the dome may not be normal. It may be elevated; there may be haemothorax or segmental lung collapse. On the left side, the bowel may herniate into the thorax; and on the right side, the liver may herniate. Rupture in blunt trauma is common on the left side.

CT in chest trauma

If a helical or multislice scanner is available, it will be useful for better demonstration of chest in sagittal and coronal planes as well as in 3D format. CT angiography could be performed to demonstrate aorta and great vessels.

BREATHLESSNESS

Asthma and acute-on-chronic airflow limitation (CAL)

- In CAL, chest X-ray shows overinflated lung, flattened domes of diaphragm, widened retrosternal space, hyper-radiolucency, a barrel-shaped chest, a relatively small and elongated heart

shadow, prominent main pulmonary arteries and pruning of peripheral pulmonary arteries (associated pulmonary artery hypertension), and thickened bronchial walls (end-on ring shadows and tramline shadows).
- In asthma, overinflation of lungs and bronchial wall thickenings may be seen. Other findings may include atelectasis caused by mucous plugging or consolidation.

High-resolution CT of 1 mm thickness is useful for investigation of CAL, especially to identify bronchiectasis, emphysematous bullae and interstitial fibrosis.

Radiological appearance in acute heart failure

Heart failure may be divided into left and right heart failure.

X-ray findings in left heart failure

- Distension of upper lobe veins (normally the upper lobe veins are smaller in calibre than the lower lobe veins).
- Interstitial pulmonary oedema. In the early stages the oedema forms around the hilar region, causing blurring of the hilar markings. Septal lines are due to accumulation of fluid along the lymphatics: 'A' lines are long and radiate from the hilar region to the periphery; 'B' lines are short and are seen in the region of the costophrenic angles.
- Alveolar pulmonary oedema. This is due to filling of the alveolar spaces with exudates. It is seen as haziness radiating from the hilar region and produces a butterfly-wing appearance. In the severe form, the alveolar oedema produces a patchy or cottonwool appearance.

X-ray appearances in right ventricular failure

- Prominence of superior vena cava (SVC) and azygous vein.
- Pleural effusion. In heart failure often more fluid is seen on the right side. In the early stages, pleural effusions are seen in the costophrenic angles as a homogeneous density demonstrating a 'meniscus sign'. The meniscus sign is seen in the erect position. The fluid in the base changes to a haziness in the supine films. This indicates mobility of the fluid. Small fluid collections are first detected in the lateral view—in the posterior costophrenic angles. In the average chest, the posterior costophrenic angle can accumulate about 150–200 mL of fluid without being seen in the PA view. In the early stages fluid can also accumulate in the fissures between the lobes. This appears as thick oblique fissures.

Pleural effusion

Pleural effusion may have various other causes, e.g. tumour. Large pleural effusions can obscure the underlying cause. If the fluid is mobile, a lateral decubitus view would be useful to demonstrate the lung bases. (Alternatively, CT scan could be performed to identify any mass in the lung base.)

Lung collapse

There are two major radiological signs:

1. Density—collapsed portion of the lung appears dense.
2. Signs of loss of volume:
   - shift of fissures—fissures are shifted towards the opacity
   - diaphragmatic elevation
   - mediastinal shift towards the side of collapse
   - splaying out of lung markings on the side of collapse due to compensatory overexpansion of the remaining lung.

CHEST PAIN

Only the causes where radiology plays a part are included in this section.

Myocardial infarction

Chest X-rays are performed to look at the heart size and shape, and also to look for evidence of heart failure. Upper limit of normal cardiothoracic ratio (CTR) is 50% (CTR = transverse diameter of the heart divided by transverse diameter of the chest).

Pericardial effusion

Chest X-ray is also useful to identify pericardial effusion. In the supine position the heart appears globular in shape, and in the erect position it produces a 'tent shape'. The angle between the right atrium and the right diaphragm is lost. On fluoroscopic examination poor pulsation may be demonstrated in cases of pericardial effusion. (For proper demonstration of pericardial effusion, echocardiography or CT scan is more useful.)

Pulmonary embolism

- Within 24–48 hours there may not be any radiological change. However, if large pulmonary arterial branches are blocked, there may be a cut-off sign (i.e. abrupt ending of an arterial branch).
- Raised hemidiaphragm—on the side of infarction.
- After about 24–48 hours an almost triangular density with its base towards the periphery of the chest may appear. (*pto*)

- There may be a small associated pleural effusion.
- Sometimes the main pulmonary artery on the affected side may enlarge.
- Later in the process, in the area of infarction there may be atelectasis or scar formation.
- Nuclear-isotope ventilation–perfusion scans are performed for diagnosis, but sometimes this is not confirmatory. However, a normal chest X-ray and abnormal isotope scan could be indicative of pulmonary embolism.
- Pulmonary arteriography is the best means of establishing or excluding pulmonary embolism. This is rarely performed because of adverse reactions and the cost. However, recently, with the introduction of multislice scanners, CT pulmonary angiograms are performed. This would be sensitive to detect emboli in pulmonary arteries up to about the 4th or 5th level of branching.
- Doppler study or venogram of the lower limb veins may show the origin of the clot.

Dissecting aneurysm

- In the PA view there may be widening of the superior mediastinum with the ascending aorta bulging to the right.
- The lateral view may show bulging of the ascending aorta anteriorly. A long-standing aneurysm of the ascending aorta can cause erosion of the posterior aspect of the sternum.
- Leakage from the aneurysm into the pericardium causes a large globular heart.
- When the dissection extends into the arch and descending thoracic aorta, the diameter widens towards the left. Sometimes a double aortic knuckle shadow can be seen. Some aneurysms leak into the pleural cavity and appear as a pleural effusion. In some patients uniform haziness can be seen in the left lung, due to blood spread along the bronchi and pulmonary arterial planes.
- CT scan can demonstrate a dissecting aneurysm and its extent.
- In order to demonstrate the exact site of rupture, some surgeons prefer an aortogram.

Pneumothorax

- Usually PA films in expiratory and inspiratory phases are obtained in the erect position.
- A large pneumothorax is well seen in a normal PA film. A small pneumothorax is usually demonstrated in the expiratory film.

- In order to identify the pneumothorax, follow the lung markings towards the periphery. The markings stop well short of the chest wall. A white visceral pleural line can be seen at this level.
- Do not confuse the accompanying shadow caused by intercostal muscles along the ribs for visceral pleura.
- Look for an associated pneumomediastinum (air can leak from bronchi in asthmatics) and subcutaneous emphysema along the chest wall and neck.

FEVER, COUGH AND PAIN

Pleurisy

- Early stages—no radiological findings.
- Later stages—small amounts of pleural fluid may be seen; there may be associated lung consolidation.

Pneumonia

- Bronchopneumonia—patchy shadows.
- Lobar or segmental pneumonia:
  - homogeneous localised shadows
  - air bronchogram may be seen
  - usually no loss of volume of lungs (this helps to differentiate from lung collapse).

HAEMOPTYSIS

Pulmonary infarction

See 'Pulmonary embolism', above.

Tumour

A mass, either solitary or multiple, can be seen in the hilar region or elsewhere in the lung. If there is any doubt about the diagnosis, CT would be useful. CT may also demonstrate any enlarged lymph nodes.

OTHER ACCIDENTS

Drowning

Pulmonary oedema is seen in cases of near-drowning in both fresh and sea water. Pulmonary oedema may not develop for up to 2 days. Therefore, negative findings in immediate chest X-rays do not exclude later development of oedema.

Inhalation of toxic gases/smoke

- In toxic gas inhalation, pulmonary oedema develops quickly—in about 4–24 hours.
- In smoke inhalation, the oedema may not develop for up to 2–4 days.

(*pto*)

- In chest X-rays oedema appears as patchy infiltrates. There may be segmental atelectasis. These changes usually resolve faster.

Ingestion of hydrocarbons (e.g. petroleum)

May develop patchy pneumonic consolidation in lung bases, usually within 1–2 hours. Severity depends on the amount ingested. Takes up to 2 weeks to resolve.

Foreign body

- Radio-opaque foreign bodies in bronchi are easily seen in chest X-rays. Foreign bodies like nuts, seeds and plastics may be difficult to see.
- Radiological signs are usually indirect, i.e. signs of obstruction.
- In children obstruction is usually ball–valve type, causing air trapping.
- PA films are obtained in inspiration and expiration. The inspiratory film may be normal, but in the expiratory film there will be hyperradiolucency and signs of increased volume on the affected side (flat diaphragm and shift of mediastinum to the opposite side).
- Chest screening is very useful to detect air trapping. Normal lungs show normal density and change of volume during breathing in comparison with the affected lung, which shows fixed volume and density.
- In adults, obstruction usually causes collapse of the lung or lobes.

Radiology in abdominal emergencies

Almost all modalities of imaging (plain X-ray, contrast study, CT and ultrasound) are used in abdominal emergencies. Of these, plain X-rays are the most commonly used.

VIEWS

- Routine views—AP in supine and erect position.
- Additional views—lateral decubitus in patients who cannot stand up, to look for fluid levels or free peritoneal gas.
- In some cases an erect chest X-ray is also performed to look for gas under the diaphragm or any pleural fluid in the lung bases.

INTERPRETATION

An inexperienced person finds it difficult to interpret an abdominal X-ray due to superimposition of various organs. This difficulty can be greatly reduced if the film is looked at in a routine manner, for example as follows.

1. Look at the bowel shadows—these are easily identifiable because of gas and faeces. Stomach, small and large bowel can be differentiated by their anatomical site and their pattern of mucosal folds and wall—valvulae conniventes in jejunal loops and haustral pattern in large bowel. Note any fluid levels and bowel dilation.
2. Look at the four major organs: liver, spleen, kidneys and bladder, for their size, position, outline and density.
3. Look at the psoas shadows and fat planes in the flank and along the pelvic walls.
4. Look for radio-opaque stones (gall and renal) and abnormal calcification (pancreatic, hepatic and abdominal aortic).
5. Look above and below the diaphragm for abnormal gas, fluid or air collections.
6. Look for any abnormal mass causing displacement of adjacent structures.
7. Look at the bony elements (lower ribs, lumbar spine and pelvis).

ACUTE ABDOMEN

In the plain X-ray of the abdomen the main aim is to identify obstruction, perforation or ileus in the bowel shadows.

Radiological signs of bowel obstruction

- There may be gaseous distension of the bowel up to the site of obstruction. In complete or almost complete obstruction, very little gas is seen in the bowel distal to the obstruction.
- Multiple fluid levels are seen in erect films.
- A step-ladder pattern of air fluid levels is seen in small-bowel obstruction. In large-bowel obstruction fluid levels are seen around the periphery. In complete obstruction of the large bowel there may be fluid levels in the small bowel as well.
- In gastric outlet or duodenal obstruction, a distended stomach with a large air–fluid level is seen.
- Volvulus. In sigmoid volvulus look for a dilated loop of bowel in the form of an inverted U in the left hypochondrium. In caecal volvulus the base of the dilated caecum usually points to the right iliac fossa. The volvulus can be confirmed by performing a limited dilute barium or diatrizoate (Gastrografin) enema.
- Intussusception. A sharp cut-off of bowel gas pattern is seen. Common intussusception is at the ileocaecal junction. There

may be dilated small bowel with multiple fluid levels. Limited barium enema examination may show a coil-spring appearance. In children the barium enema can be therapeutic and in most cases will be able to reduce the intussusception.

Radiological signs of ileus

Generalised. Slight to moderate gaseous distension of small and large bowel with multiple small fluid levels can be seen. Generalised ileus is usually seen in postoperative patients, peritonitis and retroperitoneal conditions.

Localised. The bowel loops in close proximity to an inflammatory area may show slight dilation and some fluid levels. One or two loops may be involved. This is called sentinel loop, e.g. jejunal loops and transverse colon are involved in pancreatitis and acute deep gastric ulcers. Terminal ileum is involved in conditions such as appendicitis. Hepatic flexure and some small bowel in the right hypochondrium may show fluid levels in cholecystitis. In renal colic there may be sentinel loops on the affected side.

Radiological signs in perforation

- Free peritoneal gas is usually seen under the diaphragm in the erect position. In a lateral decubitus film, free gas may be seen along the flank. The free gas is sometimes seen only after 24 hours.
- Loculated peritoneal gas, e.g. in perforation of a duodenal ulcer there may be loculated gas along the inferior liver margin. If there is a collection of gas in the lesser sac, in the plain X-ray there may be a double gas shadow projected over the fundus of the stomach.
- Retroperitoneal gas from perforation of the retroperitoneal portion of the large bowel.

In order to identify the site of perforation, diatrizoate (Gastrografin) contrast may be used (extravasated contrast is absorbed by the bloodstream and excreted by the kidney). In cases of suspected upper GI tract perforation the contrast may be given orally. In cases of colonic perforation it may be given rectally. Not all perforations can be demonstrated by this technique.

GI TRACT BLEEDING AND ISCHAEMIA

1. It is difficult to demonstrate bleeding points by barium study. However, this examination may be useful in demonstrating the presence of oesophageal varices, peptic ulcers, diverticula or tumours.

2 Highly selective coeliac, superior or inferior mesenteric arteriograms may demonstrate bleeding points. Angiography is also useful to demonstrate occluded arteries causing mesenteric ischaemia. A bleeding rate of 1 mL/min is usually required.

PANCREATITIS

1 Plain X-rays may show only indirect evidence such as sentinel loops or calcification in the region of the pancreas.
2 Barium meal may show a widened loop of duodenum due to enlargement of the pancreas.
3 Ultrasound is able to demonstrate the size and texture of the pancreas. It may also demonstrate oedematous change or any pseudocyst formation. However, sometimes it is difficult to demonstrate the pancreas by ultrasound due to obesity of the patient and presence of excessive gas.
4 A CT scan is the ideal examination to demonstrate the pancreas, especially in the obese patient. The sensitivity is such that it can demonstrate inflammatory changes, a small amount of calcification, a mass, a pseudocyst and also the state of surrounding tissues. It is also useful for follow-up study.
5 Skinny needle biopsy under CT or ultrasound control has greatly improved diagnostic ability.
6 Endoscopic retrograde cholangiopancreatography (ERCP) demonstrates the state of the pancreatic ducts.

CHOLECYSTITIS

1 Plain X-ray may demonstrate radio-opaque gallstones and sometimes demonstrates sentinel loops (localised ileus).
2 Ultrasound is the diagnostic tool of choice. It can demonstrate stones, thickness of the wall of the gall bladder and any oedematous change. It can also demonstrate the size of the bile ducts or any stones in the duct. However, demonstration of the lower common bile duct may be difficult.
3 In a post-cholecystectomy patient with symptoms of biliary colic, CT cholangiography could be useful to exclude any retained stones in the bile duct, strictures, etc.

AORTIC ANEURYSM

The majority of aneurysms are asymptomatic. However, these patients usually present to EDs when there is a rupture or leak. Severe rupture is fatal. If a slow leak is suspected, radiological investigation is carried out.

1. Plain X-rays (AP and lateral) show a soft-tissue mass, especially in the posterior abdominal wall. This is usually on the left side of the lumbar spine and is better seen in the lateral view. 50% of aortic aneurysms may have some calcification in the wall of the artery, which is very useful for identification of an aneurysm.
2. Ultrasound or CT scans are non-invasive, easier and quicker methods of diagnosing aneurysms. A CT scan is superior to ultrasound. It can demonstrate the site and length of the aneurysm. It can also demonstrate the diameter of the aneurysm and the presence of clot. CT is the study of choice in many patients, especially in obese patients. With the modern scanners CT aortography gives excellent results which also show the relationship of renal arteries to the neck of the aneurysm. This is useful for surgical planning.
3. Digital angiography is still used by surgeons to demonstrate the aneurysm and the branches of the abdominal aorta. However, this would show only the lumen and not the actual diameter of the aneurysm or the intraluminal clot.

RENAL COLIC

1. Plain X-rays may show radio-opaque calculi and may demonstrate localised ileus. CT is commonly used.
2. An IVP may demonstrate: obstruction (partial or complete), radiolucent stones, state of kidneys and collecting system.
3. If there is a non-functioning kidney and there are no radio-opaque stones, retrograde pyelography would be warranted.
4. Ultrasound may not detect all the stones in the kidney. It would demonstrate hydronephrosis in the case of ureteric obstruction.

HAEMATURIA

Severe cases of haematuria may present to the ED.

1. An IVP may reveal tumour in the kidneys, ureters or bladder.
2. CT is used to demonstrate renal and bladder tumours as well as any extension of the tumour.
3. Ultrasound can be used if CT scan is not available or if the patient is allergic to the contrast medium.

ABDOMINAL TRAUMA

Blunt trauma is more common. Radiological investigations depend on the patient's condition. The investigations include: plain abdominal X-ray, IVP, arteriograms, ultrasound and CT.

Renal contusion and laceration

1. Plain X-ray may show: loss of renal outline, loss of psoas shadow, scoliosis with concavity towards the side of injury, localised ileus on the side of injury, fracture of lower ribs, vertebrae (including transverse processes) and pelvic bones.
2. IVP may show: non-functioning kidney or delayed nephrogram; extravasation of contrast from ruptured kidney, ureter or bladder; clots, seen as filling defects within the pelvicalyceal system, ureter or bladder.
3. Arteriogram. If an IVP shows non-function and renal laceration is suspected, an emergency renal arteriogram is performed to assess the state of the renal arteries. (Renal vessel repair should be performed within a few hours.)
4. Ultrasound and CT, if available, are useful. They can demonstrate rupture, contusion and haematoma. CT is superior to ultrasound.

Renal vein thrombosis

1. An IVP shows an enlarged kidney, prolonged nephrographic phase and reduced excretion.
2. Ultrasound with Doppler may assist but helical CT in rapid sequential imaging after contrast injection has about 90% success in detecting renal vein thrombosis. Other findings include prolonged parenchymal enhancement and delayed excretion.
3. MRI is also an excellent method of demonstrating renal vein thrombosis.

Bladder trauma

- May be contusion or rupture (either intraperitoneal or extraperitoneal).
- In these cases a cystogram will be useful to demonstrate the site of the rupture.

Urethral rupture

- Usually seen in males.
- Site of rupture can be demonstrated by a retrograde urethrogram.

Spleen and liver injury

Splenic injury is more common than liver. Sometimes the plain X-ray signs may be non-specific. If there are some signs, further investigations may be necessary to confirm the diagnosis. Radiological signs depend on whether there is capsular damage or not.

Plain X-ray of abdomen and chest

- Elevation of left diaphragm in splenic injury and right in liver injury.
- Left or right effusion in spleen or liver injury, respectively.
- There may be atelectasis at the left or right base.
- There may be fracture of the lower ribs.
- Blurred liver or splenic outline.
- In splenic haematoma, the stomach may be displaced medially and the splenic flexure of colon downwards. In liver injury, the hepatic flexure may be displaced.
- In cases of rupture there may be loss of flank stripes, separation of walls of bowel loops by peritoneal fluid, obliteration of splenic or hepatic outline and general haziness of abdomen.

Ultrasound

- May show fluid (haemoperitoneum). Blood (fluid) is seen in the lateral gutters and pelvic recesses.
- May show contused areas of the organ.

CT

This is the best examination. If CT is not available, ultrasound is performed. CT can demonstrate intracapsular haematomas, laceration and haemoperitoneum.

Angiogram

Selective arteriograms would be useful to study the state of the arteries and also to demonstrate rupture.

Hollow viscus

- Rupture or perforation rarely occurs with blunt trauma, but may be seen in penetrating injury. When it occurs, there may be gas collections in the peritoneal cavity. Sometimes retroperitoneal and mediastinal gas can be seen. This can be detected in plain abdominal and chest X-rays.
- Diatrizoate (Gastrografin) study may be useful to demonstrate the site of perforation but this is not usually required.
- CT is useful to identify free peritoneal air and also any other injury to the adjacent organs.

Some obstetric emergencies

BLEEDING IN PREGNANCY

This can be due to: abortion—threatened, incomplete, complete or missed; ectopic pregnancy; placenta praevia; hydatidiform mole; placental separation (abruptio placentae).

All the above causes can be assessed by ultrasound (using transabdominal and transvaginal probes), which is the examination of choice. The fetal viability can also be assessed.

INTRAUTERINE FETAL DEATH

This can be confirmed by ultrasound.

INTRAUTERINE TRAUMA

Ultrasound is also used to assess the fetus after abdominal trauma.

Fractures of pelvis and limbs

Most fractures are easy to recognise on X-rays. However, some are difficult, e.g. hairline undisplaced fractures. In suspicious cases repeat examination by CT in 10–14 days could be performed (e.g. scaphoid fracture). In about 10–14 days some bone absorption occurs adjacent to the fracture line, which makes the fracture visible. In addition, periosteal reaction (callus) may begin to form.

Undisplaced fractures through the epiphyseal plates are also difficult to recognise. These fractures will also demonstrate bone resorption and callus in about 2 weeks time.

1. In minor fractures, look at the cortical bone for any discontinuity or dents. Also look for any irregularity in the trabecular pattern.
2. In some areas, e.g. femoral neck and scaphoid, tomogram, CT or nuclear scan may be required to demonstrate an undisplaced crack fracture.
3. If suspicious areas are encountered, oblique views should be done (thin fracture lines are visible only when the X-rays pass perpendicular to the fracture line).
4. In oblique fractures of the metaphysis, always look at the depth of the epiphyseal plates, as the fracture might extend along the plate causing widening of the growth plate.
5. In the forearm and leg, if one of the bones is shortened or dislocated, usually the other bone will have a fracture or dislocation. Therefore, in the distal limbs have a good look at the entire length of the bones, especially the proximal and distal ends and the adjacent joints.
6. In young patients look at the location of ossification centres around the joints to identify any dislocation of the epiphysis, e.g. elbow. If in doubt consult a radiologist or do a comparative view of the opposite joint.

(*pto*)

7 In the wrist, do not miss dislocation of carpal bones, e.g. lunate. Try to identify the position of carpal bones in the lateral view.
8 In the joints, look for indirect signs of haemarthrosis, i.e. displacement of adjacent fat pad. If there is haemarthrosis, always look hard to identify any hairline fracture or epiphyseal displacement. If in doubt, X-ray again in 10–14 days.
9 Look for soft-tissue swelling in the X-ray (sometimes the X-ray has to be viewed under bright light). If found, concentrate on this area to identify any fracture.
10 The pelvis is like a ring—in compression injuries it might break in two or more places. Fracture of pelvic bones may be associated with dislocation or subluxation at the sacroiliac joints or pubic symphysis.

Radiation issues

Ionising radiation can be from natural or artificial sources.

Natural radiation. Heat and light are types of radiation that we can feel or see, but there are other kinds of radiation that human senses cannot detect. We constantly receive invisible radiation from the sky (cosmic radiation), earth's crust, air and even food and drinks.

Artificial radiation. From X-rays, nuclear industries and weapons. Unlike natural radiation, these are fully controllable.

Measuring radiation. The radiation dose received by people (whole body) is measured in grays (Gy). The adverse effective dose (absorbed dose that may cause biological effects or cancer) is measured in sieverts (Sv).

RADIATION EXPOSURE AND LIMITS

- Exposure from natural radiation is about 1.5 mSv per year.
- The International Commission on Radiological Protection (ICRP) has set the following limits:
  a For radiation workers, 20 mSv per year.
  b For the general public, 1 mSv per year (over and above the natural radiation).
  c For patients, considering diagnostic benefits over radiation risk, a definite limit for dose from radiological procedures has not been set. However, scientists have calculated the possible radiation dose associated with some radiological investigations, as indicated in Table 4.1. (These figures are a

Table 4.1 Possible effective doses of radiation associated with some radiological investigations

Examination	Possible effective dose (mSv)
Dental OPG	0.01
Foot/hand (1 film)	0.02
Skull (2 films)	0.04
Chest (2 films)	0.06–0.1
Mammogram (4 films)	0.13
Cervical spine (6 films)	0.3
Abdomen/pelvis (1 film)	0.7
Thoracic spine (2 films)	1.4
Lumbar spine (5 films)	1.8
IVP (6 films)	2.5
Barium meal (11 films fluoro)	2.5–3.8
Barium enema (10 films)	6–7
Coronary angiogram	1.6–5
CT of head	2.5
CT of chest	5–8
CT of lumbar region	5
CT of abdomen	7–10
CT of coro-angio region (64-slice)	5–10
CT of whole body	15
Lung scan (nuclear)	2–3
Bone scan	3–5
Sestamibi scan	13
Radiotherapy (6 weeks)	2000
Air travel (crew)	3.8/year
Air travel (passengers)	0.05/7 h
Computer/television use	0.01/year

CT, computed tomography; IVP, intravenous pyelogram; OPG, orthopantomogram.

guide only and may vary from patient to patient, as they are highly dependent on the size of the patient and the exposure factors used. In CT, the dose also depends on the number of slices as well as the number of examinations, e.g. pre- and post-contrast studies. Thin slices produce a higher radiation dose due to more overlap between the slices.)

RADIATION RISKS

The following are suggestions and predictions only.

- Relative risk of radiation:
  - CT of abdomen (10 mSv)
- Equivalent risks
  - Smoking 140 cigarettes
  - Driving 6,000 km in a car
  - Flying 40,000 km in a jet
  - Canoeing for 5 hours

Risk of cancer per 10 mSv is 0.04% (1 in 2500 CTs of the abdomen). Some others predict that 1 in 100 patients exposed to 100 mSv (10 CTs of the abdomen) may develop cancer or leukaemia and 42 of the same 100 may eventually develop cancer from other causes.

SUMMARY

It is now known that, in diagnostic radiology, CT is a major contributor of radiation.

- Referring doctors, radiologists and radiographers should be aware that CT is a high-dose procedure. At the same time, doctors and patients must be assured that CT is a highly beneficial X-ray and should not be feared when the benefit of the examination clearly outweighs the risk.
- Doctors should order CT examination with caution, especially when ordering multiple examinations, CT with and without contrast and CT of the whole body.
- Imaging professionals should make every effort to reduce radiation as low as reasonably achievable, while obtaining adequate diagnostic information in the image.

Editorial Comment

Technology is galloping, e.g. CT coronary angiograms (320-slice), paediatric CT (256-slice)—no need for sedation as so quick—as well as the use of combinations of different modalities, e.g. PET (positron emission tomography) with CT for tumours, etc. It is hard to keep abreast, but also it means we now see lesions that we are not sure are pathological or need further tests or treatment. Ask, talk to the experts.

Chapter 5

Ultrasound in emergency medicine

Andrew Finckh and Julie Leung

Emergency department ultrasound continues to be an area of rapidly expanding importance in the practice of emergency medicine. It is a safe and reliable technology that is relatively inexpensive and easily learned.

The Australasian College for Emergency Medicine (ACEM) promotes the use of ultrasound in the ED and advocates the availability of timely ultrasound examinations 24 hours per day. Traditionally the emphasis has been on the ability of the emergency doctor and trainee to perform focused ED ultrasound examinations on trauma patients (focused assessment with sonography in trauma, or FAST) and on patients with suspected abdominal aortic aneurysm. Other applications of ultrasound in the ED include providing guidance for difficult procedures and identifying pathological conditions such as ectopic pregnancy and deep vein thrombosis (DVT).

This chapter focuses on: the basic physical principles of ultrasound; ultrasound equipment; common applications of ultrasound in the ED; training, credentialling and quality review.

Basic physical principles

'Ultrasound' is sound whose frequency is above the range of human hearing. The audible human range is 20–20,000 hertz (Hz), while diagnostic ultrasound employs frequencies of 1–20 megahertz (MHz), with the most common range being 3–12 MHz.

Propagation of sound is the transfer of energy, not matter, from one place to another within a medium.

FREQUENCY AND WAVELENGTH

Frequency and wavelength are inversely related: the higher the frequency, the shorter the wavelength. The shorter the wavelength is, the less the tissue penetration but the greater the resolution and, therefore, the clearer the image.

PIEZOELECTRIC EFFECT

Artificially grown crystals are commonly used for modern transducers. These are treated with high temperatures and strong electric fields to produce the piezoelectric properties necessary to generate sound waves.

These properties mean that when a crystal in the ultrasound transducer has a voltage applied to it, the crystal is deformed and produces a pressure, i.e. the transducer sends an ultrasound. Conversely, an applied pressure received by the transducer deforms the crystal to produce a voltage. This voltage is then analysed by the system. In essence, the piezoelectric crystal acts as both speaker and microphone.

Most transducers use many small crystal elements for the formation of each pulse.

IMAGE RESOLUTION

Resolution is the ability to distinguish between echoes. It is clearly an important characteristic of an ultrasound machine. There are three kinds of image resolution.

1. **Contrast resolution** is the ability of an ultrasound system to differentiate between tissues with varying characteristics, e.g. between liver and spleen.
2. **Temporal resolution** is the ability of an ultrasound system to show changes in the underlying anatomy over time. This is particularly important in echocardiography.
3. **Spatial resolution** is the ability of an ultrasound system to detect and display structures that are close together.
   - a **Axial resolution** is the ability to display small targets along the path of the beam as separate entities. The most important determinant of this is the length of the pulse used to form the beam. The shorter the pulse length, the better the axial resolution. Simply put, the higher-frequency probes have better axial resolution but lower penetration.
   - b **Lateral resolution** is the ability to distinguish between two separate targets perpendicular to the beam: the wider the beam, the poorer the lateral resolution. Correct positioning of the focal zones is critical to gaining the best lateral resolution for a given transducer.

INTERACTION OF SOUND WITH TISSUE

Attenuation is the term used to describe the factors affecting the echoes returning to the transducer.

The four main processes in attenuation are:

1. **Reflection.** This occurs at interfaces between soft tissues of differing acoustic impedance. Impedance is the resistance to propagation of sound. The percentage of the sound reflected is dependent on the magnitude of the impedance mismatch and the angle of approach to the interface, for example:

Soft tissue/air interface	99% reflected
Soft tissue/bone interface	40% reflected
Liver/kidney interface	2% reflected

2. **Refraction.** This is the deviation in the path of the beam that occurs when the beam passes through interfaces between tissues of differing speeds of sound when the angle of incidence is not 90°.
3. **Absorption.** This is the transfer of some of the energy of the beam to the material through which sound is travelling. It explains why high-frequency transducers cannot be used for examining deep structures within the body.
4. **Scattering.** This is the reflection of sound off objects that are irregular or smaller than the ultrasound beam. It occurs at interfaces within the sound beam path. The scatter pattern relies on the size of the interface relative to the wavelength of the sound.

ARTEFACTS

Ultrasound systems operate on the basis of certain assumptions relating to the interaction of the sound beam with soft-tissue interfaces. Some artefacts help ultrasound diagnosis. The common types of artefacts include:

Acoustic shadowing. Occurs when beam energy attenuation at a given interface is high, such as when an object of high density blocks signal transmission.

Acoustic enhancement. Occurs when there is an area of increased brightness relative to echoes from adjacent tissues.

Edge shadowing. Results from a combination of reflection and refraction occurring at the edge of rounded structures. It can be falsely interpreted as acoustic shadowing.

Reverberation artefact. Results from repeated reflections of sound between two interfaces. It is usually generated by high-level mismatch interfaces when the echo amplitude is very high.

Beam width effect. Occurs because the ultrasound beam is not a single line, although the system assumes that it is.

Velocity artefact. Occurs because various tissues have velocities that are different from the constant velocity assumed by the system. This results in incorrect placement of an object.

Mirror image. Where a single image is displayed twice due to reflection off an interface.

Ultrasound equipment

TYPES OF TRANSDUCERS

Linear and curved array transducers are most commonly used in general ultrasound.

Linear array transducer is constructed with multiple small crystal elements arranged in a straight line across the face of the probe. The beam generated by this transducer travels at 90° to the transducer face.

Curved array transducer is also constructed with multiple small crystal elements, except that the face of the transducer is convex. This results in a wider field of view at the bottom of the image and a narrower image in the near field of view.

CHOICE OF EQUIPMENT

The ultrasound requirements of individual EDs vary, depending on how the device will be used. For example, the ED that intends to limit studies to FAST and abdominal aorta scans will have different requirements from the one that wishes to perform ultrasounds to assess a first-trimester pregnancy, locate a foreign body, assess testicular blood flow or obtain central venous access. Both present and future needs of the ED need to be determined. Staff who become competent in the basic applications of ultrasound may wish to extend their skills with time.

Once the ultrasound needs and budgetary limitations of the ED have been determined, the following features of the ultrasound equipment should be considered:

- machine portability and stability
- machine size—a larger machine may offer more features but be impractical in a resuscitation situation and difficult to store when not in use
- ability to upgrade machine without replacing expensive items
- servicing of machine, including transducers and peripherals.

There are now more and more manufacturers providing machines suitable for ED ultrasound. Trial of these machines prior to purchase is an effective way of determining suitability in individual EDs.

Editorial Comment

There are several pocket-sized personal ultrasound units available for several hundred dollars. With training and appropriate indications they can be very useful and their use will quickly increase, e.g. for the urgent care of patients.

Common applications in the ED

FOCUSED ASSESSMENT FOR SONOGRAPHY IN TRAUMA (FAST)

The FAST scan is a useful diagnostic test in the evaluation of the patient with blunt abdominal trauma (see Table 5.1). The aim of FAST is to detect fluid as represented by anechoic (black) areas, particularly haemopericardium, haemoperitoneum and haemothorax. Ideally the FAST examination is performed in 5 minutes or less.

A review of 11 studies has shown FAST to be a highly specific tool, with specificity of 98%. The sensitivity in these studies was 89%. It has mostly eliminated the initial use of diagnostic peritoneal lavage

Table 5.1 Choice of equipment

Type	Essential	Optional	Specialised
Ultrasound system	Variable send-and-receive focusing Support for flat linear and curved linear transducers Measurement callipers Internal memory	Small-footprint intercostal probe Data disc Cineloop facility	Colour/amplitude mapping M-mode obstetric biometry software package Sector size control Pulsed Doppler control Continuous-wave Doppler control Transoesophageal echo facility
Transducers	Multifrequency (2.5–5.0 MHz) curved array Multifrequency (7–10 MHz) linear array (for foreign body and central line access)		Transvaginal probe Cardiac probe Transoesophageal probe
Peripherals	Video recorder hard copy device		

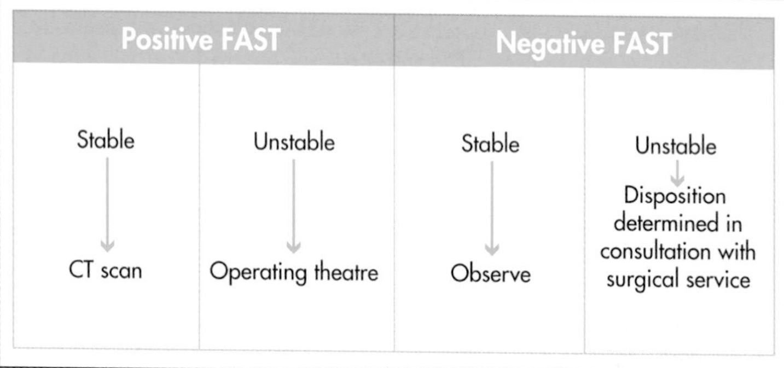

Positive FAST
Negative FAST
Stable
CT scan
Unstable
Operating theatre
Stable
Observe
Unstable
Disposition determined in consultation with surgical service

Figure 5.1 Blunt trauma algorithm

Box 5.1 Advantages and disadvantages or limitations of FAST/eFAST

Advantages	Disadvantages
• Safe to operator and patient • Rapid • Acceptable in the pregnant patient • Non-invasive • Easily performed/easily learned • Can be performed concurrently with resuscitation • Can be performed in a resuscitation area (i.e. monitored environment) • Repeatable (of particular value in the monitoring of non-operative solid organ injuries) • More cost-effective when compared with DPL or CT • Adult and paediatric applications	• Positive examination requires presence of free intraperitoneal fluid (minimum of 600 mL) • Cannot determine source of free fluid • Not reliable for excluding hollow visceral injury • Not reliable for grading solid organ injuries • Not reliable for excluding retroperitoneal haemorrhage • Patient anatomy or pathology may make exam technically difficult (obesity or subcutaneous emphysema)

in many trauma centres. The advantages and disadvantages of FAST are shown in Box 5.1.

FAST involves a minimum of four views.

1 The hepatorenal interface (Morison's pouch) and the right diaphragm. In this view, the transducer is placed at the right midaxillary line between the 11th and 12th ribs. The liver, kidney and diaphragm are viewed. Particular attention is paid to the hepatorenal interface.

2 The splenorenal interface and left diaphragm. In this view, the transducer is placed at the left posteroaxillary line between the 11th and 12th ribs. The spleen, kidney and diaphragm are viewed. The kidney usually lies more cephalad than on the right.
3 The pouch of Douglas (retrovesical or retrouterine). Ideally the bladder is full. The transducer is placed approximately 1 cm superior to the pubic symphysis. The examination is performed in both transverse and longitudinal planes.
4 Subxiphoid or intercostal views of the pericardium. With a subxiphoid view, the transducer is advanced to the xiphoid process and the beam is directed at the left shoulder. The transducer is variously tilted, swept and rotated to view the pericardial space. An effusion can be suspected when an anechoic area is seen between the liver edge and the right atrium or ventricle. A collapsed right ventricle offers evidence of pericardial tamponade. Clotting blood can be difficult to distinguish from anterior pericardial fat.

Other views include the bilateral paracolic gutters.

Extended FAST (eFAST) adds thoracic ultrasound for detection of pneumothorax and haemothorax. Ultrasound has been shown to be more sensitive than chest X-ray in the diagnosis of pneumothorax in trauma patients. Ideally the linear array probe (5–10 MHz transducer) is used. For assessment of pneumothorax the probe is placed over the anterior thorax in a sagittal orientation in the midclavicular line. Ultrasound can only detect a pneumothorax which is directly under the probe, so several sites on the anterior chest should be examined. Absence of lung sliding and the presence of the 'stratosphere' sign instead of the normal 'seashore' sign on M-mode imaging should make one suspicious of a pneumothorax.

FAST is also useful in penetrating thoracoabdominal trauma to detect pericardial effusion/cardiac tamponade, pneumothorax/haemothorax and haemoperitoneum. However, there are limitations such as detection of bowel injuries.

ABDOMINAL AORTIC SCAN

The ability to detect abdominal aortic aneurysm (AAA) can improve patient outcomes, as mortality has been shown to decrease if the diagnosis is made prior to or shortly after rupture. Ultrasound is an excellent tool for detecting the presence of AAA but can be limited in terms of the ability to assess for rupture.

This study involves scanning the aorta in both transverse and longitudinal planes continuously from the diaphragm to the aortic bifurcation. It includes measurement of the maximum aortic diameter in both planes.

If an aneurysm is present several additional items need to be assessed, including:

- proximal edge, especially relationship of aneurysm to origin of renal arteries
- distal extent, especially relationship to origin of common iliac arteries
- presence of thrombus
- presence of dissection
- true aneurysmal diameter (outside to outside edge)
- residual lumen diameter
- presence of haematoma surrounding aorta in rupture
- presence of free intraperitoneal fluid.

The presence of an AAA on ultrasound in the unstable patient confirms the need for laparotomy.

Indications for ultrasound to detect AAA include presence of syncope, shock, hypotension, abdominal pain, abdominal mass and flank pain or back pain, especially in the older patient.

Other applications

- Pregnancy:
  - First-trimester pelvic ultrasound to establish the location of the pregnancy and fetal heart rate in the symptomatic pregnant patient or the asymptomatic patient with risk factors for ectopic pregnancy.
  - Second- and third-trimester pelvic ultrasound for detection of fetal cardiac movement, location of placenta and the evaluation of the pregnant trauma patient.
- Assessment of above-calf DVT.
- ECG can be used to assess for pericardial effusion/tamponade, the presence of cardiac mechanical activity in cardiac arrest and pulmonary embolus. Rapid identification of these pathologies may lead to potentially life-saving interventions.
- Resuscitative ultrasound—assessment of hypotension in the critically ill patient. A structured ultrasound protocol evaluating the heart, IVC, abdomen, aorta and lungs can provide valuable information which can guide the clinician during the initial evaluation and stabilisation of undifferentiated shock. This provides the opportunity for improved clinical treatments and patient outcomes.

- Biliary ultrasound—cholecystitis and cholelithiasis are best imaged with ultrasound.
- Renal ultrasound—ultrasound images the kidneys well and can be a sensitive bedside test for hydronephrosis.
- Procedural uses (see Table 5.2). This includes use for vascular access and drainage of pleural effusions. Ultrasound may localise the percutaneous insertion/incision site before the procedure (static guidance) or may provide real-time guidance of the procedure with needle, catheter or other device (dynamic guidance).
- Localisation of foreign bodies.

Table 5.2 Procedural applications for ED ultrasound

Application	Strengths and uses	Limitations
Central and peripheral venous access	Body habitus Anticoagulation Lack of anatomical or palpable landmarks	Vessels may be difficult to visualise without Doppler technology
Bladder size and aspiration	Avoids dry taps Avoids urethral catheterisation	
Abscess location and aspiration	Soft-tissue infection without clear fluctuance	Other sonolucent structures
Thoracocentesis and paracentesis	Localisation of fluid and avoidance of viscera	
Pericardiocentesis	Ultrasound-guided pericardiocentesis offers a safer therapeutic alternative in the presence of pericardial tamponade than traditional 'blind' methods	
Foreign-body localisation	Excellent visualisation in fluid and uniform surrounding tissue	
Nerve blocks	More effective than blind techniques with decreased complications and lower amounts of anaesthetic required to achieve an effective block	
Lumbar puncture (LP)	Reduces number of failures of LP in difficult patients	
Arthrocentesis	Useful especially in aspirating deeper and more difficult joints such as the hip and ankle	

Training, credentialling and quality review

INITIAL TRAINING

Accurate training and experience are vital to accurate ultrasound examination. The format of courses instructing individuals in ED ultrasound depends on the number of primary applications being taught. A single-day course has proved to be adequate for those learning basic physics, knobology and how to perform FAST and abdominal aorta assessment. Sessions should include live scanning with appropriate models such as chronic ambulatory peritoneal dialysis patients (to simulate haemoperitoneum) or stable patients with aortic aneurysms.

CREDENTIALLING PROCESS AND MAINTENANCE OF STANDARDS

The ACEM has determined the credentialling process that outlines the minimum standards deemed sufficient to maintain a level of competency in ED ultrasounds. This includes the satisfactory completion of an introductory course and the performance and recording of a requisite number of accurate proctored ultrasound examinations. For example, the FAST module involves the performance of at least 25 accurate trauma examinations, with 50% of them clinically indicated and at least 5 positive for intraperitoneal, pleural or pericardial fluid. Once a level of proficiency is attained, ongoing maintenance of standards is essential. To maintain credentials, ACEM has outlined that ongoing annual ultrasound training and the performance of a specific number of ultrasound examinations for each module are required.

Individual institutions can adopt or adapt these standards as determined by local needs.

DOCUMENTATION

The results of ED ultrasound examinations that are used to facilitate patient care decisions should be documented in the patient's clinical record.

The following are basic items that should be documented:

- type of examination (e.g. FAST)
- reason for examination (e.g. blunt abdominal injury)
- views obtained—if a printer is attached, hard copies should be obtained and included in the clinical record
- adequacy of views obtained—if inadequate, state reasons
- findings and interpretation—normal, abnormal or indeterminate.

Findings incidental to the examination should also be documented and the patient informed of them.

A patient undergoing an ED ultrasound should be informed that the exam is a focused one directed at determining the presence of specific pathologies or to answer a specific clinical question. Radiologists still provide expertise in comprehensive examinations.

QUALITY REVIEW AND QUALITY IMPROVEMENT

A process of measuring and documenting performance, accuracy and image quality is essential as part of a continuous quality-improvement process. Periodic review of static images, videotapes or digital images with radiology staff will allow the identification of errors in clinical interpretation or failure to obtain appropriate images. Tracking clinical outcomes of patients by obtaining reports of follow-up imaging procedures or surgical findings can also be used to monitor the clinical interpretation of ultrasound studies.

Online resources

ACEM Policy Document. Credentialing for ED ultrasonography (Mar 2011).
www.acem.org.au

ACEP Policy Statement. Emergency ultrasound guidelines (Oct 2008).
www.acep.org

ACEM Policy Document. Use of bedside ultrasound by emergency physicians (Mar 2006).
www.acem.org.au

Chapter 6
The approach to the patient with chest pain, dyspnoea or haemoptysis

Patricia Saccasan Whelan and Anthony J Whelan

Chest pain, dyspnoea and haemoptysis are common and important symptoms which bring patients to the emergency department. The role of the emergency medical team is to rapidly identify high-risk patients, commence resuscitation if necessary, arrive at an accurate diagnosis, initiate appropriate therapies and arrange appropriate disposition. Some therapies are extremely time-dependent (e.g. reperfusion therapy for myocardial infarction) and good outcomes depend on early recognition of these seriously ill patients. However, the clinician must be aware of the tension between appropriate investigation and the costs associated with inappropriate admissions and tests.

Chest pain

The general public is increasingly aware of the importance of chest pain and the need for early presentation with this symptom. In American EDs, up to 7% of all presentations are for chest pain, prompting changes in the organisation of EDs so that many high-volume departments have specialised chest pain units where patients with this symptom are rapidly triaged and treated according to defined protocols. While there are many causes of chest pain, clinicians should be aware of disorders which are potentially life-threatening (Box 6.1). Before any chest pain patient is discharged, each of these diagnoses should at least be considered.

MYOCARDIAL ISCHAEMIA

(See also Chapter 7, 'Acute coronary syndromes'.)

History

Recognition of the symptoms of myocardial ischaemia is crucial. Modern therapies significantly improve the outcome of patients with acute ischaemia and missing this diagnosis can be disastrous. In the

Box 6.1 Causes of chest pain

Potentially life-threatening	Not life-threatening
Acute coronary syndromes	Chest wall pain
Pulmonary embolism	Gastro-oesophageal reflux
Aortic dissection	Oesophageal spasm
Tension pneumothorax	Pericarditis
Ruptured oesophagus	Mitral valve prolapse
Pneumonia	Herpes zoster

USA inappropriate discharge of patients who eventually are found to have acute coronary syndromes is the leading cause of litigation involving emergency physicians.

Take time to question the patient, using non-leading questions, to clarify the nature of the patient's pain.

- The pain of myocardial ischaemia is classically a deep visceral pain felt in the anterior chest but not localised to any part of the chest. Patients may describe heaviness, constriction, a sensation like a heavy weight or a dull ache.
- Pain usually comes on gradually, reaching a peak over a few minutes, and lasts at least a few minutes.
- Patients prefer to lie still and the pain is not exacerbated by the respiratory cycle, posture or food intake.
- Classical radiation patterns include spread to the neck, jaw or arms. Pain radiating to the left arm is more common than to the right. Heaviness (rather than pain) in both arms is also very suggestive.
- Autonomic accompaniments such as sweating, nausea and anxiety are also of concern.

While the pain of myocardial ischaemia may be severe, the severity of the pain is not consistently related to the extent of ischaemia. Angina usually lasts less than 20 minutes and there may be some benefit from oxygen and sublingual nitrates. The temporal pattern of angina is of prognostic significance (Table 6.1). Patients with a stable pattern of angina may not need admission but will need appropriate referral for follow-up.

Atypical presentations are common. Older patients, younger patients, women and diabetics are more likely to have presentations which are not immediately suggestive of myocardial ischaemia. Pain may be felt in the abdomen, jaw or arm (without chest pain), or an acute coronary syndrome may present only with dyspnoea, vomiting or syncope. Thus a high index of suspicion is necessary and the diagnosis of myocardial ischaemia should be considered (and an ECG and

Table 6.1 Braunwald classification of unstable angina

Class	Description	Risk of AMI/death in next year
I	New onset of exertional angina; angina with less effort; no rest pain	7%
II	Angina at rest within the last month but no pain in last 48 hours	10%
III	Angina at rest in the last 48 hours	11%

AMI, acute myocardial infarction

biomarkers done) in all patients in whom this diagnosis is possible.

There may be overlap with other chest pain syndromes. Some patients describe burning pain suggestive of gastro-oesophageal reflux; and while sharp, stabbing or even pleuritic-type pain makes myocardial ischaemia unlikely, it does not exclude this diagnosis. Pope et al (2000) found that up to 22% of patients with the principal complaint of sharp stabbing pain had an acute coronary syndrome.

A number of diagnostic decision tools using history and ECG findings to assist with diagnosis have been proposed (e.g. the acute cardiac ischaemia (ACI) predictive instrument, the thrombolysis in myocardial infarction (TIMI) score), which probably increase the accuracy of diagnosis. However, a high index of suspicion is the most useful safeguard.

Risk factors

A previous diagnosis of myocardial infarction, stable angina or revascularisation procedures significantly increases the risk that a new presentation with chest pain is due to myocardial ischaemia. The presence of diabetes and increasing age are also important risks. A patient with diabetes presenting with chest pain should be assumed to have coronary artery disease until it has been proven otherwise. It is not clear whether a history of other risk factors for atherosclerosis (smoking, hyperlipidaemia, family history) increases the risk that a new presentation with chest pain is due to myocardial ischaemia. This is because these findings are very common in the general population.

OTHER POTENTIALLY LIFE-THREATENING CAUSES OF CHEST PAIN

Aortic dissection

(See also Chapter 16, 'Aortic and vascular emergencies'.)

This is an important but rare disorder leading to severe chest pain associated with a significant mortality.

- Typically the pain is of abrupt onset and is of maximum intensity immediately, as opposed to the pain of myocardial ischaemia which builds up over minutes.
- The pain of aortic dissection often radiates through to the back, which is unusual in myocardial ischaemia.
- The pain may be described as 'tearing' and can be very severe, needing large doses of narcotics for control of pain.
- The appearance of a patient with severe pain and a non-specific ECG who appears shocked, yet has a high blood pressure, is a strong clue to this disorder.

Risk factors for aortic dissection include Marfan's syndrome and other inherited disorders of connective tissue, hypertension, pregnancy, bicuspid aortic valve and previous surgery involving the aorta.

Pneumothorax

(See also Chapter 9, 'Respiratory emergencies—the acutely breathless patient'.)

Pleuritic chest pain varies with the respiratory cycle and is usually worse on inspiration. Pneumothorax (air in the pleural space) is an important cause of pleuritic chest pain and is frequently associated with dyspnoea.

- Primary spontaneous pneumothorax occurs most frequently in younger males who are tall and thin but have no previous history of lung disease.
- Secondary spontaneous pneumothorax complicates chronic lung disease, especially COPD, asthma and cystic fibrosis.

Pulmonary embolism

(See also Chapter 10, 'Venous thromboembolic disease—deep venous thrombosis and pulmonary embolism'.)

Pleuritic pain can also be caused by pulmonary embolism, where there is a complicating pulmonary infarction and pleural irritation; however, massive pulmonary embolism can also cause central chest discomfort suggestive of angina. This is often associated with dyspnoea and haemodynamic collapse, and may reflect acute right ventricular dysfunction.

Pneumonia

(See also Chapter 9, 'Respiratory emergencies—the acutely breathless patient'.)

Pleuritic chest pain is a common feature of respiratory tract infections which extend to the pleura. There should be other clinical features pointing to infection.

Ruptured oesophagus

Severe anterior chest pain following vomiting is characteristic of oesophageal perforation (Boerhaave's syndrome). While vomiting may occur in myocardial infarction, it usually follows the onset of chest pain rather than preceding it. Oesophageal perforation may also follow procedures, especially oesophageal dilation.

OTHER CAUSES OF CHEST PAIN

Pericarditis

Pain is usually felt in the anterior or left chest. It has a pleuritic quality and varies according to posture. Pericarditis can occur at any age and the pain may be severe.

Reflux

The pain of reflux is usually described as burning, arising in the lower chest and 'rising' into the throat. There may be associated belching, waterbrash, dysphagia or odynophagia. Patients usually report relief with antacids but this response is not specific for reflux, and improvement with antacids or 'GI cocktails' may be seen in myocardial ischaemia. Thus, a response to antacids should not be used to rule out myocardial ischaemia.

Chest wall pain

This is the commonest cause of chest pain in outpatient practice. Pain is usually well-localised, jabbing or stabbing, lasting either for a fraction of a second or for hours or even days at a time. While a number of syndromes have been described, a precise diagnosis may not be possible. Generally pain that is described as coming from 'outside' the chest with a lancinating or knife-like quality is less likely to be due to myocardial ischaemia. Chest wall tenderness is common and pain that is reproduced by pressure on the chest wall is a non-specific finding. It should not be used to rule out myocardial ischaemia, and may co-exist with other more significant pathologies.

Anxiety

Chest pain may be associated with anxiety states and is an important component of the hyperventilation syndrome. This diagnosis should only be reached after a thorough evaluation to exclude other, possibly life-threatening, possibilities.

Abdominal disease

(See also Chapter 25, 'Gastrointestinal emergencies'.)

Upper abdominal disorders such as cholecystitis, peptic ulcer disease and pancreatitis can be associated with chest pain which dominates the presentation and may appear out of proportion to the abdominal findings. Some of these disorders may be associated with ECG abnormalities, further confusing the diagnosis. Upper abdominal pain (without chest pain) may also represent an acute coronary syndrome.

PHYSICAL EXAMINATION AND INITIAL MANAGEMENT

- Triage chest pain patients rapidly to urgent care. Important haemodynamic abnormalities should be recognised quickly.
- Commence high-flow oxygen and consider giving nitrates.
- Administer aspirin (300 mg PO stat unless there is a definite history of allergy) early, as this medication has been shown to considerably decrease the mortality rate in unstable coronary syndromes.
- Institute continuous cardiac monitoring and obtain IV access.
- Blood tests including troponins should be obtained.
- Take a focused history as all this is being implemented, as time is of the essence.
- An ECG should be done immediately.

In addition look for:

1 Impaired level of consciousness, presence of respiratory distress, diaphoresis, pallor and peripheral hypoperfusion.
2 Signs of cardiac failure. Oedema is relatively non-specific but a raised jugular venous pressure (JVP) or 3rd heart sound is very suggestive of heart failure. Signs of heart failure associated with an acute coronary syndrome place the patient in a high-risk group.
3 Peripheral pulses. Peripheral vascular disease is strongly associated with coronary artery disease. Compare pulses in both arms and measure the blood pressure in both arms if aortic dissection is possible. A difference of greater than 10 mmHg is significant but non-specific.
4 The praecordium. Clinical cardiomegaly is suggestive of left ventricular dysfunction. Similarly, a 3rd heart sound is usually abnormal. However, 4th heart sounds are common in the older population, particularly those with hypertension. Murmurs are frequently non-contributory, but features of severe aortic stenosis, mitral valve prolapse or hypertrophic cardiomyopathy may suggest a cause for chest pain. A mitral regurgitation

murmur that coincides with the patient's pain and disappears with relief of pain is highly significant for high-risk ischaemia. A pericardial rub is an important sign but may be transient or only heard in certain postures.

5 The chest. Symmetry of breath sounds and deviation of the trachea should be sought. Look also for localised chest signs, particularly crackles, rubs, features of consolidation and evidence of pleural effusion. Chest wall tenderness is non-specific and is seen in many patients with and without important cardiorespiratory disorders.
6 Abdominal examination should be done routinely, particularly to look for a non-cardiac cause for the patient's symptoms.
7 Limbs. Look for oedema, pulses and signs of deep venous thrombosis (DVT).

INVESTIGATIONS

Electrocardiogram (ECG)

All patients complaining of chest pain should have an ECG, and previous ECGs should be obtained for comparison. If the initial ECG is unhelpful and symptoms continue, a repeat ECG in 15 minutes may be diagnostic. The ECG helps to triage patients into high, intermediate and low risk for myocardial ischaemia and is crucial in the selection of treatment. ECG patterns are discussed in detail in Chapter 8, 'Clinical electrocardiography and arrhythmia management'.

Cardiac enzymes, markers

Rapid troponin assays (including point-of-care tests) have revolutionised the care of chest pain patients. Troponins are now considered the standard of care in this clinical setting. An elevated troponin confirms the diagnosis of an acute coronary syndrome and places the patient into a higher risk group. Two normal troponin values (on admission to the ED and 6 hours later) are very reassuring and may allow low-risk patients to be discharged safely from the ED, with appropriate follow-up.

Remember that chest pain can still be of cardiac origin despite a negative troponin, although the risk of an adverse outcome in this setting is less. If clinical suspicion remains, the safe approach is to keep the patient for further observation and appropriate consultation.

Other tests

A **chest X-ray** is a simple and important test in patients presenting with chest pain. As well as identifying pulmonary pathology, cardiomegaly and pulmonary venous congestion may also be found in patients with acute ischaemic syndromes.

Bedside **echocardiography** can be very helpful in the assessment of acute chest pain. Increasingly ultrasound machines are available in EDs and many emergency doctors are now skilled in echocardiography. Detection of left ventricular wall motion abnormalities strongly suggests important ischaemia or previous infarction. Echocardiography may also detect pericardial effusion, aortic dilation or even dissection, although transoesophageal echocardiography (TOE) is far superior for aortic abnormalities.

Some EDs have access to facilities for **early stress testing**. Patients presenting with chest pain who have negative troponins and non-diagnostic ECGs may undergo an exercise stress test with or without nuclear medicine myocardial perfusion scanning. Negative results improve the probability that the cause of the chest pain is not ischaemic.

CT scanning is under intense investigation as a modality to assess chest pain patients. Coronary artery calcification on CT does correlate with atherosclerosis, and recent advances in technology with rapid, multislice CT scans with contrast can accurately demonstrate coronary lesions. Recent studies suggest that a negative CT coronary angiogram can be used to identify low-risk patients who can be safely discharged from the ED. A definite role for this modality in the ED is still evolving.

DISPOSITION

Figure 6.1 summarises an integrated approach to the work-up and disposition of the chest pain patient. A combination of symptoms, examination findings, ECG results and cardiac markers often allows a precise diagnosis in many patients. Perhaps even more importantly, the risk of adverse outcomes can be assessed. High-risk features include ongoing chest pain, an abnormal ECG and elevated troponins (Box 6.2). These patients should be managed in a coronary care unit, whereas lower-risk patients might be admitted to a monitored ward bed or discharged for outpatient follow-up. Many organisations have published guidelines for the management of patients with chest pain (see 'Online resources').

Dyspnoea

Dyspnoea is the unpleasant awareness of the work of breathing. Dyspnoea may or may not be associated with hypoxaemia and tachypnoea. Accurate assessment of the dyspnoeic patient depends on

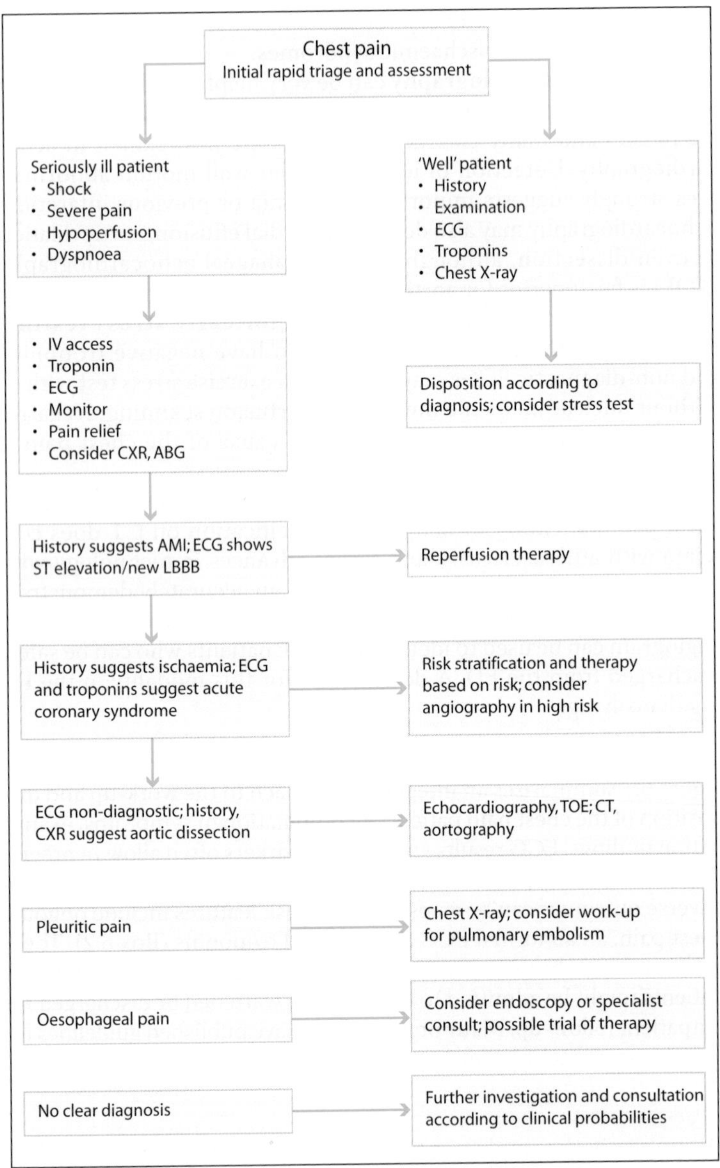

Figure 6.1 Chest pain algorithm

Box 6.2 Risk stratification in unstable angina

High risk features
- Prolonged and ongoing pain
- ECG changes, especially dynamic ST depression changes varying with pain
- Deep T wave inversion
- Elevated troponin
- Associated syncope, left ventricular failure, mitral regurgitation or gallop rhythm
- Haemodynamic instability

Intermediate risk
- Prolonged pain which has now resolved
- New-onset angina with limitation of activities of daily living
- More than 65 years old
- History of previous myocardial infarction or revascularisation procedure
- ECG normal or old Q waves, or minor ST/T changes only

Low risk features
- Angina of increased frequency, severity or at lower threshold
- New-onset angina beginning more than 2 weeks before presentation
- Normal ECG
- Negative troponin
- No high or intermediate risk features

history, physical examination and appropriate tests, especially the chest X-ray. Physical signs in the severely distressed, breathless patient may be difficult to interpret. Many patients with acute cardiogenic pulmonary oedema have prominent wheezing, but wheezing is also a cardinal physical finding in patients with airflow obstruction.

HISTORY

Important points in the history include:
- previous cardiorespiratory disease, and previous best exercise capacity
- paroxysmal nocturnal dyspnoea—seen in both asthma and left ventricular failure (LVF)
- orthopnoea—more specific for LVF
- cough and sputum production, and features such as fever or upper respiratory tract infection
- peripheral oedema
- history of atopy
- medications, especially a history of bronchodilator use
- risk factors for DVT.

PHYSICAL EXAMINATION

An immediate assessment is necessary to differentiate the critically ill patient from those who are less sick. Look for:

1 General appearance—sweating, depressed level of consciousness, extreme respiratory distress and efficacy of ventilatory effort. Immediate ventilatory support may be necessary.
2 The presence of stridor, an important clue in the diagnosis of upper airway obstruction.
3 Vital signs including respiratory rate, heart rate and oximetry. Pulsus paradoxus may be present in severe airflow obstruction.
4 Cardiac examination. The presence of a 3rd heart sound (gallop rhythm) and a raised jugular venous pulse are very suggestive of heart failure.
5 Respiratory examination. Important points include symmetry of chest movement, the presence of subcutaneous emphysema and focal signs in the chest

THE CHEST X-RAY (CXR)

Examination of a CXR is crucial in the assessment of the seriously ill patient with dyspnoea. Figure 6.2 summarises the interpretation of the CXR in the breathless patient. Recall that portable CXR machines have inherent technical limitations, in particular making assessment of heart size difficult.

OTHER TESTS

1 Arterial blood gases (ABGs). Indicated in all dyspnoeic patients to quantify the degree of hypoxaemia and demonstrate the presence of hypercarbia and acid–base abnormalities. A widened alveolar–arterial gradient may be a clue to subtle disorders such as pulmonary embolism; however, blood gas patterns are not specific for any disorder but do reflect the severity of the disease process.
2 ECG.
3 Spirometry. In patients who can cooperate, spirometry can diagnose and quantify airflow obstruction. Most modern electronic spirometers can display a flow–volume loop which can be helpful in the diagnosis of upper airway obstruction.
4 D-dimer. When combined with a clinical assessment of pre-test probability (e.g. using the Wells criteria), D-dimer can be helpful in the assessment of possible pulmonary embolism. A negative test in a patient with low pre-test probability makes pulmonary embolism unlikely. A positive test is non-specific. (*pto*)

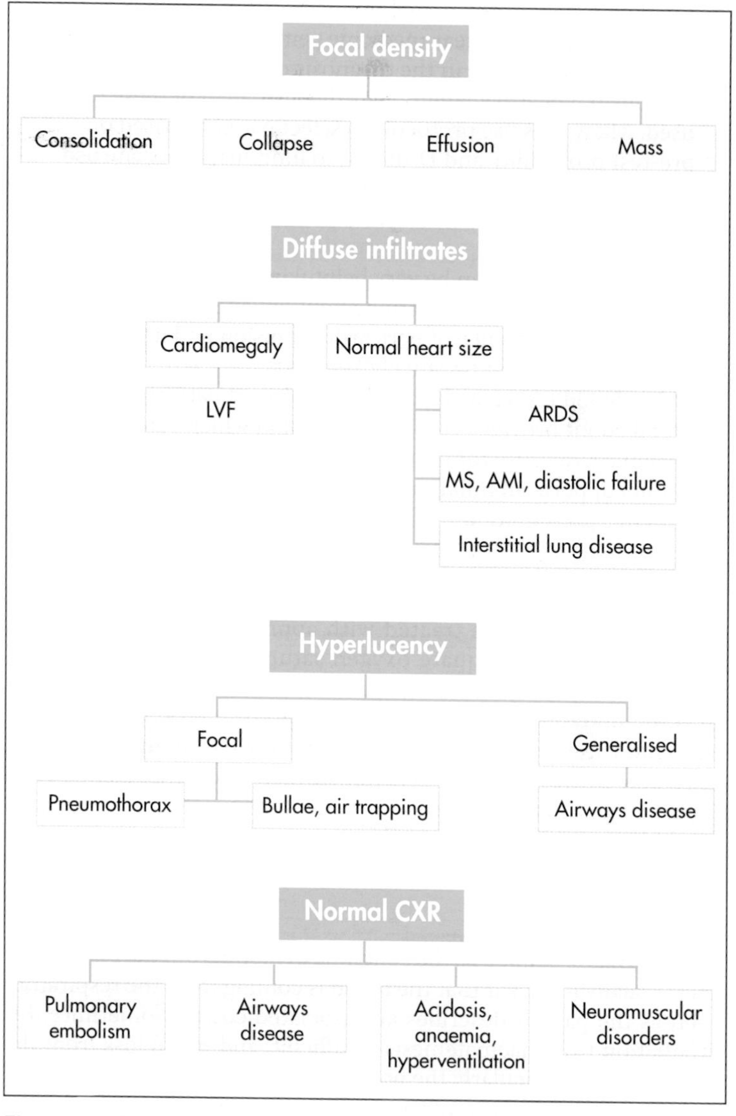

Figure 6.2 Chest X-ray interpretation in the breathless patient
AMI, acute myocardial infarction; ARDS, acute respiratory distress syndrome; LVF, left ventricular failure; MS, mitral stenosis

5 Imaging tests for pulmonary embolism. Both CT pulmonary angiography and nuclear medicine ventilation–perfusion lung scanning are valuable in the diagnosis of suspected pulmonary embolism. Local availability may dictate which of these tests is used. Many EDs use protocols to select patients, based on pre-test probability and D-dimer, to limit inappropriate use of these expensive scans. Recall the significant radiation dose associated with CT scanning and possible renal impact of IV contrast agents.
6 Echocardiography can be very helpful in the acutely breathless patient; important information about left and right ventricular function, the presence of pericardial effusion and important valvular disease can be quickly assessed.
7 Other blood tests may be helpful in selected patients. A full blood count provides crucial information which can rule out anaemia as a cause for dyspnoea, and an elevated white cell count supports an inflammatory or infective basis for the patient's presentation.

DISPOSITION AND MANAGEMENT

Disposition and management depend on the underlying cause. Hypoxaemia should be treated with appropriate oxygen therapy, aiming to achieve adequate oxygen saturation as measured with pulse oximetry. Carbon dioxide narcosis should be suspected in the seriously ill dyspnoeic patient with a depressed level of consciousness, and careful titration of oxygen therapy based on serial blood gases may be necessary. In general, correction of hypoxaemia is an important goal in these seriously ill patients. Non-invasive ventilation should be considered early in the distressed patient with impaired gas exchange.

Haemoptysis

Haemoptysis is defined as the coughing of blood from the respiratory tract. Usually it is clear that the blood is coming from the respiratory tract, as the patient describes an associated cough. Sometimes differentiation from haematemesis is difficult, and blood loss from the upper airway, particularly the nose, may be difficult to exclude.

Most haemoptysis is **minor**, and should prompt a search for the cause, usually starting with a chest X-ray. In a stable patient with minor haemoptysis, investigations may be commenced in the ED and continued as an outpatient.

Large-volume haemoptysis, defined as more than 600 mL in 24 hours, is life-threatening and frightening. It is often difficult for the patient to estimate the volume of blood loss. The immediate threat is not hypovolaemia, but hypoxaemia related to blood in the airways and lung parenchyma.

CAUSES OF HAEMOPTYSIS

- Cancer. This should always be suspected in a patient with a history of smoking. A clear chest X-ray does not rule out cancer but makes the diagnosis less likely; bronchoscopy is indicated in this setting. Massive haemoptysis is unusual in malignancy.
- Bronchiectasis. Massive bleeding can occur from abnormally dilated bronchial arteries in patients with longstanding bronchiectasis.
- Infections, particularly tuberculosis and other cavitatory lung diseases. Old cavitatory lung disease may be complicated by fungal colonisation (mycetoma), which is frequently associated with haemoptysis. Simple bronchitis may be associated with minor haemoptysis.
- Vascular disorders. Pulmonary embolism, mitral stenosis, arteriovenous malformations and aneurysms are all associated with haemoptysis of varying severity.
- Vasculitis. Systemic lupus erythematosus, Goodpasture's syndrome, granulomatosis with polyangiitis (formerly known as Wegener's granulomatosis) and other pulmonary vasculitides are associated with repeated haemoptysis, pulmonary parenchymal haemorrhage and an aggressive course.
- Other causes include anticoagulant therapy, coagulopathy and trauma.

In Australia the commoner causes of massive haemoptysis are old cavitatory lung disease, bronchiectasis and pulmonary vasculitis.

MANAGEMENT OF MASSIVE HAEMOPTYSIS

1. Assess oxygenation and the airway—urgent intubation may be necessary.
2. Arterial blood gases and appropriate oxygen therapy.
3. IV access and appropriate volume replacement.
4. Full blood count, cross-match and coagulation screen.
5. Urgent chest X-ray.
6. If there is unilateral disease and the affected side is known, nurse with the diseased lung down, to protect the healthy lung. (*pto*)

7 Bronchoscopy. This should be done with appropriate anaesthetic support; sometimes rigid bronchoscopy is necessary to provide better suction and maintenance of airway patency.
8 CT scan.
9 Urgent consultation with a thoracic surgeon.

Definitive management depends on the cause. Options include bronchoscopic techniques to control bleeding, angiography with embolisation of feeding arteries and thoracotomy with resection.

LESSER DEGREES OF HAEMOPTYSIS

Management depends on the cause, based on history, risk of malignancy and chest X-ray. If admission is not indicated, appropriate follow-up, perhaps for bronchoscopy, should be arranged.

Online resources

NSW Chest Pain Pathway
www.health.nsw.gov.au/policies/pd/2011/PD2011_037.html

Reference

Pope JH, Aufderheide TP, Ruthauser R et al (2000). Missed diagnosis of acute cardiac ischemia in the emergency department. N Englz J Med 342:1163–70.

Chapter 7
Acute coronary syndromes

Kevin Maruno and Paul Preisz

Assessing patients who may have an acute coronary syndrome (ACS) is a frequent and important part of the work performed in an emergency department. Patients most often present with 'typical' chest pain, dyspnoea, palpitations, syncope or pre-syncope. Some patients (particularly the elderly, diabetic or renal failure patients) may have atypical pain, or no pain, or just vague non-specific symptoms such as lethargy or deterioration in daily function. It is important to consider all presentations of an ACS, while also taking into consideration other life-threatening conditions.

Although many units now use a protocol approach, important alternative conditions need to be rapidly diagnosed. Some of these conditions may be immediately life-threatening, such as pulmonary embolism, aortic dissection, pneumothorax or severe pancreatitis, while others may be investigated and managed over time as an inpatient (e.g. pneumonia, cholelithiasis) or outpatient (e.g. musculoskeletal pain, gastro-oesophageal reflux disease). Alternative cardiac diagnoses (e.g. pericarditis) and non-cardiac diagnoses (e.g. peptic ulcer disease) as well as cardiac injury secondary to other illness (e.g. sepsis) should all be considered.

The acute coronary syndromes typically seen in the ED consist of the ST-elevation myocardial infarctions (STEMIs) and the second and larger group, non-ST-elevation acute coronary syndromes (NSTEACSs). NSTEACSs are then risk-stratified based on short-term prognosis as *high-risk, intermediate-risk and low-risk ACS* (Box 7.1).

Safe assessment

The patient should be assessed in a safe environment. Symptoms and signs which may indicate an ACS need to be identified as soon as possible so that treatment can be initiated to avoid or minimise myocardial damage and to avert the risk of life-threatening complications. A

Box 7.1 Initial patient assessment and stratification	
STEACS ST-elevation acute coronary syndrome *usually referred to as* **STEMI** (ST-elevation myocardial injury)	NSTEACS Non-ST-elevation acute coronary syndrome Stratify: • HIGH RISK • INTERMEDIATE RISK • LOW RISK

defibrillator must be immediately available with staff trained in its use.

- Assign a high priority at triage to patients who may have an ACS.
- Provide ECG monitoring and supplemental oxygen (if SaO_2 is less than 94% on room air) and insert an intravenous cannula as soon as possible.
- Send blood samples for testing and provide analgesia (nitrates and/or morphine) and, unless contraindicated, give oral aspirin (300 mg).
- An ECG should be performed and reviewed on presentation (within 10 minutes of arrival) to look for arrhythmias and for diagnostic changes related to acute coronary artery occlusion, most importantly **STEMI**. If no STEMI is present, then **NSTEAC** and alternative diagnoses are considered.

A chest pain pathway is given in Figure 7.1 at the end of the chapter.

DIAGNOSING ACUTE CORONARY SYNDROMES

History and examination

Typical presentations of ACS involve chest discomfort at rest or for prolonged periods (prolonged is defined as >10 minutes, not relieved by sublingual nitrates) or recurrent chest discomfort or discomfort associated with syncope or acute heart failure.

Some important points of immediate history include the ***time of onset of pain***, the character or quality of the pain, and exertion-related pain. Radiation of pain to arms and shoulder is particularly suggestive.

Risk factors and comorbidities, allergies, and contraindications to treatments should also be documented. The main cardiac risk factors include diabetes, hypertension, hyperlipidaemia, smoking, chronic renal disease and family history of premature heart disease. Note that although cardiac risk factors increase the likelihood of disease (particularly in those under 40), their absence does not exclude the diagnoses. Patients of Aboriginal descent are particularly at risk.

Physical examination is directed towards identifying signs of complications and comorbidities of ACS and finding alternative diagnoses. There may be tachycardia or bradycardia, hyper- or hypotension, sweating, nausea or evidence of heart failure (dyspnoea, basal crepitations, 3rd heart sound, poor peripheral perfusion). ***Importantly, there may be no specific physical findings in many patients with ACS.***

Cardiac myonecrosis is demonstrated by increased levels of cardiac biomarkers (such as troponins), and can occur in ACS with or without ECG changes. The testing interval to 'rule out' myocardial infarction may be reduced to 3 hours from presentation, with a second sample at least 6 hours after symptom onset (if a high-sensitivity troponin is used). Other protocols include the measurement of a single high-sensitivity troponin T level 4 or more hours from the onset of pain.

The indication for initial urgent reperfusion therapy is clinical presentation consistent with ACS and acute ECG change. This is defined as persistent ST-segment elevation of ≥1 mm in two contiguous limb leads, ST-segment elevation of ≥2 mm in two contiguous chest leads or new left bundle branch block (LBBB) pattern.

Investigation

Initial investigation

When STEMI is diagnosed on clinical and ECG criteria, revascularisation therapy is time-critical so there should be no delays waiting for investigations prior to revascularisation. In other circumstances, the tests shown in Table 7.1 should be obtained.

Management of STEMI

1 **Patients presenting within 12 hours with STEMI should have urgent time-critical reperfusion** (PCI or fibrinolysis)
   - When PCI (percutaneous coronary intervention) can be commenced without undue delay, this is the treatment of choice based on current evidence. The maximum acceptable delay is 120 minutes to balloon inflation (including transfer times), or 60 minutes if within 1 hour of symptom onset. The benefits of PCI over thrombolysis are still present up to 12 hours after the onset of symptoms if PCI can be performed within these time limits.
   - PCI is also the preferred treatment for *unstable patients* or those with *ongoing symptoms* or evidence of *failed fibrinolytic therapy* on ECG, i.e. 'rescue PCI'. This is seen as persistent (>50% of initial) ST elevation 90 minutes after administration

Table 7.1 Tests to aid in the diagnosis and stratification of patients with ACS*

Test	Comment
Full blood count	Anaemia or polycythaemia may need treatment, baseline platelet count (particularly if heparin is to be used)
Coagulation PT and APTT	Guides anticoagulant therapy
Serum chemistry	Hypokalaemia increases the risk of arrhythmia Hypomagnesaemia may be present if patient taking some diuretics or has liver/renal disease
Renal function	Creatinine (and eGFR calculation). Kidney disease is a risk factor for high- and intermediate-risk ACS Drug dosage may require adjustment if renal impairment present (e.g. heparin, sotalol)
Troponin I or T**	May take hours to rise, 2 or more measurements over time may be required (delta change); remains elevated 5–14 days Some high-sensitivity assays may be interpreted in as little 4 hours from the onset of pain
Serum lipids	Initiating treatment of hyperlipidaemia within the first few days (e.g. with statins) may be required
Blood glucose	Diabetes may be undiagnosed (especially mild NIDDM); close control of blood glucose levels improves outcomes
Chest X-ray (CXR)	May show heart failure, cardiomegaly. Do not delay urgent treatment to obtain a CXR. Do not send potentially unstable patient out of resuscitation monitoring area for CXR

APTT, activated partial thromboplastin time; eGFR, estimated glomerular filtration rate; NIDDM, non-insulin-dependent diabetes mellitus; PT, prothrombin time.
*Additional tests such as high-sensitivity C-reactive protein (CRP) and B-type natriuretic protein (BNP) or Pro-BNP are still being evaluated. In some settings bedside cardiac echocardiography can be valuable as it may be able to provide information on wall motion (myocardial ischaemia or infarction), ejection fraction (heart failure, systolic or diastolic dysfunction), valvular disease (aortic stenosis, acute mitral valve chordae disruption), free wall rupture, aortic or pericardial disease. An alternative diagnosis of pulmonary embolism can sometimes be made when significant right heart abnormality is seen on echo. Drug screening (cocaine, amphetamines) may be relevant.
**Elevated or rising troponin T and I measurements indicate myocardial damage and are predictors of increased risk of cardiac mortality. It may take several hours for troponin levels to rise and a series of tests may be required. Troponin may sometimes also be elevated in patients with heart failure, tachycardia, myocarditis, pericarditis, renal failure or other non-ischaemic cardiac injury.

of the agent. Fibrinolysis can be repeated if PCI is not available; however, benefit may be gained from early routine PCI regardless of success of pharmacological reperfusion.
— Early coronary artery bypass graft (CABG) surgery may also be considered for some patients, especially if they have anatomy that is unsuitable for stenting or have associated cardiogenic shock, valve injury or other structural complications.
— Patients who decline PCI or have contrast allergy or other contraindications to PCI should be considered for fibrinolysis. Fibrin-specific bolus agents such as tenecteplase or reteplase are now the usual choices, although streptokinase can be used unless the patient is an Indigenous Australian or Torres Strait Islander or has received streptokinase before.
— Contraindications to fibrinolysis are given below.

2 **Give anti-platelet drugs + antithrombotic drug**
Anti-platelet drugs
— Give aspirin and clopidogrel.
— The use of a potent oral antiplatelet agent (e.g. prasugrel or ticagrelor) should be considered as an alternative to clopidogrel for subgroups at high risk of recurrent ischaemic events (e.g. those with diabetes, stent thrombosis, recurrent events on clopidogrel or a high burden of disease on angiography). This may be less appropriate in patients at increased risk of bleeding (e.g. those aged >75, those with prior stroke or TIA and those with low bodyweight).
— Glycoprotein IIb/IIIa inhibitors (e.g. abciximab) are of most benefit in patients undergoing PCI, and recommended in those with recurrent ischaemia on standard medical therapy.
— *Note:* Patients who have been given clopidogrel can still have urgent CABG surgery although this is not ideal.
Antithrombotic drugs
— Give heparin as unfractionated IV heparin or subcutaneous enoxaparin (but avoid changing from one to the other).
— Among patients with STEMI undergoing primary PCI, the use of bivalirudin can be considered as an alternative to heparin and glycoprotein IIb/IIIa inhibitors.
— Patients having fibrinolysis should also receive antithrombotics (this is optional if the fibrinolytic used is streptokinase). (*pto*)

Table 7.2 **Additional treatment in STEMI**

Therapy	Dose	Comments
Oxygen	6 L (non-rebreather)	All patients when SaO_2 < 94% (room air) Issues (uncommon) with patients retaining CO_2
Aspirin	300 mg PO (soluble or rapidly absorbable)	True allergy or bleeding risks may contraindicate
Nitrates	Sublingual or spray or titrated IV	Headache, flushing, hypotension may occur with higher doses
Morphine	2.5–5.0 mg IV increments	Nausea, decreased LOC and ventilation, hypotension
Metoprolol	2.5–5.0 mg IV increments	Asthma, bradycardia, heart block, other side effects and contraindications
Clopidogrel	600 mg PO loading	Increased bleeding risk
Heparin	Low-molecular-weight or unfractionated protocols	Bleeding risk, HITS
Tenecteplase	Single dose based on body weight; 5 mg = 1000 IU < 60 kg: 30 mg 60–69 kg: 35 mg 70–79 kg: 40 mg 80–89 kg: 45 mg ≥ 90 kg: 50 mg	Bolus dosing over 5 seconds
Abciximab	IV protocol	Not with fibrinolytics (or at least reduce dose)
Frusemide	40–80 mg IV	Used when LVF present Higher doses needed if renal impairment present

HITS, heparin-induced thrombocytopenia syndrome; LVF, left ventricular failure; LOC, level of consciousness

3 **Give beta-blockers**
Beta-blockers (e.g. metoprolol 25–50 mg PO) are given unless contraindicated.

CONTRAINDICATIONS TO FIBRINOLYSIS

Absolute—acute haemorrhage is likely to cause death or severe disability

Current—

Significant uncontrollable bleeding or major bleeding diathesis

Suspected aortic dissection

Past history—

Any past proven intracranial haemorrhage

Known structural cerebral vascular lesion

Intracranial neoplasm

Major head injury within the past 3 months

Ischaemic stroke within the past 3 months

Relative—clinical judgment is required to gauge the relative risk, particularly if the alternative of PCI may be possible, even with some delay

Current—

Pregnancy

Anticoagulant therapy

Non-compressible vessel puncture

Prolonged traumatic CPR

Active peptic ulcer

Uncontrollable hypertension (systolic pressure >180 mmHg or diastolic pressure >110 mmHg)

Major surgery within the past 3 weeks

Significant internal bleeding within the past 4 weeks

Past history—

Ischaemic stroke more than 3 months ago, dementia, other intracranial abnormality that is not an absolute contraindication

Long-term poorly controlled hypertension

Editorial Comment

In general, after initial high-flow oxygen therapy further oxygen is dictated to maintain the oxygenation (SaO_2 > 90%) while avoiding further hyperoxia exposure.

ADJUNCTIVE TREATMENTS IN ACS

Reperfusion confers outcome benefit, particularly the combination of aspirin and PCI or fibrinolysis. Additional therapies also convey incremental improvement, although this is not as marked and will add to the risk of adverse events. Consider methods to reduce bleeding risk, e.g. titrate antithrombotic agents to optimal dose for weight and renal function.

Stratifying ACS without diagnostic ECG changes: NSTEACS patients

Risk stratification is now a common and useful method for guiding investigations and subsequent management in NSTEACS. History, examination and investigation direct stratification, and management based on risk group should proceed rapidly with early involvement of senior staff.

HIGH-RISK ACS

Clinical presentation suggests ACS, and any one of the following is positive:

History—

- History of LVF (or current evidence of chronic LVF)
- Chronic renal failure + typical ACS symptoms
- Diabetes + typical ACS symptoms
- Previous PCI or CABG < 6 months ago

Current presentation—

- Symptoms repetitive or prolonged (>10 minutes) and still present
- Haemodynamic compromise (systolic BP < 90 mmHg), new mitral regurgitation
- Syncope
- Elevated troponin

ECG—

- Persistent or dynamic ECG changes
- ST depression >+0.5 mm
- New T wave inversion
- Transient T wave inversion ≥ 2 mm in 2 or more contiguous leads
- Sustained VT

INTERMEDIATE-RISK ACS

Clinical presentation suggests ACS, there are no high-risk features but any one of the following is positive:

History—

- Age > 65 years
- Previous heart disease
- Chronic renal failure + atypical ACS symptoms
- Diabetes + atypical ACS symptoms
- Previous PCI or CABG >6 months ago

Any 2 or more of the following:

Family history
Hypertension
Active smoking
Hyperlipidaemia

Current presentation—

Symptoms began within the past 48 hours, occurred at rest or were repetitive or prolonged (>10 minutes)

ECG—

ECG is not normal and has changed from previous pain-free ECG but does not contain high-risk changes.

LOW-RISK ACS

Clinical presentation suggests ACS, but no high or intermediate risk features. ECG unchanged from usual for patient.

Management of NSTEACS

FOR ALL PATIENTS WITH NSTEACS

- Risk should be stratified as HIGH-, INTERMEDIATE- or LOW-risk ACS
- Initially give aspirin unless contraindicated
- All patients are treated with analgesia (nitrates, morphine) as required and oxygen to keep $SaO_2 \geq 94\%$

HIGH-RISK ACS PATIENTS

1. Anti-platelet drugs, e.g. aspirin plus clopidogrel
2. Antithrombotic drugs, e.g. unfractionated heparin or subcutaneous enoxaparin
3. Beta-blockers should be given unless contraindicated
4. Arrangements should be made for admission and coronary angiography except in those with severe comorbidities.

INTERMEDIATE-RISK ACS PATIENTS

1. Anti-platelet drugs, e.g. aspirin alone
2. Accelerated diagnostic evaluation either as an inpatient or, if considered medically safe and logistically possible, as an outpatient within 72 hours. Diagnostic and provocation tests include CTCA (CT coronary angiography), stress echo, nuclear perfusion scans (sestamibi) and exercise stress tests.

LOW-RISK ACS PATIENTS

After an appropriate period of observation and assessment, may be discharged for outpatient follow up if negative biomarkers, no high-risk ECG changes, resolved pain.

Additional management (STEMI and NSTEACS)

- Optimise the heart rate. Significant bradycardia or tachycardia—associated with poor cardiac output (e.g. hypotension, syncope/ pre-syncope heart failure or oliguria)—requires treatment with appropriate antiarrhythmics or pacing.
- Analgesia with nitrates and/or morphine should be provided as needed.
- Hypotension may require careful IV fluid volume optimisation, titration of therapeutic drugs and, in some patients, inotropes. Hypertension may resolve with analgesia or beta-blockers when appropriate but, rarely, if unresponsive consider potent agents (diazoxide, sodium nitroprusside) with close monitoring.
- Treat heart failure, if present, with diuretics, angiotensin-converting enzyme (ACE) inhibitors and other standard therapy (BiPAP).
- Medical therapy (usually a statin) is now recommended for most patients with ischaemic heart disease unless contraindicated.
- If being discharged, ensure patients diagnosed with ACS have begun an appropriate medication regimen, including aspirin (with clopidogrel in some patients), a beta-blocker, ACE inhibitor, statin and/or other treatment as required.
- Provide patients with support and advice to address the risk factors at a suitable time. A chest pain management plan is often appropriate. For all patients and their families, consider the level of social support and provide assistance for those at risk through referral to cardiac, rehabilitation and other services (e.g. social work, drug and alcohol misuse clinic). Consider patient support groups.

Cocaine-induced chest pain

Although only a minority of patients (less than 6%) with chest pain associated with cocaine use will have proven cardiac myonecrosis, cocaine (a vasoconstrictor) has multiple effects that can contribute to the development of myocardial ischaemia hours or days after ingestion. Even small doses have been associated with vasoconstriction of coronary arteries, which may be more accentuated in patients with pre-existing coronary artery disease. Cocaine users have been shown to have accelerated atherosclerosis as well as elevated levels of CRP, von Willebrand factor and fibrinogen. Anterior and inferior infarctions are equally likely and most are non-Q wave. Initial typical ischaemic ECG changes are relatively uncommon. In general, beta-blockers should be avoided in these patients and benzodiazepines are often used. Mortality overall is relatively low.

Patient transfer

Patients in a facility without specialist cardiology services and PCI facilities who have been diagnosed with STEMI and treated with fibrinolysis should be transferred to an appropriate tertiary cardiology unit. Those with a large area of at-risk myocardium, poor left ventricular function or renal failure should be transferred urgently. Adjunctive reperfusion therapies should be commenced before transfer.

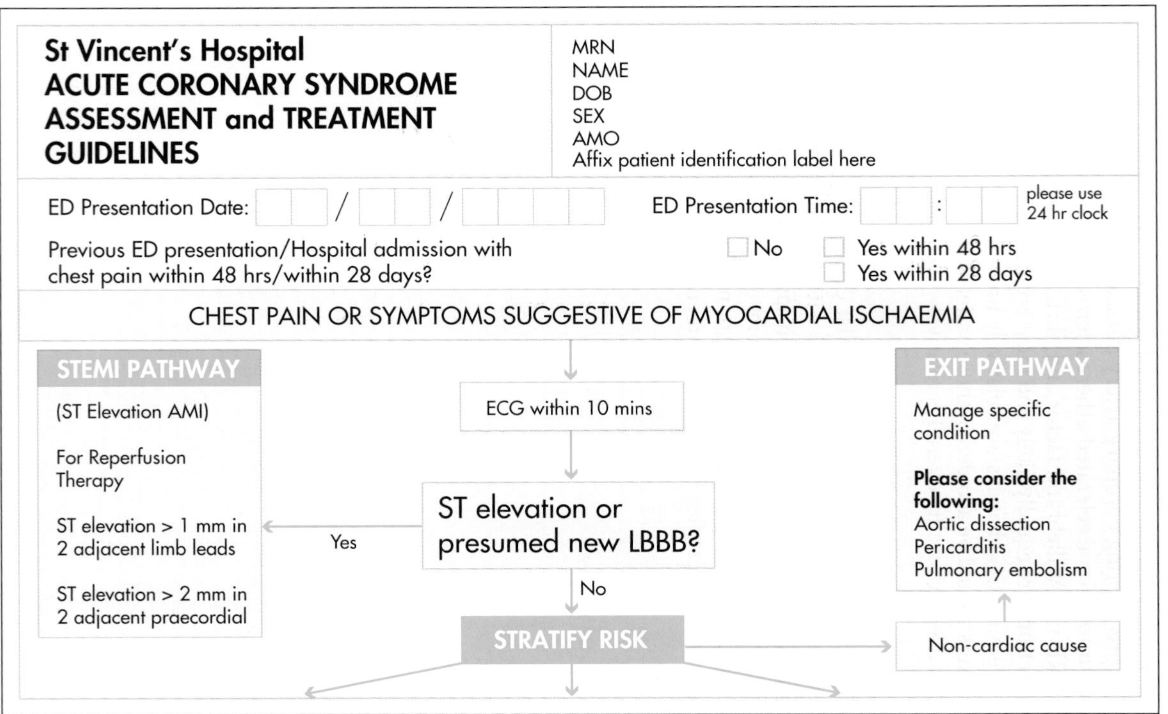
St Vincent's Hospital
ACUTE CORONARY SYNDROME ASSESSMENT and TREATMENT GUIDELINES

MRN
NAME
DOB
SEX
AMO
Affix patient identification label here

ED Presentation Date: [ ][ ] / [ ][ ] / [ ][ ][ ][ ]

ED Presentation Time: [ ][ ] : [ ][ ] please use 24 hr clock

Previous ED presentation/Hospital admission with chest pain within 48 hrs/within 28 days? ☐ No ☐ Yes within 48 hrs ☐ Yes within 28 days

CHEST PAIN OR SYMPTOMS SUGGESTIVE OF MYOCARDIAL ISCHAEMIA

ECG within 10 mins

ST elevation or presumed new LBBB?

Yes → STEMI PATHWAY

No → STRATIFY RISK

STEMI PATHWAY

(ST Elevation AMI)

For Reperfusion Therapy

ST elevation > 1 mm in 2 adjacent limb leads

ST elevation > 2 mm in 2 adjacent praecordial

EXIT PATHWAY

Manage specific condition

Please consider the following:
Aortic dissection
Pericarditis
Pulmonary embolism

Non-cardiac cause

Figure 7.1a Chest pain pathway

HIGH RISK	INTERMEDIATE RISK (no high risk features)	LOW RISK (no high or intermediate risk features)
Presentation with clinical features consistent with ACS and one or more risk features		
☐ Repetitive or prolonged > 10 mins ongoing chest pain/discomfort	☐ Chest pain or discomfort within past 48 hrs that occurred at rest or was repetitive or prolonged (but currently resolved)	☐ Onset of symptoms of angina within the last month
☐ Elevation of at least one cardiac biomarker (troponin)	☐ Age > 65 years	☐ Worsening in severity or frequency of angina
☐ Persistent or dynamic ST depression ≥ 0.5 mm or new T wave inversion ≥2 mm	☐ Known IHD: Prior MI with LVEF ≥40% or known coronary lesion > 50% stenosed	☐ Lowering in Anginal threshold
☐ Transient ST segment elevation ≥ 0.5 mm in more than 2 contiguous leads	☐ No high risk ECG changes	
☐ Haemodynamic compromise systolic BP < 90 mmHg, cool peripheries, diaphoresis, and/or new onset mitral regurgitation	☐ 2 or more of known hypertension, family history, active smoking, hyperlipidaemia	
☐ Sustained Ventricular Tachycardia	☐ Presence of known diabetes (with atypical symptoms of ACS)	
☐ LV Systolic dysfunction LVEF < 40%	☐ Chronic kidney disease; estimated GFR < 60 mL/min (with atypical symptoms of ACS)	
☐ Syncope		
☐ Chronic kidney disease estimated GFR < 60 mL/min with typical symptoms of ACS	☐ Prior aspirin use	
☐ Prior PCI within 6 months or prior CABG surgery		
☐ Presence of known diabetes (with typical symptoms of ACS)		
Recommended management on reverse page		
This tool is intended as a guideline for clinicians to provide quality patient care. It is not intended, nor should it replace, individual clinical judgement		

Figure 7.1b Chest pain pathway

St Vincent's Hospital
EMERGENCY
DEPARTMENT

MRN
NAME
DOB
SEX
AMO
Affix patient identification label here

GENERAL MANAGEMENT (Tick all relevant boxes below)

HIGH/INTERMEDIATE

- ☐ ECG baseline/Repeat ECG 6 hrs post onset of symptoms and if pain recurs
- ☐ Routine bloods (initial Troponin I + 6 hr Troponin (post onset of symptoms)) ☐ Yes ☐ No
- ☐ BSL
- ☐ Continuous cardiac monitoring — Troponin elevated ☐ Yes ☐ No
- ☐ IVC
- ☐ Pain relief ☐ SL Anginine ☐ IV GTN ☐ IV Morphine
- ☐ O_2 therapy $SaO_2 > 96\%$
- ☐ Aspirin 300 mg ☐ no ☐ Clinical indication ______
- ☐ Chest X-ray
- ☐ All cases to be discussed with senior medical officer

Recommended Management **Refer to local Drug Protocols** (tick if patient has taken prior to presentation)

Figure 7.1c Chest pain pathway

LOW RISK PATHWAY

HIGH RISK

Antiplatelet therapy

- ☐ Aspirin 300 mg
- ☐ No ☐ Clinical indication ____________
- ☐ Clopidogrel 600 mg then 75 mg dly (refer to protocol) } D/W Cardiologist
- ☐ Tirofiban
- ☐ Combination

Beta-blocker

- ☐ Yes Metoprolol (IV loading dose 5 mg. Repeat after 5 mins to total 10–15 mg) or
- ☐ No oral 25–50 mg bd
- ☐ Clinical indication ____________

Antithrombotic (Heparin)

- ☐ No
- ☐ Clinical indication ____________
- ☐ Unfractionated
- ☐ Enoxaparin (dose: 1 mg/kg bd)
- ☐ Warfarin

☐ **Refer to Cardiology**

team for admission and further management and consideration for early cath lab referral

INTERMEDIATE RISK

Antiplatelet therapy

- ☐ Aspirin 300 mg
- ☐ No ☐ Clinical indication ____________
- ☐ Clopidogrel 600 mg then 75 mg dly (D/W cardiologist)

☐ **Cardiac stress test**

Following neg troponin initial and at 6 hrs with no new ECG changes.
6 hr troponin can be taken on SSCU if first troponin negative.
Contact cardiac consultant or Registrar
Sestamibi ext 2445
(need to be caffeine free 24 hrs prior to Sestamibi)

Restratify to:

- ☐ **High risk**
  If positive stress test
- ☐ **Low risk**
  If negative stress test
- ☐ **Admit**
- ☐ **Discharge**

According to high risk/low risk protocol

LOW RISK

Antiplatelet therapy

- ☐ Aspirin 300 mg
- ☐ No ☐ Clinical indication ____________

If unlikely cardiac cause

consider alternative diagnosis exit pathway ☐

If low risk ACS

- ☐ Follow up GP within 3 days of discharge
- ☐ Stress test within 2 weeks of discharge
- ☐ Cardiology review within 2 weeks of discharge
- ☐ Consider discharge on Aspirin (discuss with SMO)
- ☐ Discharge

Figure 7.1d Chest pain pathway

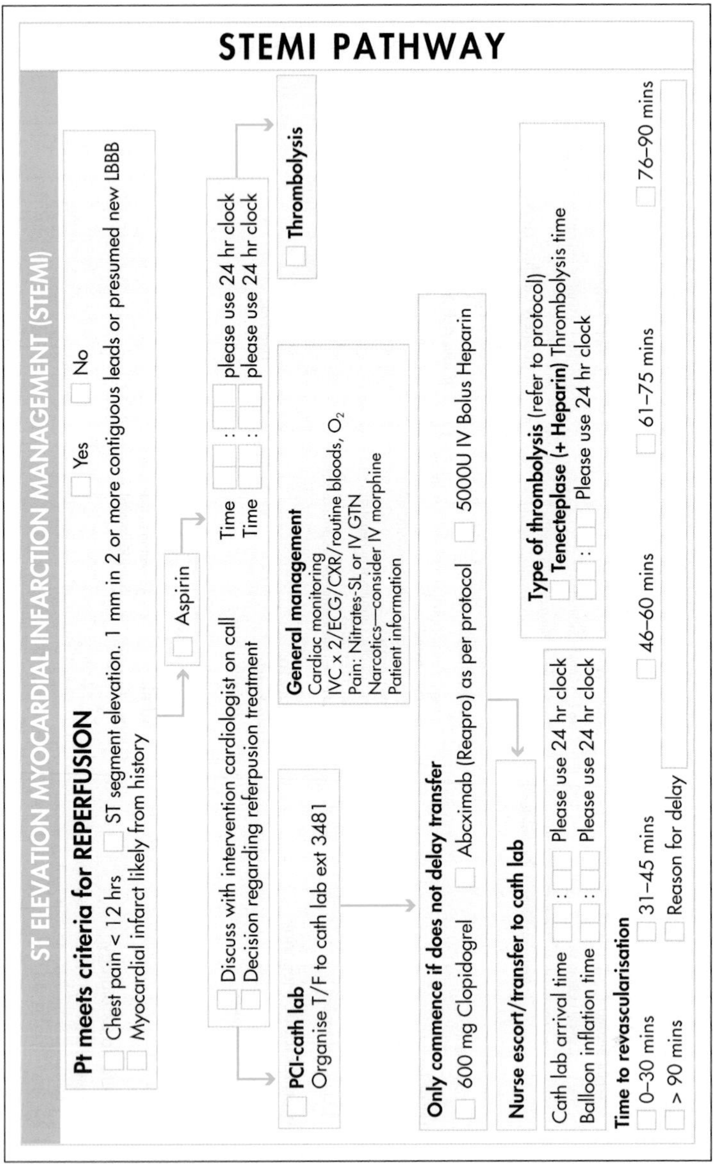

STEMI PATHWAY

ST ELEVATION MYOCARDIAL INFARCTION MANAGEMENT (STEMI)

Pt meets criteria for REPERFUSION ☐ Yes ☐ No

☐ Chest pain < 12 hrs ☐ ST segment elevation. 1 mm in 2 or more contiguous leads or presumed new LBBB
☐ Myocardial infarct likely from history

→ ☐ Aspirin

☐ Discuss with intervention cardiologist on call — Time ☐☐ : ☐☐ please use 24 hr clock
☐ Decision regarding referpusion treatment — Time ☐☐ : ☐☐ please use 24 hr clock

☐ **PCI-cath lab**
Organise T/F to cath lab ext 3481

General management
Cardiac monitoring
IVC x 2/ECG/CXR/routine bloods, O_2
Pain: Nitrates-SL or IV GTN
Narcotics—consider IV morphine
Patient information

☐ **Thrombolysis**

Only commence if does not delay transfer
☐ 600 mg Clopidogrel ☐ Abcximab (Reapro) as per protocol ☐ 5000U IV Bolus Heparin

Nurse escort/transfer to cath lab

Cath lab arrival time ☐☐ : ☐☐ Please use 24 hr clock
Balloon inflation time ☐☐ : ☐☐ Please use 24 hr clock

Type of thrombolysis (refer to protocol)
☐ **Tenecteplase (+ Heparin)** Thrombolysis time
☐☐ : ☐☐ Please use 24 hr clock

Time to revascularisation
☐ 0–30 mins ☐ 31–45 mins ☐ 46–60 mins ☐ 61–75 mins ☐ 76–90 mins
☐ > 90 mins ☐ Reason for delay

Figure 7.1e Chest pain pathway

Chapter 8
Clinical electrocardiography and arrhythmia management

Allen Yuen, Carmel Crock, Kevin Maruno and Paul Preisz

This chapter examines the clinical use of the ECG, one of the most important diagnostic tools in an emergency department. It must be stressed, however, that the ECG may appear normal, even in the presence of severe cardiac disease.

The reader should have knowledge of basic cardiac electrophysiology and anatomy, which will help in diagnosing and localising lesions from the ECG.

Indications

ECGs are indicated:

- early, to assist in diagnosis and treatment of potentially life-threatening disorders
- routinely, as part of cardiac assessment.

They should be performed in all cases of chest pain, upper abdominal pain, dyspnoea, collapse, arrest, palpitations, syncope, dizziness, non-traumatic loss of consciousness and shock; also in any patient with a history of hypertension, fluid or electrolyte imbalance, drug overdose or other conditions that may affect the heart.

ECG interpretation

This is most usefully done in the context of the presenting symptoms and signs, which fall into three main groups:

1. chest and upper abdominal pain, dyspnoea, shock
2. collapse, palpitations, syncope, dizziness, altered consciousness
3. electrolyte disturbances, drug overdose, environmental emergencies.

The ECG should be examined for rate, rhythm, P wave, PR interval, QRS morphology and axis, ST–T segment, T wave and QT interval.

With chest pain, particular attention is paid to the ST–T segment and Q waves. The underlying lesions may be determined by ECG pattern recognition. It is useful to have a previous ECG for comparison, since any changes will have more significance.

1 CHEST AND UPPER ABDOMINAL PAIN, DYSPNOEA, SHOCK

History and examination are the mainstays of assessment, with the ECG playing a complementary role. The main conditions requiring early diagnosis are acute myocardial infarction (AMI), unstable angina, aortic dissection and pulmonary embolism (PE).

Myocardial infarction

Note that the initial ECG may be normal in about half of patients with AMI.

The earliest change is ST elevation, which may occur within 30 minutes of onset of pain, and is the basis upon which a decision regarding thrombolysis or angioplasty is made.

ST elevation

- ST elevation ≥ 1 mm in LI and aVL suggests an inferior AMI (Figure 8.1), usually due to occlusion of the circumflex artery.
- ST elevation ≥ 1 mm in LII, III and aVF suggests inferior AMI, usually due to occlusion of the right coronary artery; in some cases, the left coronary system may be the site of occlusion, if the left coronary artery (LCA) is 'dominant'.
- ST elevation ≥ 2 mm in chest leads suggests anterior or anteroseptal (if only in V_1–V_3) AMI, which occurs with occlusion of the left main coronary or its branches.

If a coronary thrombus is treated early with thrombolysis or angioplasty, the ST elevation can regress and further myocardial damage may be prevented. It is therefore vital that the cardiology unit is notified at the first moment a diagnosis of suspected AMI is made, usually on the basis of a history of chest pain and the early ST–T wave changes described above.

Normal 'high ST-take-off' in anterior chest leads can confuse the diagnosis when the chest pain is atypical, but it is better to err in suspecting an acute cardiac event than to clear the patient when in doubt. Consult with an emergency doctor, cardiologist or registrar.

ST depression

ST depression > 2 mm in V_1 may indicate a posterior infarct, and this may be confirmed in ECG leads $V_{7,8,9}$. $V_{1,2}$ will also have a prominent R wave and tall T waves. Posterior infarcts are usually caused by occlusion of the right coronary artery (RCA). The RCA also supplies the sinoatrial (SA) and atrioventricular (AV) nodes and the bundle of His. Occlusion of the RCA is associated with potentially serious bradyarrhythmias.

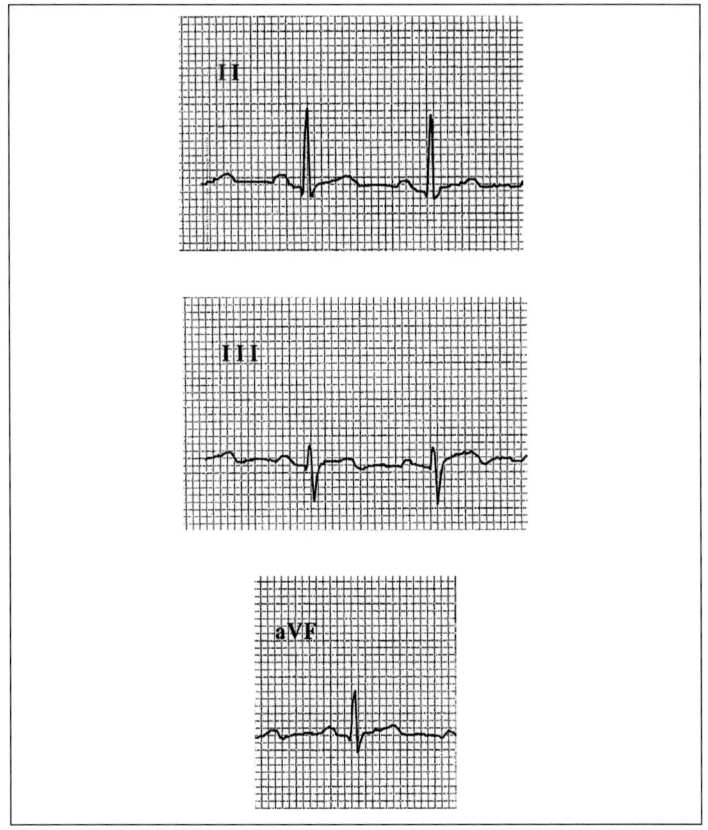

Figure 8.1 Inferior AMI, earliest changes: minimal ST elevation in leads II, III, aVF

Minor ST or Q wave changes in V_1 with signs of right ventricular failure, e.g. elevated jugular venous pressure (JVP), may point to a right ventricular infarct: right ventricular leads $RV_{3,4,5}$ may show characteristically slight ST elevation.

Q waves

- Q waves > 2 mm, > 40 ms follow in those leads showing ST elevation, if the infarct evolves (Table 8.1). They may appear within the first hour or, more commonly, within 2–6 hours (Figure 8.2). Differentiate from non-pathological septal Q waves in LI, LII, aVF or V_5,V_6, which are small (< 2 mm) and narrow.

Table 8.1 Infarct localisation—the ECG pattern distribution (early ST elevation, later Q waves)—will help to localise the site of infarction, and the usual coronary artery occluded

ECG pattern distribution	Site	Infarct-related artery
I, aVL	Lateral	Circumflex
II, III, aVF	Inferior	Right coronary, circumflex
V_2–V_4	Anterior	Left anterior descending (LAD)
V_1, V_2 (large R, ↓ ST)	Posterior	Right coronary

- A non-pathological Q wave can occur in LIII; it is narrow, < 2 mm and less than one-third the height of the QRS complex, and may disappear during deep inspiration. A small Q wave in LIII is significant if associated with one in LII.
- Sometimes Q waves do not develop, but AMI can still be suspected if there are small R waves with 'lack of progression of R waves' across the anterior leads (normally the R wave increases in amplitude from V_2 to V_4). These infarcts are often associated with inverted T waves.
- Non-Q AMI refers to subendocardial infarcts. Up to 40% of infarcts are not transmural, but they predispose to reinfarction. Blood should be sent for cardiac enzymes on arrival of the patient with chest pain so that, where there is no ECG evidence of AMI, the diagnosis is not missed.

R wave

A prominent R wave in V_1, and often V_2, suggests a posterior infarct, as well as incomplete right bundle branch block (RBBB), right ventricular hypertrophy (RVH) or left accessory pathway.

T waves

Hyperacute peaked T waves in V leads may be the only sign of AMI; they may occur in hyperkalaemia or without a known cause.

Left bundle branch block (LBBB)

New LBBB, with chest pain, indicates AMI. The location may be diagnosed by inspecting the affected leads to see whether there is concordance of ST segments with QRS complexes (in non-AMI LBBB the ST segments are discordant with the QRS, i.e. they point in opposite directions).

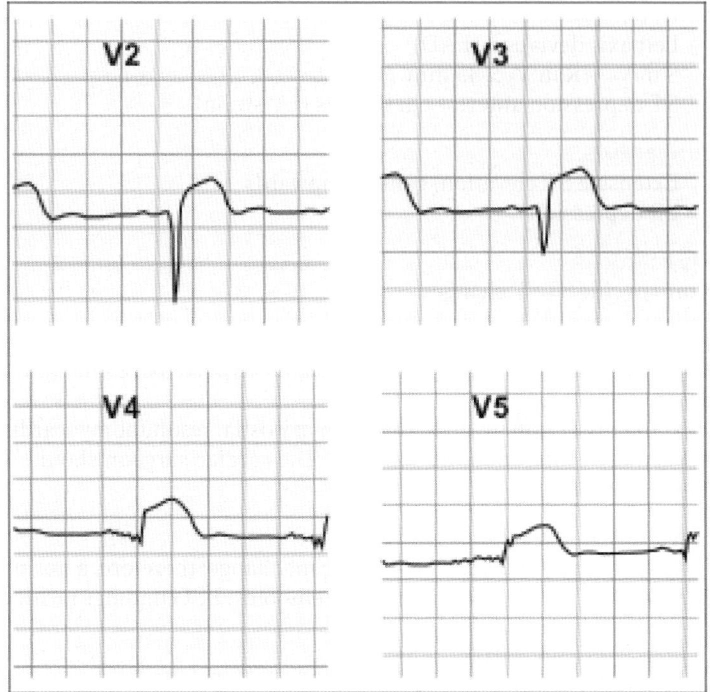

Figure 8.2 Anterior AMI, later changes: Q waves, prominent coved ST elevation V_2–V_5

In LBBB, AMI is present if:

- the QRS is upright and the ST is elevated > 5 mm
- the QRS is depressed and the ST is also depressed
- there are Q waves in LI and aVL, which indicate a lateral AMI.

Right bundle branch block (RBBB)

RBBB does not mask AMI, as ST elevation does not occur in non-AMI RBBB.

Unstable angina, acute coronary syndrome, acute ischaemia

The ECG may be normal, but acute ischaemia is confirmed by 2 mm or more ST depression in anterior or standard leads. This may be induced by exercise. If angina is prolonged greater than 20 minutes, then this can be regarded as pre-infarctional.

Left ventricular hypertrophy

- Left axis deviation (LAD)
- S in V_2 + R in $V_5 > 35$ mm
- ST depression anterior chest leads (LV strain)

Pericarditis

- Extensive ST elevation, concave upwards
- PR depression

Myocarditis

Non-specific ST–T changes.

Aortic dissection

The ECG is non-specific, with associated hypertensive changes in the majority.

If the dissection involves the coronary ostia, resultant myocardial ischaemia or infarction may be seen. The cardiac surgeon should be notified urgently.

Pulmonary embolus (PE)

Over 40% of patients show no significant change; therefore, a normal ECG does *NOT* rule out a pulmonary embolus. ECG findings include:

- sinus tachycardia
- RBBB, usually partial
- R axis deviation
- $S_1Q_3T_3$ (acute cor pulmonale)
- ST elevation in aVR
- anterior T wave inversion V_1–V_4 (Figure 8.3); differentiate from the normal T-wave inversion found in some youths, athletes and Black people in V_1–V_3.

Anticoagulation is indicated (see Chapter 11, 'Venous thromboembolic disease ...'). Consult urgently for compromised patients following massive PE as they may need urgent thrombolysis or embolectomy.

2 COLLAPSE, PALPITATIONS, SYNCOPE, DIZZINESS, ALTERED CONSCIOUSNESS

The ECG can help to determine a cardiac cause.

AMI, acute ischaemia, unstable angina or acute coronary syndrome

These can cause syncope or coma as a result of vasovagal reaction, cardiogenic shock, tamponade or any of the following arrhythmias.

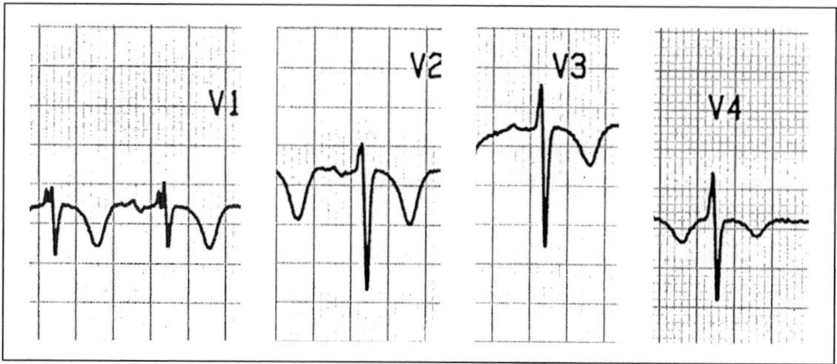

Figure 8.3 Acute pulmonary embolism: partial RBBB, inverted T waves V_1–V_4

Ventricular asystole

Absence of any electrical activity with a 'flat' ECG is asystole requiring cardiac massage, full CPR and the use of adrenaline as in advanced life support (ALS) guidelines.

Ensure that leads are attached and recording amplitude is correct, as low-voltage VF may be misinterpreted as asystole. Direct current reversion should be tried, if there is any doubt.

Ventricular fibrillation (VF)

This grossly irregular and variable amplitude arrhythmia is easy to recognise (Figure 8.4), unless it is low in amplitude, when it can be mistaken for asystole (if in doubt, treat as VF). It requires:

- immediate defibrillation beginning with 200 J biphasic or 360 J monophasic according to full CPR and ALS protocols, with
- adrenaline 1 mg IV, repeated every 3 minutes as required, and
- lignocaine 1–1.5 mg/kg or 100 mg bolus IV or amiodarone 5 mg/kg or 300 mg bolus IV as the mainstays of drug therapy.
- Magnesium 5 mmol should also be considered.

Lack of response to treatment will lead to deterioration, agonal rhythm with a sine-wave pattern, asystole and death. (*pto*)

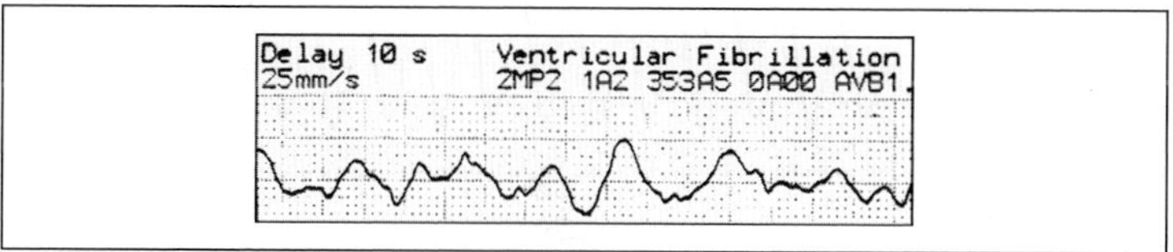

Figure 8.4 Ventricular fibrillation

Rarely, continued ALS may still rescue a patient with a preterminal rhythm.

Ventricular tachycardia (VT)

A wide-complex tachycardia represents VT (Figure 8.5) in over 90% of cases, approaching 100% in patients with prior AMI. If in doubt, treat as VT.

Most VT occurs in the setting of structural heart disease, usually ischaemic.

- If the patient is not haemodynamically compromised, chemical cardioversion should be attempted, with lignocaine 1–1.5 mg/kg (or standard 100 mg bolus), procainamide 1 mg/kg (or 100 mg bolus) IV over 1 minute or amiodarone 150 mg over 1–2 minutes.
- If the patient is unstable (chest pain, hypotension or acute pulmonary oedema), prompt synchronised electrical cardioversion beginning with 50–100 J biphasic should be performed (once sedated, or consciousness lost).
- Pulseless VT is treated as for VF with immediate (unsynchronised) defibrillation (200 J biphasic) with CPR and ALS.

VT can occur in the absence of structural heart disease, and this type of VT may last for seconds to weeks and generally has a benign prognosis. Cardiology consultation regarding medical management is advised.

Diagnostic difficulty occurs in cases of supraventricular tachycardia (SVT) with aberrancy/intraventricular conduction defect, which can mimic the ECG appearances of VT. There should be typical LBBB or RBBB changes; otherwise it is not SVT with aberrancy, and must be regarded as VT.

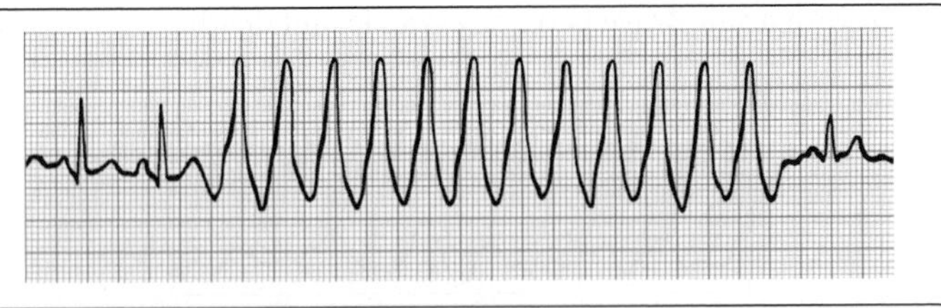

Figure 8.5 Ventricular tachycardia: onset from sinus rhythm

Prolonged QTc interval

A QTc (corrected for the rate) of over 0.44 s predisposes to VT and torsades, and should be corrected as soon as possible. Table 8.2 lists the causes of a prolonged QTc, which may progress to torsades de pointes.

Table 8.2 Causes of prolonged QT interval and torsades de pointes

Cause	Specific drugs, conditions
Antiarrhythmics	Quinidine, procainamide, disopyramide, amiodarone, sotalol
Antipsychotics	Risperidone, fluphenazine, droperidol, pimozide, clozapine, olanzapine, thioridazine, haloperidol, chlorpromazine
Antidepressants	Tricyclics: amitriptyline, imipramine, clomipramine, dothiepin, doxepin
Anti-infective	Macrolides: erythromycin, clarithromycin, azithromycin, roxithromycin Quinolones: ciprofloxacin, moxifloxacin, norfloxacin Antifungals: fluconazole, ketoconazole Antimalarials: hydroxychloroquine, mefloquine, quinine
Miscellaneous drugs	Cisapride, cocaine, methadone, lithium, sumatriptan, organophosphates
Cardiac disease	Ischaemia, complete heart block
Electrolyte disturbances	Hypomagnesaemia, hypocalcaemia, hypokalaemia
Hypothyroidism	
Congenital long QT syndrome	

Any serious tachycardia associated with prolonged QTc should be treated by correcting the underlying cause, magnesium or cardioversion. Class 1B antiarrhythmics such as phenytoin (but not Class 1A drugs) and Class II antiarrhythmics such as propranolol may also be effective, particularly for the congenital type. Pacing may be needed.

Torsades de pointes

This is a polymorphic broad-complex VT with 'twisting of the axes', often several complexes alternating above and below the isoelectric line. The danger is it may degenerate into VF, but it is more often self-limiting. Causes include drugs which prolong the QT interval, electrolyte disturbances and ischaemia.

- Treatment involves drug withdrawal, IV magnesium sulfate 2 g bolus over 1 minute, followed by an infusion, and correction of electrolytes and ischaemia.

(*pto*)

- An isoprenaline infusion or transcutaneous pacing may be used to accelerate the heart rate and terminate the arrhythmia.
- Unsynchronised cardioversion 50–100 J biphasic is recommended for haemodynamic instability; however, torsades may be resistant to electrical therapy.

Brugada syndrome

This is a disorder which causes VF and polymorphic VT, and which can be inherited in an autosomal dominant pattern. It is more common in South-East Asians and males, and there may be a family history of sudden cardiac death. There is an abnormality in the cardiac sodium (Na^+) channel. It should be considered in any young male presenting with syncope, seizures, chest pain, sudden cardiac arrest, a family history of unexplained death or the incidental finding of a Brugada pattern on routine ECG.

The ECG features of Brugada are ST elevation and T wave inversion in leads V_1–V_3, mimicking a RBBB. Figure 8.6 (opposite) shows a type 1. These changes may be transient. The rarer types 2 and 3 have 'saddleback' ST segments with upright T waves.

- Treatment is insertion of an implantable cardiac defibrillator (ICD).
- Drug therapy with sotalol may be tried if the patient is assessed by a cardiologist as low risk.

Heart block

High-degree heart block, particularly if associated with AMI, may deteriorate to complete heart block requiring urgent pacing. Incomplete occlusions can cause intermittent blocks.

First-degree AV block

The PR interval is > 0.2 s.

Second-degree, Möbitz type I, Wenckebach

The PR interval increases progressively until a 'dropped beat', with no QRS/ventricular response, occurs. The subsequent PR interval is shorter than the PR before the dropped beat.

Second-degree, Möbitz type II

The PR interval is constant, in association with frequent dropped beats, often regular, e.g. 1 in 3. Deterioration results in a high rate of progression to complete heart block.

No treatment is indicated for first- and second-degree blocks unless there is ischaemia or poor cardiac output, when atropine 0.3–0.6 mg IV may be given with supplementary oxygen.

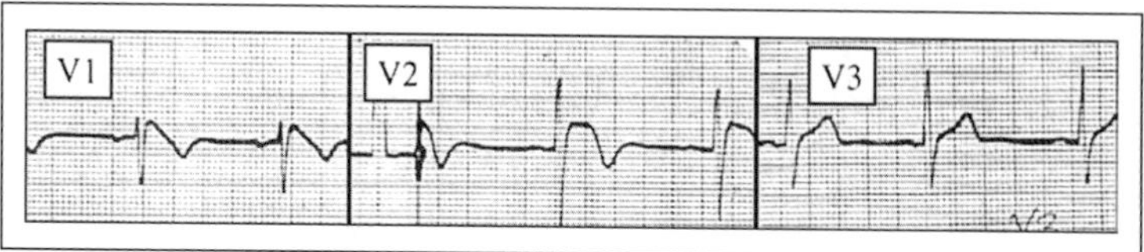

Figure 8.6 Brugada syndrome type 1
Courtesy Dr Jitu Vohra, Cardiologist, Epworth & Royal Melbourne Hospitals, Victoria.

Third-degree, complete AV/heart block (CHB)

There is no P to QRS relationship; all of the atrial impulses are blocked at the AV node, so that regular P waves (rate > 50) are seen with an independent, idioventricular, QRS with a rate of around 30–40. If the QRS complex arises just below the AV node, the QRS may be narrow and normal in appearance (junctional AV block). More-distal rhythms are relatively wide (> 0.12 s). In general, the broader escape rhythms are more unstable, and more likely to progress to ventricular standstill.

Patients with complete heart block (CHB) may decompensate with poor cardiac output, hypotension or loss of consciousness (Stokes-Adams attack).

- Urgent treatment with atropine 0.3–0.6 mg IV, isoprenaline infusion and/or pacing are indicated.
- Atropine appears to be more effective for narrow-complex CHB, and may worsen the block in broad-complex CHB.

Bundle branch block (BBB)

BBB generally indicates disease in the main conducting system, and syncope can result from an associated AMI with decompensation, progression to CHB and asystole.

LBBB (Figure 8.7), due to functional or anatomical block of the LBB and delayed depolarisation of the left ventricle, is seen as an rS in V_1 and a broad RR^1 in V_5, V_6 with a wide QRS (> 0.12 s). It can be benign, but it is more commonly associated with ischaemic heart disease (IHD) and hypertension. It is important to note that evidence of AMI may still be seen on the ECG (see above, under 'Myocardial infarction').

RBBB (Figure 8.8), due to functional or anatomical block of the RBB and delayed depolarisation of the right ventricle, is seen as an RSR^1 pattern in V_1 $V_{,2}$ with a wide QRS (> 0.12 s) and is often benign, but can also be a sign of acute right heart strain, such as acute pulmonary embolism. AMI is not disguised by a RBBB.

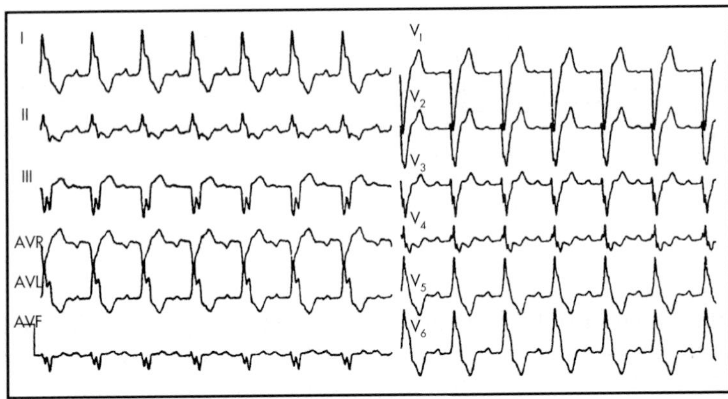

Figure 8.7 Left bundle branch block

Left anterior fascicular block, anterior hemiblock (LAFB) is seen as left-axis deviation ($q_1R_1S_3$) and a normal-duration QRS. In patients with chest pain, it signifies partial occlusion of the left anterior descending artery and occurs in about half of anterior infarctions. If the LAD occlusion is more extensive, RBBB will also be present.

Left posterior fascicular block, posterior hemiblock (LPFB) is rare and seen as right-axis deviation (S_1R_3) and a normal-duration QRS. Since the posterior fascicle is broad, its occurrence indicates a widespread lesion such as an inferolateral infarct, cardiomyopathy or cor pulmonale. If associated with RBBB, this signifies extensive coronary artery disease with high risk of complete AV block.

Atrial fibrillation (AF)

In atrial fibrillation, there are no P waves, and the rhythm is irregular (Figure 8.9). It is the most common supraventricular tachycardia and its incidence increases with age.

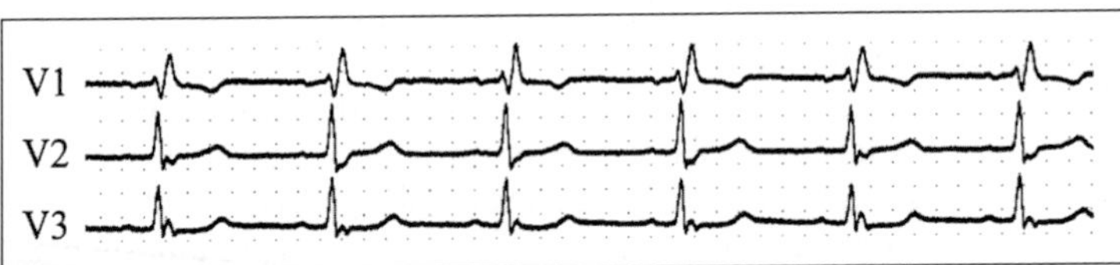

Figure 8.8 Right bundle branch block

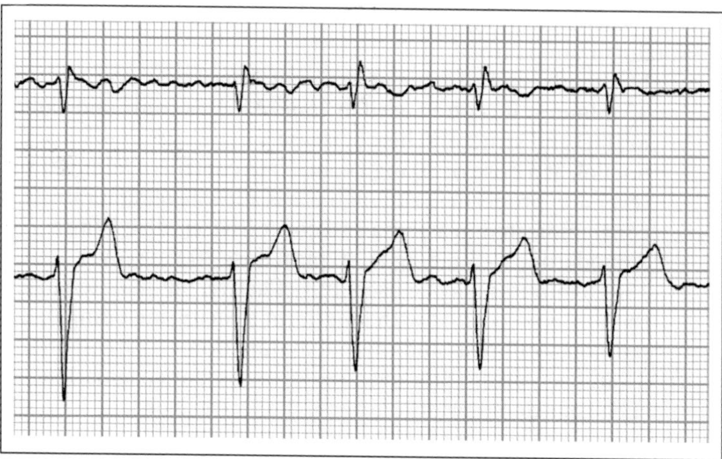

Figure 8.9 Atrial fibrillation

In acute AF, precipitating factors such as fever, pneumonia, recent cardiac surgery, alcohol or caffeine use and thyrotoxicosis should be sought. When caused by AMI or PE, with rapid ventricular response (130–180 bpm), AF may result in poor cardiac output with palpitations and syncope. It usually co-exists with hypertensive, dilated, valvular or rheumatic heart disease, though up to 25% of patients have 'lone' AF with no structural heart disease.

Acute management involves ventricular rate control or reversion to sinus rhythm and will often require consultation with the cardiology unit. Asymptomatic AF may not need any emergency management. Rate control is best achieved with drugs which prolong AV nodal conduction, such as IV beta-blockers (e.g. metoprolol), calcium-channel blockers (e.g. verapamil) or digoxin.

- Digoxin has long been the mainstay of therapy, but while it slows the rate, it may prolong the arrhythmia. Ensure the arrhythmia is not a Wolff-Parkinson-White (WPW) syndrome, as digoxin may precipitate VF in WPW.
- Reversion to sinus rhythm ('rhythm control') may be achieved by synchronised electrical cardioversion or by pharmacological means.
- Patients with haemodynamic instability due to rapid AF require sedation and synchronised cardioversion starting at 50–100 J biphasic. Synchronised cardioversion is often used in new-onset AF, if a trial of an antiarrhythmic agent has not been successful.

- Pharmacological reversion may be achieved using flecainide, sotalol or amiodarone.
  - Flecainide may be given at a dose of 2 mg/kg IV over 30 minutes. It is often used in 'lone' AF. It is contraindicated in IHD and structural heart disease.
  - Sotalol, at a dose of 80 mg IV, has rate control in addition to reversion properties, although it has a low reversion rate. It is contraindicated in asthma and congestive cardiac failure.
  - Amiodarone 4–5 mg/kg IV (typical dose 300 mg) over 15–20 minutes may be used. It is effective, but maintenance therapy is associated with long-term toxicity, including pulmonary fibrosis and thyroid dysfunction.
- If AF has been present for over 48–72 hours, anticoagulation must be considered prior to reversion (electrical or pharmacological). This is to prevent systemic embolus (cerebral, mesenteric, peripheral) from left atrial thrombus. In many instances, it will be difficult to ascertain the exact duration/time of onset of AF.
- Transoesophageal echocardiography (TOE) is used to detect left atrial or left atrial appendage thrombus prior to reversion in AF of >48–72 hours' duration.
- If left atrial thrombus is detected on TOE (or if TOE is unavailable), a period of 3 weeks anticoagulation prior to reversion followed by 4–6 weeks anticoagulation after reversion is advised. Anticoagulation consists of enoxaparin followed by warfarin.
- In patients in permanent AF, long-term antithrombotic therapy is given to prevent thromboembolism. The selection of antithrombotic agent (aspirin or warfarin) is based on the risk of stroke versus the risk of bleeding in a particular patient.

Editorial Comment

Selected ED cardioversion for AF less than 48 hours makes sense for the patient and the hospital and is supported by the literature.

ED cardioversion of atrial fibrillation

(Kevin Maruno and Paul Preisz)

The commonest clinically significant cardiac arrhythmia seen in emergency departments is AF. This may be a first episode or recurrent, which is then subclassified as *paroxysmal* (self-terminating,

< 24 hours), *persistent* (sustained > 7 days) or *permanent*. There are many causes and clinical settings for AF, and investigation should be initiated either urgently or as an outpatient depending on the clinical context.

AF may be asymptomatic, or be associated with palpitations, dyspnoea, chest discomfort, decreased exercise tolerance or feelings of anxiety or pre-syncope. Apart from an irregularly irregular pulse, usually with a fast rate, additional physical findings vary. Heart failure may be present. Signs of associated cardiovascular disease, e.g. mitral valve disease, ischaemic heart disease or hypertension, may be present. Signs of the underlying cause, e.g. anaemia, sepsis or thyrotoxicosis, may be present. AF with a very rapid ventricular rate (>200 bpm) suggests the possibility of an underlying accessory pathway.

Acute AF may be associated with alcohol (and some other drugs), surgery, electrocution, myocardial infarction, myopericarditis, pulmonary embolism, lung diseases, hyperthyroidism, metabolic conditions and many other causes. Treatment of these may lead to resolution.

Up to two-thirds of new or recurrent episodic AF may resolve without treatment within the first 24 hours. When associated with another illness, treatment of the primary problem may lead to reversion to sinus rhythm. Investigation for both cardiac disease, particularly structural or ischaemic disease, and underlying causes should be undertaken. Echocardiography, particularly transoesophageal echocardiography (TOE), is very useful. The risk of stroke should be considered in each patient.

Box 8.1 Objectives in atrial fibrillation

1. Identify and treat causative factor
2. Decide on rate or rhythm control, and implement treatment to slow rate or revert to sinus rhythm
3. Prevent thromboembolism, balancing the risk of stroke against the risk of bleeding on anticoagulants

Management to give symptomatic relief and to prevent tachycardia-induced cardiomyopathy is either by rate control or by rhythm control (Table 8.3).

- Rate control can be best achieved with drugs such as beta-blockers, verapamil or diltiazem. Digoxin, while no longer considered first choice, may be useful in those with heart failure due to its inotropic effects. Drugs that slow atrioventricular conduction are contraindicated in those with accessory pathway.

Table 8.3 Indications for rate or rhythm control in persistent AF

	Consider rate control	Consider rhythm control
Age	Older people (> 65 years)	Younger people (< 65 years)
Symptoms	Few or no symptoms	Severe symptoms
AF type	Permanent	Lone AF or new-onset
Complications	People without congestive heart failure	People with congestive heart failure
Contraindications	People with contraindications to antiarrhythmic drugs or cardioversion	People eligible for antiarrhythmic drugs or cardioversion
Comorbidities	People with coronary artery disease	AF secondary to treated/ corrected precipitant

Adapted from NHMRC Clinical Practice Guideline.

- Rhythm control can be achieved by either electrical cardioversion or pharmacotherapy. Pharmacological restoration to sinus rhythm may be achieved by agents such as flecainide or amiodarone, however careful assessment of safety and likely efficacy of the chosen agent is required for each patient. Flecainide is contraindicated in those with structural heart disease.

Electrical cardioversion in the ED requires most importantly a safe environment. A resuscitation area and staff trained in airway and resuscitation equipment is essential.

- The need for cardioversion may be immediate (e.g. hypotension, worsening heart failure) or semi-elective.
- Patients require procedural sedation, e.g. propofol, midazolam or other agents with airway management and monitoring.
- Energy delivery at 200 J DC (synchronised mono- or biphasic) is usually adequate, with the higher energy levels recommended to increase the likelihood of initial success and avoid the possible conversion to VF (which may be more common at lower energy levels).
- Conversion to VF is a rare event but necessitates immediate unsynchronised defibrillation with usual advanced ALS management.
- Cardioversion also carries a risk of thromboembolism, with this risk greatest when the arrhythmia has been present for greater than 48 hours. Following cardioversion, atrial 'stunning' may occur, and anticoagulation may need to be continued for 4 weeks afterwards in high-risk patients.

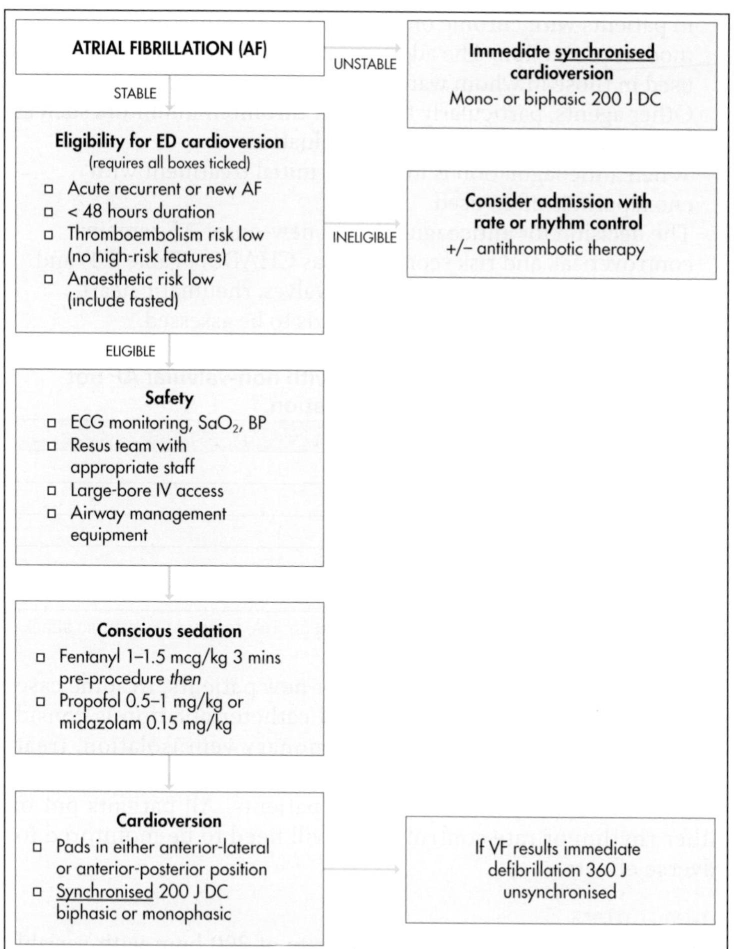

Figure 8.10 Pathway for electrical defibrillation of atrial fibrillation
Adapted from American College of Cardiology/American Heart Association/European Society for Cardiology Guidelines for the management of patients with atrial fibrillation, 2006

Independent of rate or rhythm control strategy, thromboembolism risk requires addressing. This will include the intrinsic risk of thromboembolism, choice of treatment, risk of major haemorrhage and patient preference.

- Multiple studies have demonstrated that oral anticoagulation with warfarin is effective for prevention of thromboembolism in patients with chronic or recurrent AF. Aspirin offers only modest protection. The addition of clopidogrel to aspirin may be used in those in whom warfarin is contraindicated or unreliable.

- Other agents, particularly the direct thrombin inhibitors such as dabigatran, are currently under evaluation.
- When anticoagulation is indicated, initial treatment with enoxaparin is often used.
- The decision for anticoagulation in new-onset AF remains controversial, and risk scores such as $CHADS_2$ (Table 8.4) and high-risk features such as metallic valves, rheumatic heart disease or recent stroke or TIA needs to be assessed.

Table 8.4 Stroke risk in patients with non-valvular AF not treated with anticoagulation

		$CHADS_2$ score
C	CCF (EF < 35%)	1
H	Hypertension	1
A	Age ≥ 75	1
D	Diabetes mellitus	1
S	Past stroke or TIA	2

CCF, congestive cardiac failure; EF, ejection fraction; TIA, transient ischaemic attack

Cardiac follow-up is important for new patients. In some cases electrophysiological study (EPS) and catheter ablation is considered. Atrial appendage closure, pulmonary vein isolation, treatment for valvular heart disease and other surgical management may also be appropriate in selected patients. All patients put on either rhythm or rate control drugs will need to be monitored for adverse effects.

Atrial flutter

Generally, atrial flutter has an atrial rate of 300 bpm with variable block (commonly 2:1 or 3:1). It has the same causes as AF, and may be treated similarly. Despite its regular rate, it may still result in atrial thrombus.

Flutter waves may be most obvious in the inferior leads, and are described as having a sawtooth appearance. Rate control is as for AF. The most effective treatment is synchronised cardioversion, beginning with 25–50 J biphasic. Pharmacological agents are less effective in reverting atrial flutter than atrial fibrillation. The same precautions regarding anticoagulation apply for atrial flutter.

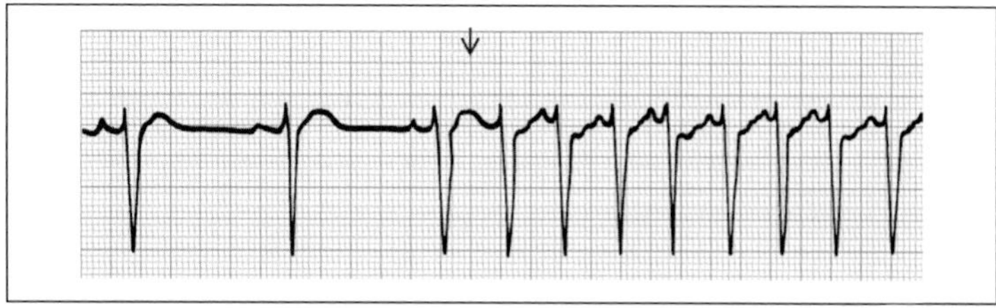

Figure 8.11 Paroxysmal supraventricular tachycardia

Paroxysmal supraventricular tachycardia (PSVT)

PSVT has a regular rate, usually 150–200 bpm (range 100–280 bpm; see Figure 8.11). It is a junctional tachycardia, where the AV node is an integral part of the arrhythmia circuit.

AV nodal re-entry tachycardia (AVNRT) is where the circuit is within the AV node itself, while AV re-entry tachycardia (AVRT) is where an additional (accessory) pathway is involved.

- Vagal manoeuvres such as carotid sinus massage may terminate PSVT.
- Adenosine is effective and relatively safe to use for chemical reversion, given as IV boluses through a wide-bore (e.g. 18-gauge in cubital fossa) IV cannula of 6 mg, 12 mg or up to 18 mg if needed. In some patients, it causes a feeling of impending doom which may be prevented or treated with a small dose of midazolam, 0.01 mg/kg IV.
- Verapamil 5 mg IV slowly at 1 mg/minute may be used with care, but it can cause intractable hypotension, CHB and asystole, especially if the patient is also on a beta-blocker or digoxin.
- Radiofrequency ablation (RA) may be needed if adenosine is unsuccessful.

SVT with intraventricular conduction defect (aberrant conduction), such as when there is a concurrent BBB or WPW syndrome causing a broad QRS complex, is difficult to differentiate from VT. Adenosine is safe for SVT with BBB, but in WPW it may cause hypotension and unstable VT.

Wolff-Parkinson-White syndrome (WPW)

WPW is due to pre-excitation of the ventricles by an accessory pathway, bypassing the AV node, resulting in a short PR interval and a slurred upstroke or 'delta wave' on the R wave, best seen in V_2–V_6 (see Figure 8.12).

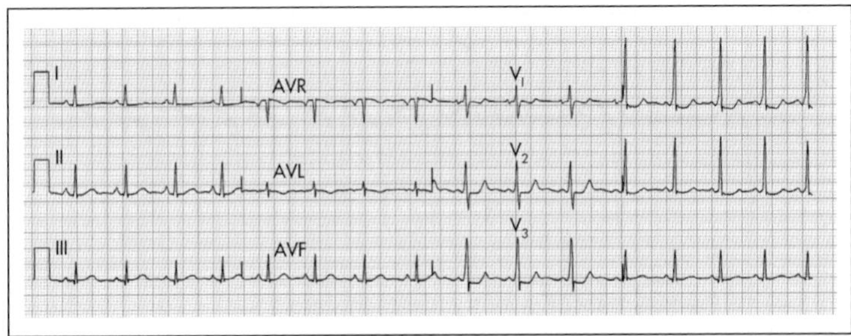

Figure 8.12 Wolff-Parkinson-White type A with typical delta waves

If associated with a dominant R in V_1 and inverted T waves in V_1–V_4, this is due to a left accessory path (type A WPW); otherwise the accessory path is on the right (type B WPW). The ECG of type A WPW can be mistaken for a posterior AMI.

Serious paroxysmal tachyarrhythmias can occur by retrograde re-entry mechanisms or by rapid conduction of superimposed AF/atrial flutter, such as when digoxin is used for treating AF when WPW is unrecognised. Impulses may be rapidly conducted down the accessory path and cause a bizarre ECG with variable width QRS tachycardia, hypotension and eventual VF arrest.

- Treat WPW tachyarrhythmias with IV procainamide 100 mg over 2–5 minutes, up to a total dose of 1 g, if stable (watch for and suspend if hypotension or QRS widening) or cardioversion if decompensated.
- Other drugs (but not digoxin) may be used, but there is risk of exacerbating aberrant conduction.
- Radiofrequency ablation or surgery may be needed.

Holter monitoring

Despite a history suggestive of an abnormal rhythm, none may be detected during ED assessment. The patient should be considered for admission for cardiac monitoring or Holter monitoring as an outpatient.

Holter monitoring involves attaching a patient to a portable personal ECG monitor, which records usually two ECG channels on tape or computer for 24 hours. A technician then scans the recordings by computer and identifies periods of arrhythmia, which are then presented to the cardiologist for review to see if episodes of palpitations, syncope, angina, etc can be explained.

- Sinus bradycardia < 35 bpm, sinus pauses < 3 s, Wenckebach, brief runs of AF, multiple atrial ectopics and isolated ventricular ectopic beats may all be found in otherwise normal persons, and do not warrant treatment.
- Sustained arrhythmias are more significant, particularly in symptomatic patients.
- Holter monitoring is also useful in checking response to antiarrhythmics.

3 ELECTROLYTE IMBALANCE, DRUG OVERDOSE, ENVIRONMENTAL EMERGENCIES

Arrhythmias can arise as a result of any of these conditions.

Potassium or magnesium imbalance

Potassium or magnesium imbalance cause similar effects and are important to recognise early, as each may progress to serious arrhythmias if uncorrected.

Hyperkalaemia or hypermagnesaemia

Hyperkalaemia or hypermagnesaemia may cause tall, peaked T waves, flat P waves, wide QRS and undefined ST–T changes. Higher levels will cause various tachyarrhythmias including VT and, eventually, asystole.

Hypokalaemia or hypomagnesaemia

Hypokalaemia or hypomagnesaemia may result in a prolonged QT, flattened T waves and small U waves; note that U waves may occur in healthy people in V_2–V_4, but the T waves are normal. ST depression and first- or second-degree heart block may also be seen. Lower levels can cause atrial and ventricular arrhythmias, notably torsades de pointes.

Calcium imbalance

Hypercalcaemia

Hypercalcaemia shortens the ST and the Q–T intervals, but widens the T wave. Bradycardias, BBB, second-degree heart block and CHB can deteriorate to asystole if levels are markedly elevated.

Hypocalcaemia

Hypocalcaemia lengthens the ST and therefore the Q–T interval, with risk of VT and torsades. A prolonged QTc may be caused by any drug which causes hypocalcaemia, hypokalaemia and hypomagnesaemia.

Environmental emergencies

Hypothermia and electrocution are examples causing cardiac effects.

Hypothermia

With severe hypothermia, cardiac effects can be related to the temperature. The initial response is a sinus tachycardia for temperatures down to 32°C, then bradycardia for temperatures down to about 30°C. Osborn waves, which are deflections at the end of the QRS complex and in the same direction as the QRS, appear at around 30°C and increase in height as the temperature falls. Various arrhythmias occur down to 27°C, when VF may occur and cause death. In some patients, VF does not occur, and the temperature can fall as low as 22°C, culminating in fatal asystole. Gradual rewarming and ALS should be instituted early to avoid this.

See also Chapter 29, 'Drowning'.

Electrocution

Cardiac effects can vary from nil to ST changes, transient arrhythmias, BBB, heart block, myocardial necrosis and cardiac asystole. If the route from entry to exit points traverses the torso, cardiac damage is more likely.

- A low current of 10–100 microamps, resulting from stray currents or earthing faults in household equipment, can cause a microshock, which can result in VF arrest.
- If the skin resistance is lowered by moisture, a 0.24 milliamp (mA) current from a 240 volt source can be increased to a current of 240 mA and cause a macroshock, with resultant VF.
- Contact with high-tension power lines (> 1000 A) or a lightning strike (> 12,000 A) can cause cardiorespiratory arrest from asystole (more commonly) or VF. Early ALS may save these patients, but the severity of their burns will determine their fate.

See also Chapter 31, 'Electrical injuries'.

Axis (electrical pathway mapping)

Axis generally refers to the QRS axis and the direction of depolarisation in the ventricles as reflected in the frontal plane (the anterior chest wall). It is best illustrated by a clock face with each numerical division representing 30° (see Figure 8.13).

- The horizontal direction can be determined by inspecting LI, to see whether the QRS deflection is mainly *up* (positive impulse moving from right to left) or *down* (negative impulse from left to right).

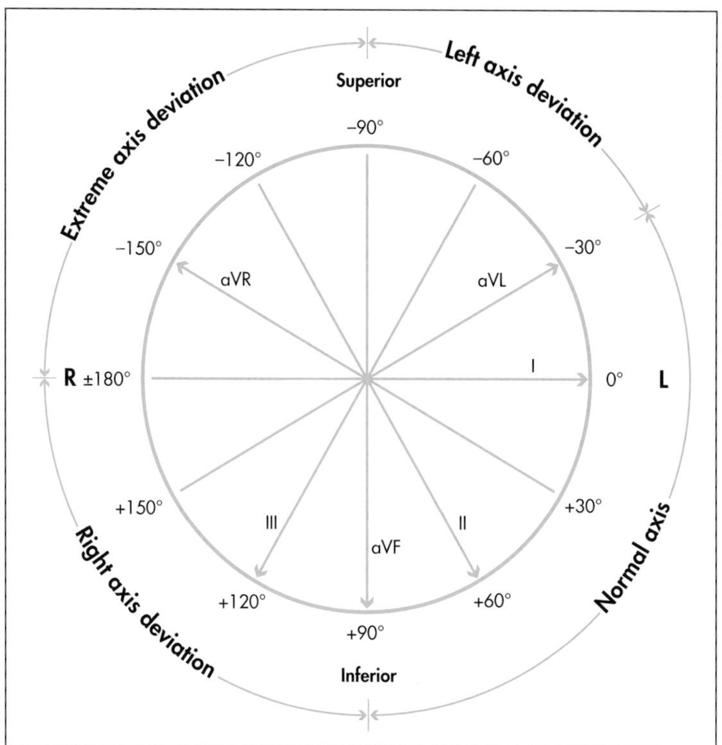

Figure 8.13 The QRS frontal plane cardiac axial reference system
Yuen Derek, after Fisch C, Mirvis D, Goldberg A. Electrocardiography. In: Libby P, Bonow R et al (eds). Braunwald's Heart disease. 8th edn. Philadelphia: WB Saunders; 2007

- The vertical direction is reflected in aVF (the vertical axis). If the QRS deflection is mainly up, the impulse is travelling towards the foot, and if the QRS is down, the impulse is towards the head.

Combining this information, the quadrant in which the QRS vector lies can be determined.

- QRS in LI up, in aVF up—vector in left lower quadrant (normal axis)
- QRS in LI up, in aVF down—vector in left upper quadrant (left axis deviation—LAD)
- QRS in LI down, in aVF up—vector in right lower quadrant (right axis deviation—RAD)

(*pto*)

- QRS in LI down, in aVF down—vector in right upper quadrant (indeterminate or extreme RAD).

To determine the axis more accurately (within 30°), note which limb or standard lead has the most isoelectric QRS (equally up and down); the axis is at 90° to this in the predetermined quadrant (use Figure 8.13). The range of normal axis can extend from –30° to +90°, as patients who are obese can have a more horizontal heart (vector in left upper quadrant), while those who are asthenic have a more vertical heart (90° axis). Thus, if the QRS is isoelectric in lead aVR, and the above criteria point to the left upper quadrant (LAD), then a perpendicular (90°) to the aVR axis gives an axis of –60° in the left upper quadrant. The QRS axis is then –60° in the frontal plane.

While the above are more accurate, a simple summary is:

- QRS in LI negative = RAD
- QRS in LII negative = LAD.

Significance

Left axis deviation. LAD should raise the suspicion of anterior hemiblock (left anterior fascicular block—LAFB), often as a result of occlusive disease of the left anterior descending artery or cardiomyopathy.

Right axis deviation. RAD suggests posterior hemiblock (right posterior fascicular block—RPFB) and usually right (occasionally, left) coronary artery disease, right ventricular hypertrophy, acute cor pulmonale (as in massive pulmonary embolus) or cardiomyopathy.

Note: In general, the vector moves towards hypertrophy, and away from infarction.

QRS axis. QRS axis can also be described in the horizontal plane, looking up. Using the chest leads, the QRS is normally isoelectric in V_3 or V_4. If the QRS is isoelectric over V_1 or V_2, this is counterclockwise rotation; and if in V_5 or V_6, it is clockwise rotation.

Chapter 9
Respiratory emergencies: the acutely breathless patient

Craig Hore and John Roberts

General principles

Exclude airway compromise, which may be subtle, as the cause of acute breathlessness. Management of airway problems always comes first. Dyspnoea is a sensation which has multiple aetiologies and can be difficult to assess.

There may be several reasons why the patient with comorbidities experiences dyspnoea. This patient may require comprehensive treatment strategies to optimise their condition and thus relieve their symptoms.

Initial goals in assessment and management are:

1. To identify and treat life-threatening abnormalities of gas exchange, acute onset or deterioration of hypoxia and hypercarbia.
2. To commence non-invasive ventilation in the form of bi-level positive airway pressure (BiPAP) or continuous positive airway pressure (CPAP) where indicated.
3. To identify when intubation and ventilation is required and initiate this therapy.
4. To identify and commence specific treatment to relieve respiratory distress based on initial history and examination.
5. To formulate a plan of investigation and management of cases where the exact cause of respiratory distress is unknown or uncertain.

Triage all patients presenting with a respiratory system emergency to a monitored acute bed. Obtain IV access. Arterial blood gases (ABGs), chest X-ray (CXR) and BiPAP services should be available.

Oxygen therapy

(Craig Hore)

Delivery of oxygen is one of the most common therapies in the ED and an important component of resuscitation. Acute hypoxaemia is immediately life-threatening, and the 'first-line drug' for hypoxaemia is oxygen! It is a safe drug: the complications of oxygen therapy are concentration- and time-dependent, uncommon and take time to develop. Other aspects of oxygen delivery may also need to be improved in the hypoxaemic patient, especially cardiac output, haemoglobin, tissue perfusion and reducing tissue O_2 requirements.

Table 9.1 The haemoglobin–oxygen (Hb–O_2) dissociation curve

SaO_2 (%)	PaO_2 (mmHg)	Level
98	100	Arterial blood
90	60	
75	40	Venous blood
50	26	
~33	~20	Tissue

SaO_2, oxygen saturation; PaO_2, partial pressure of oxygen in arterial or venous blood or tissue
Note: When $SaO_2 \approx$ 60–90%, there is a linear relationship between SaO_2 and PaO_2.

Essentially, oxygen should be delivered to all patients who have acute respiratory failure to maintain a partial arterial pressure (PaO_2) of 60–80 mmHg (or a $PaO_2 > 55$ mmHg in chronic respiratory failure). The lowest fraction of inspired oxygen (FiO_2) that provides an acceptable PaO_2 should be chosen. Choosing the right mode of delivery is also important.

OXYGEN DELIVERY SYSTEMS

Simple delivery systems

These are variable performance systems—the FiO_2 delivered not only depends upon the oxygen flow rate, but also on the rate and depth of respiration. The FiO_2 delivered by various systems can be estimated (Table 9.2).

Nasal prongs. These are easy to use and usually well tolerated by the patient, allowing them to eat, drink and talk without interrupting oxygen delivery. They are ineffective if the patient has blocked nasal passages or is an obligate mouth breather. Flow rates > 4 L/min can lead to mucosal drying and are less well tolerated.

Hudson mask. A simple and easy way to deliver oxygen but delivery is variable (see above). Flow rates < 4 L/min are not recommended as rebreathing can occur.

Entrainment systems

Venturi masks. This system uses the Bernoulli effect to entrain a fixed amount of air to mix with oxygen. This is an example

Table 9.2 **Estimation of the fraction of inspired oxygen (FiO_2) achieved by simple delivery systems**

Flow rate (L/min)	FiO_2
2 (nasal prongs)	0.25
3 (nasal prongs)	0.28
4 (nasal prongs)	0.30
6	0.40
8	0.45
15	0.65
15 (reservoir mask)*	0.70

*If a double wall supply is used, a flow rate of 30 L/min and FiO_2 up to 0.90 can be achieved.

of a fixed performance system—the FiO_2 delivered is more independent of patient factors. Nonetheless, it may vary in patients with very high peak inspiratory flow rates. One commonly used system delivers the following options: 24/28/35/40/50/60% oxygen. The lower concentrations are especially useful for patients with chronic obstructive pulmonary disease (COPD) and CO_2 retention.

Partial rebreathing systems

Reservoir masks. These can achieve a higher FiO_2 than simple masks, but it is essential to keep the reservoir inflated with O_2. This can require high flow rates. This is a good initial choice for most conscious, unwell, hypoxaemic patients in the ED.

Anaesthetic circuits. Mentioned for completeness; rarely used in the ED setting.

Non-rebreathing systems

Resuscitation bags (e.g. Laerdal, Baxter). The commonly used bags are self-inflating, and have a series of one-way valves and a reservoir bag. The aim is to keep the reservoir bag at least 75% inflated with O_2. An FiO_2 of close to 100% can be delivered if 15 L/min O_2 is used and the reservoir bag is inflated (50% without a reservoir bag). There is a growing trend to use disposable, single-use bags to help overcome the problem of incorrect assembly and sterilisation. The ability to use a bag–mask system is a vital skill that should be learned and mastered early!

Gas-driven inflating valves (e.g. Oxy-viva).

Others

- Positive-pressure ventilators
- Non-invasive positive-pressure ventilation (e.g. CPAP, BiPAP)
- Hyperbaric oxygen (HBO) therapy

Other delivery systems are dealt with in more detail in other chapters of this text.

Investigations in respiratory emergencies

(Craig Hore)

ARTERIAL BLOOD GASES (ABGs): OXYGENATION AND VENTILATION

ABGs reflect oxygenation (PaO_2), ventilation ($PaCO_2$) and acid–base status. The last is dealt with in more detail in Chapter 27, 'Acid–base and electrolyte disorders'.

Oxygenation

Remember that, even for 'normal' lungs, the PaO_2 varies with the following parameters.

The inspired O_2 concentration (FiO_2). Never take ABGs, or try to interpret ABGs, without noting the FiO_2. If room air, this is 21% (i.e. $FiO_2 = 0.21$).

Age. PaO_2 falls with age. As a rough guide to what to expect at a given age, use the following estimation:

$$PaO_2 \approx 105 - (1/3 \times \text{age})$$

Altitude. PaO_2 falls by ~3 mmHg for each 1000 feet (~300 m) above sea level.

Temperature. For each degree Celsius rise (or fall) in temperature, the PaO_2 will rise (or fall) by ~5%.

pH. For each 0.1 decrease (or increase) in pH, the PaO_2 will increase (or decrease) by ~10%.

Do not take oxygen off a hypoxic patient to perform ABGs. Perform the ABGs with the patient on oxygen and note the FiO_2. The A–a gradient (the difference between alveolar and arterial oxygen pressure, $P_{A-a}O_2$) is calculated from the alveolar gas equation:

$$PAO_2 = PiO_2 - (PaCO_2/R)$$

PAO_2 is the alveolar oxygen tension and R is the respiratory quotient (usually 0.8). The partial pressure of inspired oxygen (PiO_2) is determined by the atmospheric pressure, which varies with altitude. Usually, it is assumed that the patient is breathing at sea level, that atmospheric pressure is 760 mmHg and that the water vapour pressure is 47 mmHg. There is usually a small difference between the PAO_2 and the PaO_2—the A–a gradient or $P_{A-a}O_2$.

- $P_{A-a}O_2 < 15$ mmHg is normal.
- $P_{A-a}O_2 = 20$–30 mmHg reflects mild pulmonary dysfunction.
- $P_{A-a}O_2 > 50$ mmHg reflects severe pulmonary dysfunction. Note that pulmonary embolism is only one of many causes of an increased $P_{A-a}O_2$.

The gradient varies with age: add 3 for each decade over the age of 30 years.

The PAO_2 can also be quickly estimated using one of the following rules of thumb:

- If breathing room air,

$$PAO_2 \approx 145 - PaCO_2$$

- If breathing supplemental O_2,

$$PAO_2 \approx 6 \times \%O_2 \qquad \textit{or}$$

$$PAO_2 \approx (7 \times \%O_2) - PaCO_2$$

The causes of hypoxia

There are four main types of hypoxia:

1. **stagnant hypoxia** resulting from decreased cardiac output
2. **anaemic hypoxia** resulting from decreased haemoglobin
3. **histotoxic hypoxia** resulting from decreased oxygen-binding capacity
4. **hypoxaemic hypoxia** resulting from decreased O_2 saturation.

The take-home message from this list is that the patient can be 'hypoxic' with a normal O_2 saturation. Perhaps the most obvious example is histotoxic hypoxia resulting from CO poisoning.

Acute respiratory failure is generally associated with hypoxaemic hypoxia. The problem is getting the oxygen from the lungs into the capillaries. **Ventilation/perfusion (V/Q) mismatch** is the commonest cause.

- At one extreme of V/Q mismatching, there is normal ventilation but *abnormal perfusion* (**dead space ventilation**). This mismatching affects the exchange of O_2, resulting in hypoxaemia. Hypercarbia occurs to a lesser extent, as CO_2 diffuses more easily than O_2. The classic example is pulmonary embolism.

- At the other extreme, there is normal blood flow but *abnormal ventilation* (**shunt**). This is most commonly a result of **venous admixture** where capillary blood and alveolar gas do not equilibrate, such as when blood is flowing through a consolidated lung. The larger the shunt, the less responsive it is to supplemental O_2.

Ventilation

Hypercarbia (↑ $PaCO_2$)

The commonest cause of hypercarbia is alveolar hypoventilation. This can be due to a variety of problems, e.g. airway obstruction, narcotics, CNS disorders, PNS disorders, chest wall disorders. Remember there are other uncommon causes of hypercarbia, including V/Q inequality (e.g. COPD, emphysema); increased CO_2 production (e.g. hyperpyrexia, hypercatabolism, thyrotoxicosis, inappropriate carbohydrate load); and increased dead space (e.g. physiological—V/Q mismatch or 'dead space ventilation', equipment—long ventilator tubing and circuitry).

The clinical effects of hypercarbia

- Respiratory drive will typically be increased, unless it is suppressed due to the underlying cause of the hypercarbia (e.g. CNS disorders, narcotics).
- There is a rise in endogenous catecholamines leading to tachycardia, hypertension, increased CO, increased cerebral blood flow and raised intracranial pressure (ICP).
- Peripheral vasodilation typically occurs.
- The patient initially becomes anxious and restless, followed by a decreased level of consciousness and eventually coma if it remains uncorrected.

The 'chronic CO_2 retainer'

Some patients with chronic respiratory disorders (e.g. COPD) have a chronically elevated $PaCO_2$. The chemoreceptors adjust to this elevated level and essentially become less 'sensitive' to fluctuations in $PaCO_2$, relying more on changes in PaO_2—the so-called 'hypoxic drive'. A high FiO_2 could depress ventilation by decreasing this hypoxic stimulus. This is the theory, but clinically it actually rarely occurs in patients with acute respiratory failure.

Hypoxia can kill quickly, so give oxygen to the hypoxaemic patient. If the patient may have chronic CO_2 retention, still give oxygen, accepting a PaO_2 of 50–60 mmHg or even less.

OTHER INVESTIGATIONS IN RESPIRATORY EMERGENCIES

The chest X-ray (CXR)

The CXR is one of the most useful investigations in the patient with respiratory failure. In order to interpret the film correctly, and to avoid missing important findings, a good routine for assessing the CXR is a must. The principles of chest radiography, and other chest imaging modalities, are dealt with in more detail in Chapter 4, 'Diagnostic imaging in emergency patients'.

The lung can react in a similar fashion to a variety of insults. Therefore, there are no absolute rules in terms of radiological patterns that allow us to distinguish between these insults with 100% accuracy. *It is important to always interpret the CXR in the light of your clinical history and examination findings!* There will be times when an acutely short-of-breath patient presents to the ED and is found to be hypoxaemic without any significant changes seen on CXR. The differential here includes pulmonary vascular disease (e.g. emboli), respiratory problems (e.g. asthma, early COPD, early chronic lung disease, early pneumonia) and non-respiratory problems (e.g. compromised airway, high oxygen consumption, hyperthermia, intracardiac shunt).

Tests of forced expiration

These tests are effort- and technique-dependent and may not be able to be properly performed when the patient is acutely breathless.

Peak expiratory flow rate (PEFR) is measurable using a simple, portable flow meter. It is reproducible by most patients after several practice efforts. PEFR may be reduced in COPD, asthma and respiratory muscle weakness. PEFR may be normal or increased in restrictive lung diseases such as fibrosis. It is perhaps most useful as a monitor for asthmatic patients in the outpatient/home setting. It may also be helpful in the ED as one of the means to assess discharge suitability of asthmatic patients (e.g. PEFR should be at least 75% of predicted or best).

Forced vital capacity (FVC) is the volume of air that can be exhaled with maximum force following a full inspiration. It varies with age, sex, height and general physique.

Forced expiratory volume in 1 second (FEV_1) is the maximum amount of air that can be forcibly exhaled in 1 second following a full inspiration. FEV_1 is reduced in disease that affects airflow, lung elasticity and/or the state of the chest wall, including respiratory musculature. If FEV_1 improves by > 15–20% following bronchodilator therapy, there is said to be reversible airway obstruction. FEV_1 normally accounts for > 75% of the FVC. In obstructive airway disease, FEV_1/FVC is classically < 70%. In restrictive lung disease, FEV_1/FVC is classically normal or increased.

Microbiological methods

Treatment of suspected severe respiratory infections should not be delayed while awaiting the results of laboratory tests. A causal pathogen is found in less than 50% of cases of community-acquired pneumonia. This percentage decreases even further if the cultures are taken after antimicrobials have been given.

Blood cultures can often be collected in the ED before antimicrobial therapy is commenced. Ideally, 2 sets should be taken at least 1 hour apart. The second set may not be possible when rapid empirical therapy is indicated.

The value of **sputum culture** is limited but may be improved if the sputum is purulent, properly collected—not contaminated by the upper respiratory tract (e.g. saliva, epithelial cells) and, where possible, taken before antibiotics are given—and transported to the lab within 2 hours of collection. Where bacterial infection is not likely (e.g. many upper respiratory tract infections), cultures are usually not indicated. Respiratory syncytial virus (RSV) immunofluorescent-labelled antibody examination of exfoliated cells in nasopharyngeal secretions may be undertaken in paediatric acute bronchiolitis.

The **nature of the sputum** may be helpful: copious, pink frothy sputum is characteristic of acute left ventricular failure; copious, purulent, pungent sputum of lung abscess; clear, watery sputum of alveolar cell carcinoma; and rusty, mucoid sputum of pneumococcal pneumonia.

Invasive respiratory investigations

Invasive techniques such as percutaneous needle biopsy, diagnostic bronchoscopy, transbronchial biopsy and bronchoalveolar lavage are rarely undertaken in Australasian EDs. An exception is diagnostic and/or therapeutic **thoracentesis**.

Pleural fluid is normally a pale yellow colour. It is turbid in the setting of empyema or parapneumonic effusion. Blood in pleural fluid may be due to trauma, malignancy or pulmonary infarction. Other common analyses of pleural fluid include:

- protein (pleural fluid protein < 30 g/L represents a transudate; > 30 g/L represents an exudate)

- lactate dehydrogenase (LDH) (pleural fluid : serum LDH ratio < 0.6 represents a transudate; > 0.6 represents an exudate)
- white cell count (leukocytes may be due to a parapneumonic effusion, pulmonary embolus or empyema; lymphocytes may be due to tuberculosis, malignancy or a vasculitis)
- glucose (pleural fluid glucose may be < 50% serum glucose levels in bacterial infections, malignancy, rheumatoid arthritis and systemic lupus erythematosus (SLE))
- cytology (malignant cells, mesothelial cells), and
- culture.

Life-threatening conditions presenting with breathlessness

(John Roberts)

ACUTE ASTHMA

Initial management

1 Give oxygen and salbutamol or other short-acting beta-2-agonist immediately, if not already commenced, after taking a brief history and physical examination.
2 Focus on delivering oxygen, reversing the bronchospasm and relieving symptoms as soon as possible in a high-acuity, well-supervised, monitored area with IV access.

Assess severity

Assess severity as mild, moderate or severe and life-threatening using signs of physical exhaustion, cyanosis, speech, PEFR, spirometry (the most accurate test, but may not be possible initially), oxygen saturation, heart rate, respiratory rate and pulsus paradoxus (abnormal decrease in blood pressure on inspiration). Refer to Table 9.3.

Features of severe and life-threatening asthma include: paradoxical chest wall movement, exhaustion, sweating, vomiting, panic, speaking in short phases or words only, pulse rate > 120/min, pulsus paradoxus > 12 mmHg, central cyanosis, quiet, *NOT* wheezy chest, PEFR < 50% of predicted or < 100 L/min, FEV_1 < 50% of predicted or < 1 L, pulse oximetry < 90%.

Editorial Comment

In acute severe asthma, intravenous magnesium is now increasingly being used.

Table 9.3 Initial assessment of acute asthma in adults

Findings	Mild	Moderate	Severe and life-threatening*
Physical exhaustion	No	No	Yes Paradoxical chest wall movement
Talks in:	Sentences	Phrases	Words
Pulse rate	<100/min	100–120/min	> 120/min†
Pulsus paradoxus	Not palpable	May be palpable	Palpable‡
Central cyanosis	Absent	May be present	Likely to be present
Wheeze intensity	Variable	Moderate to loud	Often quiet
PEFR	More than 75% of predicted (or best if known)	50–70% of predicted (or best if known)	Less than 50% of predicted (or best if known) or less than 100 L/min#
FEV_1	More than 75% of predicted	50–75% of predicted	Less than 50% of predicted or less than 1 L
Oximetry on presentation			Less than 90% Cyanosis may be present**
Arterial blood gases (assay)	Not necessary	Necessary if initial response poor	Necessary††
Other investigations	Not required	May be required	Check for hypokalaemia Chest X-ray to exclude other pathology (e.g. infection, pneumothorax)

* Any of these features indicates that the episode is severe. The absence of any feature does not exclude a severe attack.
† Bradycardia may be seen when respiratory arrest is imminent.
‡ Paradoxical pulse is more reliable in severe obstruction. Its presence (especially if > 12 mmHg) can identify patients who need admission. Its absence in those with severe exacerbations suggests respiratory muscle fatigue.
# Patient may be incapable of performing test.
**Measurement of oxygen saturation is required: many patients look well clinically and may not appear cyanosed despite desaturation.
†† $PaCO_2$ > 50 mmHg indicates respiratory failure. PaO_2 < 60 mmHg indicates respiratory failure.
Reproduced with permission from 'Initial Assessment of Acute Asthma In Adults', page 50 of The Asthma Management Handbook 2006 published by The National Asthma Council Australia. www.nationalasthma.org.au/handbook

Difficult-to-treat patients are usually those who have delayed presentation and/or deteriorated despite outpatient steroid treatment.

Also observe carefully the patient who has childhood onset of asthma, is steroid-dependent, has previously been intubated or has a history of severe episodes, especially requiring ICU admission, as they are at increased risk.

Further treatment

1 Hydrocortisone 250 mg IV or equivalent (maximum adult dose) in severe and life-threatening cases; repeat 6-hourly and review at 24 hours.
2 Oral steroids for moderate severity, e.g. prednisolone at 0.5–1.0 mg/kg daily.
3 Salbutamol nebulised, 1 mL of 5 mg/mL solution + 3 mL saline every 15–30 minutes.
4 If not responding, give salbutamol 250 microg (0.5 mL of 500 microg/mL solution) IV bolus over 1 minute, then IV infusion at 5–10 microg/kg/hour.
5 Ipratropium bromide 2 mL (500 microg) with salbutamol 2-hourly (optional in moderate severity, not required in mild cases).
6 Adrenaline 0.5 mg IM or slowly IV in severe, prearrest cases or where anaphylaxis may be present. In these circumstances, adrenaline is best administered in 0.1 mg boluses (1 mL of 1 : 10,000 solution) or 1 mg in 100 mL burette titrated slowly. Subsequent adrenaline infusions should be prepared and titrated based on local hospital protocols.

Intubation and ventilation, while often seen as a last resort, are required for respiratory arrest or exhaustion leading to an immediate prearrest state. Asthmatic patients who are intubated are at risk of barotrauma and are ventilated using permissive hypercapnoea.

Assess response to therapy

- Use the same criteria used to assess severity.
- Severe and life-threatening cases require ABGs, CXR and electrolytes.
- Observed deteriorations in oxygen saturation monitoring require prompt treatment.
- Continuous metered-dose inhaler (MDI) or nebulised salbutamol can result in blood levels equivalent to therapeutic salbutamol infusions. Patients who are hypoventilating, have

mucus-obstructed airways or are not responding to nebulised salbutamol may require parenteral therapy.
- Patients with COPD may begin to deteriorate due to hypercarbia associated with high oxygen flow and reduced hypoxic drive, signalling the need for reduced FiO_2 and/or BiPAP support.

Admission, discharge, follow-up

Observe until the patient is clearly fit for discharge. Longer periods of observation may be required if the patient presents at night or if review, follow-up and compliance with therapy may be compromised.

Every patient discharged following an acute asthma episode should have a clear follow-up plan, including a review of medications, precipitating factors and need for an asthma action plan.

ACUTE EXACERBATION OF COPD

Patients with COPD, because of their marginal lung function at diagnosis, are prone to significant symptoms with minor precipitants. The precipitant may include acute infection (most commonly), small pneumothoraces, deteriorations in cardiac performance and arrhythmias and may be complicated by acute anxiety and increasing O_2 consumption.

Smoking is the commonest cause of COPD and acute interventional counselling is as effective as any other measure in reducing smoking in all ED patients.

Indigenous Australians continue to lose significantly more quality life years because of smoking and COPD.

Initial stabilisation

1. Give oxygen initially, titrated to O_2 saturation > 90%. Monitor carefully for hypercarbia and intervene before significant decrease in LOC or loss of hypoxic drive.
2. Commence nebulised bronchodilator therapy with salbutamol and ipratropium bromide.
3. Give IV hydrocortisone 200 mg.
4. Monitor respiratory rate, ECG, pulse oximetry.
5. Obtain IV access.
6. Assess sputum volume, colour, ABGs, spirometry and CXR.
7. If patient febrile or appears septic, sputum and blood cultures.

Further treatment

1. Regular nebulised salbutamol 5 mg q4h and ipratropium bromide 500 microg q6h.

2 Antibiotics per *Therapeutic Guidelines* if evidence of infection. If IV antibiotics are required due to severity, inability to safely swallow, use guidelines for community-acquired pneumonia, usually Class III or IV.
3 Hydrocortisone IV maximum 400 mg/day. Long-term steroid therapy is only indicated where reversible bronchospasm has been identified.
4 Consider additional treatment with nitrates and diuretics if pulmonary oedema is also a factor. Crackles on auscultation may be pre-existing due to pulmonary fibrosis rather than pulmonary oedema; check old records.
5 BiPAP is highly effective in acute symptom relief, treatment of hypercarbia and exhaustion. Many intubations have been prevented by early institution of BiPAP. BiPAP should be initialised with care and with consideration of the fact that many of these patients become acutely claustrophobic and take time to adjust to their face being covered and the sensation of the pressure changes.

Patients who have reported good quality of life despite home O_2 therapy may request intubation in the event of respiratory arrest or BiPAP failure, if there is a reversible precipitating factor.

Advance directives should be checked and respected.

Admission, discharge, follow-up

All but the most minor exacerbations presenting to hospital will require admission.

GP liaison, multidisciplinary community care, pulmonary rehabilitation programs, influenza vaccination and establishment of advance directives continue to improve patient outcomes and reduce length of stay and readmission rates.

ACUTE PULMONARY OEDEMA

This topic is covered in Chapter 10, 'Acute pulmonary oedema'.

PNEUMONIA

- Initially, presentation may be subtle, with fever and malaise.
- Pleuritic chest pain, sputum and dyspnoea may not occur until more advanced, unless there is a significant pre-existing respiratory comorbidity.
- Pneumonia presenting with respiratory distress generally represents a severe case likely to require ICU monitoring and management.

(*pto*)

- CXR may not be helpful until later in the course of the illness and after rehydration.
- The immediate threats to life are hypoxaemia and systemic sepsis.

Management

1. Initiate high-flow oxygen.
2. Obtain IV access.
3. Initiate goal-directed sepsis management if examination reveals signs of severe sepsis.
4. Blood culture from a minimum of 2 sites and sputum culture are helpful to potentially rationalise and target antibiotic therapy.
5. Commence antibiotic therapy as soon as cultures taken in high parenteral doses using antibiotic guidelines and Pneumonia Severity Index Score (Figure 9.1, over the page).

Consider that respiratory symptoms may be secondary to severe sepsis from another source.

Be aware of the aggressive therapy required for the immunosuppressed patient or hospital-acquired pneumonia.

Consider severe acute respiratory syndrome (SARS) and *Legionella* as potential causes, particularly in rapidly deteriorating cases associated with respiratory failure.

SPONTANEOUS PNEUMOTHORAX

Traumatic pneumothoraces are treated more aggressively and are covered in Chapter 3, 'Resuscitation and emergency procedures'.

The classic presentation of spontaneous pneumothorax is that of the thin, tall young man with pleuritic chest pain and dyspnoea. Spontaneous pneumothoraces occur in families and can be recurrent.

Illness such as COPD and asthma may be associated with spontaneous pneumothorax, especially in association with acute exacerbations where the pneumothorax may have precipitated the presentation.

Initial stabilisation

The immediate threat to life is the tension pneumothorax which, if untreated, will lead to circulatory collapse. Circulatory collapse is preceded by extreme and rapidly deteriorating respiratory distress.

Tension pneumothorax leading to significant compromise will be obvious clinically.

The presence of tension is independent of the size of the pneumothorax, although it will progressively enlarge unless there is marked gas trapping in the affected lung. The patient may be agitated and confused and appear restless with dyspnoea, tachypnoea and cyanosis. The affected hemithorax will appear hyperinflated, neck veins distended.

The patient will be tachycardic and hypotensive. Tracheal shift, if palpable, will be away from the side of the pneumothorax. Auscultation reveals reduced or absent breath sounds on the affected side. The affected hemithorax is hyperresonant to percussion. Subcutaneous emphysema, if present, may become suddenly worse.

- Identify the affected hemithorax and place a 12-gauge IV cannula in the 2nd intercostal space, midclavicular line. Attach it to a flutter valve or leave it open to air.
- Needle thoracostomies with IV cannulae are prone to block or kink and may be too short to drain reliably unless a longer than standard cannula is used.
- Placement of the cannula commits to a formal tube thoracostomy.
- Experienced practitioners adept at rapid insertion of tube thoracostomy will be less likely to need needle thoracostomy. Nonetheless, the patient must not be allowed to deteriorate or remain untreated if a slow process of tube thoracostomy is anticipated.
- Initiate high-flow oxygen.
- Obtain IV access for sedation and analgesia in the case of tube thoracostomy.

Specific treatment

Treatment options are available, depending on the patient's underlying condition and the response of the pneumothorax.

1. **Conservative management as an outpatient**
   - Suitable for patients with a small pneumothorax, no pre-existing lung disease, mild symptoms and no hypoxia. The pneumothorax is treated with high-flow oxygen while being assessed, but is not drained. The patient is discharged after remaining stable for 4–6 hours of observation.
   - The patient is advised to seek follow up X-rays (12–48 hours, shorter if a repeat X-ray is not taken prior to discharge), and full resolution and clearance is required before flying or diving. Discharge is not advised if any doubts exist as to the patient's ability to return promptly to hospital.
2. **Aspiration of pneumothorax**
   - Suitable for patients with moderate symptoms and a 20–40% pneumothorax with no underlying lung disease (secondary spontaneous pneumothorax). (*continues on p. 184*)

CHARACTERISTIC	NO. OF POINTS ASSIGNED
Demographic factors	
Age	
Men	Age (in years)
Women	Age (in years) – 10
Nursing home resident	+10
Coexisting illnesses	
Neoplastic disease	+30
Liver disease	+20
Congestive heart failure	+10
Cerebrovascular disease	+10
Renal disease	+10
Findings on physical examination	
Altered mental status	+20
Respiratory rate ≥ 30/min	+20
Systolic blood pressure < 90 mmHg	+20
Temperature < 35°C or ≥ 40°C	+15
Pulse ≥ 125 beats/min	+10
Laboratory and radiographic findings	
Arterial pH < 7.35	+30
Blood urea nitrogen ≥ 30 mg/dL (11 mmol/litre)	+20
Sodium < 130 mmol/litre	+20
Glucose ≥ 250 mg/dL (14 mmol/litre)	+10
Haematocrit < 30%	+10
Partial pressure of arterial oxygen < 60 mmHg or oxygen saturation < 90%	+10
Pleural effusion	+10

Stratification of risk score

RISK	RISK CLASS	SCORE	MORTALITY
Low	I	Based on algorithm	0.1%
Low	II	≤ 70	0.6%
Low	III	71–90	0.9%
Moderate	IV	91–130	9.3%
High	V	>130	27.0%

Figure 9.1 The Pneumonia Severity Index, used to determine a patient's risk of death. The total score is obtained by adding to the patient's age (in years for men or in (years – 10) for women) the points assigned for each additional applicable characteristic

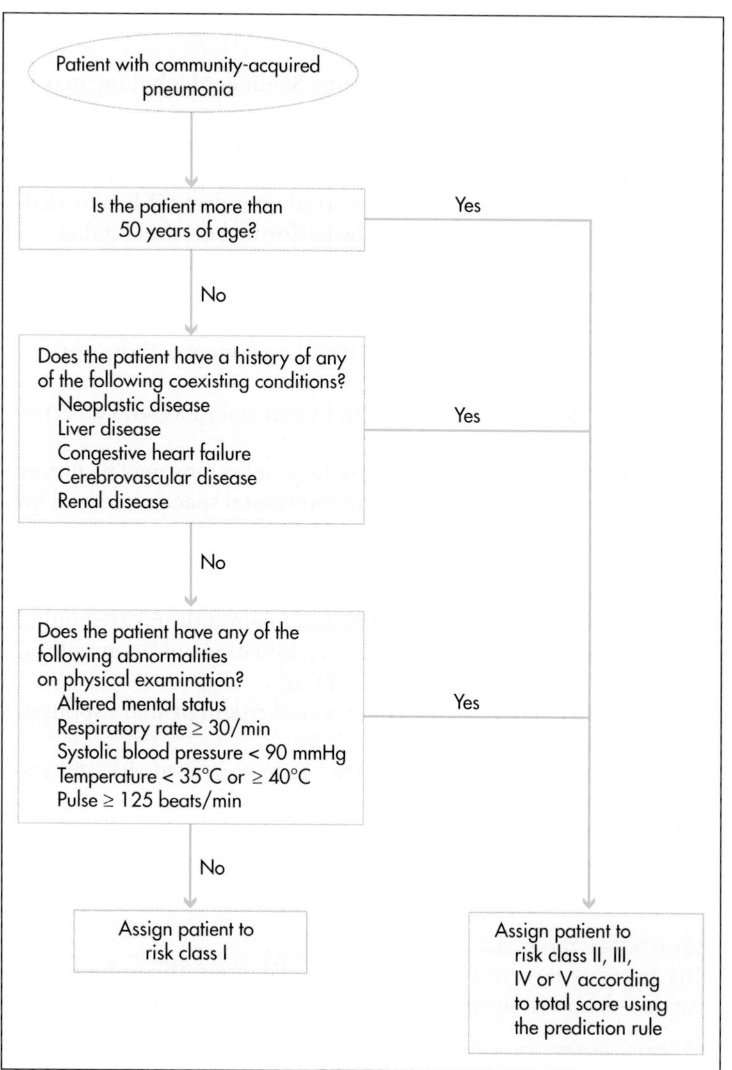

Figure 9.1 Continued

Based on Fine MJ, Auble TE, Yealy DM et al. A prediction rule to identify low-risk patients with community-acquired pneumonia. N Engl J Med 1997; 336:243–50, as presented in Halm EA, Teirstein AS. Management of community-acquired pneumonia. N Engl J Med 2002; 347(25):2039–44

- An IV cannula and three-way tap or other catheters designed for the purpose may be used.
- A pigtail catheter inserted using Seldinger technique may be safer and also effective if continuous drainage is required.
- The pneumothorax is aspirated using a three-way tap and then X-rays are repeated.
- If the pneumothorax has recurred on repeat CXR, a formal tube thoracostomy should be performed or, if a suitable catheter was used initially, it may be connected to an underwater drain and low suction.

3 **Tube thoracostomy**
- The best choice for those with a large pneumothorax or significant underlying lung disease.
- Place the tube in the 4th–5th intercostal space and directed superiorly.
- Avoid placing the tube where lung adhesions may be present as seen on CXR. Use the 2nd intercostal space midcostal line if necessary. Connect to low suction.

Large pneumothoraces are regarded as > 2–3 cm of collapse; however, treatment decisions regarding 'smaller' pneumothoraces should be based on the patient's stability, as determinations of pneumothorax size from CXR are notoriously inaccurate.

Male smokers have a 20-fold increased risk of primary spontaneous pneumothorax.

COPD and cystic fibrosis patients have increased risk and associated mortality.

Recurrent spontaneous pneumothoraces (i.e. same hemithorax) should be referred to a thoracic surgeon for possible thorascopic treatment.

PULMONARY EMBOLISM

This topic is covered in Chapter 11, 'Venous thromboembolic disease—deep venous thrombosis and pulmonary embolism.'

ACUTE LUNG INJURY (NON-CARDIOGENIC PULMONARY OEDEMA)

- This represents a range of conditions characterised by inflammation or injury causing increased permeability of lung tissue and exudation of fluid into the alveoli.
- Wet, stiff lungs make gas exchange and ventilation difficult.

- The condition may not become apparent until the patient starts to decompensate and tire, hours after the initial insult. Further decompensation is likely and should be anticipated.
- Respiratory dysfunction may become apparent as late as 48 hours or longer after the initial insult and may take weeks or months to resolve.
- Causes include pulmonary contusion, aspiration, chemical pneumonitis, narcotic overdose, near drowning, transfusion of blood products, SARS, avian influenza and severe sepsis.
- When invasive ventilation is required, care should be taken to avoid further ventilator-associated lung injury, as these patients are particularly at risk, especially from barotrauma.

ANAPHYLAXIS WITH BRONCHOSPASM

(See also Chapter 40, 'Dermatological presentations to emergency'.)

- Anaphylaxis may present with respiratory distress with or without shock as a result of the type 1 hypersensitivity reaction.
- Initial management is as for acute severe asthma; however, these patients require adrenaline, at least subcutaneous 0.3 mg for mild cases and IM 0.5 mg and/or titrated IV adrenaline for more severe cases.
- They can be identified by known history of allergy and precipitants, airway involvement with signs of oedema and voice changes, urticaria and pruritus. Suspect also when 'asthma' is of sudden onset without obvious precipitant.
- Following this initial therapy the patient should also receive IV hydrocortisone 200 mg and antihistamine therapy.
- Observe the patient for up to 12 hours because of the risk of late relapse.

HYPERVENTILATION

- Organic causes of hyperpnoea and hypocapnia must be considered and excluded initially.
- A CXR will be normal and ABGs will show respiratory alkalosis.
- Patients may present with non-exertional chest pain, blurred vision, palpitations, paraesthesiae, carpopedal spasm, fear, panic and hysteria.
- Treatment is with patient education and relaxation techniques, the goal being to achieve self-control.
- A short course of benzodiazepines may be useful. (*pto*)

- Antidepressants possibly have a role in recurrent cases but should not be initiated in the ED.
- Mitral valve prolapse may present with atypical chest pain, palpitations, dyspnoea, anxiety and panic attacks—so, if a typical click is heard and associated ECG changes seen, an outpatient echocardiogram should be arranged.
- 'Paper bag breathing' is not recommended.

Editorial Comment

ABC (airway, breathing, circulation)—beware of breathing, as deterioration can be subtle; look for trends in observations and tests.

Respiratory rates are very good measures of the degree of respiratory compromise.

Pulse oximetry—respond if low or drops.

For ventilated patients with high and increasing oxygen requirements and reversible conditions, early consultation with retrieval ECMO (extracorporeal membrane oxygenation) services, where available, is advised.

Chapter 10
Acute pulmonary oedema

Anthony F T Brown

Overview

Acute pulmonary oedema (APO) is one of the acute heart failure (AHF) syndromes that include a spectrum of conditions ranging from acute decompensated chronic heart failure (ADHF), hypertensive AHF, high-output HF and right heart failure, to the more dramatic APO and cardiogenic shock.

APO accounts for up to 1% of emergency department visits, with a 7.4–15% in-hospital mortality and around a 25% 1-year mortality.

Although the classical gasping, frail, elderly patient may dominate the doctor's perspective, APO presents to the ED in a diverse population, from those suffering from an underlying acute coronary syndrome (ACS), whether an ST-elevation myocardial infarct (STEMI) or non-ST-elevation myocardial infarct (NSTEMI), those with an acute hypertensive event, to those with chronic decompensated heart failure or a non-cardiogenic cause.

All have subtly different historical, examination and investigation findings, and may require a wide variety of urgent treatment modalities.

Pathophysiology

APO may be divided into cardiogenic and non-cardiogenic causes.

ACUTE CARDIOGENIC PULMONARY OEDEMA

Acute cardiogenic pulmonary oedema is the most severe manifestation of congestive heart failure, and is associated with an increase in lung fluid secondary to hydrostatic leakage from pulmonary capillaries into the alveoli and interstitium of the lungs. Underlying this is an abrupt rise in left ventricular end-diastolic pressure and left atrial pressure related to left ventricular dysfunction.

The causative heart disease leading to left ventricular failure may be predominantly systolic failure with impaired cardiac contractility, i.e. with an ejection fraction (EF) under 40%, diastolic failure with impaired myocardial relaxation and distensibility (but with a normal or even supranormal EF), or a combination of both.

APO may develop out of the blue, or be precipitated in patients with existing heart disease as a result of an acute cause such as ischaemia, an arrhythmia or medication change.

Box 10.1 lists the potential causes of cardiogenic pulmonary oedema, whether related to predominant systolic or to diastolic dysfunction, with common precipitating factors.

Box 10.1 Causes of cardiogenic pulmonary oedema

Precipitating factors

- Myocardial ischaemia
- Cardiac arrhythmia:
  — tachycardia, including atrial fibrillation
  — bradycardia, conduction abnormality
- Volume overload, including blood transfusion
- Hypertensive crisis
- Systemic infection, including septic shock
- Cardiac infection—myocarditis, endocarditis
- Pulmonary embolism
- Medication-related:
  — inappropriate reduction of therapy
  — drug non-compliance
  — cardiac depressant (beta-blocker)
  — salt-retaining (non-steroidal anti-inflammatory drug, NSAID)
- High output state—anaemia, thyrotoxicosis, beriberi
- Alcohol excess or withdrawal

Predominant systolic heart failure

- Acute coronary syndrome
- Hypertension
- Cardiomyopathy
- Myocarditis
- Valvular disease, particularly acute aortic or mitral regurgitation

Predominant diastolic heart failure (one-third to one-half of all patients)

- Hypertension, including renovascular disease
- Aortic stenosis (indicates critical disease)
- Cardiomyopathy—hypertrophic (HCM) or restrictive
- Acute coronary syndrome

NON-CARDIOGENIC PULMONARY OEDEMA

Non-cardiogenic pulmonary oedema occurs without a rise in pulmonary capillary wedge pressure > 18 mmHg, and may result from a wide variety of mechanisms that include:

- increased capillary permeability in acute respiratory distress syndrome (ARDS), septicaemia, aspiration of gastric contents, inhaled toxins, pancreatitis, uraemia or near-drowning
- decreased oncotic pressure such as in hypoalbuminaemia, but usually in combination with another cause
- mixed or unknown causes such as neurogenic pulmonary oedema, high-altitude pulmonary oedema (HAPE), transfusion-related acute lung injury (TRALI), heroin overdose, smoking freebase cocaine, eclampsia, pulmonary embolism and post lung re-expansion.

NEUROGENIC PULMONARY OEDEMA

This is a rare cause of APO developing within a few hours of an acute neurological insult associated with sympathetic over-reactivity and intracranial hypertension. Typical causes include prolonged seizures, head injury or a subarachnoid or intracerebral haemorrhage.

It usually resolves over 48–72 hours, determined by the management and course of the underlying primary neurological insult.

Clinical features

HISTORY

Patients may be too distressed to give a history until after aggressive medical management, but may report chest pain, palpitations, a change in medication or recent fever (see Box 10.1) as a precipitating cause, or remember previous flash episodes of 'fluid on the lung'.

Acute breathlessness is universal, and may occur precipitately or on the background of cough, exertional dyspnoea, orthopnoea, paroxysmal nocturnal dyspnoea (PND) and dyspnoea at rest.

Other non-specific features such as fatigue and nocturia may occur in those with previously compensated heart failure. Finally, confusion, coma and respiratory arrest can ensue.

EXAMINATION

- Patients with APO are frightened, sweaty, restless, unwilling to lie down, and may wheeze or froth pink sputum in extreme cases.
- Tachypnoea, tachycardia, reduced oxygen saturation, hyper- or hypotension and cyanosis all occur.
- Inspiratory basal crackles, a raised jugular venous pressure (JVP) from secondary right-heart failure and a 3rd heart sound S_3 gallop are typical; whereas in non-cardiogenic pulmonary

oedema, patients may have a warm periphery, bounding pulse and usually absence of an S_3 gallop or jugular venous distension.

- A new systolic murmur can indicate an acute mechanical complication such as papillary muscle rupture or an acquired ventricular septal defect (VSD) in the setting of an acute myocardial infarction (AMI).

Differential diagnosis

Pulmonary embolism (PE) and acute pneumonia must be excluded, although PE becomes more common in heart failure, and severe pneumonia may in itself lead to non-cardiogenic pulmonary oedema.

Investigations

ELECTROCARDIOGRAM (ECG)

This is essential to diagnose an AMI, arrhythmia or heart block, and may determine the need for time-critical reperfusion therapy in the presence of chest pain particularly with STEMI. See Chapter 7, 'Acute coronary syndromes'.

It may also indicate underlying heart disease with left ventricular strain or hypertrophy, pre-existing coronary artery disease or even an electrolyte disturbance.

CHEST X-RAY (CXR)

CXR can confirm the presence of APO, but due to its relatively poor sensitivity, it should not be used to rule out the diagnosis even when oedema fluid is not visible, or in the presence of technical issues particularly with a portable film.

The CXR may help to differentiate APO from an exacerbation of chronic obstructive pulmonary disease (COPD) or asthma.

1. Typical features of cardiogenic pulmonary oedema include cardiomegaly, pulmonary venous congestion with upper lobe diversion, perihilar 'bat's wing' infiltrates, Kerley B engorged subpleural lymphatics, interstitial oedema and small pleural effusions.
2. A normal heart size may occur in acute valvular rupture, diastolic dysfunction, myocarditis or non-cardiogenic causes of pulmonary oedema.
3. Non-cardiogenic pulmonary oedema will also show patchy or peripheral oedema, rather than even and central. Kerley B lines and pleural effusions are usually not present.

LABORATORY TESTS

A full blood count, electrolyte and liver function tests, cardiac enzyme biomarkers including troponin, coagulation profile and thyroid function test should be sent, but usually add little to the immediate management.

Biomarkers

Troponin

An elevated troponin may indicate myocardial damage from an ACS, particularly in the presence of new ECG changes, but also occurs in the absence of ACS, for instance in severe sepsis or from a PE.

B-type natriuretic polypeptide (BNP)

Other biomarkers such as BNP and *N*-terminal (NT) pro-BNP are of most value when the diagnosis is uncertain in a patient with acute dyspnoea. A BNP level under 100 pg/mL makes heart failure unlikely (approximate negative likelihood ratio (LR) = 0.1), and above 400 pg/mL makes heart failure likely (approximate positive LR = 6).

However, between 100 and 400 pg/mL is an 'indiscriminate zone' that necessitates clinical judgment with further testing. In addition, both markers may be raised in the presence of renal disease, PE and cor pulmonale, and conversely both may be low in 'flash' APO, acute papillary muscle rupture and the obese.

Thus BNP use in the ED is still uncommon, and in the ICU can be problematic, and may be better suited to assessing progress in response to therapy.

Arterial blood gases

As with laboratory tests, ABGs add nothing to the immediate management and serve only to delay therapy. They may be useful to monitor hypercapnoea in the non-responding patient.

Management of APO

1 Sit the patient upright, apply high-flow oxygen via a non-rebreathing mask and commence non-invasive monitoring in a resuscitation area.

2 Commence vasodilator therapy with nitrates to reduce preload, particularly in patients with systolic blood pressure (SBP) above 140 mmHg.

   a Give glyceryl trinitrate (GTN) 150–300 microg sublingually. This dose may be repeated. Remove the tablet or cease if hypotension (SBP below 100 mmHg) occurs.

   b Change to a GTN infusion in resistant cases, particularly those associated with ischaemic chest pain. Add 200 mg GTN to 500 mL 5% dextrose (i.e. 400 microg/mL) in a glass bottle with low-absorption polyethylene infusion set. Commence at 1 mL/h (6.66 microg/min) and gradually increase to 20 mL/h or more, taking care to maintain SBP above 100 mmHg.
3. Give frusemide 40 mg IV or twice the usual oral daily dose if already taking frusemide tablets, which may be repeated after 20–30 minutes.
   a Avoid overdiuresis, as this may activate neurohormonal systems with a deterioration in renal function and a worsened outcome, particularly in those presenting hypertensive with predominant diastolic dysfunction.
   b Surprisingly, no randomised controlled trial has shown a mortality benefit with the use of frusemide alone in acute decompensated heart failure, whether as a bolus or as an infusion.
4. Give small increments of morphine only if there is chest pain with dyspnoea, starting at 0.5 mg IV in the elderly up to 2.5 mg in younger patients.
   a Do not use morphine routinely, particularly if the patient is tired, may have COLD/asthma or is becoming obtunded with a rising arterial partial pressure of CO_2 ($PaCO_2$).
   b Again morphine does not lessen mortality and may worsen acidosis.
5. Commence non-invasive ventilation (NIV) in those who do not respond to the above standard pharmacological therapy.
   a Use continuous positive airway pressure (CPAP) via a tight-fitting face mask, high-flow gas circuit and starting with 10–15 cmH_2O.
   b CPAP improves lung mechanics and enhances left ventricular performance, reducing the need for endotracheal intubation (relative risk [RR] 0.44) and the in-hospital mortality (RR 0.64).
   c Consider bi-level positive airway pressure (BiPAP) non-invasive positive-pressure ventilation (NIPPV) as an alternative. However, it is more complex to set up and costly, and although it reduces the need for intubation (RR 0.54) it does not reduce the in-hospital mortality of cardiogenic pulmonary oedema, possibly relating to a negative association with an increased rate of AMI.

Disposal

1. Patients who present hypotensive with SBP < 90 mmHg, or deteriorate and/or do not tolerate pharmacological vasodilation, have a poor prognosis, with mortality up to 80%.
   a. Call for senior help if you have not already done so! Manage the patient as for cardiogenic shock with intubation and mechanical ventilation, applying 5–10 cmH_2O positive end-expiratory pressure (PEEP).
   b. Support the circulation with inotropes such as dopamine 2–20 microg/kg/min and dobutamine 2–30 microg/kg/min. Noradrenaline or adrenaline may be required for extreme hypotension, but the higher myocardial oxygen demand may ultimately be deleterious.
   c. Look for a treatable mechanical cause with an urgent transthoracic echocardiogram, such as an acute valvular rupture or VSD, and organise immediate cardiac surgical referral if one of these is found.
   d. Admit the patient to intensive care. An intra-aortic balloon pump may be used as a temporising measure while reperfusion therapy—such as acute angioplasty or coronary revascularisation—is performed in the setting of an ST-elevation myocardial infarction, or while valvular or VSD repair is organised (see above).
2. The majority of patients respond to standard pharmacological therapy plus NIV.
   a. Arrange admission to a coronary care or telemetry unit if there are ongoing cardiac issues such as pain, ischaemia, arrhythmias or an electrolyte disturbance and close monitoring or respiratory support are necessary.
   b. Otherwise, particularly in the elderly patient with brief decompensation of chronic heart failure, admit the patient to a non-monitored medical bed.
3. Non-cardiogenic pulmonary oedema is managed according to the underlying primary cause, e.g. antibiotics for infection, and with non-invasive or invasive respiratory support as necessary.

Online resources

UpToDate: multiple topics, updated Apr 2010 to Mar 2012. www.uptodate.com/home

Chapter 11

Venous thromboembolic disease—deep venous thrombosis and pulmonary embolism

Tim Green

Introduction

Deep venous thrombosis (DVT) and pulmonary embolism (PE) are both manifestations of a single pathological entity, venous thromboembolic (VTE) disease, and are best considered as points on a continuum of a single pathological process. VTE is the third most common cardiovascular disease after ischaemic heart disease and stroke. A West Australian study in 2008 recorded the annual event rate of VTE as 0.85 cases per 1000 population and extrapolated up to 17,400 cases per year in Australia.[1]

VTE has a significant untreated mortality of up to 30%.[2] Mortality within a month of diagnosis is 6% for DVT and 12% for PE.[3] While hospitalisation or recent hospitalisation itself is the major risk factor for developing VTE, up to 43% of cases are acquired in the community and commonly present to emergency departments.[4]

While both DVT and PE have a number of characteristic clinical features, these are neither sensitive nor specific and clinical diagnosis is difficult. ED evaluation involves a structured approach of risk stratification, screening investigations, a search for alternative diagnoses and selection of an appropriate imaging strategy. The approach taken in an individual ED will depend on its case-mix and the availability of key modalities of investigation, and a balance must be struck between the harms of undiagnosed disease and the adverse events associated with both invasive investigations and anticoagulation.

While VTE is increasingly safely treated in the community, often in a hospital in the home (HITH) setting, it is important to identify patients who may need invasive therapies such as thrombolysis or surgery. While parenteral and oral anticoagulation effectively decrease morbidity and mortality from VTE, they pose a not inconsiderable cost, inconvenience and risk of harm, so it is critical that a firm diagnosis of VTE is made before committing a patient to long-term therapy.

Pathophysiology

Predisposition to VTE is best understood by analysis of Virchow's triad of *venous stasis, vessel wall injury* and *hypercoagulable states* and forms the basis of most clinical decision rules for VTE.

- Stasis may result from immobility (particularly in hospital), external compression by pelvic tumours or lower limb plaster splints.
- Vessel wall injury may be the result of trauma, surgery or intravascular device.
- Hypercoagulability is a feature of pregnancy, oral contraceptive pill or HRT use, cancer and a number of thrombophilic disorders[5] (see Box 11.1).

Age is an important risk factor for VTE, via a number of mechanisms: increasing venous valve incompetence, acquired thrombophilia such as malignancy, increased risk of comorbid diseases such as cardiac failure, renal disease or the need for surgery, particularly joint replacement.

Venous thrombi, particularly when fresh, may dislodge and embolise centrally to the right ventricle and pulmonary arterial circulation or paradoxically via a patent foramen ovale or atrial septal defect into the systemic circulation. Patients with proximal leg or pelvic vein DVT will develop PE in approximately 50% of cases. Calf vein DVT are much less likely to embolise to the lungs, but are the most common source of paradoxical emboli.[6]

Pulmonary emboli lead to hypoxaemia by increasing both anatomical and physiological dead space. Multiple or large emboli will lead to an increase in pulmonary vascular resistance, which in turn leads to increasing right ventricular wall tension and may lead to right ventricular dysfunction. Increased right ventricular wall pressure may

Box 11.1 Thrombophilic disorders associated with VTE

Antithrombin III deficiency
Protein C deficiency
Protein S deficiency
Factor V Leiden
Prothrombin G20210A
Homocysteinaemia
Antiphospholipid syndrome
Elevated factor VIII
Elevated factor IX
Elevated factor XI
Elevated fibrinogen

compress the right coronary artery as well as impairing subendocardial blood flow, and precipitate myocardial ischaemia. This may be accompanied by micro-infarction and elevation of cardiac biomarkers such as troponin. Massive PE will eventually cause paradoxical interventricular septal motion, left ventricular diastolic dysfunction and impaired cardiac output. Death is the result of circulatory shock and myocardial ischaemia.

Therapeutic anticoagulation inhibits formation of new clot. Fresh clot is more friable and prone to embolise. In time, existing clot ages and becomes more stable, decreasing the risk of embolism. With therapeutic anticoagulation the fibrinolytic pathway is able to partially or completely remove pre-existing clot. The success of this process will be measured in the incidence of post-phlebitic complications such as oedema and venous ulcers in the lower limb following DVT or chronic pulmonary hypertension and cor pulmonale complicating PE.

Clinical features

DVT may cause calf and/or thigh pain and lower limb swelling but is frequently asymptomatic. Typical signs of DVT, including unilateral swelling, oedema, erythema, local warmth and tenderness along the distribution of deep veins, are variable in frequency and examination may be entirely normal. Extensive pelvic or proximal DVT may present with a grossly swollen, painful limb of pale or dusky blue appearance (phlegmasia alba dolens and phlegmasia cerulea dolens, respectively). These presentations represent an acute limb threat and mandate aggressive inpatient therapy, frequently with catheter-delivered thrombolysis or thrombectomy.

Patients with **PE** may or may not have clinical evidence of concomitant DVT. Common but non-specific symptoms of PE include dyspnoea, pleuritic chest pain, apprehension and cough (> 50%). Haemoptysis, sweats, syncope and non-pleuritic pain are less common (15–30%).[7] Apart from tachycardia and tachypnoea, physical signs of PE such as pleural rubs, loud P2 or gallop rhythm are relatively rarely found. Massive PE should be considered in patients who present with sudden cardiovascular decompensation, syncope, unexplained hypoxia, shock or pulseless electrical activity (PEA) cardiac arrest.

DIFFERENTIAL DIAGNOSES

DVT—ruptured Baker's cyst, cellulitis, muscle strain/haematoma, superficial venous thrombophlebitis, chronic venous insufficiency

PE—

Pulmonary: pneumonia, asthma, COPD, pneumothorax, pleurisy
Cardiovascular: ACS, pericarditis, CCF, aortic dissection
Musculoskeletal: chest wall strain, rib fracture
Anxiety

Diagnostic approach and clinical decision rules

ED assessment for patients presenting with symptoms of possible VTE is focused on searching for and ruling out alternative diagnoses, establishing the clinical likelihood for VTE and determining whether diagnostic imaging is required. Clinical impression, or pre-test probability (PTP), is best guided by one of many validated clinical decision rules that have been produced for both DVT and PE. Such risk stratification combined with the measurement of D-dimer can either rule out significant risk of VTE or mandate specific imaging.

Table 11.1 **Clinical model for predicting the pre-test probability of DVT**

Clinical characteristic	Score
Active cancer (patient receiving treatment for cancer within the previous 6 months or currently receiving palliative treatment)	1
Paralysis, paresis or recent plaster immobilisation of the lower extremities	1
Recently bedridden for 3 days or more, or major surgery within the previous 12 weeks requiring general or regional anaesthesia	1
Localised tenderness along the distribution of the deep venous system	1
Entire leg swollen	1
Calf swelling at least 3 cm larger than that on the asymptomatic side (measured 10 cm below tibial tuberosity)	1
Pitting oedema confined to the symptomatic leg	1
Collateral superficial veins (non-varicose)	1
Previously documented DVT	1
Alternative diagnosis at least as likely as DVT	–2

A score of 2 or higher indicates that the probability of DVT is likely; a score of less than 2 indicates that the probability of DVT is unlikely. In patients with symptoms in both legs, the more symptomatic leg is used.

Reproduced from Wells PS, Anderson DR, Rodger M et al. Evaluation of D-dimer in the diagnosis of suspected deep-vein thrombosis. N Engl J Med 2003;349:1227–35, with permission.

DVT

Wells et al have published clinical decision rules for both DVT and PE.[8,9] Wells' criteria for DVT are listed in Table 11.1.

- For patients with a score of < 2 and a negative D-dimer, VTE is effectively ruled out.
- Patients scoring ≥ 2 have an approximate risk of VTE of 28% and require further assessment with ultrasonography. If ultrasonography is negative but D-dimer is positive, repeat ultrasound in 1 week should be recommended.[8]

Pregnant and postpartum women should not be assessed with these criteria and should generally all have ultrasonography if DVT is suspected.

PE

For patients in whom the clinical 'gestalt' for PE is low (< 15%), the PE Rule-out Criteria (PERC Rule) can be applied prior to ordering D-dimer or imaging.[10] The mnemonic HADCLOTS represents 8 clinical criteria which if all met can effectively rule out PE without further investigation.

H Hormone: no oestrogen use/pregnancy
A Age < 50 years
D DVT/PE: no previous history
C Coughing blood: no haemoptysis
L Leg swelling: absence of unilateral limb swelling
O Oxygen: $SaO_2 > 95\%$
T Tachycardia (absence): HR < 100 bpm
S Surgery: nil recent (< 28 days)

A myriad of clinical decision rules have been described for evaluation of PE.[11] The Wells PE Score remains the most commonly used[9,12] (Table 11.2).

- Low pre-test probability as judged by a Wells score ≤ 4 combined with a negative D-dimer effectively rules out PE without requiring imaging.
- Patients with positive D-dimer or a Wells score > 4 may have PE diagnosed or ruled out with CT pulmonary angiography.[9,13,14]
- V/Q scanning can be considered in patients with a normal chest X-ray when contrast and radiation exposure need to be avoided/ minimised. An alternative strategy is to perform lower limb ultrasound first, with a positive diagnosis of DVT obviating the need for further investigation.

Table 11.2 **Wells PE Score**

Clinical feature	Points
Suspected DVT	3
Alternative diagnosis less likely than PE	3
Heart rate > 100 bpm	1.5
Prior VTE	1.5
Immobilisation within prior 4 weeks	1.5
Active malignancy	1
Haemoptysis	

Score < 2: low risk (3.4%)
Score 2–6: moderate risk (27.8%)
Score > 6: high risk (78.4%)
Adapted from Wells PS, Anderson DR, Rodger M et al. Excluding pulmonary embolism at the bedside without diagnostic imaging: management of patients with suspected pulmonary embolism presenting to the emergency department by using a simple clinical model and D-dimer. Ann Intern Med 2001;135:98–107.

Investigations

ECG: mainly performed to exclude acute myocardial ischaemia or pericarditis, ECG may reveal signs of right ventricular strain. Sinus tachycardia is common, as is anterior T wave inversion. The classical S_1, Q_3, T_3 pattern is relatively specific for PE but quite rarely seen.

Chest X-ray: the main purpose of chest radiography is to establish alternative diagnoses such as pneumonia or pneumothorax. In cases of PE, chest X-ray is often normal or near-normal. Signs of focal oligaemia (focal decrease in vascular markings) or pulmonary infarction (such as the Hampton's hump, a peripheral wedge-shaped density above the diaphragm) are not common. Atelectasis and small pleural effusions are often non-specific markers of PE.

Blood gases: although blood gas analysis may provide useful information of acidosis in moderate to severe PE, the diagnostic utility of identifying hypoxaemia, hypocarbia or elevated A–a gradient is not great and is not helpful in determining whether imaging is necessary. Evidence of hypoxaemia is easily diagnosed using non-invasive pulse oximetry.

D-dimer: D-dimer is produced during the breakdown of fibrin by plasmin and is a marker of the presence of clot and in vivo thrombolysis. A good-quality quantitative D-dimer ELISA has a sensitivity of about 80% for DVT and 95% for PE, and is subsequently a useful test to rule out VTE, particularly if the assessment of clinical likelihood is low. Unfortunately the specificity of D-dimer is low, and it is frequently elevated in patients with acute illness (such as ACS, cancer or sepsis), in the postoperative period and during and after pregnancy.

Troponin: elevation in cardiac biomarkers such as troponin, while not diagnostic of VTE, is a marker of severity of PE and may predict complications and mortality.

Ultrasound: Doppler ultrasound has almost completely replaced contrast venography in the diagnosis of DVT. DVT is manifest by lack of vein compressibility, direct visualisation of thrombus and abnormal Doppler flow response to compression. Whole-leg colour-flow Doppler ultrasound is performed by radiology departments and vascular laboratories, and has a sensitivity of 91–96% and a specificity of 98–100%.[15,16] Bedside ultrasound in the ED, using a limited technique of 2-point compression of the femoral and popliteal veins, is being increasingly used to exclude proximal vein DVT and is a skill that can be readily acquired by competent ED sonographers.[17]

CT pulmonary angiography (CTPA): modern multi-detector spiral CT scanners are able to obtain images with a resolution of less than 1 mm and are able to diagnose very small peripheral emboli. CTPA has now completely replaced conventional pulmonary angiography. In addition to diagnosing or ruling out PE, CT may establish an alternative diagnosis by imaging pathology in the lung or aorta. Modern CTPA has a sensitivity of 83% and a specificity of 96%.[18] CTPA may not be readily available in smaller centres or after hours. Contrast allergy and renal impairment limit its safety in some groups, and the cumulative radiation burden of modern medicine remains a concern.

Ventilation–perfusion scan: V/Q scanning is now a second-line test for PE, but still has a role in patients intolerant to iodine-containing contrast and by virtue of its lower radiation dose in pregnant patients. V/Q scanning is of most utility in patients without underlying acute or chronic lung disease. High-probability V/Q scans and normal V/Q scans are able to diagnose or exclude PE. Intermediate-probability scans are common and necessitate another diagnostic approach.

Other imaging:

CT contrast venography may be performed immediately after CTPA without requiring further IV contrast to diagnose proximal DVT.[19]

DVT may also be diagnosed as an incidental finding during abdominal/pelvic contrast CT.

Gadolinium-enhanced contrast magnetic resonance angiography (MRA) may be used in cases where ultrasound is not diagnostic.

Bedside echocardiography is of particular use in evaluating critically ill patients in the ED resuscitation room with right ventricular dilation, hypokinesis, and rarely direct clot visualisation may diagnose massive PE or one of its mimics (AMI, pericardial tamponade, aortic dissection).

Tests for underlying thrombophilia in confirmed cases of VTE: while testing for underlying thrombophilic disorders has traditionally been advocated, some now question the cost–benefit of this. Idiopathic (versus provoked) VTE is associated with a similar risk of recurrence as VTE associated with a thrombophilic disorder, and it is argued that a decision about the duration of anticoagulation can be made for all idiopathic VTE without extensive testing. An exception is the antiphospholipid syndrome, which if diagnosed in a patient with VTE mandates lifelong anticoagulation.[4]

Treatment

ANTICOAGULATION

Standard treatment for all VTE includes initial anticoagulation with heparin and warfarin, with heparin being discontinued when the INR is therapeutic.

- Low-molecular-weight heparin (LMWH) such as enoxaparin is usually preferred to unfractionated heparin.[20] LMWH allows outpatient treatment in selected patients in a typical dosage of enoxaparin 1.0 mg/kg BD or 1.5 mg/kg daily.
- Caution should be exercised in obese patients and in patients with renal impairment. Patients weighing > 100 kg should have LMWH dose calculated for 100 kg.
- Unfractionated heparin remains the treatment of choice for hospitalised patients at high risk of bleeding, requiring invasive procedures or with renal failure.
- Oral anticoagulation with warfarin may be started concurrently with heparin with a target INR in the range of 2–3.
- Warfarin is usually continued for 3–6 months but may be recommended as lifelong treatment in patients with a high risk of recurrence.[21, 22]

GRADUATED COMPRESSION STOCKINGS

Use of stockings reduces the risk of post-phlebitic syndrome following DVT and is recommended for all unless pre-existing leg ulceration or extensive varicosities contraindicate it.[23]

VENA CAVAL FILTERS

May be considered in cases where anticoagulation is contraindicated or where PE has recurred despite therapeutic anticoagulation.[24]

THROMBOLYSIS/SURGERY

There is little high-level evidence for the use of thrombolysis or surgical embolectomy in massive PE (defined by blood pressure < 90 mmHg for > 15 minutes) or submassive PE. However, there is widespread consensus opinion to consider these treatments in haemodynamically unstable patients with confirmed PE.[25] Tissue plasminogen activator (rTPA) is the recommended thrombolytic agent.

Limb-threatening proximal DVT may be treated with local thrombolytic therapy using urokinase infused into a distal cannula.

Disposition

Most patients with DVT can be managed as outpatients. Exceptions include extensive proximal DVT, limited cardiorespiratory reserve, high risk of bleeding, risk of poor compliance with therapy, inadequate social supports and a contraindication to LMWH that necessitates IV unfractionated heparin.[26] Patients with confirmed PE are usually admitted to hospital. Recent studies argue that carefully selected patients with PE may be safely discharged from the ED or after a short period of in-hospital observation.[27]

Editorial Comment

The literature and clinical practice are allowing for increasing treatment of patients at home with follow-up after discharge. The management of this important clinical group will change markedly with newer anticoagulant therapy and refinement of at-risk groups.

Pearls and pitfalls in venous thromboembolic disease are given opposite.

Pearls and Pitfalls

- If high clinical suspicion of DVT, and initial Doppler ultrasound is negative, consider a progress study in 7 days.
- Compartment syndrome secondary to calf haematoma is an increasingly recognised complication of LMWH treatment for lower-limb DVT. Ensure the diagnosis is well established before committing a patient to anticoagulation, and have a high index of suspicion when a patient being treated for DVT re-presents with increasing lower-limb pain.
- Point of care ultrasound screening for lower-limb DVT and echocardiography are increasingly within the competence of emergency doctors, but appropriate training, credentialling and cooperation with local echo and ultrasound services is essential.
- Upper-limb DVT are much less common than lower-limb DVT. They are commonly the complication of central venous lines or associated with cervical ribs and thoracic outlet syndrome, and are commonly misdiagnosed initially. While less likely to embolise, they may lead to disabling upper-limb oedema. These are more commonly managed with thrombolytic or surgical therapies, so referral is mandatory.
- The best management of isolated calf vein DVT is controversial. Some advocate avoiding anticoagulation and performing serial ultrasound at 7 and 14 days to detect propagation, which would then mandate treatment. Alternatively, LMWH alone may be started with repeat ultrasound in 7 days. Anticoagulation is then ceased if there is not propagation, and a further ultrasound done in a further 7 days to ensure propagation hasn't occurred. Compression stockings should be recommended for all.

Acknowledgements

The author acknowledges George Jelinek and Martin Duffy who contributed previous versions of this chapter.

References

1. Ho WK, Hankey GJ, Eikelboom JW. The incidence of venous thromboembolism: a prospective, community-based study in Perth, Western Australia. Med J Aust 2008; 189(3):144–7.
2. Dunmire SM. Pulmonary embolism. Emergency Medicine Clinics of North America 1989; 7:339–54.
3. White RH. The epidemiology of venous thromboembolism. Circulation. 2003 Jun 17;107(23 Suppl 1):I4–8.
4. Cohen AT, Agnelli G, Anderson FA et al for the VTE Impact Assessment Group in Europe (VITAE). Venous thromboembolism (VTE) in Europe: The number of VTE events and associated morbidity and mortality. Thromb Haemost 2007;98:756–76.

5. Dalen JE. Should patients with venous thromboembolism be screened for thrombophilia? Am J Med 2008;121:458–63.
6. Kearon C. Natural history of venous thromboembolism. Circulation 2003;107:I-22–I-30.
7. Miniati M, Prediletto R, Formichi B et al. Accuracy of clinical assessment in the diagnosis of pulmonary embolism. Am J Respir Crit Care Med 1999;159:864–71.
8. Wells PS, Anderson DR, Rodger M et al. Evaluation of D-dimer in the diagnosis of suspected deep-vein thrombosis. N Engl J Med 2003;349:1227–35.
9. Wells PS, Ginsberg JS, Anderson DR et al. Use of a clinical model for safe management of patients with suspected pulmonary embolism. Ann Intern Med 1998;129:997–1005.
10. Kline JA, Courtney DM, Kabrhel C et al. Prospective multicenter evaluation of the pulmonary embolism rule-out criteria. J Thromb Haemost 2008;6:772–80.
11. Lucassen W, Geersing GJ, Erkens PM et al. Clinical decision rules for excluding pulmonary embolism: A meta-analysis. Ann Intern Med 2011;155:448–60.
12. Klok FA, Kruisman E, Spaan J et al. Comparison of the revised Geneva score with the Wells rule for assessing clinical probability of pulmonary embolism. J Thromb Haemost 2008;6:40–4.
13. Van Belle A, Buller HR, Huisman MV et al. Effectiveness of managing suspected pulmonary embolism using an algorithm combining clinical probability, D-dimer testing, and computed tomography. JAMA 2006;295:172–9.
14. Righini M, Le Gal G, Aujesky D et al. Diagnosis of pulmonary embolism by multidetector CT alone or combined with venous ultrasonography of the leg: a randomised non-inferiority trial. Lancet 2008;371:1343–52.
15. Lensing AW, Prandoni P, Brandjes D, et al. Detection of deep-venous thrombosis by real-time B-mode ultrasonography. N Engl J Med 1989;320:342–5.
16. Gaitini D. Current approaches and controversial issues in the diagnosis of deep venous thrombosis via duplex Doppler ultrasound. J Clin Ultrasound 2006;34:289–97.
17. Crisp JG, Lovato LM, Jang TB. Compression ultrasonography of the lower extremity with portable vascular ultrasonography can accurately detect deep venous thrombosis in the emergency department. Ann Emerg Med 2010:56:601–10.
18. Stein PD, Fowler SE, Goodman LR et al. Multidetector computed tomography for acute pulmonary embolism. N Engl J Med 2006;354:2317–27.

19. Loud, PA, Katz DS, Bruce DA et al. Deep venous thrombosis with suspected pulmonary embolism: detection with combined CT venography and pulmonary angiography. Radiology 2001;219:498–50.
20. Kearon C, Kahn SR, Agnelli G et al. Antithrombotic therapy for venous thromboembolic disease. Chest 2008; 133:454S.
21. Ho WK, Hankey GJ, Lee CH, Eikelboom JW. Venous thromboembolism: diagnosis and management of deep venous thrombosis. Med J Aust 2005;182:476–81.
22. Lee CH, Hanky GJ, Ho WK, Eikelboom JW. Venous thromboembolism: diagnosis and management of pulmonary embolism. Med J Aust 2005;182(11):569–74.
23. Brandjes DP, Büller HR, Heijboer H, et al. Randomised trial of effect of compression stockings in patients with symptomatic proximal-vein thrombosis. Lancet 1997;349:759–62.
24. Streiff MB. Vena caval filters: a comprehensive review. Blood 2000;95:3669–77.
25. Fesmire FM, Brown MD, Espinosa JA et al. Critical issues in the evaluation and management of adult patients presenting to the emergency department with suspected pulmonary embolism. Ann Emerg Med 2011;57:628–52.
26. Bates SM, Ginsberg JS. Treatment of deep-vein thrombosis. N Engl J Med 2004;351:268–77.
27. Aujesky D, Roy P-M, Verschuren F et al. Outpatient versus inpatient treatment for patients with acute pulmonary embolism: an international, open-label, randomised, non-inferiority trial. Lancet 2011;378:41–8.

Chapter 12
Shock

Steve Dunjey

Shock is a clinical condition, commonly encountered in practice, with multiple causes which share the final common pathway of inadequate tissue perfusion. The consequence of inadequate perfusion is that insufficient metabolic substrates (primarily oxygen) are provided to sustain cellular homeostasis. The challenge for the clinician is to manage the shock, and to simultaneously seek and treat the cause.

It seems clear that reducing the time to recognition of this state of inadequate perfusion will significantly reduce mortality, but recent publications have strongly made the point that vital-sign abnormalities (decreased BP, increased pulse/respiratory rate) are insensitive markers of early hypotension. While a search for the best early marker of shock continues, it seems that we can improve detection by searching for altered mental status, poor skin perfusion and oliguria and by recognition of an elevated lactate level.

Causes and effects

Causes of shock are loosely grouped as follows:

- hypovolaemic (inadequate circulating volume)
- cardiogenic (inadequate myocardial contractility)
- distributive (adequate volume, which is maldistributed)
- obstructive (adequate volume, with impedance of flow).

A more complete list of causes is given in Table 12.1. A patient in shock will manifest signs of:

- the cause of the shock
- inadequate tissue perfusion, with end-organ dysfunction (e.g. confusion, agitation, acidosis, decreased urine output, reduced capillary return, etc); see Box 12.1
- compensation. The cardiovascular response predominates, and is marked by tachycardia, peripheral vasoconstriction (sweaty, pale, cold peripheries with decreased capillary return), central vasoconstriction (narrowed pulse pressure) and decreased blood flow through non-vital structures, such as abdominal viscera (manifested by decreased urine output, decreased bowel sounds).

Table 12.1 Causes of shock

Type of shock	Causes	Signs
Hypovolaemic	Haemorrhage Vomiting/diarrhoea Dehydration Addisonian crisis	Obvious external blood loss/signs of trauma/signs of concealed blood loss Skin turgor Dry mucous membranes ↓ JVP
Cardiogenic	Myocardial infarction (especially anterior, R ventricular) Myocardial contusion Acute valvular lesion Cardiomyopathies Arrhythmias	Extremes of pulse rate ↑ JVP ECG evidence of AMI, arrhythmias New murmurs
Distributive	Neurogenic/spinal cord injury Anaphylaxis Sepsis	Flaccid paralysis, warm peripheries, relative bradycardia, priapism Urticaria, angio-oedema, wheezes Febrile, warm peripheries, evidence of focus
Obstructive	Pulmonary embolism Cardiac tamponade Tension pneumothorax	Evidence of DVT, pulmonary hypertension, ↑ JVP Distant muffled heart sounds, pulsus paradoxus, electrical alternans Subcutaneous emphysema, midline shift trachea, ↓ breath sounds

AMI, acute myocardial infarction; DVT, deep vein thrombosis; JVP, jugular venous pressure

Box 12.1 Adverse effects of shock

- CNS: confusion, restlessness and decreased level of consciousness
- Myocardium: may impair myocardial function in severe shock
- Lung: hypoxia, and sustained shock may induce adult respiratory distress syndrome in survivors
- Liver: elevation of hepatic transaminases and bilirubin
- Gastrointestinal tract: ischaemia, ileus, diarrhoea, stress ulceration and bacterial translocation into the systemic circulation
- Kidney: oliguria and renal failure
- Coagulopathy
- Other tissue damage: all tissues are impaired by sustained underperfusion, but the processes involved are difficult to quantify

Compensation can be so effective in young patients that the underlying shock state is manifest only by tachycardia, and more fully revealed by measuring postural BP drop (greater than 20 mmHg systolic). Younger patients are able to maintain an increased heart rate and cardiac output, but may suddenly deteriorate when they are unable to compensate further. Elderly patients may be incapable of mounting a tachycardic response to shock because of medications (especially beta-blockers) or underlying heart disease.

Overview of management

Shocked patients should be managed in a fully monitored area. The assessment and treatment of the shocked patient should occur in parallel. Initial treatment focuses on resuscitation, monitoring (to assess response to treatment) and seeking a specific cause (history, examination and investigations). Once the cause of shock has been determined, specific therapy should be considered. What follows is a description of initial management, then a description of specific therapies once the cause is known.

AIRWAY AND BREATHING

1. Secure the airway.
2. Enhance oxygenation. All patients will benefit from supplemental oxygen: initially provide the highest level of inspired O_2 available.
3. Support ventilation if necessary.

CIRCULATION

1. Control accessible haemorrhage.
2. Gain intravenous access with a minimum of 2 large-bore peripheral IV lines.
3. Begin fluid replacement. The volume of fluid replacement required will depend to a great degree on the type of shock being treated. Hypovolaemic shock commonly requires large volumes of fluid replacement, whereas patients with cardiogenic shock may require very little, if any at all. It is reasonable to begin with 250–500 mL boluses of fluid, and to review the response.
4. If the patient demonstrates ongoing signs of shock despite adequate volume replacement, the use of inotropic/vasopressor support should be considered.

MONITORING

Monitoring may include pulse rate, non-invasive blood pressure, urine output, temperature, central venous pressure (CVP), pulse oximetry and ECG. If the blood pressure remains low, or the patient is perceived to be unstable, invasive arterial monitoring should be considered.

INVESTIGATIONS

The cause of shock should be sought, and investigations appropriate to make a diagnosis should be performed on the basis of the history and exam findings.

- In general terms, patients will often have baseline blood tests performed (FBC, electrolytes, group and hold or cross-match if blood loss is the likely cause, coagulation profile), ECG and CXR.
- In modern emergency departments, it is generally easy to access a blood-gas machine, and frequent assessment of lactate is most helpful. A lactate level above 4 mmol/L is significantly elevated, and in most circumstances is a sign of tissue hypoperfusion.
- Bedside ultrasound is becoming an essential tool in the assessment of shocked patients in the ED. It is useful both in rapid evaluation of the cause of shock and in ongoing management (assessment of IVC diameter and RV filling give some indication of volume status). It is cheap, non-invasive, and easy to repeat, and current literature supports the view that bedside ultrasound plays a crucial role.

Hypovolaemic shock

Hypovolaemic shock involves the loss of intravascular volume. Among the most common causes in patients presenting to the ED are blood loss (external, internal) and dehydration. The aims of management are to limit further fluid loss and replenish circulating intravascular volume.

External haemorrhage is best controlled with direct pressure. Currently the use of military antishock trousers (MAST) is controversial and appears limited to patients with major pelvic and lower-limb injuries where the device stabilises fractures and produces pelvic compression, which limits further blood loss.

Adequacy of fluid resuscitation can be judged by the response of measured cardiovascular parameters (pulse rate, blood pressure, central venous pressure, urine output) and by a reduction in serum lactate. Fluids used include crystalloids and colloids, although currently crystalloids are used more frequently.

MANAGEMENT

1. Assess and treat airway, breathing and circulation (ABCs).
2. The initial fluid of choice is usually an isotonic crystalloid (normal saline/Hartmann's), which is best delivered as 250–500 mL aliquots rapidly infused (or 20 mL/kg aliquots for children).
3. Consider the use of blood products if blood loss is the primary cause of shock. If necessary (e.g. in established shock, with ongoing loss of blood) transfuse O-negative blood until either group-specific or fully cross-matched blood is available.
4. Large-bore peripheral lines are preferred. Central venous catheters (CVCs) can be time-consuming, difficult to insert and have the potential to cause injury. CVCs can be used if peripheral access proves impossible, or at a later stage when resuscitation is well established. Intraosseous access is an important alternative route in the shocked patient, and should be attempted if normal peripheral access is difficult or impossible.
5. Surgically correctible sources of blood loss should be sought, and haemorrhage arrested. Some sources of haemorrhage may be controlled medically (e.g. oesophageal varices with infusion of IV octreotide).
6. The endpoint of fluid therapy is still the subject of debate. Normal parameters may be detrimental in patients with some conditions which require surgical control of a bleeding source (examples include ruptured abdominal aneurysm, ectopic pregnancy, truncal stab wounds). Inadequate fluid resuscitation is, however, still a cause of preventable death, particularly in younger shocked patients, and the aim of therapy in most patients is return of near-normal blood pressure. A sustained low pressure in bleeding patients is known to produce the triad of hypothermia, acidosis and coagulopathy.
7. Ongoing blood loss may produce coagulopathy, requiring treatment with appropriate doses of cryoprecipitate, fresh frozen plasma, platelets. etc.

Cardiogenic shock

Cardiogenic shock results from cardiac dysfunction with decreased cardiac output. With increasing ventricular dysfunction, florid pulmonary oedema may develop. There are often prominent signs of right ventricular failure, such as jugular venous distension.

The most common initiating event for cardiogenic shock is acute ischaemic damage to the myocardium. Once more than 40% of the myocardium is affected, ejection fraction falls and cardiogenic shock results from the reduced cardiac output. Ischaemia can also trigger cardiogenic shock by producing papillary muscle dysfunction, septal defects, free-wall rupture or right ventricular infarction. Traditionally, tachy- and bradyarrhythmias are listed separately although both can cause shock.

Cardiogenic shock is a highly lethal condition with a mortality rate in excess of 80% if a non-invasive, supportive approach is used. Preventing cardiogenic shock from developing is the most effective therapy, and every effort should be made to limit infarct size in patients with acute myocardial infarction (AMI). It seems clear that percutaneous transluminal coronary angioplasty (PTCA) or emergency coronary artery bypass is more effective than thrombolytic therapy.

MANAGEMENT

1 Assess and treat ABCs.
2 Maintaining an adequate blood pressure can be difficult, particularly because the volumes of fluid used in normal resuscitation can have an adverse effect, causing further dilation of the compromised ventricle. The patient's condition does not always allow time for institution of sophisticated monitoring (e.g. Swan-Ganz catheter) and may force the clinician to administer empirical therapy. If the patient is already in pulmonary oedema, a fluid bolus should be avoided, but for other patients it is acceptable to try incremental small boluses of crystalloid as a first step (100–250 mL).
3 If there is no response to a fluid challenge, a vasopressor is required. Commonly used agents include dobutamine and dopamine.
4 Afterload reduction leads to improved cardiac function, but further reduction in blood pressure may compromise the function of other vital organs. Afterload reduction is therefore something to institute with caution to prevent exacerbation of hypotension.
5 Specific therapy includes aspirin, control of arrhythmias and reperfusion of the infarcted area.
6 Consider the use of intra-aortic balloon pump for patients who remain haemodynamically unstable.

Distributive shock

A number of pathological conditions cause distributive shock, the hallmarks of which are maldistribution of intravascular fluid through microvascular leak and/or vasodilation.

SEPTIC SHOCK

(See also 'Sepsis' in Chapter 41, 'Infectious diseases'.)

Septic shock results from a host response to infection with triggering of an immunological cascade. While the microbiological products are harmful, the widespread and unregulated host response produces chemical mediators which harm the host as well as the infecting organism. Chemical mediators involved include the complement system, leukotrienes, prostaglandins, thromboxanes, histamine, bradykinins, tumour necrosis factor (TNF) and interleukin-1.

Septic shock occurs in approximately 50% of those with Gram-negative bacteraemia, and in about 20% of those with *Staphylococcus aureus* bacteraemia. The Gram-negative organisms most often implicated are *Escherichia coli, Klebsiella, Pseudomonas, Enterobacter* and *Proteus* species.

Septic shock is marked clinically by signs of infection (although this may not be obvious in the immunocompromised or those at extremes of age) and vasodilation (warm peripheries despite hypotension). Eventually, myocardial dysfunction adds to the instability caused by microvascular leak and vasodilation.

Management

1. Assess and treat ABCs.
2. Large volumes of IV fluid may be required.
3. In addition to fluids, inotropes are likely to be necessary, and should be chosen to address the twin problems of decreased systemic vascular resistance and decreased myocardial function. Noradrenaline is an appropriate agent.
4. Sophisticated, invasive monitoring is usually required, including an arterial blood pressure monitor and central pressure monitoring. Current thinking is that better outcomes are reached with early goal-directed therapy, which follows set guidelines for physiological parameters, including
   - central venous pressure (CVP) 8–12 mmHg
   - mean arterial pressure (MAP) > 65 mmHg
   - central venous oxygen saturation (SvO_2) > 70%
   - urine output > 0.5 mL/kg/h.

5 The source of sepsis should be aggressively and rapidly sought. It is appropriate to administer empirical antibiotic therapy unless a focus can be established. Other treatments may include surgical drainage, debridement or laparotomy.

ANAPHYLACTIC SHOCK

(See also anaphylaxis flow chart, Figure 40.1.)

Anaphylactic shock results from the release of chemical mediators from mast cells and basophils. These chemicals (including histamine, leukotrienes, TNF, various cytokines, etc) cause vasodilation and capillary leakage, and subsequently hypotension. In addition, they can cause life-threatening compromise of the upper airway (angio-oedema) and ventilation (bronchospasm).

Clinically the syndrome is marked by a recent exposure to an allergen, the presence of urticaria/angio-oedema (90% of patients), bronchospasm, rhinitis, conjunctivitis and gastrointestinal cramping.

Management

1 Place the patient in the supine position (or left lateral position for vomiting patients).
2 Give IM adrenaline 1:1000, at a dose of 0.01 mg/kg bodyweight to a maximum dose of 0.5 mg (0.5 mL), injected into the lateral thigh.
3 All patients will benefit from supplemental oxygen and IV fluids. Use normal saline.
4 Support airway and ventilation. Be ready to deal with rapid progressive loss of airway. Be ready for resistant bronchospasm.
5 Remove the offending agent if possible.
6 Re-examine the patient frequently to assess progress. If resuscitation with IM adrenaline and IV normal saline is not effective, an infusion of IV adrenaline may be required: 1 mg of adrenaline added to 100 mL of normal saline can be run at 30–100 mL/h (5–15 microg/min).
7 Medications such as corticosteroids, antihistamines (H_1 and H_2) and antileukotrienes have no proven impact on the dangerous effects of anaphylaxis. They may have some benefit in treating mild allergic reactions involving skin. Promethazine can make vasodilation and hypotension worse.

NEUROGENIC SHOCK

Neurogenic shock occurs when sympathetic tone is lost following spinal cord transection above the T6 level (T4–T8). Loss of sympathetic tone causes peripheral vasodilation and is classically associated with bradycardia.

Management

1 Assess and treat ABCs. If the level of injury is high enough (e.g. high cervical), there may be compromised ventilatory effort.
2 Engage in a thorough search for other causes of hypotension. Blood loss should be sought and confidently excluded before hypotension is attributed to neurogenic causes alone.
3 If neurogenic shock does need to be treated, it is relatively unresponsive to fluid resuscitation, and overhydration is to be discouraged. Patients may require treatment with inotropic/vasopressor agents to effectively raise blood pressure.

Obstructive shock

Obstructive shock is hypotension due to impeded venous return. Circulatory volume is normal, but blood flow through the heart is compromised.

Specific clinical signs are of impeded venous return (distended neck veins) and also of the cause.

PERICARDIAL TAMPONADE

Pericardial tamponade occurs when fluid accumulates in the pericardial space, compressing the heart and eventually impairing cardiac filling. Classically, patients manifest Beck's triad (hypotension, elevated JVP and muffled heart sounds), and may have marked pulsus paradoxus. Clinical deterioration can be rapid. ECG may show electrical alternans, and the diagnosis can be established definitively with echocardiography.

Management

1 Assess and treat ABCs.
2 All patients benefit from IV fluids and oxygen.
3 Specific therapy is emergent pericardiocentesis (which ideally should be done with echo and ECG guidance) or open thoracotomy.
4 Other specific therapies depend on the cause of the effusion.

TENSION PNEUMOTHORAX

Obstructive shock results from a tension pneumothorax when raised intrathoracic pressure induces collapse of cardiac chambers and subsequent impaired cardiac filling. Specific signs include respiratory distress, with shift of the trachea from the midline and a hyperresonant, quiet chest on the side of the pneumothorax. The diagnosis is clinical, and should not depend on a confirmatory chest X-ray.

Management

1 Assess and treat ABCs.
2 Specific therapy is to drain the pneumothorax, initially by needle thoracostomy, immediately followed by a formal intercostal catheter.
3 Sucking chest wounds can cause a tension pneumothorax and should be covered with a non-permeable dressing stuck down on three sides, in addition to draining the pneumothorax.
4 A pneumothorax that resists drainage and continues to bubble vigorously may represent an injury to a major airway. Cardiothoracic help should be sought.

PULMONARY EMBOLISM

Massive pulmonary embolism can cause obstructive shock (see Chapter 11, 'Venous thromboembolic disease...').

Summary

There are many causes of shock, but the initial approach is always the same. Secure an airway, supplement ventilation if necessary, provide oxygen and resuscitate with IV fluids (except for cardiogenic shock). The cause of the shock should be sought, and specifically treated as appropriate.

Chapter 13
Pain management in the emergency department

John Vinen

Staff providing emergency care should be competent in the assessment and management of pain. The early relief of pain is a right and an expectation for all patients. The management of pain can be compromised by misunderstandings, myths, prejudice and inappropriate reliance on inflexible cookbook formulas. Good patient care demands timely and effective pain relief; failure to effectively manage pain is a failure in the quality of care.

A significant proportion of patients presenting to the ED are in pain, with pain the major reason for presentation.

Time-to-analgesia (from arrival/triage time) is a key aspect of quality of care in EDs. Studies have demonstrated that delayed and subtherapeutic pain relief remains a problem, with a median of 58 minutes or more (up to 107 minutes for less-urgent triage categories) for time-to-analgesia.

A range of strategies, including nurse-initiated analgesia, can be implemented in order to achieve the time-to-analgesia benchmark of < 20 minutes.

Patients in severe pain should be allocated triage category 2 (to be seen by a doctor within 10 minutes of arrival) to ensure that analgesia is administered early. Alternatively, where nurse-initiated analgesia is available, patients in pain may be allocated lower triage categories unless their condition requires otherwise.

The approach to pain management

Acute pain is a symptom, not a diagnosis.

While it is important to treat the pain, the *cause* should always be identified and treated. It is unsafe to treat the patient's pain and discharge them after their pain has been controlled without a clear cause of the pain being identified and treated.

Frequently the cause is obvious, such as acute appendicitis or trauma. Many times, however, the underlying aetiology is not clear and a diagnostic work-up is required. A history from the patient or a parent and a thorough physical examination is essential to determine the aetiology. The history and examination should include the following items.

HISTORY

- History of present illness (HPI)
- Current medications
- Medication allergies
- Past medical history
- Social history
- Family history

PAIN HISTORY

- Onset
- Character
- Duration
- Radiation
- Associated symptoms
- Quality
- Ameliorating and provoking factors
- Patient rating, if possible, using a standard pain scoring system (see Figure 13.1, below)

CLINICAL EXAMINATION

- Observation of response to pain (particularly pre-verbal or cognitively impaired patients), e.g. rubbing a particular area, guarding, facial expression, vital signs (tachycardia, hypertension, tachypnoea).
- Focused physical examination (part of body or region in pain) to include vital signs. Increases in pulse, respiratory rate and blood pressure are often but not always noted in the presence of acute pain. However, vital signs may be normal as a result of other physiological factors.
- Functional assessment.

Note: Pain medications should not be withheld during initial evaluation for an acute abdomen or any other acute painful condition.

FURTHER DIAGNOSTIC WORK-UP

Pathology studies, X-rays or other diagnostic tests may be needed, directed by the findings of the history and physical examination.

SPECIALTY CONSULTATION

Specialty consultation may be required, particularly for patients with chronic pain syndromes.

Establishing a pain management process in the ED

Up to 70% of patients presenting to the ED have pain as part of their presenting complaint.

It is important to ensure that there is an efficient and effective process of patient care in the ED that includes a sub-process focusing on pain management.

In order to ensure rapid and adequate analgesia for patients presenting with pain, a process of pain assessment and management needs to be in place. Key components of this process are:

- an alerting/activation process (commonly performed by the triage nurse)
- a uniform method of assessment utilising a standardised pain scoring system
  - commonly performed by the triage nurse
  - use of a nurse-initiated medication policy can minimise delays in administering analgesia.

The triage process and triage form (electronic and/or hard copy) should incorporate assessment of pain and allocation of a pain score in addition to prescribing and administering analgesia (and other essential medications), with provision for monitoring vital signs including the pain score and response to treatment.

1 Use of a pain pathway or guideline (can be incorporated into a specific condition guideline/pathway/SOP)
2 Documentation
3 Ready access to the required equipment and medications
4 Ongoing monitoring of the patient including their response to analgesia (including use of a pain score and, where indicated, a sedation score)
5 Quality-of-care monitoring using quality indicators such as time-to-analgesia (from time of triage to time of administration)

Assessment of pain

- The assessment of pain with the allocation of a pain score should be considered as one of the 7 vital signs.
- Accurate assessment of severity and character of the pain and the individual's response to it is essential in order to decide on

the pain management required. Analgesia is most effective when the patient's medications are tailored to their requirements.
- Different levels of distress from similar degrees of pain stem from variations in a range of factors, including culture, ethnicity, environment, beliefs, perceptions of pain, religious beliefs, age, illness, duration of pain and associated symptoms.
- Adequate pain assessment begins with the history and physical examination.

There are a range of factors that should be used in assessing the **severity of pain** and the **response to treatment**. These include:
- physiological factors
  - pulse rate
  - blood pressure
  - respiratory rate
- behavioural features
- pain scales.

A visual analogue scale (VAS) in centimetres may be used to evaluate the patient's subjective sensation of pain (Figure 13.1).

Alternatively, a numerical rating scale (NRS) from 0 to 10 (0 = no pain, 10 = worst possible pain, see Figure 13.1) has been demonstrated to correlate closely with the VAS in measuring pain, with the VAS and the NRS having almost identical minimum clinically significant differences.

Pain response is unique to each individual. A good guide to adequate analgesia is the dozing patient who opens the eyes when his or her name is called. (*pto*)

Table 13.1 **Suggested analgesia for acute pain in adults based on the VAS or NRS**

Pain score	Suggested analgesic
1–2	Paracetamol 500 mg PO 2 tabs 4-hourly PRN
3–4	Paracetamol and codeine 30 mg PO 2 tabs 4-hourly PRN
5–7	Oxycodone 5 mg 6-hourly PRN or Tramadol 50–100 mg IV injection
8–10	Morphine IV, titrated to response

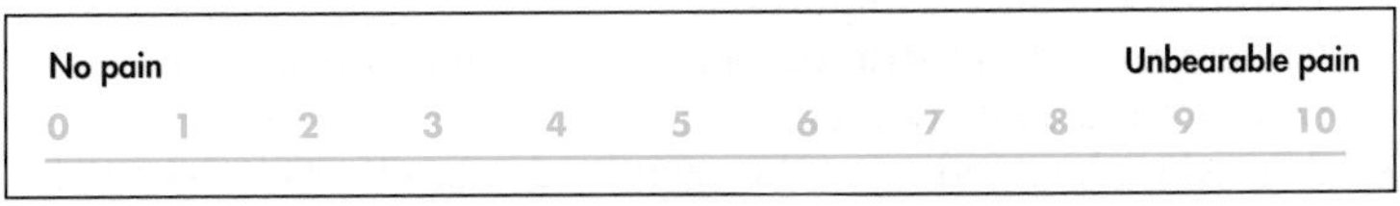

No pain										**Unbearable pain**
0	1	2	3	4	5	6	7	8	9	10

Figure 13.1 Visual analogue scale assessment of pain

In the evaluation of acute pain, a difference in the VAS of < 20 mm is unlikely to be clinically significant.

Ongoing monitoring and assessment of pain severity should take place every 2 hours (more frequently where pain is a major feature of the patient's condition), in addition to requests from the patient for analgesia, and every 8 hours once the pain is controlled.

It is useful to determine the **type of pain** the patient is experiencing, as this can guide the selection of analgesics (more than one type of pain may be present (see Table 13.2)). Pain may be one of three types: somatic, visceral or neuropathic.

1. Somatic pain is well localised and may be responsive to paracetamol, cold packs, corticosteroids, localised anaesthetic (topical or infiltrate), non-steroidal anti-inflammatory drugs (NSAIDs), opioids and tactile stimulation.
2. Visceral pain is more generalised and is most responsive to opioid treatment.
3. Neuropathic pain may be resistant to opioid therapy and consideration should be given to adjuvant therapy such as tricyclic antidepressants and anticonvulsants.

The rational use of analgesics and sedatives

A large number of pharmacological agents for the management of pain exist, each with their own indications, contraindications, modes of action and routes of administration. In order to select the correct agent, an understanding of the principles that determine the use of analgesics and sedatives in the ED is required.

Always refer to the drug's product information (PI) before prescribing or administration.

GUIDING PRINCIPLES

- Rapid onset of action is required.
- Agents need to be effective, i.e. potent.
- Judicious intravenous administration, either bolus or by an infusion (titration to effect desired), is the most effective way to achieve the desired result.
- Duration of effect is important.
- Concurrent administration of a sedative enhances patient comfort and cooperation.
- A good understanding of the agent's adverse effects is essential for safe use.

Table 13.2 Tool for determining type of pain

	Type of pain		
	Somatic pain	**Visceral pain**	**Neuropathic pain**
Location	Localised	Generalised	Radiating or specific
Patient description	Pin prick, stabbing or sharp	Ache, pressure or sharp	Burning, prickling, tingling, electric shock-like or lancinating
Mechanism of pain	A-delta fibre activity Located in the periphery*	C fibre activity Involved, deeper innervation*	Dermatomal*** (peripheral) or non-dermatomal (central)
Clinical examples	Superficial laceration Superficial burns Intramuscular injections, venous access Otitis media Stomatitis Extensive abrasion	Periosteum, joints, muscles Colic and muscle spasm pain** Sickle cell Appendicitis Kidney stone	Trigeminal Avulsion neuralgia Post-traumatic neuralgia Peripheral neuropathy (diabetes, HIV) Limb amputation Herpetic neuralgia
Most responsive treatments	Paracetamol Cold packs Corticosteroids Local anaesthetic either topically or by infiltration NSAIDs Opioids Tactile stimulation	Corticosteroids Intraspinal local anaesthetic agents NSAIDs Opioids via any route	Anticonvulsants Corticosteroids Neural blockade NSAIDs Opioids via any route Tricyclic antidepressants

HIV, human immunodeficiency virus; NSAIDs, non-steroidal anti-inflammatory drugs

* Most postoperative patients experience A-delta and C fibre pain and respond best to narcotics via any route and NSAIDs.

** Colic and muscle spasm may be less responsive to opioids and respond best to antispasmodics, NSAIDs, benzodiazepines, baclofen.

*** Segmental distribution follows a dermatome chart. This traces the pathway of sensation to its nerve root.

Modified from Assessment and management of acute pain. ARHQ Guideline Clearing House. March 2006.

- Resuscitation skills, including airway management, together with a full range of resuscitation equipment, are essential to deal with the occasional situation that occurs as a result of excessive sedation or an allergic reaction. Administration of naloxone may be required. (*pto*)

- Administration of oxygen via mask or nasal cannula with monitoring by oximetry should be considered. (Capnography should also be considered and should be used where there is a risk of hypoventilation leading to hypercapnia.) Patients with known respiratory and cardiovascular disease should be given supplemental oxygen and their oxygen saturation should be monitored; cardiac monitoring may also be necessary.

PHARMACOLOGICAL AGENTS

Simple analgesics

Aspirin (acetylsalicylic acid) with or without codeine, and paracetamol with or without codeine, are commonly used for mild pain. Both are also used as antipyretics; aspirin also has an anti-inflammatory action. Non-steroidal anti-inflammatory drugs (NSAIDs) are also commonly used as analgesics. NSAIDs are more-potent analgesics than paracetamol and aspirin. Table 13.3 lists the commonly used agents and their properties.

Table 13.3 **Adult sedatives, muscle relaxants and analgesics**

Drug	Dose	Frequency	Route
Sedatives/muscle relaxants			
Diazepam	0.1–0.3 mg/kg	A total dose of < 5 mg is usually adequate	IV injection
Midazolam	0.1–0.2 mg/kg		IV injection, IM injection
Orphenadrine citrate	100 mg	Twice daily	PO
Non-steroidal anti-inflammatory drugs (NSAIDs)			
Aspirin	325–650 mg	Every 4 h PRN	PO
Ibuprofen	200–400 mg	Every 4–6 h	PO
Indomethacin	25–50 mg	2 or 3 times daily up to 150–200 mg/day	PO
Naproxen	250 mg	Every 6–8 h	PO
Sulindac	200 mg	Twice daily	PO
Ketorolac	15–30 mg	6-hourly	IM injection

Narcotics and opioid analgesics

Natural and synthetic opioids are the most commonly use analgesic agents in the ED. Opiates should be administered IV and titrated to desired effect. Onset of action is rapid. They may also be administered IM or subcutaneously (SC). Respiratory depression, nausea and vomiting are the most common side effects. Concurrent administration of an anti-emetic PRN as necessary (such as metoclopramide) should

Table 13.4 Opioid comparative table

Drug	Approximate dose equivalent to 10 mg IM/SC morphine[1]	Approximate duration of action (hours)[2]	Comments
Agonists			
Codeine[3] (analgesic only)	120–130 mg SC/IM; 200 mg oral	3–4	Mild-to-moderate pain; not recommended
Dextro-propoxyphene[4]	Unknown	4–6	Mild-to-moderate pain; not recommended
Fentanyl	100–150 microg SC	1–2 (IM)	Moderate-to-severe acute or chronic pain; preferred in renal impairment
Hydromorphone[4]	1.5–2 mg SC/IM; 6–7.5 mg oral	2–4; 24 (controlled release)	Moderate-to-severe acute or chronic pain
Methadone (analgesic only)	Complex; discuss conversion with a pain or palliative care specialist	8–24 (chronic dosing)	Severe chronic pain
Morphine[4]	30 mg oral	2–3; 12–24 (controlled release)	Moderate-to-severe acute or chronic pain
Oxycodone	15–20 mg oral	3–4; 12–24 (controlled release)	Moderate-to-severe acute or chronic pain; preferred in renal impairment (adjust dose)
Pethidine[4]	75–100 mg IM	2–3	Not recommended
Tramadol[4]	100–120 mg IM/IV; 150 mg oral	3–6; 12–24 (controlled release)	Moderate-to-severe acute or chronic pain
Partial agonists			
Buprenorphine (analgesic only)	0.4 mg IM; 0.8 mg sublingual	6–8	Not first-line for analgesia

1 Dose equivalents are a guide only and may be greater than the maximum dose.
2 Duration of action depends on dose and route of administration.
3 Inactive, must be metabolised to morphine.
4 Has an active metabolite.
From Australian Medicines Handbook, Jan 2012.

be considered, except in children under 10 years of age because of the high incidence of extrapyramidal reactions. Ondansetron is a suitable alternative for adults and children. Supplemental oxygen and oximetry monitoring should be used in patients with cardiac and lung disease. Cardiac monitoring may also be necessary.

Opiates should not be withheld because of a perceived risk of addiction. The dangers of addiction have been exaggerated. Respiratory depression can be reversed by the opioid antagonist naloxone (0.8–2.0 mg IV repeated as necessary). *Note:* Naloxone has a short half-life compared with narcotic analgesics. Repeat doses may be required.

Morphine should be used in preference to pethidine because:

- Duration of action of pethidine is shorter.
- Pethidine has no additional analgesic benefit.
- Pethidine has a similar side-effect profile to morphine, including bronchospasm and increased biliary pressure.
- Pethidine is metabolised to norpethidine which is associated with toxic effects, especially seizures, particularly in association with renal dysfunction.
- Pethidine has a range of serious interactions with other drugs.
- Pethidine is the most commonly abused medical narcotic because of its euphoric effects.

In fact, there is very little evidence supporting the continued use of pethidine.

Morphine releases histamine resulting in 'morphine itch', a distressing side effect that can be treated with H_1 and H_2 antagonists.

Tramadol is frequently used as an alternative to morphine and pethidine because it lacks their addictive properties. It can be administered orally or by IM or IV injection. Dose reductions are required in patients with impaired hepatic or renal function. Look out for side effects and drug interactions.

Skeletal muscle relaxants

These drugs are used to treat pain due to ligamentous strains, tension myalgias and radiculopathies in combination with rest, splinting and application of heat. Drugs in this group include orphenadrine citrate and benzodiazepines such as diazepam and midazolam.

Nitrous oxide (N_2O)

A colourless gas with a sweet taste and odour, this is a good analgesic agent frequently used as a 50% N_2O mixture with 50% oxygen (Entonox). It is often used by supervised self-administration. Analgesia occurs within 20 seconds, peaking in 1–2 minutes. It also has potent sedative and anxiolytic properties. It can cause euphoria, dysphoria, drowsiness, light-headedness and nausea.

Contraindications include the presence of gas-containing cavities, especially a pneumothorax.

Nitrous oxide is particularly useful to use with children.

Sedating agents

Benzodiazepines are commonly used in the ED, usually in combination with an opioid to treat pain, most commonly during procedures requiring sedation and muscle relaxation (reduction of dislocations and fractures, cardioversion). Hypoventilation, airway obstruction and apnoea can occur with even small doses, particularly in the elderly.

Midazolam has ideal properties for use during procedures requiring short-term sedation because of its short half-life. The dose of midazolam is 0.01–0.15 mg/kg (titrated cautiously to response).

Flumazenil, a benzodiazepine antagonist, can be used to reverse the sedative effects of benzodiazepines. It is particularly useful after procedures where midazolam has been used, in order to speed up recovery. The dose is 0.2 mg followed by 0.1 mg increments up to a total of 1 mg: the usual dose is 0.3–0.6 mg. Care should be taken not to produce an acute benzodiazepine withdrawal syndrome. Seizures may occur as a result of its use.

Ketamine

Ketamine is a dissociative anaesthetic. It induces a state of analgesia, amnesia and unresponsiveness to noxious stimuli while at the same time preserving airway and breathing reflexes. With care, it is a safe alternative to general anaesthesia for minor procedures on children in the ED. Ketamine should only be administered by staff with advanced airway and resuscitation skills. Patients should be fasting for at least 3 hours and fully monitored during the procedure. For doses and effects, see Table 2.1.

Local anaesthesia

INTRAVENOUS REGIONAL ANAESTHESIA (BIER'S BLOCK)

Intravenous regional anaesthesia is a rapid and effective technique suitable for fracture reduction and extremity wound repair. The technique requires the use of a double blood-pressure cuff, drainage of blood from the limb and IV administration of prilocaine (2.5 mg/kg). Prilocaine, because of its high level of tissue binding, is safer to use than lignocaine.

LOCAL INFILTRATION

Lignocaine, with or without adrenaline, is the agent of choice for the majority of local anaesthetic procedures in the ED.

Note: Adrenaline should not be used in situations where end arteries are involved, i.e. fingers, toes, nose, ears, penis.

A 0.5–1.0% lignocaine solution is recommended, and when adrenaline is used it should be used as a 1:200,000 solution. The size of the needle and the speed of injection are important in minimising pain associated with the injection of the local anaesthetic agent. Buffering lignocaine with the addition of sodium bicarbonate (1 mEq/mL per 10 mL lignocaine) decreases the pain associated with lignocaine infiltration. A 25-gauge needle should be used, at least with the initial infiltration, with the rate of injection being as slow as possible.

The dose of lignocaine should not exceed 3 mg/kg for plain lignocaine and 7 mg/kg for lignocaine with adrenaline. Adrenaline-containing solutions should not be used for end arteries. Care should be taken to avoid intravascular injection.

TOPICAL APPLICATION

EMLA patches or cream can be used to anaesthetise small areas in children. They are frequently used in preparation for insertion of an intravenous cannula or lumbar puncture. EMLA is a mixture of 2.5% lignocaine and 2.5% prilocaine. It should not be applied to mucosal surfaces and, where the cream is used, an occlusive dressing should be utilised. The major disadvantage of EMLA in the ED is that it takes at least 60 minutes to achieve adequate analgesia.

Topical analgesia using a local anaesthetic agent such as amethocaine (often in combination with a cycloplegic such as homatropine) is commonly used to relieve ophthalmic pain.

LOCAL ANAESTHETIC BLOCKS

A variety of peripheral nerve blocks are possible. Nerve blocks are generally less painful than local infiltration, especially in sensitive areas, including the palm and sole. A useful block is a femoral nerve block which is used for analgesia (usually in combination with a narcotic) for fractured shaft of femur. Either lignocaine or bupivacaine, individually or in combination, is used for femoral nerve blocks.

The dose of lignocaine in the adult is 20 mL 1% with adrenaline (not more than 7 mg/kg).

A combination of 10 mL 1% lignocaine and 10 mL 0.25% bupivacaine with adrenaline (maximum of 2 mg/kg lignocaine) can be used for rapid onset and long duration of action.

Non-pharmacological methods

Patients presenting to the ED in pain focus on the painful stimuli in what is to them an unfamiliar, threatening environment. Establishing a patient–doctor relationship and reassuring the patient at the same time lessens anxiety and fear and can also mitigate the patient's reaction to pain. The initial encounter with the patient sets the tone for the rest of the patient–doctor interaction; reassurance and empathy go a long way towards managing the situation.

Elevation, the application of ice to the injured area and splinting are effective analgesic techniques, especially for traumatic limb injuries. Using these techniques either singly or in combination can reduce or even obviate the need for pharmacological analgesic agents.

Paediatric analgesia and sedation

Children have an exaggerated response to painful stimuli. Adequate analgesia and sedation are essential in managing children in what to them is a terrifying environment. Verbal reassurance and parental assistance and distraction are important, though in most situations pharmacological intervention will be required. As with adults, the treating doctor must be adept in advanced airway management and life support.

The assessment of the degree of pain in children can be difficult.

Patients may have pain where communication is difficult or impossible, with physiological or behavioural clues the only indication of the pain. This is usually the case with children where behaviour and physiological responses (pulse rate, respiratory rate and blood pressure) can be useful.

Children as young as 5 years have been shown to be capable of using the visual analogue scale (VAS). Recently the usefulness of a coloured analogue scale (CAS) and a facial affective scale (FAS, see Figure 13.2) were assessed. Both scales have numerical values on the reverse side to assist in documenting the pain severity. Almost all children are easily able to use both the CAS and the VAS. A visual analogue scale, facial affective scale or a colour analogue scale should be used in assessing and monitoring pain in children.

APPROACH TO THE CHILD

Non-pharmacological techniques including distraction, reassurance, elevation, application of ice and splinting are just as important, if not more so, in children as in adults. Children lend themselves to alternative routes of analgesic/sedative drug administration: oral,

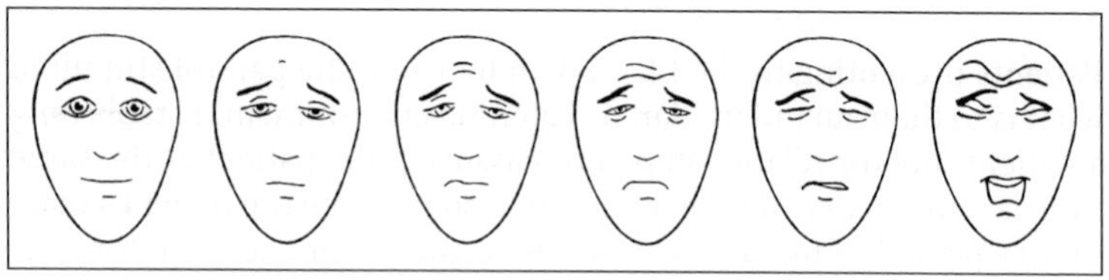

Figure 13.2 Facial affective scale to assist children in indicating the severity of their pain
Hicks CL, von Baeyer CL, Spafford PA et al. Faces Pain Scale—Revised: toward a common metric in pediatric pain measurement. Pain 2001; 93(2):173–83. Used with permission from IASP®. See www.iasp-pain.org/Content/NavigationMenu/GeneralResourceLinks/FacesPainScaleRevised/default.htm for instructions on use of the scale

nasal, topical and rectal. The easiest manner of drug administration in children is transmucosally (either orally, nasally or rectally). While the effect of a drug administered this way is less predictable, and higher doses are required compared with parenteral administration, it is a very effective and useful way of administering drugs to apprehensive children (Table 13.5).

Three main analgesics are routinely used for treating pain in children: paracetamol, ibuprofen and codeine. Paracetamol and ibuprofen are equally effective, though paracetamol has fewer side effects. Codeine has variable effectiveness and is less commonly used.

Intranasal (IN) midazolam has been found to be easy to administer, well tolerated, safe and effective for the sedation of children.

No one drug is ideal for all situations—a combination of agents may be required to produce the desired effect. Consideration should be given to using a general anaesthetic in operating theatres if a prolonged or difficult procedure is required.

Editorial Comment

Intranasal fentanyl is very effective, rapidly absorbed across mucous membranes with an onset of 2–3 minutes. Dose needs to be modified according to age.

NEONATAL ANALGESIA

The use of oral glucose administered with a dummy has been demonstrated to provide a degree of analgesia in neonates.

Painful injuries or procedures, however, require the careful use of opioids.

Table 13.5 **Paediatric sedatives and analgesics**

Drug	Route	Paediatric dose (mg/kg)	Maximum daily dose (mg)
Aspirin[1]	PO	10–15 q4h	975
Paracetamol[2]	PO	10–15 q4h	975
Ibuprofen	PO	5–10 q6h or q8h	1200
Codeine[3]	PO	0.5 q4h to q6h	3/kg/day
Morphine	IV, IM	0.1–0.15 q3h to q4h	10
Fentanyl[4]	IV, IM	1 microg/kg	
Pethidine	IV, IM	0.1–2.0 q3h to q4h	100
Diazepam	IV	0.05–0.2, titrate over 3 minutes to desired effect	10
	PR	0.5	
Midazolam	IV, IM	0.01–0.15	4
	IN, PR	0.2–0.4, titrate over 3 minutes to desired effect in 0.02 mg/kg increments	
	PO	0.5	
Ketamine[5]	IV, IM	0.5–4 mg/kg administered during 30–60 seconds	

IM, intramuscularly; IN, nasally; IV, intravenously; PO, orally; PR, rectally

1 Remember Reye's syndrome in young children. Do not use aspirin for children under 12 years of age.

2 Can be given orally, rectally or intravenously.

3 Can be given orally, rectally or by intramuscular injection.

4 Do not use in children under 2 years.

5 Pre-administration of atropine (10 microg/kg–100 microg minimum, maximum 500 microg IV).

Analgesia in the elderly

Elderly patients are at increased risk of medication-related adverse events, so the risks of administering analgesia must be carefully considered.

Increased potential for drug interactions and adverse effects of pain medication increase the challenge of pain management in the elderly due to the presence of comorbidities and need for polypharmacy that increases the risk of drug interactions.

Pain relief is a common and important factor in the quality of life of the elderly.

The comorbidity of pain, sleep disturbance and psychological distress is well-recognised in all age groups. (*pto*)

Where possible, because of the associated adverse events, NSAIDs should be avoided in the elderly.

Analgesia in pregnancy and breastfeeding

Used appropriately, common analgesics such as paracetamol, NSAIDs (including aspirin) and opioids are relatively safe.

The use of NSAIDs (including aspirin) in the third trimester is not recommended. NSAIDs are also associated with increased risk of miscarriage, therefore should be used with caution.

Paracetamol and NSAIDs are safe during breastfeeding; aspirin should not be used.

Drug-seeking patients

Staff working in EDs frequently express concern that patients may feign illness in an effort to receive opioid analgesics. There is no doubt that there are patients whose patterns of use of emergency services support a diagnosis of drug addiction and drug seeking.

Suspicion of drug seeking can result in failure to provide adequate analgesia when required.

Mistrust of a patient with severe pain has been associated with failure to diagnose serious conditions associated with intravenous drug use. The identification of obviously painful conditions should preclude any concern about drug seeking or addiction.

Inadequate knowledge of the pharmacology of opioids contributes to inadequate pain management in opioid-tolerant patients, such as those in methadone maintenance programs—large doses of narcotic analgesics titrated to effect are required to control pain in patients who are physically tolerant to opioids.

Consultation with the pain management service is indicated in the management of opioid-dependent patients.

Analgesia in special situations

There are a number of common clinical situations in the ED where a combination of agents or a different approach is required to achieve the desired analgesic and sedative effect (Table 13.6).

Analgesia can safely be administered in patients with acute abdominal pain without affecting the physical examination findings.

- Jellyfish stings—hot water (not so hot as to cause burns) is recommended.
- Multiple trauma—a general anaesthetic may need to be administered in order to safely and effectively manage patients with serious injuries.

Table 13.6 Emergency department approach to analgesia in special situations

Indication	Analgesic(s) of choice	Adjuncts
Cardioversion	IV fentanyl IV midazolam	
Renal colic	IV morphine	Indomethacin suppositories PR
Headache	PO soluble aspirin plus metoclopramide 10 mg IV Chlorpromazine 12.5–25 mg IV/IM Sumatriptan 6 mg IM	IV morphine
Fractured shaft of femur	IV morphine	Femoral nerve block
Ophthalmic pain due to ciliary muscle spasm	Topical tropicamide* *and/or* IV morphine *or* Oral analgesics	Cyclopentolate hydrochloride* Homatropine hydrobromide

IM, intramuscularly; IV, intravenously; PO, orally; PR, rectally
*Contraindication: glaucoma

- Pain due to envenomation—frequently requires the administration of antivenom to relieve the pain.

Patient monitoring

Monitoring of the patient's vital signs (temperature, pulse rate, blood pressure, respiratory rate, level of consciousness, oximetry, pain score) should begin before and continue throughout the recovery phase. The intensity of monitoring will depend on the level of sedation/analgesia, pre-existing illness (cardiac or respiratory disease) and the patient's general condition.

The greatest risk associated with pain management is excessive sedation and its resultant complications, particularly hypoxia.

Capnography should also be used where there is a risk of hypercapnia.

Patient discharge

Full recovery from the side effects of analgesia should take place prior to discharge (Box 13.1). Patients, or their parents in the case of children, should be given both verbal and written instructions (Box 13.2).

Box 13.1 Discharge criteria after sedation and analgesia

- Return to baseline verbal skills*
  - Can understand and follow directions
  - Can verbalise, including correct diction
- Return to baseline muscular control function*
  - If an infant, can sit unattended
  - If a child or adult, can walk unassisted
- Return of sensation and muscle function where a nerve block has been used
- Return to baseline mental status
- Patient or responsible person with the patient can understand emergency department discharge instructions about specific conscious sedation and/or analgesia

* These items may need to be modified to account for the patient's visit to the ED.

Box 13.2 Paediatric discharge instructions

Your child has been given a sedative or pain medication as part of their emergency department visit today. Medications of this type can cause the child to be sleepy, to be less aware, not to think clearly or to be more likely to stumble or fall. Because of this they should be watched closely for the next 8 hours. In addition, please observe the following precautions:

- No eating or drinking for the next 2 hours. If your child is an infant, he/she may be fed half a normal feed 1 hour after discharge.
- No play that requires normal childhood coordination, such as bike riding, skating or use of swings or monkey bars for the next 24 hours.
- No playing without adult supervision for the next 8 hours. This is especially important with children who are normally allowed to play outside alone.
- No baths, showers, cooking or using possibly dangerous electrical devices (such as curling irons) without adult supervision for the next 8 hours.
- If you notice anything unusual about your child or have any questions, please call the emergency department immediately.
- Side effects of analgesics are common, predictable and manageable.
- The extremes of age require careful attention to and management of the requirements for analgesia.

Key Principles of Acute Pain Management

- Early assessment
- Assess and monitor severity
- Use guideline-based dosing
- Titrate to response
- Monitor for adverse effects

Pearls and Pitfalls

- Delay in administration of analgesia is common. Time-to-analgesia is a quality indicator.
- The presence of pain and the requirement for analgesia should be an integral component of the triage process, with the nurse-initiated medication policy incorporating analgesics.
- Analgesia should be provided in an anticipatory rather than a reactive fashion.
- Regular assessment of pain results in improved pain management.
- Patients at risk of inadequate analgesia include: the elderly, children, patients with diminished cognitive function and opioid-dependent/resistant patients.
- There is good correlation between visual analogue and numerical rating scales.
- Uncontrolled, unresponsive, unusual or unexpected pain requires reassessment of the diagnosis and consideration of alternative causes of the pain.
- Inadequate analgesia is a common problem.
- Patients should not be discharged with fentanyl patches unless prescribed by the pain management service
- A combination of non-pharmacological and pharmacological analgesia can be very effective and reduce the dose and frequency of pharmacological agents.

Summary

- Assessment of pain severity, analgesia requirement and administration of analgesia should be integral components of the triage process, coupled with a nurse-initiated medication policy.
- An analgesia policy should also be built into the overall patient care process of the ED, with specific patient care guidelines incorporating pain management.
- Time-to-analgesia should be utilised as a continuously monitored ED quality indicator.
- An understanding of the causes of pain and its effect on patients, together with a detailed history and physical examination, forms the basis of the administration of timely and effective analgesia.
- All analgesics have a role in pain management in the ED. What is required is a good understanding of the indications, dose, contraindications, side effects and interactions of each analgesic and when to co-administer analgesics in order to achieve maximal effect.
- Non-pharmacological strategies should also be utilised where appropriate.

- Special attention needs to be given to unresponsive or unusual pain and to the very young and elderly.
- Patients presenting with pain should not be discharged until the cause of the pain has been identified and pain controlled.

Definitions

Adjuvant analgesic—a drug that has a primary indication other than to treat pain but has analgesic effect in some painful conditions or is capable of decreasing the side effects of analgesics; commonly administered in combination with one of the primary analgesics (e.g. opioids).

Analgesia—absence of pain; commonly used to mean adequate pain relief.

Drug tolerance—this occurs when a fixed dose of a drug produces a decreasing effect so that a dose increase is required to maintain a stable effect; the effect occurs particularly with opioids.

SOP—standard operating procedure.

Online resources

American College of Emergency Physicians. ACEP Clinical Policy: Critical issues in the prescribing of opioids for adult patients in the emergency department
www.acep.org/clinicalpolicies

American Society of Anesthesiologists
www.asahq.org

Australian and New Zealand College of Anaesthetists (ANZCA)
www.anzca.edu.au

Australian College for Emergency Medicine. Guidelines for implementation of the Australian triage scale in emergency departments.
www.acem.org.au/media/policies_and_guidelines/G24_Implementation__ATS.pdf

International Association for the Study of Pain (IASP)
www.iasp-pain.org

National Guideline Clearinghouse website
www.guidelines.gov

National Health and Medical Research Council
www.nhmrc.gov.au/guidelines-publications

New South Wales Department of Health
www.health.nsw.gov.au

Chapter 14
Trauma

Martin Duffy, Karon McDonell
and Anthony Grabs

Trauma in Australia and New Zealand is the leading cause of death in the first 4 decades of life. Fortunately, injury-related deaths have declined over the past 20 years; however, they continue to be a significant burden on health resources. The identification and management of seriously ill patients requires a coordinated approach that includes pre-hospital management, emergency management and definitive surgical care. The development of the Early Management of Severe Trauma Course and the Definitive Surgical Trauma Course, both available in Australia and New Zealand, has provided the platform for improved trauma management.

Definition of major injury

Numerous trauma scoring systems are presently used throughout the world in an attempt to define the severely injured patient. Unfortunately, all have their advantages and disadvantages, with one of the key problems being the need to collect data 'after the fact'. Scoring at the time of presentation may underestimate the severity of the injury and lead to under-triage. Major injury has previously been defined as having an Injury Severity Score (ISS) in excess of 15, as it was associated with a chance of dying in excess of 10%. Most trauma centres would now define major injury as:

- ISS > 15
- requirement for urgent surgery
- intensive-care admission
- inpatient stay longer than 3 days
- head injury requiring assisted ventilation for more than 24 hours
- death.

Patients with major injuries need to be triaged early, with activation of a coordinated trauma response from emergency, anaesthetics, intensive care and surgery.

Pre-hospital triage

Pre-hospital assessment and management by ambulance services now enables the initial triage of patients to regional or major trauma services. The overriding goal is to get the *right patient* to the *right hospital* at the *right time*. Patients meeting the criteria should be considered as having potentially life-threatening injuries requiring the services of an appropriately designated trauma centre and thus allowing a trauma call to be put out pre-arrival after notification by the ambulance. Major trauma centres are able to talk directly via radio with the paramedics.

On arrival at the ED, these features indicate a potentially critically ill trauma patient:

- respiratory distress—rate < 10/min or >30/min, or cyanosis
- systolic BP < 90 mmHg or no palpable radial pulse in children
- reduced level of consciousness (LOC)
- serious trauma to any region of the body
- burns (partial or full thickness) > 20% in adults or > 10% in children.

The definition of **serious trauma** to any body region includes:

- Penetrating injury of:
  - head
  - neck
  - chest
  - abdomen
  - perineum
  - back
- Head injury with:
  - one or both pupils dilated
  - open head injury
  - severe facial injury
- Abdominal injury with:
  - distension
  - rigidity
- Spinal injury with:
  - weakness
  - sensory loss
- Limb injury with:
  - vascular injury with ischaemia of limb
  - amputation
  - crush injury
  - bilateral femur fractures

YES ← **IS A STAFF SPECIALIST PRESENT IN ED?** → NO

YES	NO
Page on **mechanism only** **= STABLE Triage Cat 2** If patient meets any other criteria **= MAJOR Triage Cat 1**	**All** Trauma Page Activations **= MAJOR = Triage Cat 1**

- Head injury with documented GCS < 13

MECHANISM

- Fall ≥ 3 metres (6 stairs = 1 metre approx)
- Ejection from vehicle or known fatality to other occupants
- Motor vehicle accident (MVA) with vehicle rollover or significant vehicle deformation
- Medium to High Speed MVA (≥ 60 kph)
- Extrication time > 20 minutes
- Pedestrian impact ≥ 30 kmh
- Motorcycle/pedal cyclist impact ≥ 30 kmh
- Fall from a **moving** horse
- Consider other suspicious mechanism involving significant force (e.g. explosion or hanging)
- **Consider patients > 65 years with minor/moderate mechanism**
- Inter-hospital trauma transfers within 24 hours of injury

INJURIES

- Penetrating injury to **any body region**
- Flail chest
- Paralysis or **potential spinal injury** (sensory deficit or paraesthesia)
- Pelvic instability
- Major crush injury to torso, upper thigh or **amputation** of a limb
- Pregnant patients with injury post trauma
- Two or more long bone fractures (adjacent tibia/fibula or radius/ulna do not count as two)
- Burns > 20% BSA/> 10% BSA in children
- Injuries to > two body regions
- Multiple admissions arriving simultaneously

SIGNS

- Airway problems including burns and **inhalation injury**
- Intubated or attempted intubated, fitting
- Breathing difficulties including shallow or retractive breathing
- Respiratory rate < 10 or > 30 breaths/min
- Cyanosis/Capillary refill > 2 secs
- Pulse rate < 50 or > 130 bpm
- Systolic BP < 90 mmHg
- Pupil(s) dilated or unreactive

Does the **Code Crimson** policy apply?

If a MAJOR trauma call is **OVERRIDDEN** by an **ED CONSULTANT** this must be documented in the patient's notes

Figure 14.1 Trauma page criteria

Preparation

Effective communication between the pre-hospital personnel and the receiving hospital is paramount. The history of the injury and pre-hospital management is extremely important and this should be relayed via the IMIST-AMBO system:

I	IDENTIFICATION	Patient's name and details
M	MECHANISM	Mechanism of injury
I	INJURIES	ABCDEF
S	SIGNS	Vital signs and GCS
T	TREATMENT/TRENDS	Interventions Response to treatment
A	ALLERGIES	Does the patient have any allergies?
M	MEDICATIONS	Are the medications with the patient?
B	BACKGROUND	Medical history
O	OTHER ISSUES	Characteristics of the scene Social Advance care order Belongings/valuables

Adapted from the Centre for Health Communication Ambulance/ED Handover Protocol.

This information enables the trauma team to prepare and focus their attention on specific early interventions that may be life-saving for the given situation. For example, the multi-trauma victim with abdominal injuries who remains hypotensive after 2 L of intravenous fluids in the field will need un-cross-matched group O blood, warmed via a rapid infuser to be available on arrival and will probably require early transfer to the operating suite for definitive care.

Editorial Comment

If a massive transfusion (i.e. > 1 whole blood volume in 24 hours or > 50% of blood volume loss in 3 hours) is required, the local massive transfusion guideline (see Figure 14.2) should be implemented immediately to avoid morbidity and mortality.

It is often best to prepare for the incoming trauma patient by mentally working your way through the airway, breathing and circulation management (ABCs) and thinking about what equipment/personnel may be necessary for each area of concern. Knowledge of the mechanism of injury enables some prediction of possible

St Vincent's Hospital

MASSIVE TRANSFUSION GUIDELINE

Definition	**Massive Transfusion** is when greater than one whole blood volume is given to a patient within 24 hours, or replacement of >50% blood volume loss in 3h.
Notify Blood Bank	**Phone 9148 or 9150** As soon as a patient is recognised as potentially requiring massive transfusion and baseline bloods have been taken, the **blood bank should be notified** of the clinical situation and the anticipated demand, so that they can plan and call for help as required. A **named senior clinician** must take responsibility for communication with the blood bank and completing the tally sheet.
Maintain Homeostasis	Consider early definitive haemostasis eg surgery or interventional radiology. Measures should be taken to prevent and correct hypothermia (with the use of fluid warmers and external warming devices), acidosis and electrolyte abnormalities eg: aim ionised Ca > 1.1.
Pre-Treatment Status	It is important to recognise patients on anti-platelet drugs, warfarin or other anticoagulants or those who have a known coagulopathy, as clotting components and adjuvants may be required immediately. Trauma patients arriving in ED may have already lost a significant blood volume and may also require clotting components as soon as they are available.

Order 4 units of Packed Red Blood Cells (PRBC).

In an **emergency**, if there is **no current group and hold**, uncrossmatched group 0 blood may be issued

(Rh –ve for **premenopausal females**, otherwise Rh +ve is acceptable).

If bleeding is considered to be severe and ongoing, blood components other than PRBC should generally be given after 4 units have been transfused.

Order subsequent products as required in groups alternating as follows:

4–6 units PRBC 4 units Fresh Frozen Plasma (FFP) 1 pooled Platelets	4–6 units PRBC 4 units Fresh Frozen Plasma (FFP) 6 units Cryoprecipitate

Mixture of components may vary aiming for:

- Platelet count >50 x 10^9/L or >100 x 10^9/L with head injury
- Fibrinogen >1g/L
- PT, APTT <1.5 x mean control
- Hb > 80g/L (may vary depending on scenario)

Monitor:

- Arterial or venous blood gases every 60–90 min during the resuscitation
- Monitor FBC, EUC, Coags and Fibrinogen every 3h
- Samples should be labelled urgent and sent immediately to the lab.

Consider adjunct medications:

- Protamine (Heparin reversal)
- Vit K (Warfarin reversal)
- Prothrombinex (Warfarin reversal)
- Antifibrinolytics
- Desmopressin
- Recombinant Factor VIIa

Consider seeking advice via switch, of the haematologist-on-call at any time.

Figure 14.2 Massive transfusion guideline

injury/injuries. Standard precautions are a must—goggles, mask, impervious gown and gloves. The early donning of lead gowns enables potentially crucial X-rays to be performed in a timely and appropriate fashion without significant interruption to resuscitation efforts once the patient arrives.

Editorial Comment

Code Crimson

A badly injured trauma patient can exsanguinate from major internal bleeding quickly. It has been shown that a direct transfer of the patient to a waiting operating theatre suite, with anaesthetics, ICU, etc ready to receive the patient and get the patient into theatre for the surgeon to stem the blood loss, saves lives and morbidity, e.g. major vessel, cardiac injury. It also allows prompt, effective resuscitation, e.g. avoids hypovolaemic arrest with its poor results, avoids massive transfusions, etc. It is a criteria-based, practised organisational innovation, at times even avoiding stopping in the ED. It must be called and supervised by senior staff. It works.

Systematic assessment and management

The care of an injured patient by a trauma team is somewhat different to traditional medicine, with diagnosis, investigations and management frequently occurring simultaneously and performed by more than one doctor. A team leader should direct the overall management, including:

1 primary survey
2 resuscitation
3 history
4 secondary survey
5 definitive care.

When caring for the paediatric trauma patient, the priorities are the same as for the adult patient. Allowances must be made for the child's size and physiology, but the approach to assessment and management is otherwise identical. Beware of differences in injury patterns and the child's ability to compensate. Don't forget the parents—modify your approach to include family in the resuscitation room.

Care of the pregnant patient follows a similar line. Again, allowing for differences due to the anatomical and physiological changes of pregnancy, assessment and management are the same as for the non-pregnant patient. Positioning of the mid–late pregnant woman is important, as the gravid uterus may compress the vena cava. To avoid this position, try tilting the pelvis to the left side using a rolled towel underneath, if not contraindicated. Early use of fetal monitoring is important, but good care of the mother equals good care of the fetus, so remain focused on the following priorities as outlined for the adult patient.

Primary survey

During the primary survey you need to simultaneously identify and manage immediately life-threatening injuries. The priorities of the primary survey, in order, are:

1 Airway maintenance with cervical spine protection

2 Breathing and oxygenation
3 Circulation and control of external haemorrhage
4 Disability—brief neurological examination
5 Exposure with environment control.

The primary survey needs to be continually repeated throughout the initial phase of management. The key to good trauma care is directed assessment, followed by appropriate and timely intervention and subsequent directed reassessment—the AIR (assessment, intervention, reassessment) approach.

Six key injuries that need to be excluded during the primary survey can be remembered by the mnemonic **A**t **T**his **M**oment **F**ind **O**minous **C**onditions:

A Airway obstruction
T Tension pneumothorax
M Massive haemothorax
F Flail chest
O Open pneumothorax
C Cardiac tamponade

1 AIRWAY MAINTENANCE WITH CERVICAL SPINE PROTECTION

Patients with a decreased level of consciousness or inadequacy of protective reflexes are prone to airway obstruction and aspiration. All patients should be considered to have a cervical spine injury until proved negative—this has significant implications for airway management. The head and neck should be supported at all times, especially during log-rolling.

The first priority is to establish a patent and protected airway. This may require:

- the removal of blood, vomitus and foreign bodies by posturing, suction or Magill's forceps
- jaw thrust and chin lift manoeuvres
- the insertion of an oropharyngeal/nasopharyngeal airway
- endotracheal intubation
- establishment of a surgical airway.

A high concentration of oxygen should be administered to all patients. Patients with a decreased LOC associated with a traumatic brain injury should be considered for early endotracheal intubation.

Nasotracheal intubation is rarely required in acute management and should only be performed by staff experienced in the procedure. A surgical airway is only indicated if there is an inability to perform bag–mask ventilation or failure to intubate.

2 BREATHING AND OXYGENATION

Once the airway has been deemed patent and protected, the adequacy of ventilation should be assessed. This is achieved by:

- exposure of the chest
- inspection for cyanosis, tachypnoea, chest movement and chest wall integrity
- palpation of the tracheal position, subcutaneous emphysema and chest wall integrity
- percussion
- auscultation for the presence and symmetry of air entry
- oxygen saturation ± arterial blood gases.

The team should identify and provide immediate management for the following life-threatening injuries well before a chest X-ray has been obtained:

- tension pneumothorax
- large haemothorax
- large flail segment
- open pneumothorax.

However, early chest X-ray may provide vital warning of a potentially life-threatening chest injury not yet detected by clinical examination.

3 CIRCULATION AND CONTROL OF EXTERNAL HAEMORRHAGE

The maintenance of adequate tissue perfusion, especially of the brain, is the primary objective of the circulation component of the primary survey. Hypotension is almost always due to blood loss in the trauma setting. The common sites for bleeding include the thoracic cavity, the peritoneal cavity, the retroperitoneum or the pelvis. You must **stop the bleeding**. This may simply require the application of pressure to a site of external haemorrhage, or it may necessitate transfer to the operating suite for an immediate laparotomy. Early application of a pelvic binder in the appropriate setting may be life-saving.

Examination

Assessment of a patient's circulatory status does not require waiting for the blood pressure reading. Information gained from examination of the patient's pulse, skin and level of consciousness is enough to make immediate resuscitation decisions, and the only equipment required is your eyes and your fingers. Remember to interpret your findings in the context of each individual you are assessing—the young, fit male who can compensate well despite considerable blood loss versus the elderly female with multiple comorbidities on numerous physiology-altering medications are two entirely different scenarios. Beware of patients who are hypotensive in the supine position—they have lost in excess of 30–40% of their blood volume and will require urgent resuscitation (Table 14.1).

Pulse. The pulse rate and character should be determined as an initial assessment of the circulatory status. Tachycardia with a small volume pulse is due to hypovolaemia until proven otherwise. Patients with systolic BP less than 80 mmHg frequently have absent peripheral pulses.

Skin perfusion. Pale, cool, clammy skin with a capillary refill time greater than 2 seconds is an early indicator of hypovolaemia.

Level of consciousness. A decreased LOC is an indicator of poor cerebral perfusion and, again, is presumed to be due to hypovolaemia until proven otherwise.

Priorities

1 **Control of external haemorrhage.**
This may require direct digital pressure over a wound, suturing/stapling of briskly bleeding scalp wounds, the reduction of facial fractures and nasopharyngeal packing.

2 **Establishment of intravenous access.**
Two large-bore cannulas (14- or 16-gauge) should be inserted, usually into the cubital fossa of each arm. In patients with severe upper limb or chest trauma, one large-bore cannula

Table 14.1 Estimated fluid and blood losses based on patient's initial presentation (for a 70 kg patient)

	Class 1	Class 2	Class 3	Class 4
Blood loss (mL)	Up to 750	750–1500	1500–2000	> 2000
Blood loss (% blood volume)	Up to 15%	15–30%	30–40%	> 40%
Pulse rate (bpm)	< 100	> 100	> 120	> 140
Blood pressure	Normal	Normal	Decreased	Decreased
Pulse pressure	Normal or increased	Decreased	Decreased	Decreased
Respiratory rate (breaths/minute)	14–20	20–30	30–40	> 35
Urine output (mL/h)	> 30	20–30	5–15	Negligible
CNS/mental status	Slightly anxious	Mildly anxious	Anxious, confused	Confused, lethargic
Fluid replacement (3:1 rule)	Crystalloid	Crystalloid	Crystalloid and blood	Crystalloid and blood

should be above the diaphragm and one below the diaphragm. Intraosseous needles have traditionally been used in children under 8 years old with life-threatening injury if venous access cannot be established within an appropriate timeframe. Purpose-made intraosseous needles for adult patients are now commonly available.
Large-bore cannulas may also be placed in the subclavian or jugular position or into the femoral vein if necessary. The use of ultrasound to find appropriate intravenous access in the difficult patient is becoming more common.

3 **Resuscitation fluids.**
Warmed intravenous fluids should be given at a rate appropriate for the clinical situation at hand. Minimal volume resuscitation may be appropriate in some circumstances in an attempt to avoid 'popping the clot' before surgical control of bleeding has been achieved. Anticipate the need for transfusion early, as fully cross-matched blood takes at least 40 minutes to organise. Be prepared to use group-specific or un-cross-matched group O blood in urgent cases.

4 **Stop the bleeding.**
Fluid resuscitation does not replace the need to control ongoing bleeding—get the patient to the operating suite at the **right time**.

'Code Crimson' is a protocol designed to facilitate the rapid transfer to operating theatres (OTs) of massive exsanguinating trauma or vascular emergencies. This involves bypassing resuscitation cubicles, where valuable time may be wasted while carrying out monitoring and radiology. It has been shown that, although each minor task may individually consume barely minutes, together they accumulate some 20 minutes to ready the patient.

Deteriorating haemodynamic status may be due to:

- ongoing blood loss
- tension pneumothorax
- cardiac tamponade.

Immediate directed re-examination for tension pneumothorax and cardiac tamponade should be performed. Frequently neck veins will be collapsed in hypovolaemia; however, if the jugular venous pressure is raised, this suggests increased intrathoracic pressure. Having clinically ruled out these two conditions, you are then faced with the challenge of determining the source of ongoing blood loss.

Major blood loss can occur from the following five sites:

1 external haemorrhage

2 long-bone fracture/s
3 chest
4 pelvis
5 abdomen/retroperitoneum.

Focus on these sites, particularly when dealing with the trauma patient who remains hypotensive despite intravenous fluid resuscitation and other appropriate measures. It is imperative to remember that, at this stage of the resuscitation, determining the site of blood loss is far more important than trying to determine which specific organ is bleeding.

External haemorrhage can be visualised and then controlled with appropriate pressure. Long-bone fractures can be determined by clinical examination and then splinted to limit further blood loss. Significant blood loss into the chest can be ruled out by clinical examination and with the aid of an early chest X-ray. Likewise, significant blood loss from the pelvis can be ruled out by clinical examination and with the aid of an early pelvic X-ray. The abdomen/retroperitoneum is, by default, the only other site of blood loss left to contend with and, in the context of haemodynamic instability, this usually means an emergency laparotomy is in order.

Always remember, however, that the patient may bleed into multiple sites simultaneously, making such an 'orderly' assessment difficult in practical terms. The role of bedside ultrasonography as an adjunct to the clinical examination in the trauma patient has been developing for many years throughout the world and is rapidly expanding in Australia, replacing diagnostic peritoneal lavage in many centres. It has the advantage of being rapid, safe, non-invasive and, most importantly, repeatable.

Code Crimson activation can be simplified to four steps:

1 Pre-hospital notification by ambulance service of major trauma ('batphone').
2 Switchboard sends a major trauma page to trauma team.
3 Team leader (most senior emergency doctor) upgrades to Code Crimson on patient arrival, in consultation with surgical registrar.
4 Switchboard sends Code Crimson page to surgical and anaesthetic teams.

The use of **ultrasound** in a directed and limited manner by performing a focused assessment with sonography in trauma (FAST) examination is now commonplace. Its primary role is to look for free fluid in the abdomen by examining the hepatorenal, splenorenal and retrovesical regions. In the appropriate circumstances, examination for fluid in the pericardial sac may also be carried out. It should be performed by an experienced team member and should not distract the trauma team from the other components of the primary survey. Extended FAST examination continues to evolve, detecting thoracic injuries such as pneumothorax/haemothorax with potentially greater accuracy than plain chest radiography, not to mention its role in assessment of a patient's volume status and response to resuscitation. *Remember:* It is a **rule-in** test—if it is negative all bets are off.

4 DISABILITY: BRIEF NEUROLOGICAL EXAMINATION

A decreased level of consciousness is due to hypoxia or hypovolaemia until proven otherwise. Beware of hypoglycaemia. However, once these issues have been addressed, the priority is to determine the presence or absence of an intracranial injury that requires urgent neurosurgical intervention. The pupils should be assessed for size, symmetry and response to light and the patient's level of consciousness should be quickly assessed using the **AVPU** method—i.e. is the patient:

- A Alert?
- V responding to Verbal stimuli only?
- P responding to Painful stimuli only?
- U Unresponsive?

The **Glasgow Coma Scale (GCS)** may also be used to assess the LOC at this stage, or can be deferred until the secondary survey is performed. In conscious patients, all limbs should be assessed for movement and sensation to detect possible spinal injury.

All patients with a GCS score of less than 12 should have aggressive ABC management, including consideration for early intubation. This will enable controlled ventilation/oxygenation and allow the team to focus on the circulatory status, thus attending to two key factors responsible for adverse outcomes in traumatic brain injury—hypoxaemia and hypotension.

5 EXPOSURE WITH ENVIRONMENT CONTROL

Patients who have sustained a major injury should have all their clothing cut off without delay to allow adequate assessment of the entire body. Remember, however, that hypothermia kills trauma patients. Unless your resuscitation room has dedicated temperature-control capabilities, as soon as your examination and any required procedures have been performed the patient needs to be covered. A warming mattress and a Bair Hugger may also be needed to control the patient's temperature.

Resuscitation

As the initial assessment is performed and airway and breathing issues are attended to, **intravenous fluids** should be given in volumes appropriate for the estimated extent of hypovolaemia. In general, hypotensive patients should have 20 mL/kg of warmed IV fluids infused rapidly. An adult patient who requires more than 2 L of IV fluids and remains hypotensive should have blood as the next resuscitation fluid. Ideally, cross-matched blood should be given, but group-specific or un-cross-matched group O blood may need to be given, depending on the patient's clinical status.

The above traditional approach is being challenged, particularly with regard to the critically ill trauma patient who is shocked and has an acute coagulopathy on arrival at the ED, with some suggesting 'damage-control resuscitation' using plasma/blood products and minimal volume resuscitation until surgical control of bleeding is achieved. Adjunctive therapy with the early administration of tranexamic acid has been shown to decrease mortality; however, the role of factor VIIa remains to be determined. Fortunately, such complex patients are a small percentage of trauma admissions.

While placing intravenous lines, **draw blood** for the following investigations. Note that not all will be necessary in every situation.

- Full blood count
- Electrolytes/urea/creatinine
- Glucose
- Liver function tests
- Amylase/lipase
- Coagulation studies
- Group and hold/cross-match
- Blood alcohol level—including an appropriate sample for the police when required
- Beta-human chorionic gonadotrophin (hCG)

The timing of **radiological studies** will vary depending on the urgency of the situation. In major trauma patients, however, the early performance of a trauma series (chest X-ray/pelvis/lateral C-spine) is appropriate and usually takes place as the team is performing the primary survey. The most logical order for the films is:

1. chest X-ray—as an adjunct to 'B' and 'C' assessment
2. pelvis—as an adjunct to 'C' assessment
3. lateral C-spine—because this film on its own will not exclude a cervical spine injury, it may be delayed if necessary while continuing immobilisation measures (and is often replaced by CT).

During the resuscitation phase, a **urinary catheter** should be passed to assess urine output. A urinary catheter is contraindicated if there is blood at the external meatus, blood in the scrotum or rectum, the prostate cannot be palpated or is high riding. In general, a urethrogram is indicated in these circumstances and an urgent urological opinion should be sought. A suprapubic bladder catheter is an option in the presence of significant urethral trauma.

A **nasogastric tube** should be placed in all intubated patients and patients who have sustained significant abdominal trauma. This is to prevent gastric aspiration and the development of acute gastric dilation. In the presence of head or facial injuries the tube should be placed via the mouth.

The **relief of discomfort** is an important component of trauma care, and analgesia should be provided in an appropriate form and amount depending on the clinical state of the patient. In most circumstances this will equate to the provision of an intravenous opioid delivered in small aliquots and titrated to effect while monitoring for adverse events.

Consider tetanus immunisation and prophylactic antibiotics as required.

The **ongoing resuscitation status** should be monitored by:

- respiratory rate and effort
- pulse oximetry
- peripheral perfusion
- pulse rate/ECG rhythm
- blood pressure—with particular attention to pulse pressure
- GCS score
- arterial blood gases (ABGs)—base deficit and lactate
- urine output.

Persistent haemodynamic instability should again raise the possibility of:

- continued blood loss
- tension pneumothorax
- cardiac tamponade
- other conditions—e.g. myocardial injury, spinal cord injury, etc
- equipment problems—e.g. blocked or displaced intercostal catheter, dislodged peripheral or central access resulting in extravasation of fluids, malfunction of ventilation equipment, etc.

At this stage the trauma team leader should decide whether the patient should be transferred immediately to the operating suite for a resuscitative thoracotomy and/or laparotomy.

Management of life-threatening conditions

As previously stated, life-threatening conditions should be suspected and identified during the primary survey. The management of these conditions may be based in the ED or may require immediate transfer to the operating suite.

TENSION PNEUMOTHORAX

The critical initial step is to decompress the pleural space. Classic teaching is to insert a 12- or 14-gauge cannula into the 2nd intercostal space in the mid-clavicular line. Quoted success/failure rates have generated controversy, prompting recommendations to instead perform blunt thoracostomy via a lateral approach. The bottom line—regardless of method used—is to make sure you have *decompressed* the chest! This should be followed by an intercostal catheter in the 4th or 5th intercostal space just anterior to the mid-axillary line.

OPEN PNEUMOTHORAX

A large combine should be placed over the defect and secured in position with a transparent dressing (Opsite). At the same time, a large intercostal catheter needs to be inserted to treat the now 'closed' pneumothorax and to prevent the possible development of a tension pneumothorax.

MASSIVE HAEMOTHORAX

A large intercostal catheter (minimum 28 Fr) should be inserted into the 4th or 5th intercostal space just anterior to the mid-axillary line and directed posteriorly. An initial drainage of greater than 1500 mL should signal the team to consider early thoracotomy, especially in penetrating trauma.

All intercostal catheters should be connected to an underwater sealed drain and have low wall suction applied. A stat dose of prophylactic antibiotics (a 1st-generation cephalosporin for the non-allergic patient) should reduce the risk of an infective complication.

FLAIL SEGMENT

Flail segments frequently result in inadequate ventilation/oxygenation and are prone to the collection of air or blood in the pleural cavity. Associated pulmonary contusions are the major cause of morbidity and can result in progressive deterioration in respiratory function. Adequate drainage of the pleural cavities should be ensured by a large intercostal catheter; otherwise the management remains largely supportive with adequate analgesia via an appropriate route (including such options as a thoracic epidural) and assisted ventilation/oxygenation (ranging from non-invasive techniques such as bi-level positive airway pressure (BiPAP) to endotracheal intubation).

ONGOING BLOOD LOSS

These patients should be considered for early transfer to the operating suite for a resuscitative thoracotomy and/or laparotomy. If pelvic bleeding is suspected, the immediate application of a pelvic binder for pelvic stabilisation and early angiography should be considered.

CARDIAC TAMPONADE

The diagnosis should be suspected clinically and confirmed with FAST if possible. Management revolves around adequate resuscitation and performing a left anterolateral thoracotomy to release the fluid within the pericardial sac. This should be undertaken by the most experienced trauma team member.

Needle pericardiocentesis should only be considered in smaller hospitals if experienced staff are not available. Needle pericardiocentesis may be life-saving but rarely drains the pericardial sac adequately and is associated with significant complications.

PULSELESS ELECTRICAL ACTIVITY (PEA)

This is sometimes called electromechanical dissociation and in the context of trauma is usually caused by exsanguination, tension pneumothorax, massive haemothorax or cardiac tamponade. PEA should be managed by immediate intubation, ventilation, bilateral chest drains, the administration of at least 3 L of intravenous fluids and consideration for an open thoracotomy and pericardial release. This is of special importance in penetrating chest injuries.

History

A nominated member of the trauma team should obtain further information that will allow the acute event to be managed in the context of the patient's pre-morbid state. A simple way to cover most of the important areas is to use the AMPLE approach:

- **A** Allergies
- **M** Medications—particularly anticoagulants!
- **P** Past history—particularly diseases that alter clotting ability; pregnancy
- **L** Last food/fluid; last tetanus injection
- **E** Event details

This history may not be available directly from the patient and other sources may need to be questioned, e.g. pre-hospital personnel, relatives, friends, the local doctor, old medical records, etc. In the unconscious patient always remember to look for a medical alert bracelet or any pertinent information on the person or in a wallet/ handbag.

Details of the **mechanism of injury** are vitally important. Conceptually, injury is the result of a transfer of energy to the body's tissues. The severity of injury is dependent on the amount and speed of energy transmission, the surface area over which the energy is applied and the elastic properties of the tissues to which the energy transfer is applied. In the Australian setting, the most common cause is blunt trauma; however, penetrating trauma is on the increase. Common causes of blunt trauma include:

1 motor vehicle crashes
2 pedestrian–motor vehicle accidents
3 falls
4 industrial accidents
5 assaults.

Specific injuries may be predicted from the mechanism of injury.

1 Injuries in motor vehicle crashes

- Frontal impact—cervical spine fracture, anterior flail chest, traumatic aortic disruption, pneumothorax, myocardial contusion, ruptured spleen or liver, posterior dislocation/fracture of hip/knee.
- Lateral impact—cervical spine fracture, lateral flail chest, traumatic aortic disruption, pneumothorax, diaphragmatic injury, ruptured spleen or liver, renal injury, fractured pelvis.
- Rear impact—cervical spine injury.
- Ejection—increased risk for any injury.
- Rollover—increased risk for any injury.

Important information from pre-hospital personnel that provides some idea of the energy transfer involved includes details of the estimated speed, impact, damage to vehicle, entrapment, use of restraint devices, deployment of airbags, etc. Nowadays, digital photos of the scene are an invaluable source of information.

2 Injuries in pedestrian–motor vehicle accidents

Remember the injury triad—impact with the bumper, impact with the bonnet and windscreen, and subsequent impact with the ground.

- Bumper—lower limb fractures, fractured pelvis, torso injuries in children.
- Bonnet/windscreen—head injury, torso injuries.
- Ground—head injury, spinal injuries.

(*pto*)

Again, pre-hospital information that gives some idea of the energy transfer involved is important.

3 Injuries in falls

- The predominant underlying mechanism of injury is deceleration.
- Important considerations include the height of the fall, the landing surface and the position of the patient on impact.
- Injuries include head, spine, torso, pelvis and multiple fractures (calcaneus, ankle, tibial plateau, hip and vertebral column).

4 Injuries in industrial accidents

- May be blunt or penetrating.
- Other mechanisms need to be considered—blast, thermal, chemical.
- Injuries will depend on the above mechanisms.

5 Injuries in assaults

- Unfortunately a common cause.
- May be blunt or penetrating.
- Determine the energy transfer—weapon, fists, stomping.
- Injuries will depend on the above mechanisms.
- Stabbings are low-energy injuries—severity determined by organs injured, e.g. major vascular injury versus muscle.
- Gunshot injuries vary in energy level—increased bullet velocity equals increased injuries secondary to cavitation.

Knowledge of the mechanism of injury provides 'advance warning' regarding possible injuries—it is a useful guide, but remember there are always exceptions.

Secondary survey

The secondary survey is a detailed systematic head-to-toe examination in order to detect all injuries and enable planning of definitive care. This should not commence until the primary assessment and management have stabilised the patient. During the secondary survey all components of the primary survey should be repeated and the team should be responsive to any new findings. Unless the patient has been transferred immediately to the operating suite, the secondary survey should be undertaken in the ED.

Head. Assess the scalp for lacerations, contusions, fractures and burns. Examine the ears for haemotympanum and cerebrospinal fluid (CSF) leakage. Check the eyes for visual acuity, pupil symmetry and response to light, movements, lens injury; always check for the presence of contact lenses and remove them early.

Face. Assess for lacerations, contusions, fractures and burns. Check cranial nerve function. Examine the mouth for bleeding, loose teeth and soft-tissue injuries.

Cervical spine and neck. Assess for tenderness, bruising, swelling, deformity, subcutaneous emphysema and tracheal deviation. Beware of carotid dissection.

Chest. Assess for evidence of rib fracture, subcutaneous emphysema, open wounds, haemothorax and pneumothorax. Check for evidence of myocardial injury, and perform a 12-lead ECG.

Abdomen. Assess for bruising of the anterior abdominal wall, distension, tenderness and guarding, rebound, rectal and vaginal examinations.

Back. All trauma patients need to undergo a log-roll with cervical spine immobilisation to examine the entire length of the spine, looking for tenderness, bruising or deformity. This should be done early so the patient can be removed from the spinal board, improving patient comfort and decreasing the risk of pressure injuries in patients with spinal cord injuries and altered sensation/awareness. A rectal examination should be done at this time.

Limbs. All limbs need to be examined for fractures, lacerations, haematomas, peripheral pulses and neurological deficits. All fractures should be reduced and splinted and consideration given for intravenous antibiotics and tetanus prophylaxis.

Specific injuries

HEAD TRAUMA

(See also Chapter 15, 'Neurosurgical emergencies'.)

Traumatic brain injury is common. Unfortunately, despite this fact, there is limited good evidence in the literature upon which to base investigation and management decisions, particularly with regard to the patient with mild head injury. The NSW Health Institute of Trauma and Injury Management has recently published the adult trauma clinical practice guideline *Initial Management of Closed Head Injury in Adults,* 2nd edition, in an ongoing effort to fill this void and provide clinicians with evidence-based advice.

It is important to determine at an early stage whether your facility can provide the appropriate care necessary for the patient's severity of injury or whether urgent transfer to another hospital will provide the best possible care. There has been the re-release of the ITIM guidelines which advocates the use of the Abbreviated Westmead Post Traumatic Amnesia Screen (A-WPTAS). Recent studies have shown this to be an effective screening tool to identify a brain injury being present.

Classification systems abound and all have their limitations, but the following GCS-based system is a useful guide:

- mild head injury—GCS 14–15
- moderate head injury—GCS 9–13
- severe head injury—GCS 3–8

Editorial Comment

The management of concussion is complex and still evolving. There is increasing awareness, especially in sports injury and research using amnesia scales. Doctors need to keep up to date on recommendations as to when people can return to sports/contact sports/work after a concussive episode.

Mild head injury

Fortunately the majority of patients you deal with will have only a mild injury, usually characterised by an awake patient who may have a history of a brief loss of consciousness and some degree of amnesia about events surrounding the injury. Often the history of loss of consciousness is unclear and, despite information from bystanders and pre-hospital personnel, it can be difficult to determine the true details of the event.

In general, if there is a history of more than a brief loss of consciousness, persistent post-traumatic amnesia, significant headache or vomiting following the injury, then a CT scan of the head should be performed. If the CT scan is normal, subsequent deterioration is unlikely and the majority of patients can expect an uneventful recovery.

Importantly, all patients with mild head injury should be screened for post-traumatic amnesia with the abbreviated Westmead PTA Scale (see Figure 14.3). Persistent post-traumatic amnesia not only raises the suspicion for significant intracranial injury (prompting CT imaging if not already performed), but may also signal an increased risk for post-concussion symptoms, prompting appropriate referral.

Most patients with mild head injury may be discharged to the care of a responsible adult provided the home circumstances are adequate. Prior to discharge a discussion with the patient and carer regarding important symptoms and signs to look out for should take place—and this information should also be provided in written form by way of a head injury advice card.

Moderate head injury

Patients with this degree of head injury require more-aggressive management and further investigation. Remember to keep in mind the different needs of patients, depending on where they lie on the disease spectrum.

Early endotracheal intubation and controlled ventilation/oxygenation should be considered. Appropriately aggressive fluid resuscitation in the hypovolaemic patient is also vitally important. Having performed a primary and secondary survey and responded appropriately to the findings, the next priority is to determine whether a neurosurgically correctable lesion is present by proceeding to urgent CT scanning.

Further management will depend on the findings, with a number of patients requiring urgent transfer to the operating suite for evacuation of a haematoma. The majority of other patients will require admission for ongoing neurological observations.

Severe head injury

Patients with severe head injury are fortunately in the minority. However, when faced with such a patient a coordinated team approach with meticulous attention to the prevention of secondary brain injury is paramount. Early notification of the neurosurgical team is important. The ABCs must be appropriately and aggressively resuscitated. Key points in the management include:

1 Endotracheal intubation with controlled ventilation/oxygenation. Prior to sedating and paralysing the patient, every attempt should be made to perform and document a limited neurological examination—the GCS and pupillary responses. It is important to note these findings in the context of the patient's blood pressure at the time because of its potential influence on cerebral perfusion/function. Also, remember it is the best motor response that is the more accurate predictor of outcome.

2 Mild hyperventilation to a PCO_2 of 30–35 mmHg in the patient showing signs of raised intracranial pressure from an expanding haematoma—as a 'stop gap' to make it to the operating suite. The patient's end-tidal CO_2 should be monitored closely, having confirmed the accuracy of the readings by performing a formal ABG measurement.

3 Fluid resuscitation with normal saline, Hartmann's or blood (no glucose-containing solutions) as required to maintain a mean arterial pressure of greater than 90 mmHg in the patient suspected of raised intracranial pressure. (*pto*)

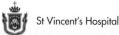

St Vincent's Hospital

ABBREVIATED WESTMEAD PTA SCALE (A-WPTAS)
GCS & PTA TESTING OF PATIENTS
WITH MTBI FOLLOWING MILD HEAD INJURY

MRN			SURNAME
OTHER NAMES			
DOB	SEX	AMO	WARD/CLINIC

(Please enter information or affix Patient Information Label)

USE OF A-WPTAS AND GCS FOR PATIENTS WITH MTBI

The A-WPTAS combined with a standardised GCS assessment is an objective measure of post traumatic amnesia (PTA). Only for patients with **current GCS of 13–15 (<24 hrs post injury)** with impact to the head resulting in confusion, disorientation, anterograde or retrograde amnesia, or brief LOC. **Administer both tests at hourly intervals** to gauge patient's capacity for full orientation and ability to retain new information. **NB:** *This is a screening device, so exercise clinical judgment. In cases where doubt exists, more thorough assessment may be necessary. If GCS deteriorates by >2 then cease A-WPTAS and commence neurological observations on emergency patient assessment sheet.*

ABBREVIATED WESTMEAD PTA SCALE (A-WPTAS) AND GLASGOW COMA SCALE (GCS)

ADMINISTRATION AND SCORING

1. ORIENTATION QUESTIONS

Question 1: WHAT IS YOUR NAME?

The patient must provide their full name.

Question 2: WHAT IS THE NAME OF THIS PLACE?

The patient has to be able to give the name of the hospital. For example: St Vincent's Hospital. (NB: The patient does not get any points for just saying 'hospital'.) If the patient can not name the hospital, give them a choice of 3 options. To do this, pick 2 other similar sized hospitals in your local area or neighbouring region. The three choices are 'Royal Prince Alfred, Royal North Shore or Prince of Wales'.

Question 3: WHY ARE YOU HERE?

The patient must know why they were brought into hospital, e.g. they were injured in a car accident, fell, assaulted or injured playing sport. If the patient does not know, give them three options, including the correct reason.

Question 4: WHAT MONTH ARE WE IN?

For emphasis the examiner can ask what month are we in now? The patient must name the month. For example, if the patient answers 'the 6th month', the examiner must ask the further question 'What is the 6th month called?'.

Question 5: WHAT YEAR ARE WE IN?

It is considered correct for patients to answer in the short form '08', instead of '2008'. Also, an acceptable alternative prompt (for the rest of the 2000's) is 'The year is 2000 and what?'

2. PICTURE RECOGNITION

Straight after administering the GCS (standardised questions), administer the A-WPTAS by presenting the 3 Westmead PTA cards. Picture Cards the first time—T1: Show patients the target set of picture cards for about 5 seconds and ensure that they can repeat the names of each card. Tell the patient to remember the pictures for the next testing in about one hour. Picture Cards at each subsequent time T2–T5: Ask patient, 'What were the three pictures that I showed you earlier?'.

SCORING

- For patients who free recall all 3 pictures correctly, assign a score of 1 per picture and add up the patient's GCS (out of 15) and A-WPTAS memory component to give the A-WPTAS score (total = 18). Present the 3 target pictures again and re-test in 1 hour.
- For patients who can not free recall, or only partially free recall, the 3 correct pictures, present the 9-object recognition chart. If patient can recognise any correctly, score 1 per correct item and record their GCS and A-WPTAS score (total = 18). Present the target set of pictures again and re-test in 1 hour.
- For patients who neither remember any pictures by free recall nor recognition, show the patient the target set of 3 picture cards again for re-test in 1 hour.

ADMISSION AND DISCHARGE CRITERIA

A patient is considered to be out of PTA when they score 18/18. Both the GCS and A-WPTAS should be used in conjunction with clinical judgment. Patients scoring 18/18 can be considered for discharge. For patients who do not obtain 18/18 re-assess after a further hour. Patients with persistent score <18/18 at 6 hours post time of injury should be considered for admission. If abnormal PTA was present or patient's pain score is greater than 4.5/10 on discharge please refer patient to the Friday mild brain injury rehabilitation clinic. Patients who reside in outer metropolitan or rural areas refer to their GP. Please provide patient with a head injury advice sheet.

Figure 14.3 Westmead Post Traumatic Amnesia (PTA) Scale

4 Mannitol 0.5–1 g/kg given as an infusion over approximately 5 minutes in the patient showing signs of raised intracranial pressure from an expanding haematoma—as a 'stop gap' to make it to the operating suite; frusemide 20–40 mg IV may also be used, often in addition to mannitol.

St Vincent's Hospital

ABBREVIATED WESTMEAD PTA SCALE (A-WPTAS)
GCS & PTA TESTING OF PATIENTS
WITH MTBI FOLLOWING MILD HEAD INJURY

MRN		SURNAME	
OTHER NAMES			
DOB	SEX	AMO	WARD/CLINIC

(Please enter information or affix Patient Information Label)

Date: Time:		T1	T2	T3	T4	T5	T6	T7	T8	T9	T10	T11	T12
Motor	Obeys commands	6	6	6	6	6	6	6	6	6	6	6	6
	Localises	5	5	5	5	5	5	5	5	5	5	5	5
	Withdraws	4	4	4	4	4	4	4	4	4	4	4	4
	Abnormal flexion	3	3	3	3	3	3	3	3	3	3	3	3
	Extension	2	2	2	2	2	2	2	2	2	2	2	2
	None	1	1	1	1	1	1	1	1	1	1	1	1
Eye Opening	Spontaneously	4	4	4	4	4	4	4	4	4	4	4	4
	To speech	3	3	3	3	3	3	3	3	3	3	3	3
	To pain	2	2	2	2	2	2	2	2	2	2	2	2
	None	1	1	1	1	1	1	1	1	1	1	1	1
Verbal	Oriented ** (tick if correct)	5	5	5	5	5	5	5	5	5	5	5	5
	Name	❑	❑	❑	❑	❑	❑	❑	❑	❑	❑	❑	❑
	Place	❑	❑	❑	❑	❑	❑	❑	❑	❑	❑	❑	❑
	Why are you here	❑	❑	❑	❑	❑	❑	❑	❑	❑	❑	❑	❑
	Month	❑	❑	❑	❑	❑	❑	❑	❑	❑	❑	❑	❑
	Year	❑	❑	❑	❑	❑	❑	❑	❑	❑	❑	❑	❑
	Confused	4	4	4	4	4	4	4	4	4	4	4	4
	Inappropriate words	3	3	3	3	3	3	3	3	3	3	3	3
	Incomprehensible sounds	2	2	2	2	2	2	2	2	2	2	2	2
	None	1	1	1	1	1	1	1	1	1	1	1	1
GCS	Score out of 15	/15	/15	/15	/15	/15	/15	/15	/15	/15	/15	/15	/15
	Picture 1												
	Picture 2												
	Picture 3												
A-WPTAS	Score out of 18	/18	/18	/18	/18	/18	/18	/18	/18	/18	/18	/18	/18

** must have all 5 orientation questions correct to score 5 on verbal score for GCS, otherwise the score is 4 (or less).

Pain Score on Discharge
No pain = 0
Worst Pain Imaginable = 10
Patient Score ______

PUPIL ASSESSMENT	T1		T2		T3		T4		T5		T6		T7		T8		T9		T10		T11		T12	
	R	L	R	L	R	L	R	L	R	L	R	L	R	L	R	L	R	L	R	L	R	L	R	L
Size																								
Reaction																								

+	REACTS BRISKLY
SL	SLUGGISH
C	CLOSED
–	NIL

TARGET SET OF PICTURE CARDS

PUPIL SIZE

2 3 4 5 6 7 8

5 Prophylactic anticonvulsants. At the discretion of the treating neurosurgeon—usually phenytoin 15 mg/kg administered intravenously at a rate no faster than 50 mg/min in adult patients.

6 Meticulous nursing care. Positioned head up 30°. Avoidance of constricting endotracheal ties, etc.

The management of the patient with head injury with intercurrent hypotension can be a real challenge. Therefore, it is important to keep a few key principles in mind:

1 Head injury + hypotension = worse outcome.
2 Determine the cause of the hypotension.
3 Treat the cause of the hypotension.
then
4 Treat the head injury.

NECK INJURIES

The accurate assessment and management of neck injuries is important, not only because of the potentially devastating effects of cervical spine/spinal cord injuries, but also because of the life-threatening potential of injuries to other vital structures such as the airway/larynx and vascular anatomy. A detailed search for swelling, expanding haematoma formation, subcutaneous emphysema, tracheal deviation, hoarseness, stridor and carotid bruits should be performed.

Key points in management include:

1 Ensure airway patency. Repeated examinations are essential and early intubation may be life-saving.
2 Blunt injury to vascular structures can be 'occult'. Maintain a high degree of suspicion and proceed to further investigation, e.g. ultrasound, angiography.
3 Beware of penetrating injuries. If the platysma is breached, the right place for the patient to be further examined and treated is in the operating suite with on-table angiography facilities.
4 Clear the cervical spine. Patients suffering blunt trauma who meet the following 5 criteria can be classified as having a low probability of cervical spine injury and can be cleared on clinical grounds. No radiological imaging is required if the patient has:
   — normal alertness
   — no intoxication
   — no painful, distracting injury
   — no midline cervical tenderness
   — no focal neurological deficit.

An alternative guideline for clearing the cervical spine is the Canadian C-spine rule; see Figure 14.4.

ABDOMINAL TRAUMA

The abdomen is renowned for its reputation as an 'occult' source of blood loss in the trauma victim. Add to this reputation the poor sensitivity and specificity of the physical examination in this setting,

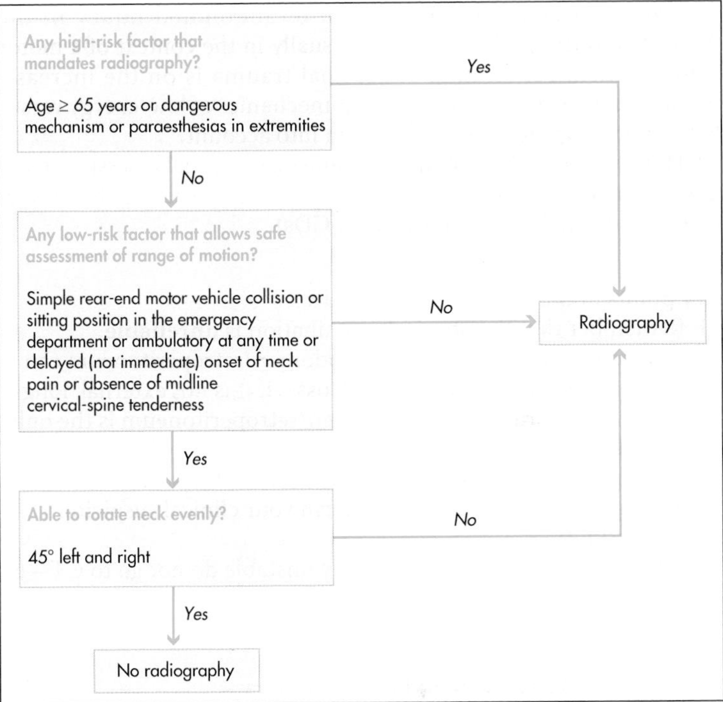

Figure 14.4 The Canadian C-spine rule
For patients with trauma who are alert (as indicated by a score of 15 on the Glasgow Coma Scale) and in a stable condition and in whom cervical-spine injury is a concern, the determination of risk factors guides the use of cervical-spine radiography. A dangerous mechanism is considered to be a fall from an elevation of ≥ 3 feet (1 metre) or 5 stairs; an axial load to the head (e.g. diving); a motor vehicle collision at high speed (> 100 km/h) or with rollover or ejection; a collision involving a motorised recreational vehicle; or a bicycle collision. A simple rear-end motor vehicle collision excludes being pushed into oncoming traffic, being hit by a bus or a large truck, a rollover and being hit by a high-speed vehicle

and it is not hard to see why investigation and management decisions can seem daunting.

As stated previously, during the initial assessment of such patients it is important to keep in mind that it is more important to determine the site of bleeding as opposed to the specific organ injured. Remember the full 'extent' of the abdomen when assessing a patient—the anterior borders are the trans-nipple line superiorly, the inguinal ligaments and pubic symphysis inferiorly and the anterior axillary lines laterally.

The most common mechanism of abdominal injury in the Australian setting is blunt trauma, usually in the context of a motor vehicle crash. Penetrating abdominal trauma is on the increase, though, and the differences in the biomechanics of low-energy versus high-energy injuries need to be taken into account.

However, regardless of the mechanism, the initial assessment and management need to follow the same principles of airway, breathing, cardiovascular, drug therapy (the ABCDs).

Blunt abdominal trauma

Key points in the management include:

1. Remember that the physical examination is **unreliable**.
2. By a process of elimination the abdomen/retroperitoneum can be diagnosed as the site of blood loss—if it is not external, long bones, chest or pelvis, the abdomen/retroperitoneum is the only site left.
3. If the patient is haemodynamically stable, a CT scan is an appropriate investigation to confirm your clinical suspicion (Table 14.2).
4. If the patient is haemodynamically unstable do not go to CT—go to the operating suite!

Table 14.2 Imaging in abdominal trauma

	Ultrasound	Diagnostic peritoneal lavage	Computed tomography
Indication	Document free fluid if decreased BP	Document bleeding if decreased BP	Document organ injury if BP normal
Advantages	Early diagnosis; performed at the bedside; non-invasive; repeatable; 86–97% accurate	Early diagnosis; performed at the bedside; 98% accurate	Most specific for injury; 92–98% accurate
Disadvantages	Operator dependent; bowel gas and subcutaneous air distortion; misses diaphragm, bowel and some pancreatic injuries	Invasive; misses injury to diaphragm and retroperitoneum	Cost and time; transfer to medical imaging department; misses diaphragm, bowel tract and some pancreatic injuries

5 For the patient 'in between', a FAST examination or a diagnostic peritoneal lavage may be invaluable (Table 14.2).
6 Remember that a FAST examination can only *rule in* the presence of free fluid. If it is negative, all bets are off.
7 Be appropriately aggressive with resuscitation fluids—the **right amount** for the **right patient** at the **right temperature**.
8 **Stop the bleeding**—for some patients this will mean immediate transfer to the operating suite.

Penetrating abdominal trauma

Advice regarding resuscitation and imaging is as for blunt trauma (see above). Other important points include:

- The entry wound can be a misleading predictor of the trajectory of penetration and potential underlying injury/ies—**do not** rely on it.
- Anterior abdominal stab wounds with hypotension, peritonitis or evisceration of omentum or small bowel require no further imaging or investigation—they need to go to the operating suite for a laparotomy.
- Local exploration of stab wounds under sterile conditions and local anaesthesia may be performed by the skilled surgeon in stable patients, searching for a breach in the anterior fascia. If a breach is present the patient is at increased risk of an intraperitoneal injury, and common practice in Australia is to proceed to laparoscopy.
- The value of repeated examinations should not be underestimated.

THORACIC TRAUMA

The majority of chest injuries can be managed in the ED with the use of supplemental oxygen, an appropriately placed intercostal catheter and the judicious use of analgesics via an appropriate route. Hence, it is important that doctors working in such an environment develop the skills to assess and manage these patients correctly.

Often when the patient first arrives, the examination and chest X-ray are performed in the supine position, and allowances must be made for this in terms of exam technique and film interpretation. For example, percussion should be performed in an anterior to posterior direction for detecting the presence of a haemothorax—and the chest X-ray will have a generalised increase in radiodensity on the affected side as compared to the usual meniscus on an erect film. Watch out for the patient with a widened mediastinum on chest X-ray suspicious for a contained rupture of the aorta—if you don't have cardiothoracic facilities, transfer the patient without delay so further investigation and treatment can take place at the right hospital.

Keep in mind the presence of common intercurrent diagnoses that may impact on a patient's ability to cope with their chest injury, such as chronic airflow limitation and asthma, not to mention smoking status.

Given the important structures within the chest, it is not surprising that patients can suffer a large number of possible life-threatening injuries, including those previously discussed under the primary survey, as well as the following:

Pulmonary contusion. Commonly associated with many of the other injuries and is often the main cause of deteriorating lung function. Develops over hours to days. May require increasing supplemental oxygen, non-invasive ventilatory support or subsequent intubation/ventilation.

Haemothorax. Drainage via an appropriately sized and placed intercostal catheter is important, as noted previously. Transfer to the operating theatre needs to be considered in any patient who drains more than 1500 mL immediately or continues to drain more than approximately 200 mL/h for 2–4 hours.

Simple pneumothorax. There is some controversy as to how some of these injuries should be managed depending on such factors as the size of the pneumothorax, associated injuries, need for positive-pressure ventilation, need for transfer to another facility, and co-existent respiratory diseases; most would still advocate drainage via an appropriately sized intercostal catheter.

Blunt cardiac injury. Suspect in the patient who remains haemodynamically unstable. There is no single clear diagnostic test—the ECG, cardiac markers and other imaging modalities such as echocardiography are all adjuncts to the clinical examination.

Traumatic aortic disruption. Most patients die at the scene. If they survive to reach hospital, there is a window of opportunity to investigate and treat them at a facility with cardiothoracic capabilities. Signs to look for on the chest X-ray include a widened mediastinum, obliteration of the aortic knob, deviation of the trachea to the right, obscuration of the aortopulmonary window, depression of the left main stem bronchus, deviation of the oesophagus (nasogastric tube) to the right, widened paratracheal stripe, widened paraspinal interfaces, presence of a pleural or apical cap, left haemothorax or fractures of the first and second ribs or the scapula. Early surgical consultation is important.

Tracheobronchial tree disruption. An unusual injury; patients usually die at the scene. Suspect if a large air leak persists after placement of an intercostal catheter for a pneumothorax. Early surgical consultation is important.

Traumatic diaphragmatic injury. Often missed; interpret X-rays with care. Early surgical consultation is important.

Traumatic oesophageal disruption. Rare; fatal if missed because of subsequent mediastinitis. Suspect if there is a left pneumothorax or haemothorax without a rib fracture, pain or shock out of proportion to the injury (usually a blow to the lower sternum or epigastrium) or if there is particulate matter in the intercostal catheter. Early surgical consultation is important.

However, having noted the above injuries, do not underestimate the significant morbidity and potential mortality associated with the most common of chest injuries—**rib fractures**! Important points in the management of this everyday problem include:

1 The ability of X-rays to detect rib fractures is poor—even if the films are read accurately!
2 If the patient has a good history and significant pain, rib fracture is probably the diagnosis.
3 The role of the chest X-ray is to help exclude complications such as a pneumothorax, haemothorax, pulmonary contusion, atelectasis, subsequent pneumonia.
4 It is clear from the above that 'rib views' are not necessary.
5 The presence of intercurrent disease may influence management decisions.
6 Adequate analgesia that allows deep breathing and coughing is paramount to the successful management of patients with these injuries:
   - Start with simple oral therapy—paracetamol.
   - Add other oral options—NSAIDs/oxycodone, being alert for respiratory depression.
   - Use parenteral therapy—opioids, again being alert for respiratory depression.
   - The use of patient-controlled analgesia may be appropriate in many circumstances.
   - Consultation with the anaesthetic/pain management service with the view to other alternatives—intercostal blocks/epidural anaesthesia.

(*pto*)

7 Paramedical services play an important role—physiotherapy.
8 Use non-invasive ventilatory support such as BiPAP early.
9 Closely monitor the patient's progress—respiratory rate and effort, pulse oximetry, ABGs.
10 Be prepared for the patient who, despite the above measures, continues to struggle—intubation with controlled ventilation/oxygenation may be necessary.
11 With few exceptions, elderly patients with fractured ribs require inpatient care.

PELVIC TRAUMA

Pelvic injuries can range in severity from simple pubic rami fractures to unstable injuries with associated life-threatening exsanguination. It is important to appreciate the magnitude of the force required to fracture the pelvis—and hence the high association with other potentially life-threatening injuries.

Three common mechanisms of injury are:

1. anteroposterior compression, e.g. crushing injury
2. lateral compression, e.g. motor vehicle crash
3. vertical shear, e.g. fall from a height.

Be suspicious of significant pelvic injury with the above mechanisms and perform a careful clinical examination, noting any lower-limb shortening or rotation (in the absence of a lower-limb fracture) and any pain or movement on palpation of the pelvic ring. Compression-distraction of the pelvic ring is controversial and at most should be performed *once* ***with compression*** *only* as part of this examination because of the risk of exacerbating any bleeding. The early performance of a pelvic X-ray as part of the trauma series will assist decision making.

Important points in the management of these injuries include:

1. Major pelvic disruption with haemorrhage should be suspected from the mechanism of injury, e.g. motorcycle crash, pedestrian–motor vehicle accident, fall from a height or a direct crushing injury.
2. Significant injuries are usually clinically apparent.
3. Be alert for and understand the potential for major blood loss—from the ends of fractured bones, from injured pelvic muscles and from the pelvic veins/arteries—and fluid-resuscitate the patient appropriately.
4. Simple measures to control bleeding in the ED include:
   - bringing the lower limbs back out to length with traction
   - internally rotating the lower limbs and strapping them together

— the application of a pelvic binder—this may be as simple as wrapping a sheet around the pelvis.

5 Early consultation with the angiography/orthopaedic teams is paramount.

Always remember the possibility of associated **urological injury**. Suspicious examination findings include blood at the external urethral meatus, scrotal or perineal bruising and an impalpable or high riding prostate on rectal exam (all contraindications to catheterisation, as previously noted). In the multi-injured patient with a significant pelvic fracture, the bladder and/or urethra may be injured. In this setting the urethra is more commonly injured above the urogenital diaphragm. The patient is often in 'retention.' The usual approach to management includes:

1 Assess and treat for other life-threatening conditions.
2 Perform a urethrogram and treat accordingly.
3 Suprapubic catheterisation in selected patients.
4 Urological consultation.

MUSCULOSKELETAL TRAUMA

Musculoskeletal trauma is very common. Fortunately most injuries are neither limb- nor life-threatening, although they can on occasion look very dramatic. It is important not to be distracted by the injury and to manage all these patients in an orderly fashion with meticulous attention to the ABCs first. Some important points in the management of such injuries include:

1 Musculoskeletal injuries that are potentially life-threatening need to be recognised early and managed appropriately:

Major arterial haemorrhage. These injuries may be as obvious as an avulsed limb or as subtle as the bleeding associated with a long-bone injury or major joint dislocation. Do not blindly clamp open injuries—use direct pressure. Limb realignment and splinting are important measures that help reduce blood loss. Carefully assess the limb for the presence of distal pulses—absence equals arterial injury until proven otherwise. It is important to contact the surgical team early with a view to transfer to the operating suite for urgent exploration and/or angiography on the operating table.

Crush syndrome. Be alert for this potential problem in any patient who has had a significant portion of a limb trapped for a period of time. The associated rhabdomyolysis and release of toxic by-products can lead to life-threatening hyperkalaemia, hypovolaemia, metabolic acidosis, hypocalcaemia and disseminated intravascular coagulation (DIC). Resuscitate the patient with large volumes of normal saline, aiming for a urine output of approximately 200 mL/h in an adult. Alkalinisation with sodium bicarbonate and the use of osmotic diuretics have also been advocated, although evidence is limited.

2. Most other injuries can be diagnosed and treated as part of the secondary survey.
3. Carefully examine the limb—skin integrity, colour, bruising, haematoma formation, neurovascular status, bony tenderness, function.
4. Be thorough—it is easy to overlook extremity injuries; therefore repeated examination is important.
5. Only proceed to imaging once the patient is stable and all life/limb threats have been addressed. Image the joints above and below the suspected fracture site.
6. Limb realignment and splinting reduces movement at the injury site, limits further bleeding and reduces pain. Always re-examine the neurovascular status of a limb if you have performed manipulation or applied a splint.
7. Early elevation of the injured limb reduces oedema formation.
8. Provide adequate analgesia, usually in the form of intravenous opioids titrated to effect.
9. Consider tetanus and antibiotic prophylaxis for open injuries.
10. Always be on the alert for complications—any site where muscle is contained within a closed fascial space has the potential to develop compartment syndrome.

Compartment syndrome

- This is a time-critical diagnosis—you have 4–6 hours at most to save the ischaemic contents of the compartment! It is potentially devastating if missed.
- Commonly occurs in the leg, forearm, foot, hand, gluteal region and thigh.
- Suspect the diagnosis in any patient who has pain greater than expected and that typically increases when the involved muscles are passively stretched—most of the other clinical signs are insensitive or develop late in the disease process.
- Warning—the distal pulse is usually present!
- Measure compartment pressures—greater than 35 mmHg in a normotensive patient is abnormal (lower pressures in the

hypotensive patient may be significant). The trend in repeated measurements is generally more helpful than a one-off reading.

Treatment

1 Release any constricting bandages, casts, etc.
2 Urgent fasciotomy if no improvement.
3 Treat complications, e.g. rhabdomyolysis.

Definitive care

Definitive care in all trauma patients needs to be directed by the trauma surgeon or the team leader.

Definitive care involves:

1 specific investigations, e.g. CT scan of the head/chest
2 consultation with specialty teams
3 documentation of all injuries and treatment
4 specific management plans from all appropriate teams
5 definitive placement to appropriate specialty team.

TERTIARY SURVEY

The tertiary survey is a complete review of the patient performed within the first 24 hours of their admission to hospital, aimed at detecting any further injuries or problems that may have been overlooked in the excitement of the initial resuscitation. It includes a further thorough head-to-toe clinical examination as well as a complete review of all investigations and treatments performed thus far.

Trauma service performance improvement

Care of the injured patient requires the services and skills of many different individuals. Trauma service performance improvement refers to the evaluation of the quality of care provided by a trauma service. Hospital-based performance improvement programs generally focus on the following aspects of health care.

- Safety—the extent to which risks and inadvertent harm are minimised
- Effectiveness of care—does the treatment/intervention achieve the desired outcomes?
- Appropriateness—is the selected treatment/intervention likely to produce the desired outcome?
- Consumer participation—engaging consumers in planning and evaluating healthcare services
- Efficiency—maximal total benefit is derived from the available treatments/resources

- Access—the extent to which an individual or population can obtain healthcare services

Performance improvement in trauma relies on the continual efforts of the multidisciplinary trauma team to measure, monitor, assess and improve both processes and outcomes of care. Trauma performance improvement programs are based on the following elements:

- a trauma registry/database to identify problems and the results of corrective actions
- multidisciplinary peer review of care, including morbidity and mortality analysis
- incident monitoring
- use of specific statistical methods for mortality analysis (e.g. Revised Trauma Score and Injury Severity Score—TRISS and A Severity Characterisation of Trauma—ASCOT)
- classification of deaths and complications as preventable, potentially preventable, non-preventable
- clinical indicators to measure current practice against accepted benchmarks
- use of evidence-based clinical guidelines, protocols and pathways
- evidence of 'loop closure'—that is, evidence that the process/ outcome needing improvement is remeasured following corrective action and that improvement is demonstrated.

CLINICAL PRACTICE GUIDELINES AND PROTOCOLS

Clinical practice guidelines and protocols are outlines of accepted management approaches based on best available evidence and are designed to assist clinical decision making. Clinical pathways are multidisciplinary plans of best clinical practice for specified groups of patients with a particular diagnosis that aid the coordination and delivery of high-quality care.

CLINICAL INDICATORS

Clinical indicators are measures of the process or outcomes of care. They are not designed to be exact standards, but rather act as 'flags' to alert clinicians to possible problems in the system or opportunities for improvement. For clinical indicators to be effective they must be relevant and clearly defined. Development of a set of clinical indicators is interactive. Indicators are reviewed on an ongoing basis with reference to the usefulness of the data and the resources required to collect it. Trauma service indicators are used to monitor process and outcomes of care from the pre-hospital phase through to rehabilitation and discharge. Close analysis of data is required, as there may be valid reasons why an event occurs differently from an expectation.

Examples of trauma service clinical indicators are:

- proportion of patients with a documented GCS < 9 who do not receive an endotracheal tube (ETT) within 10 minutes of documentation of that score
- proportion of head-injured patients with a documented GCS < 12 who do not have a CT scan of the head within 4 hours of arrival in the ED
- proportion of trauma patients transported to hospital by ambulance (not entrapped at the scene) who have a documented scene time of > 20 minutes.

OUTCOME MEASURES

Historically, trauma services have focused on the issue of preventable deaths as the main outcome measure. Outcome analysis in trauma is slowly expanding. Trauma services are now beginning to analyse other outcomes such as morbidity, functional impairment, quality of life and patient satisfaction. Comparison of outcomes across different sites relies on use of standardised, reliable outcome measures. Similarly, morbidity analysis requires tight definitions of problems, with rate comparisons potentially confounded by demographic differences between hospitals.

A large number of measures exist for outcomes analysis in trauma. These include:

- Glasgow Outcome Scale (GOS) for head-injured patients
- Disability Rating Scale (DRS)
- Short Form (SF)-36 survey
- sickness impact profile
- Hospital Anxiety and Depression Scale (HADS)
- functional independence measure (FIM).

Conclusion

The patient suffering multiple injuries is often a distressing sight and can at times seem like an overwhelming challenge to manage. By approaching care of such patients in a directed manner, prioritising the assessment and management of life-threatening injuries as outlined above, hopefully both you and your patients can look forward to the best outcomes possible. Appropriate and timely intervention is the key.

Online resources

American College of Surgeons. Trauma performance improvement: A reference manual. http://ncrtac-wi.org/uploads/ACS_Trauma_Performance_Improvement_Manual.pdf

American Trauma Service www.amtrauma.org

Australasian Trauma Society www.traumasociety.com.au

Brain Trauma Foundation www.braintrauma.org

Eastern Association for Surgery of Trauma www.east.org

Liverpool Hospital Trauma Department www.sswahs.nsw.gov.au/Liverpool/Trauma

National Trauma Research Institute www.ntri.org.au

NSW Institute of Trauma and Injury Management (ITIM) www.itim.nsw.gov.au/wiki/Home

Paediatric Trauma Assessment and Management http://depts.washington.edu/pedtraum

The Alfred Trauma Service www.alfredhealth.org.au/traumaservice

Trauma Care UK www.trauma.myzen.co.uk

Trauma.org www.trauma.org

Youth and Road Trauma Forum at Westmead www.bstreetsmart.org/index.php

Chapter 15
Neurosurgical emergencies

Rob Edwards

This chapter covers the approach to the patient who presents with headache as well as the following neurosurgical emergencies, both traumatic and non traumatic:

- traumatic brain injury (TBI)
- subdural haematoma
- cervical spine injury and spinal cord injuries
- intracranial haemorrhages such as subarachnoid haemorrhage (SAH), subdural haemorrhage (SDH) and intracerebral haemorrhage (ICH)
- emergency presentations of patients with space-occupying lesions (SOLs)
- complications of ventriculoperitoneal shunts
- epidural abscess.

Before examining each of these individually, it is instructive to consider some important concepts and principles that are relevant irrespective of the actual pathology involved.

General concepts

PRIMARY VERSUS SECONDARY BRAIN INJURY

Primary brain injury is the injury that occurs at the time of the trauma. Interventions that affect primary brain injury are obviously out of the immediate control of the emergency doctor, but are very important and include public health measures aimed at prevention. Some measures that have reduced TBI include compulsory use of seat belts in cars and helmets for motorcycle riders and pedal cyclists.

Secondary brain injury occurs after the initial injury and is due to the sequelae of the original injury, such as raised intracranial pressure, hypoxia, hypercarbia or hypotension. Its effects can therefore be either minimised or prevented with good management. Many of the management strategies in the emergency department revolve around minimising secondary brain injury.

Cerebral perfusion pressure (CPP) is the pressure that drives perfusion of the brain and is defined by the equation

CPP = Mean arterial pressure (MAP) – Intracranial pressure (ICP)

Normally ICP is between 5 and 10 mmHg. Autoregulatory mechanisms will maintain constant cerebral blood flow when the cerebral perfusion varies between 50 and 150 mmHg. In some patients, such as those with severe head injury, cerebral autoregulation may be lost, thus making the brain more susceptible to hypotension. Any process that reduces MAP (e.g. hypovolaemic shock) or increases ICP (post-injury oedema, expanding intracranial haematoma or mass, hypercarbia) will compromise cerebral perfusion, leading to secondary brain injury.

Editorial Comment

The management of concussion is complex and still evolving. There is increasing awareness of issues related to concussion, especially in sports and in research using amnesia scales. Doctors need to keep up to date on recommendations as to when people can return to sports/contact sports/work after a concussive episode.

HEADACHE

Headache is a common symptom of a neurosurgical emergency (e.g. any of the intracranial haemorrhages, space-occupying lesion). It may also be a symptom of a life-threatening non-surgical emergency (e.g. meningitis, encephalitis), a symptom of many other less serious disease processes (e.g. migraine) or a non-specific manifestation of a non-neurological process (e.g. any serious infection such as pneumonia, influenza, pyelonephritis).

As headache is a frequent complaint of patients presenting to the ED, the problem is to differentiate the patients who harbour a serious cause from those who do not. The fact that some conditions are relatively uncommon (e.g. the incidence of subarachnoid haemorrhage is about 12 cases per 100,000 per year) cannot be relied upon as these patients select EDs, through either referral from their primary doctor or self-referral.

Boxes 15.1 and 15.2 outline some criteria for computed tomography (CT) of the brain of both trauma and non-trauma patients, respectively. Further information regarding the features of different types of headaches is given under the heading of each specific diagnosis.

Box 15.1 Indications for cerebral CT in mild head injury

- Glasgow Coma Scale (GCS) score < 15 at 2 hours after injury
- Persistent abnormal alertness/behaviour or cognition despite 'normal' GCS
- Deteriorating GCS score
- Suspected open, or a depressed, skull fracture
- Age ≥ 65 years
- Vomiting (2 or more episodes)
- Major mechanism of injury with significant force
- Focal neurological signs
- Persistent headache
- Anticoagulant therapy or coagulopathy
- Loss of consciousness > 5 minutes
- Persistent post-traumatic amnesia
- Consider CT if any of the following are present: large scalp haematoma or laceration, multisystem trauma, delayed presentation or re-presentation

Box 15.2 Indications for urgent cerebral CT in non-trauma patients with headache

- Focal neurological signs
- Altered mental status or change in behaviour
- Age > 60 years
- Nausea and vomiting
- Severe or sudden onset suggestive of subarachnoid haemorrhage (SAH)
- Absence of other demonstrable cause for headache
- History of cerebral tumour, warfarin use or other condition (e.g. shunt, hydrocephalus, recent craniotomy)

Features which indicate that a headache is due to raised ICP are associated nausea and vomiting and headache worse on awakening in the morning and on lying down.

GLASGOW COMA SCALE (GCS)

The GCS is a widely accepted scale for assessing alterations to a patient's level of consciousness. A score is given based on 3 components—eye opening, verbal response and motor response (see Table 15.1). In adults, the score achieved correlates well with the severity of the underlying condition. It is also useful for objectively following a patient's progress. Maximum score is 15 and minimum is 3.

HERNIATION SYNDROMES

The cranial cavity is divided into compartments by fibrous dura mater (the falx cerebri and tentorium cerebelli). The tentorium separates the

Table 15.1 Glasgow Coma Scale

Eye opening	Spontaneous	4
	To voice	3
	To pain	2
	None	1
Best verbal response	Alert	5
	Confused	4
	Inappropriate words only	3
	Incomprehensible sounds	2
	Nil	1
Best motor response	Obeys commands	6
	Localises pain	5
	Withdraws to pain	4
	Abnormal flexion	3
	Abnormal extension	2
	None	1

cerebrum above from the cerebellum and brainstem below. Because of the rigidity and non-expansible nature of the cranial vault, significant increases in ICP can lead to herniation syndromes where the contents of one compartment herniate across an opening in these dural structures, causing specific neurological signs. The significance of a herniation syndrome is that ICP has increased beyond the capacity of the brain to compensate, and death will ensue if emergency treatment is not undertaken. Raised ICP above the tentorium leads to herniation of the uncus of the temporal lobe. This manifests as dilation of the ipsilateral pupil (later bilateral), contralateral pyramidal weakness and increased tone.

Raised ICP will also lead to high blood pressure and bradycardia (Cushing response).

MANAGEMENT PRINCIPLES

The aims of treatment are to prevent secondary brain injury, treat the underlying condition, minimise symptoms and optimise neurological and functional recovery. ED management is concerned with the first 3 of these.

Airway, breathing and circulation (ABCs)

A patent airway is the first priority (see Chapter 2, 'Securing the airway, ventilation and procedural sedation'). Simple manoeuvres to maintain patency may prevent secondary brain injury from hypoxia. Airway protection is also important—patients with a GCS of 8 or less will not be able to protect their airway from *aspiration* or maintain a patent airway, and need intubation. Adequate ventilation is required to avoid *hypoxia* and *hypercarbia*. Treatment measures vary from oxygen therapy by mask to full mechanical ventilation if required. Adequate CPP relies in part on a normal blood pressure. *Hypotension* should therefore be treated with prevention of further blood loss and volume expansion.

Measures to decrease ICP

A number of interventions can reduce ICP.

- Adequate sedation and paralysis of the intubated patient with neurosurgical emergency, including at the time of rapid-sequence induction.
- Osmotic agent. Administration of a hyperosmolar solution to use osmotic pressure to draw water out of the brain decreases ICP. Traditionally, mannitol infusion of 1 g/kg (equates to 5 mL of 20% mannitol per kg) has been used; however, a recent meta-analysis of 5 small studies comparing mannitol with hypertonic saline has suggested that hypertonic saline solution (e.g. 7.5% saline) is more effective and has fewer adverse effects than mannitol. Indicated when there is severe increase in ICP (e.g. evidence of herniation syndrome, significant mass effect on CT or high ICP as measured by ICP monitor).
- Steroids (dexamethasone) help to reduce oedema associated with space-occupying lesions. They are not shown to be useful in traumatic brain injury.
- Barbiturates. Bolus therapy with thiopentone can reduce increases in ICP. Should be given only when there is an ICP monitor to guide therapy.
- Maintain normal PCO_2. Hyperventilation to lower than normal PCO_2 is not recommended, as this causes cerebral vasoconstriction and does not improve outcome. In ventilated patients, target PCO_2 should be in the normal range.
- Elevate the head of the bed 30° if the spinal column has been cleared.

Surgery

The indications for surgery will be discussed specifically for each condition.

Traumatic neurosurgical emergencies

TRAUMATIC BRAIN INJURY (TBI)

TBI is a major cause of morbidity and mortality in Australia. Of all trauma-related deaths, TBI is a major factor in a significant proportion. Of those who survive TBI, some are left with neurological impairment that often requires lengthy rehabilitation and may result in inability to return to work or function normally. The social and financial costs of this morbidity are very high. It is a relatively high-prevalence injury, and it has been estimated that in Australia there are about 150 admissions to hospital per year with TBI per 100,000 population and that peak incidence is in the age group 15–35 years.

Classification and pathophysiology

There are different ways of classifying TBI. Each is useful in that there is some relationship to treatment and prognosis. Table 15.2 outlines a classification according to the actual pathology of the injury. TBI can also be classified according to severity based on GCS (GCS 8 = severe, GCS 9–13 = moderate, and GCS 14–15 = mild or minor).

Table 15.2 Pathological lesions seen in traumatic brain injury

Type of injury	Lesion
Skull fractures	Depressed
	Base of skull
	Linear
Cerebral contusion	
Haemorrhage	Intracerebral
	Subarachnoid
	Subdural
	Extradural
Diffuse axonal injury	

Assessment and diagnosis

Assessment should be performed according to advanced trauma life support principles, which use a prioritised and systematised approach (for general principles of trauma management, see Chapter 14, 'Trauma'). The diagnosis of TBI per se is usually obvious from the history. Markers of a significant injury that need to be considered for CT scan are *any one* of:

- loss of consciousness (though not always present)
- amnesia for event
- mechanism of injury involving major force.

The occasional patient presents with an altered conscious state without a definite history of trauma. In cases where the patient may have been drinking alcohol, it is sometimes misdiagnosed as alcohol or drug intoxication. This is a classic misdiagnosis that can have lethal consequences. Where alcohol use and head injury co-exist, always assume that any alteration in mental state is due to the head injury.

Clinical features

The severity of the mechanism of injury, a history of loss of consciousness and the duration of loss of consciousness are important. Did the patient regain consciousness? The patient may be experiencing symptoms such as headache, nausea and vomiting. There may be amnesia concerning the events around the time of injury, or for a period before the injury (retrograde amnesia). Anterograde amnesia is the inability to remember information acquired since the injury. This often manifests as the patient asking the same questions over and over again.

On examination, local head trauma (lacerations, haematomas) may be present. The GCS should be measured (Table 15.1). Focal neurological signs such as pupillary dilation with or without hemiparesis with increased tone and reflexes indicate an uncal herniation syndrome requiring emergency management. Where there is significant increase in ICP, the Cushing reflex will lead to hypertension and bradycardia. Clues to a fractured skull base are cerebrospinal fluid (CSF) leak from the nose, bilateral periorbital bruising (raccoon eyes), CSF leak from the ear, haemotympanum and bruising behind the ear (Battle's sign).

Investigations

Definitive investigation is a CT scan of the head. This should be done urgently for severe and moderate head injuries. For mild head injury (GCS 14–15), the indications are listed in Box 15.1, above.

Blood tests such as white cell count (WCC), haemoglobin and serum chemistries are relevant though not diagnostic. Coagulation studies should be done if there is intracranial haemorrhage or if the patient is on anticoagulants. A blood group and hold should be done if the patient requires evacuation of a haematoma, as there may be significant blood loss in this procedure.

Management

A systematic trauma approach that identifies and prioritises injuries is mandatory. As outlined above under 'General concepts', this will allow immediate management of life-threatening problems such as airway obstruction, lack of airway protection, hypoxia, blood loss and hypotension, thus avoiding secondary brain injury. Specific management includes the following.

Measures to reduce ICP

The specific measures mentioned above are appropriate for all patients with severe TBI. An osmotic agent such as hypertonic saline 7.5% or 20% mannitol (see 'Management principles' above) is usually reserved for those who have evidence of a herniation syndrome, evidence of mass effect on CT or high ICP as measured on an ICP monitor.

Surgical intervention

Surgery is required for drainage of extradural (see Fig 15.1) and subdural hematomas. This may be required emergently if they are causing mass effect with raised ICP. Supportive therapy is required for contusions, subarachnoid haemorrhage and diffuse axonal injury. Surgery is also required for depressed skull fracture (see Fig 15.2). In severe head injuries, insertion of an ICP monitor and monitoring of intra-arterial blood pressure to direct therapy (see above) is aimed at reducing raised ICP. To maintain adequate cerebral blood flow, a CPP of above 70 mmHg is ideal.

Analgesia

In a setting where patients with TBI can be closely monitored and CT scanning performed, sensible use of opiate analgesia to relieve

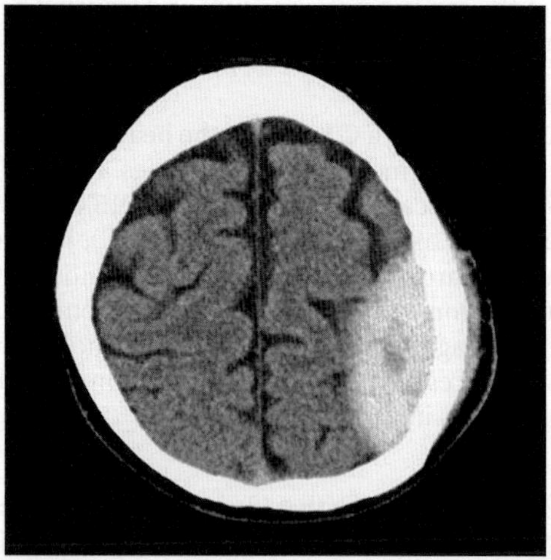

Figure 15.1 CT scan showing a left-sided extradural haematoma

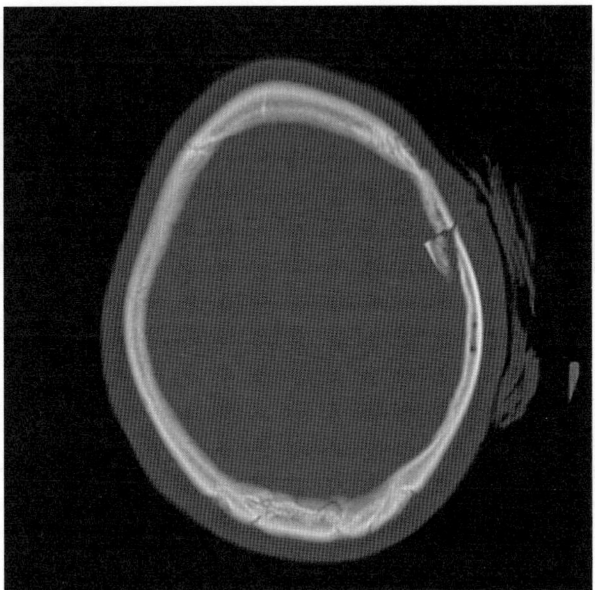

Figure 15.2 Depressed skull fracture. Bone windows of CT brain in a patient who was noted to have dysphasia after being hit on the head with a bat, due to local pressure to the speech centre of the brain

headache and pain is indicated. Codeine is not a good analgesic as it can cause a lot of nausea. Carefully titrated doses of morphine are preferable. Paracetamol (IV or orally for patients who can swallow) can be used. Aspirin is contraindicated because of its antiplatelet effect.

Other acute treatments

If seizures occur during the acute phase, phenytoin (loading dose 15 mg/kg IV infusion) can be given to prevent further seizures.

Patients with mild but significant head injury not having a CT scan should be observed until they have been normal and symptom-free for an appropriate length of time. In most EDs, 4 hours is the period used. When discharged, these patients should be provided with written head injury advice.

About one-third of patients with so-called minor head injury have disabling symptoms for several days to weeks after the head injury, including headaches, difficulty concentrating and dizziness. Patients should be warned about this.

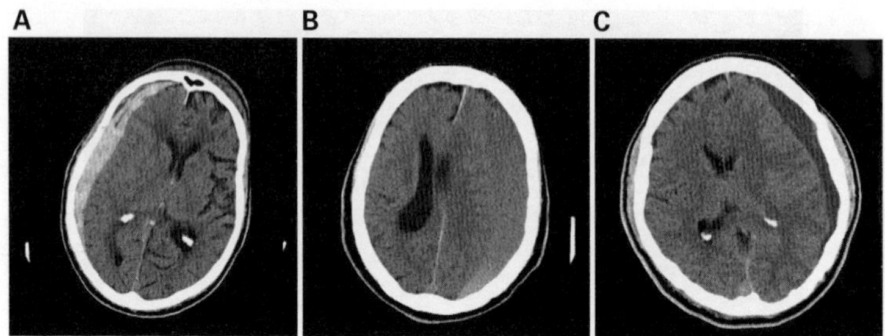

Figure 15.3 Non-contrast cerebral CT scans showing subdural haematomas of varying age. A: Acute right subdural. B: Left isodense, 10- to 14-day-old subdural with mass effect showing compression of the ventricle and midline shift to the right. C: Chronic left subdural

SUBDURAL HAEMATOMA

Subdural haematoma can present without a definite history of trauma; however, it is usually traumatic in origin. Subdural haematomas arise from injury to the bridging veins in the subdural space (between the dura mater which follows the contour of the bony skull, and the pia mater which follows the contour of the cortex of the brain). Where there is cortical atrophy this space is prominent and more at risk of subdural haematoma from an injury.

Clinical features

Depending on the time course of the bleed, a subdural haematoma can be acute, subacute or chronic (see Fig 15.3). When large, it presents with symptoms of mass effect (see 'Space-occupying lesions,' below). Other symptoms include headache, confusion and ataxia. The clinical picture can be non-specific.

Investigation

Definitive diagnosis is by cerebral CT scan. Full blood count, coagulation studies and blood group and hold should also be ordered.

Treatment

Appropriately manage the airway, breathing and circulation. Any coagulopathy should be reversed. Drainage is indicated if there is significant mass effect or neurological impairment.

CERVICAL SPINE AND SPINAL CORD INJURIES

Vertebral column injury refers to injury of any of the bones, joints and ligaments that make up the vertebral column. This may or may not be associated with spinal cord injury, which refers to injury of the spinal cord itself and is associated with neurological deficit.

The types of trauma that are high risk for spinal injury include high-speed motor vehicle crashes (particularly if there has been ejection from the vehicle), diving injuries, rugby football injuries and falls. In the elderly, falls from the standing position can easily result in cervical spine injury, especially at the C2 level. In this group, mortality is significantly higher than in younger patients.

Clinical features

Assessment of presence of vertebral column injury

The features of vertebral column injury are midline pain, particularly on attempted movement, and local tenderness. It may or may not be associated with a spinal cord injury (see below), which is manifest by neurological deficit.

NEXUS Criteria for clinical clearance of cervical spine

The NEXUS (National Emergency X-radiography Utilization Study) criteria are a set of criteria for clearing the cervical spine clinically that have been developed and prospectively validated in a cohort of over 34,000 patients. Patients who are alert and lucid, have no midline neck tenderness, have no other significant distracting injuries (or have not received significant doses of opiates for pain) and have no neurological signs of spinal cord injury can be cleared of a cervical spine injury without X-ray. All other patients require a radiological evaluation of the cervical spine (See 'Imaging the cervical spine', below).

Assessment of presence of spinal cord injury

The neurological deficit can be classified according to *function* (motor, sensory or autonomic), its *distribution* (level and, in partial cord lesions, which part of the body is affected) and whether the loss of function is *complete or incomplete.*

An evaluation of motor tone, power and reflexes should be done. The initial screening sensory examination is with light touch or pinprick. If there is other evidence of neurological deficit, test temperature and proprioception (posterior column).

When sensory loss is present, a sensory level below which sensation is lost can define the level of the injury. A working knowledge of the dermatomes of the body is required. It helps to remember that the junction of shoulder and neck is at C4, the nipple at T4, the umbilicus at T10 and the inguinal region at L1. When the patient is log-rolled to examine the back, perianal and buttock sensory testing should be done, as well as assessment of anal tone. Sparing perianal sensation and anal tone may be evidence that the lesion is not complete and there may be some functional recovery.

Other clinical clues that suggest spinal cord injury are diaphragmatic breathing in high-mid to lower cervical spine injury (loss of intercostal power supplied by the thoracic cord with intact diaphragm supplied by C4, C5 and C6). In males, priapism may be present, due to loss of sympathetic tone. There may also be hypotension and bradycardia due to loss of sympathetic vascular tone. Other causes of shock from trauma (haemorrhage, pericardial tamponade and tension pneumothorax) must be ruled out.

Whether or not the cord lesion is complete or partial is obviously vital for prognosis. Complete lesions have total loss of all three modalities (motor, sensory and autonomic). Partial lesions can have some residual function in any of the modalities. There are some syndromes with typical patterns of deficit indicating injury to certain parts of the cord (Table 15.3).

It should also be remembered that, in patients with a vertebral column injury, between 5% and 7% will have a second injury.

Table 15.3 Partial spinal cord syndromes

Syndrome	Part of cord affected	Motor	Sensory
Brown-Séquard	Hemisection of cord	Ipsilateral loss	Loss of ipsilateral proprioception, contralateral pain/ temperature
Anterior cord	Anterior half of cord	Bilateral motor loss	Bilateral temperature loss; intact proprioception/vibration
Central cord		Weakness in upper limbs, sparing of lower limbs	Loss of sensation in upper limbs, lower limbs spared

Imaging the cervical spine

In patients who cannot be cleared clinically (see NEXUS criteria above), radiological assessment should be done.

Plain radiology

Plain films have limited utility in assessment of the cervical spine. Anatomical detail is lacking, interpretation is difficult especially for inexperienced doctors, films are frequently technically inadequate and sensitivity is not acceptable. A meta-analysis of studies comparing plain radiography with CT showed that plain radiology had a pooled sensitivity of 52% versus 98% for CT scan for the detection of cervical spine injury.

In the past, plain cervical X-rays have been recommended as an initial screening investigation; however, many authors recommend that CT scan be the initial imaging modality of choice. While they are still commonly used in Australian EDs, the clear indications for CT scan (without plain films) are:

1 Clinically unevaluable patients. Patients with decreased level of consciousness or who are intubated, uncooperative or who have multiple painful and distracting injuries (e.g. severe multiple trauma).
2 High clinical suspicion of cervical spine injury, including
   a Neurological deficit
   b Significant pain and tenderness in the cervical spine.
3 Technical considerations likely to impair ability to perform adequate plain radiography. For example, body habitus.

In patients who are alert, cooperative and do not have any of the high-risk features above, the combination of plain radiography plus repeated clinical assessment is commonly used as first-line screening. Any abnormalities suggesting a cervical spine injury need to be elucidated with a CT. Patients with significant pain or midline tenderness despite normal plain films also require a CT.

At a minimum, 3 views should be taken of the cervical spine. These are lateral, anteroposterior (AP) and odontoid peg (open-mouth) views. The lateral view must show down to the cervicothoracic junction (C7 and at least the upper part of the body of T1). If it does not, a swimmer's view can be obtained to better show the cervicothoracic junction. This view needs to show both the alignment and some detail of the C7/T1 area.

Other films may be useful in certain situations. Oblique views of the cervical spine can be used to evaluate the pedicles and facet joints on each side. They can also be used as an alternative to swimmer's view in imaging the cervicothoracic junction. Flexion and extension views are indicated to detect instability in an otherwise normal cervical spine with symptoms.

Table 15.4 outlines a system for reviewing cervical spine X-rays. Figure 15.4 illustrates some common cervical spine fractures and dislocations.

Table 15.4 System for review of cervical spine X-rays

Quality of film	Includes all of C7 and at least part of T1
Alignment	Check for smooth continuity of four 'lines': anterior alignment of vertebral bodies, posterior alignment of vertebral bodies, the spinolaminal line (junction of lamina and spinous process) and tips of spinous processes
Prevertebral soft tissue swelling	Best judged in upper cervical spine. 5 mm allowed at C2, 7 mm allowed at C3, 15–20 mm at C4 and below
Predental space (between dens and anterior arch of C1)	< 2–4 mm in adults and < 4–5 mm in children
Relationship of adjacent vertebral bodies	E.g. movement of one body on another, angulation
Integrity of the elements of each vertebral body	E.g. loss of height, visible fracture lines, abnormalities in bony architecture
Facet joints between adjacent vertebrae	Subluxation or dislocation
Integrity of posterior elements	Pedicles, laminae and spinous processes
Integrity of odontoid peg	On lateral and peg views
Subluxation of either atlantoaxial joint	On peg view
Alignment and integrity of all elements on anteroposterior (AP) film	Particularly look for alignment of spinous processes in midline and alignment of facet joints

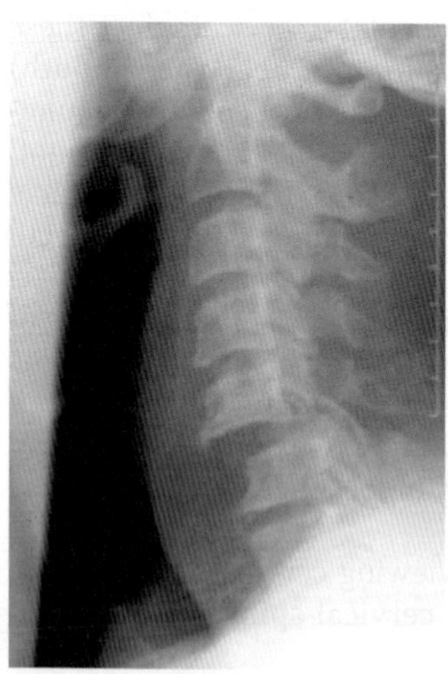

Figure 15.4A Bilateral facet joint dislocation between C5/C6 showing displacement of C6 posteriorly relative to C5, and prevertebral soft-tissue swelling at that level

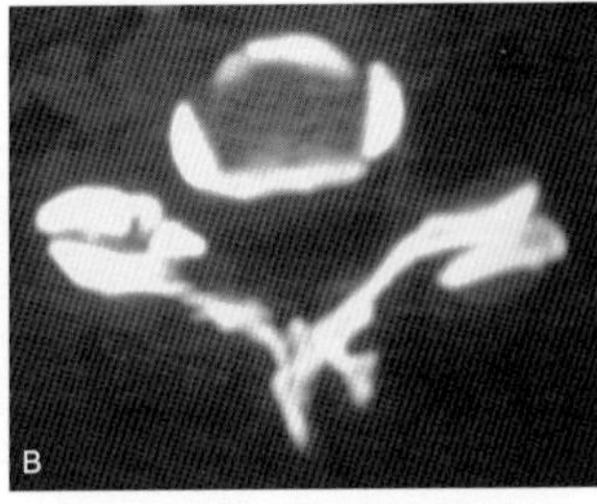

Figure 15.4B Unifacet joint dislocation between C4/C5. X-ray shows angulation and posterior displacement of C5 relative to C4 and splaying of the spinous processes.

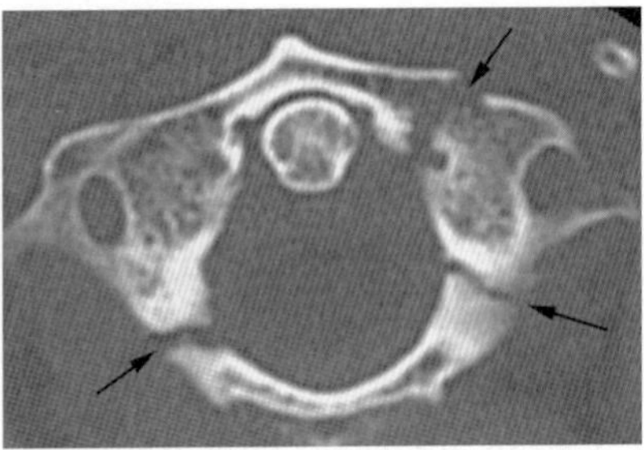

Figure 15.4C Fracture of posterior arch of C1 (Jefferson fracture)

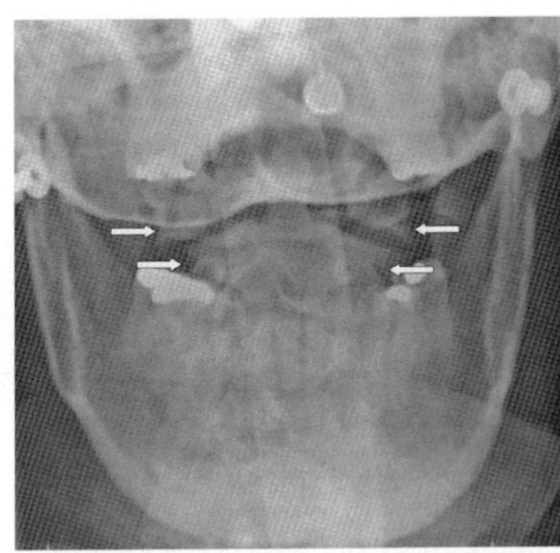

Figure 15.4D Odontoid view of C1/C2 showing instability of C1 relative to C2

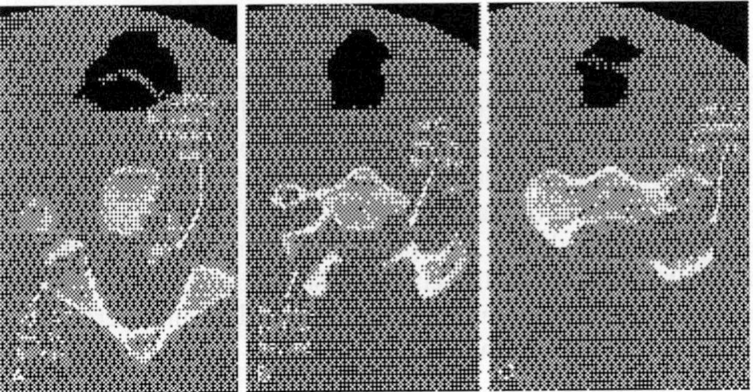

Figure 15.4E Fracture of pedicle of C2 (Hangman's fracture)

Editorial Comment

Clearing a neck is a very common task in the ED. Most head CT trauma patients should have a neck CT at the same time. Get formal radiological/neurosurgical opinion readily as these can be difficult and easily missed, e.g. facet joint dislocation on CT resulting in paraplegia.

Magnetic resonance imaging (MRI)

CT scans are particularly useful for identifying bony injury. Clinical and radiological assessment as described above will pick up the vast majority of fractures and dislocations. MRI is better for identifying ligamentous injury, however, and is useful in the further assessment of known injuries or the investigation of spinal cord injury without radiological abnormality (SCIWORA).

Determination of stability of vertebral column injury

The ability of the vertebral column to protect the spinal cord from abnormal movement and, therefore, injury should be evaluated. This should be done by a spinal surgeon.

The vertebral column can be considered to consist of three structural components: the anterior, middle and posterior columns.

- The anterior column consists of bone and ligaments from the anterior half of the vertebral bodies forward.
- The posterior column is made up of the neural arch (laminae and pedicles), spinous processes and posterior ligamentous complex.
- The remainder, the middle column, is from the posterior longitudinal ligament and posterior half of the vertebral body.

If at least two out of three of these columns are disrupted, the injury is considered unstable.

Treatment

In the patient with multiple injuries, vertebral column and spinal cord injuries should be managed as part of a prioritised management plan that addresses other serious injuries in context (see Chapter 14 for general principles of trauma management). The consequences of injury to the spinal cord in a patient with an unstable vertebral column injury are of major life-changing significance for the patient. Precautions to prevent further injury to the cord should therefore be instituted from the beginning.

Immobilisation of vertebral column

Precautions to prevent movement of the vertebral column should be instituted until it has been cleared. Patient transfers should be carried out while maintaining the position of the vertebral column. In hospital, this means use of specialised lifting frames (e.g. Jordan frame) or techniques (e.g. log-rolling, spinal lifting technique). In each of these manoeuvres, a designated person needs to continuously maintain the position of the cervical spine.

Numerous orthoses are available to minimise vertebral column movements. There is no perfect splint that prevents all vertebral column movements, particularly in uncooperative patients. Cervical collars restrict but do not completely prevent cervical spine movement. Soft collars are very poor at preventing movement; hard collars are better. At a minimum, any patient with a suspected cervical spine fracture should wear a hard cervical collar and the techniques for transfer outlined above should be used. Additional immobilisation with 'sandbags' may be used. Imaging should be expedited, as prolonged periods in hard collars and lying supine without moving are uncomfortable and painful.

Airway management may be problematical. Mask ventilation has been shown to result in inadvertent neck extension. If intubation is required, in-line immobilisation of the cervical spine by a person designated purely for that role and intubation by an experienced operator during rapid-sequence induction has been shown to be a safe technique.

Referral and supportive care

Patients with high cervical lesions may have respiratory muscle weakness that may lead to respiratory failure. Depending on the severity, treatment for this may vary from supplemental oxygen to mechanical ventilation. Elderly patients in particular are at risk of delayed respiratory complications if left lying supine for long periods immobilised in cervical collars.

Patients with spinal cord injury should also have a gastric tube passed and an indwelling urinary catheter placed. Early transfer to a specialised spinal unit within 24 hours of injury has been shown to positively affect outcomes.

Early referral to a spinal surgeon (neurosurgeon or orthopaedic surgeon) should happen as soon as diagnosis is made. Decisions regarding the stability of a vertebral column lesion should be made by the spinal surgeon. Additionally, patients may require long-term immobilisation with skeletal traction.

Non-traumatic neurosurgical emergencies

SUBARACHNOID HAEMORRHAGE (SAH)

(See also Chapter 24, 'Neurological emergencies'.)

Early diagnosis of SAH can improve chance of survival. However, the morbidity and mortality are still significant. Up to 50% of SAH patients die and a third of survivors are left permanently disabled and dependent. While a proportion die from the initial haemorrhage, a group of patients will die from re-bleeding. The size of this latter group suffering repeat haemorrhages can be minimised if there is prompt diagnosis and treatment. Despite this, diagnosis of SAH is often missed or delayed.

In two-thirds of patients with SAH the source of bleeding is a rupture of a cerebral aneurysm. The commonest site is the anterior communicating artery.

In about 20% of patients no identifiable cause is found, and a small number have an arteriovenous malformation (AVM). A family history of aneurysmal haemorrhage increases the patient's risk of the same.

Clinical features

Sudden onset of severe headache is the hallmark of SAH. This is often associated with nausea, vomiting and symptoms and signs of meningism (photophobia, neck stiffness). Neurological deficit ranges from none to coma. Absence of meningism or neurological signs *does not* exclude the diagnosis.

There are different scoring systems available for grading the severity of SAH, all of which do a reasonable job in predicting mortality, functional outcome for survivors and length of hospital stay. Table 15.5 outlines the World Federation of Neurological Surgeons (WFNS) grading system for subarachnoid haemorrhage and its relation to mortality.

Patients may occasionally present with effects of the aneurysm before it has bled, such as warning headaches and occasionally oculomotor nerve palsy (ptosis, dilated pupil and diplopia with the eye in the down and out position).

Investigations

Diagnosis of the bleed is usually by cerebral CT scan (see Figure 15.5). The ability of a cerebral CT to pick up an SAH degrades over time. If scanned with a third-generation CT scanner within the first 24 hours, it has been reported that between 92.9% and 98% will be visible; however, by 1 week post-bleed only 50% are visible.

Table 15.5 The World Federation of Neurological Surgeons (WFNS) grading system for subarachnoid haemorrhage

Grade	GCS score and motor deficit	Mortality (%)
I	GCS 15	5
II	GCS 13–14, no motor deficit	9
III	GCS 13–14, with motor deficit	20
IV	GCS 7–12	33
V	GCS 3–6	77

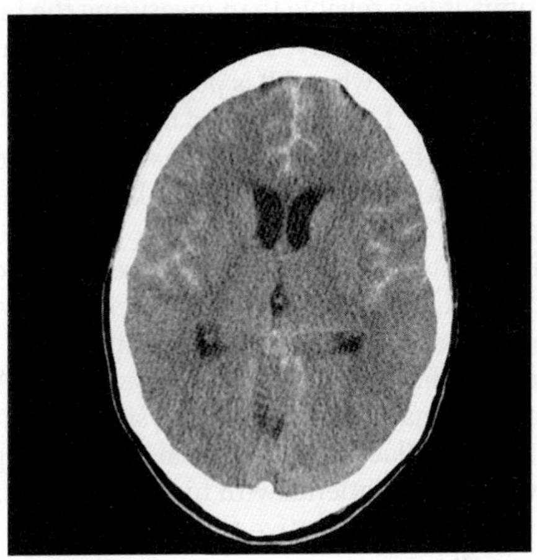

Figure 15.5 Non-contrast CT brain showing extensive subarachnoid haemorrhage

Because the consequences of a missed diagnosis of SAH are potentially lethal, it has been routinely recommended that a lumbar puncture (LP) should be performed in patients with a negative CT so that those with a false-negative CT can be picked up. There has been recent debate in the literature as to whether or not routine LP on all patients with negative CT is required, owing to the fact that most of the LPs done in this circumstance are normal and also because there has been recent evidence that if the scan is done within 6 hours of the bleed then the sensitivity is 100%. Certainly if the patient presents after 6 hours of onset or there is a high degree of clinical suspicion, LP should be performed.

- The LP should be examined for the presence of blood (either macroscopic or microscopic). If red blood cells are present, it is difficult to differentiate a traumatic tap from a subarachnoid haemorrhage. The CSF should be examined for breakdown products of red blood cells (oxyhaemoglobin and bilirubin) by CSF spectrophotometry.

- Oxyhaemoglobin takes 2 or more hours to develop, but bilirubin takes 12 hours to develop. A traumatic tap can give rise to oxyhaemoglobin only, but the presence of both bilirubin and oxyhaemoglobin peaks on spectrophotometry is suggestive of SAH.
- Xanthochromia is the yellow appearance to the naked eye of the supernatant of the centrifuged CSF specimen. The yellow colour is due to the presence of bilirubin. Inspection of the CSF for xanthochromia is less reliable than measuring the bilirubin peak with CSF spectrophotometry. Therefore, CSF spectrophotometry should always be done when LP is performed to rule out SAH.
- Because it does take 12 hours for red blood cells in CSF to break down to bilirubin, it is theoretically possible that performing an LP too soon after the occurrence of the haemorrhage may lead to false-negative LP.

Once a SAH is detected, further imaging is required to demonstrate the source of the bleed. This is done with either 4-vessel cerebral angiography or CT angiogram (circle of Willis). The latter is a less invasive alternative that can identify aneurysms and AVMs. It has a sensitivity of approximately 96% for aneurysms of greater than 3 mm diameter. It has not replaced conventional cerebral angiography, but is useful in investigating patients with high clinical suspicion of SAH but who have equivocal or negative CT and LP.

Treatment

1. Urgent measures to ensure adequacy of the airway and breathing may be required if the patient has a significantly reduced level of consciousness.
2. Definitive treatment is to prevent re-bleeding either by early surgery to clip the aneurysm or by endovascular occlusion with a coil. The latter is done by angiographic placement of a detachable coil.
3. Spasm of cerebral vessels is a delayed complication of SAH that may lead to cerebral ischaemia. The risk of this can be minimised by using nimodipine, which should be started intravenously within 72 hours of the SAH. The patient needs to be kept adequately hydrated with IV fluids.
4. In the ED, effective analgesia and treatment of nausea and vomiting with antiemetics is important. Acute elevation in blood pressure should be treated to minimise risk of re-bleeding.

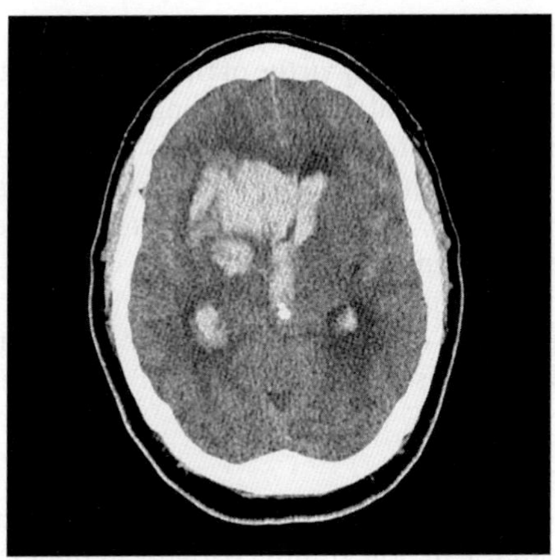

Figure 15.6 Non-contrast cerebral CT scan with large intracerebral bleed with blood extending into ventricles

SPONTANEOUS INTRACEREBRAL HAEMORRHAGE

Spontaneous intracerebral haemorrhage is usually related to poorly controlled hypertension. Patients who are on anticoagulated warfarin or newer anticoagulants are also at risk of intracerebral haemorrhage.

Patients usually present with sudden-onset headache and neurological impairment. Focal neurological signs are usually related to the location of the bleed. In larger bleeds (see Figure 15.6), especially where there is mass effect, there is usually reduced level of consciousness or coma. Herniation syndromes may be seen, especially with posterior intracranial fossa bleeds.

Most intracerebral bleeds are treated medically with attention to the priorities of airway, breathing and circulation as well as correction of any coagulopathy (e.g. reversal of anticoagulation).

Indications for surgery include:

- posterior fossa haemorrhage with mass effect
- intraventricular blood causing acute hydrocephalus.

SPACE-OCCUPYING LESIONS

A number of non-traumatic conditions can present to the ED with the acute effects of a space-occupying lesion (SOL). These include tumours (primary and secondary tumours). Subdural haematomas may occur without a definite history of trauma. Large cerebellar infarcts can be complicated by significant swelling, rapid increase in ICP and a herniation syndrome.

Clinical features

The clinical presentation is by virtue of the enlarging size of the lesion, mass effect (local or general) or surrounding oedema (see Figure 15.7). Symptoms vary greatly from just headaches, with features suggestive of raised ICP (worse on lying and in the morning, associated with nausea and vomiting), to patients with coma and herniation syndromes at the severe end of the spectrum.

The patient may present with seizures (focal or generalised). Persistent depression of GCS post-ictally or development of status epilepticus should raise clinical suspicion and necessitate urgent cerebral CT.

Investigations

Definitive diagnosis is usually by CT scan. Box 15.2 outlines the indications for brain CT in non-trauma patients in the ED.

Management

The ED management of these conditions is guided by the same principles outlined at the beginning of this chapter. Raised ICP from tumours is often responsive to treatment with bed rest and dexamethasone. Further seizures can be prevented with phenytoin (15 mg/kg slow IV infusion).

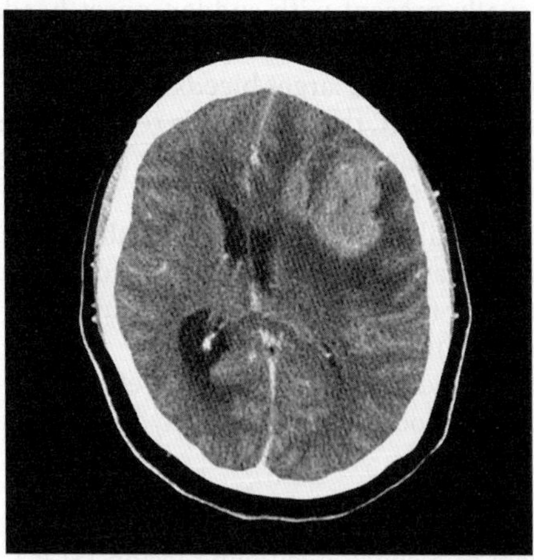

Figure 15.7 Cerebral CT scan with contrast showing left frontal enhancing space-occupying lesion with surrounding oedema resulting in marked mass effect (shift of midline to right, compression of ventricles). Patient had presented with status epilepticus and dilation of left pupil due to herniation syndrome with no previous history of seizures

COMPLICATIONS OF VENTRICULAR DRAINAGE DEVICES

Patients with a ventriculoperitoneal (VP) shunt not infrequently present to the ED with shunt malfunction or complications. The commonest of these are shunt obstruction and shunt infection. Less commonly, disconnection and migration of drainage catheter may occur. It is important to recognise these complications when they occur as, untreated, they can lead to significant morbidity or mortality.

Clinical features

The patient will usually have a clear history of having had a VP shunt inserted. Often there is a history of a similar presentation in the past. Symptoms and signs are variable, but include one or more of the following: headache, decreased level of consciousness, ataxia, nausea and vomiting.

On examination the patient may have a decreased level of consciousness and, in severe cases, focal neurological signs may indicate a herniation syndrome. Papilloedema may be present and paralysis of upward gaze may be seen. If a shunt reservoir is palpable, inability to empty it by pressing on it would suggest a distal obstruction; if it can be compressed but is slow to refill, this suggests a distal proximal obstruction.

Investigation

- Plain X-rays over the course of the shunt (shunt series) will show fractured tubing, disconnections, fluid collections, migration of the shunt tubing.
- A non-contrast cerebral CT will demonstrate ventricular size (hydrocephalus, slit ventricles), other evidence of increased ICP and the position of the proximal shunt components.
- A radioisotope nuclear scan using technetium-99 can confirm obstruction and isolate its location.

Management

The general principles of management are as outlined for other neurosurgical emergencies, namely attention to the airway, breathing and circulation, and specific measures to reduce ICP. Definitive treatment for a shunt blockage is shunt revision.

EPIDURAL ABSCESS

Epidural abscess is a rare but devastating condition that is often diagnosed late, resulting in permanent neurological disability. It is estimated to account for 0.2–1.2 cases per 10,000 hospital admissions per year. Modern-day mortality is less than 10%, but persistent neurological disability is common in survivors, especially if diagnosis is delayed or the patient is elderly.

Risk factors

The pathogenesis is thought to be related to a coincidence of risk factors. These are compromised immunity (e.g. diabetes, IV drug use, chronic medical illnesses), disruption to the spinal column (e.g. degenerative disease, surgery, epidural anaesthesia) and a source of infection (e.g. soft-tissue infections, intravenous drug use). Overall, diabetes and IVDU are the most frequent risks. Staphylococci are by far the commonest group of causative organisms.

Clinical features

Initially fever associated with back pain, and later neurological deficit. Meningism may be present on examination. There may be tenderness over the spine. Variable degrees of motor weakness, sensory loss and loss of reflexes may be observed.

Investigation

MRI is the imaging modality of choice. The white cell count is only raised in two-thirds of cases. The erythrocyte sedimentation rate (ESR) and C-reactive protein (CRP) are usually elevated, however.

Management

Urgent surgical decompression and drainage followed by a prolonged course of antibiotics.

Editorial Comment

Not all neurosurgical presentations are an emergency, fortunately. The common presentation of low back pain is difficult to assess. Serious causes can be excluded by the use of red flags (see Figure 15.8, 'Low back pain assessment and treatment guidelines'). As with low back pain, a systematic approach to diagnosis and management allows the clinician to safely manage a distressing and often difficult presenting condition.

Online resources

Initial management of closed head injury in adults, 2nd ed. NSW Institute of Trauma and Injury management. 2011. www.itim.nsw.gov.au/wiki/Head_injury_CPG

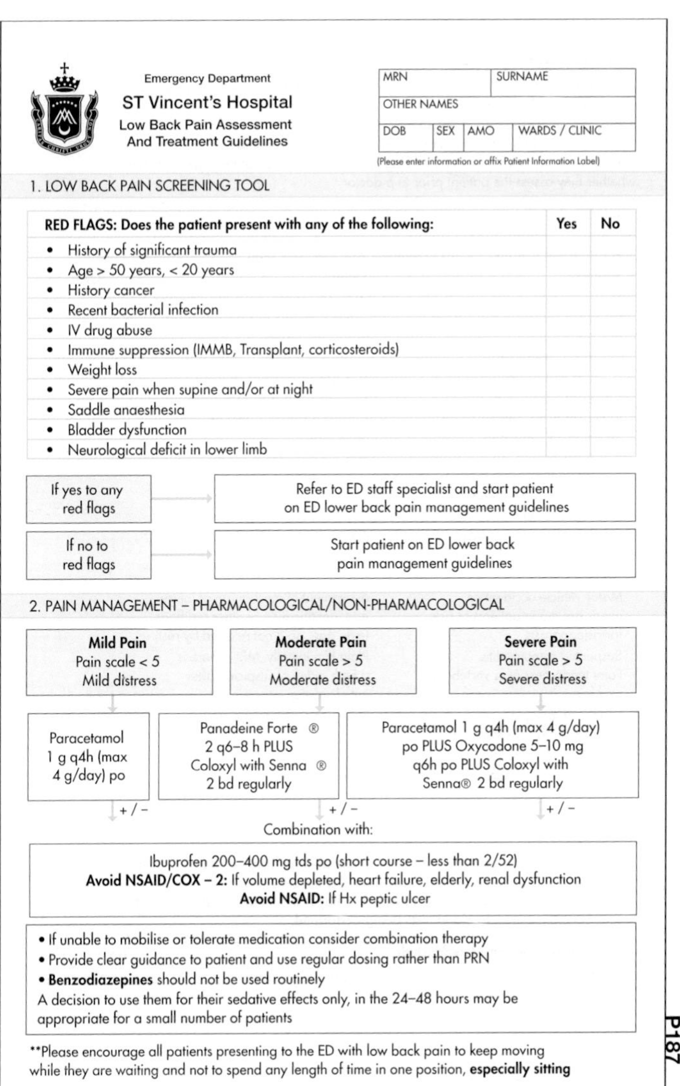

Emergency Department
ST Vincent's Hospital
Low Back Pain Assessment
And Treatment Guidelines

MRN			SURNAME
OTHER NAMES			
DOB	SEX	AMO	WARDS / CLINIC

(Please enter information or affix Patient Information Label)

1. LOW BACK PAIN SCREENING TOOL

RED FLAGS: Does the patient present with any of the following:	**Yes**	**No**
• History of significant trauma		
• Age > 50 years, < 20 years		
• History cancer		
• Recent bacterial infection		
• IV drug abuse		
• Immune suppression (IMMB, Transplant, corticosteroids)		
• Weight loss		
• Severe pain when supine and/or at night		
• Saddle anaesthesia		
• Bladder dysfunction		
• Neurological deficit in lower limb		

If yes to any red flags → Refer to ED staff specialist and start patient on ED lower back pain management guidelines

If no to red flags → Start patient on ED lower back pain management guidelines

2. PAIN MANAGEMENT – PHARMACOLOGICAL/NON-PHARMACOLOGICAL

Mild Pain Pain scale < 5 Mild distress	**Moderate Pain** Pain scale > 5 Moderate distress	**Severe Pain** Pain scale > 5 Severe distress
Paracetamol 1 g q4h (max 4 g/day) po	Panadeine Forte ® 2 q6–8 h PLUS Coloxyl with Senna ® 2 bd regularly	Paracetamol 1 g q4h (max 4 g/day) po PLUS Oxycodone 5–10 mg q6h po PLUS Coloxyl with Senna® 2 bd regularly
+/–	+/–	+/–

Combination with:

Ibuprofen 200–400 mg tds po (short course – less than 2/52)
Avoid NSAID/COX – 2: If volume depleted, heart failure, elderly, renal dysfunction
Avoid NSAID: If Hx peptic ulcer

• If unable to mobilise or tolerate medication consider combination therapy
• Provide clear guidance to patient and use regular dosing rather than PRN
• **Benzodiazepines** should not be used routinely
A decision to use them for their sedative effects only, in the 24–48 hours may be appropriate for a small number of patients

Please encourage all patients presenting to the ED with low back pain to keep moving while they are waiting and not to spend any length of time in one position, **especially sitting

St. Vincent's Hospital Sydney Limited ABN 77054 038 872

P187

Figure 15.8 St Vincent's Hospital Emergency Department low back pain assessment and treatment guidelines (*continues overleaf*)

3. REFERRAL TO PHYSIOTHERAPIST

Mon–Fri 8 am–4 pm, please text page the physiotherapist to make them aware of the patient if they fulfil the following criteria:

- If the patient is clear of red flags
- If the patient's only Red Flag is neurological deficit in lower limb

If the patient has more than one Red Flag, it is at the discretion of the physiotherapist whether they assess the patient prior to a doctor

4. IMAGING

Appropriate imaging studies in patients with low back pain		
Findings	**Study**	**Ordered**
Nonradicular pain No history of trauma or red flags	Wait 4 weeks for back films (limit to anteroposterior and lateral views)	
Occult infection or neoplasm suspected	Bone scan or MRI	
Spondylolisthesis that does not respond to conservative treatment or accompanied by neurological symptoms	Consider surgical consultation regarding selection of flexion-extension films, CT, MRI or bone scan	
Radicular pain Persistent sciatic symptoms with obvious level of nerve root impingement	MRI or referral to surgeon	
Sciatic symptom but nerve root dysfunction ambiguous	EMG, CT, MRI or surgical consultation	
Trauma Motor vehicle accident or minor trauma in patients at risk for osteoporosis	Lumbar spine film after careful assessment of mechanism of injury and identification of other red flags (e.g.: age, pain not relieved by rest)	
Suspected osteomyelitis Point tenderness over vertebrae and fever	Plain film initially, MRI if there is a high index of suspicion after initial workup	
History of malignancy Abnormalities consistent with metastatic disease	Plain film, bone scan or MRI	
CT, computed tomography; EMG, electromyography; MRI, magnetic resonance imaging		

5. PATHOLOGY

Blood test should only be performed on those people who have 'red flags'. Exactly which blood tests to be performed depends on the clinical scenario.
As with imaging studies, any patient with 'red flags' should be discussed with the senior ED clinical prior to blood tests being performed.

Blood tests to be considered include:	**Yes**	**No**
ESR. Probably the most helpful test to screen for malignancy or infection when the suspicion is low		
FBC		
UEC		
LFT		
CALCIUM / PHOSPHATE / MAGNESIUM		

Figure 15.8 St Vincent's Hospital Emergency Department low back pain assessment and treatment guidelines (continued)

BSL		
EPG/IEPG		
Blood cultures		
Coagulation studies		

6. REFERRAL TO NEUROSURGEON – After consultation with ED staff specialist

1. Any patient with 'red flags'
2. Any patient without 'red flags' who has not responded to standard management

References

Steven J. Atlas MD, MPH, Richard A. Deyo MD (2001)
Evaluating and Managing Acute Low Back Pain in the Primary Care Setting
Journal of General Internal medicine 16(2), 120–231
Thomas O. Staiger, MD Douglas S. Paauw, MD; Richard A. Deyo, MD; Jeffrey G Jarvik, MD Imaging Studies for acute low back pain
When and when not to order them
Vol.5/no.4/April 1999/Postgraduate Medicine
NSW Therapeutic Assessment Group Inc. (TAG)
Prescribing Guidelines for Primary Care Clinicians – Low back Pain. Published 1998, Revised 2002

7. DISCHARGE PLANNING

Once there is diagnosis of Mechanical Back Pain, Mon–Fri 8 am–4 pm, please ensure the patient has been reviewed by the ED physiotherapist. If not available, or is out of hours, please follow the following steps:

Provide the patient with the 'Management of Non-specific Low Back Pain' information sheet from EDIS (clinical screen protocols)

AND

1. If the patient has private insurance or the injury is work cover, please refer them for follow up with a private physio
   - If the patient has a private physio they know already, please provide a referral letter
   - If they don't have a private physio, you can give the patient the following website address: www.physiotherapy.asn.au which is on the discharge information sheet and follow the 'Find a physio' cue in the left side menu bar to find a local physio

OR

2. If the patient has no private insurance, it is not a workcover injury and they live in SESIAHS, refer them to outpatient physiotherapy by placing a patient sticker, patient contact phone number and your diagnosis in the Out of Hours Physiotherapy Out-patient referral book (kept in the Write Up room on the shelf under the photocopier) and provide the patient with a referral letter

OR

3. If the patient requires Outpatient Physiotherapy follow-up and lives outside SESIAHS, please refer them back to the GP, so they can refer them onto their nearest provider

Medications on Discharge: Dr. can give prescription (within hours) or use prepacks in the ED accessed via prescription (after hours)

8. PROGRESS NOTES

Figure 15.8 continued

Chapter 16
Aortic and vascular emergencies

Mark Gillett

Acute aortic dissection

OVERVIEW

Aortic dissection is the commonest aortic catastrophe, with a peak incidence between 50 and 70 years. Males are affected twice as often as females. The condition can be rapidly fatal without immediate treatment. However, diagnosis can be difficult and is often delayed.

Acute aortic dissection refers to a tear in the aortic intima that results in separation between the intima and the media. Blood flows into this space, creating a false lumen. The tear in the aortic wall may propagate proximally and/or distally, potentially involving any arterial branches from the aorta. The Stanford classification system is widely accepted, with type A (proximal) involving the ascending aorta (plus or minus the descending aorta) and type B (distal) involving the descending aorta alone. Type A generally presents at between 50 and 60 years with Type B typically occurring a decade later.

Factors associated with the condition include hypertension, stimulant abuse, genetic conditions including Marfan's syndrome, inflammatory vasculitides and pregnancy.

DIAGNOSIS

- Aortic dissection may mimic other common clinical presentations, therefore a high index of suspicion for the condition is required.
- Typically, patients present with pain in the chest, back or abdomen which is of sudden onset and tearing in quality.
- On examination, patients are typically agitated, pale and sweaty. Discernible discrepancies in limb pulses and blood pressures occurs in only approximately 30% of cases. Aortic valve regurgitation is detected in 45% of cases but is commoner in proximal dissections than in distal.
- Associated presentations may include syncope, coronary artery occlusion, cardiac tamponade, cardiac failure due to acute aortic regurgitation, stroke, limb ischaemia or mesenteric infarction.

- Chest X-ray often shows widening of the superior mediastinum and irregularity of the aortic shadow, but can be normal in 15% of cases.
- D-dimer levels are frequently elevated in aortic dissection; however, they are neither sensitive nor specific enough to be relied on as a stand-alone diagnostic test.
- Definitive diagnosis is by either contrast CT scanning or transoesophageal echocardiography (TOE). CT is the preferred technique in stable patients, whereas bedside TOE is ideal for critically unwell patients.

MANAGEMENT

Treatment should be instituted rapidly, as the death rate may be as high as 1% per hour for the first 24 hours. Type A dissections generally require surgery whereas type B are usually managed medically. All patients should be managed in a tertiary centre experienced in dealing with the condition.

- Pain is treated with IV morphine but is often very severe and difficult to control.
- Blood-pressure reduction is instituted with a beta-blocker to reduce vessel-wall shear pressure. Intravenous esmolol is an ideal agent due to its rapid onset and offset of action. Alternatively, repeat boluses of IV atenolol will suffice. Sodium nitroprusside can be used as an adjuvant agent to achieve further reductions in blood pressure, but should not be used without prior beta-blockade. Target parameters are pulse rate 60 bpm and systolic BP of 100–120 mmHg.
- Open surgery is indicated in type A dissections due to the high risk of life-threatening cardiac tamponade, stroke and cardiac failure related to aortic valve regurgitation. Type B dissections are generally managed medically but may be candidates for endovascular stenting in cases associated with mesenteric, renal or lower limb ischaemia.

Ruptured abdominal aortic aneurysm

OVERVIEW

Abdominal aortic aneurysm (AAA) affects approximately 2% of the population, with a peak incidence between 70 and 75 years of age and a significant male predominance. 95% of AAAs occur below the level of the renal arteries. The most common life-threatening complications of AAA seen in the emergency department are rupture or threatened rupture.

The risk of rupture increases with aneurysmal size. The 5-year risk is 1–2% when the aneurysm is < 5 cm in diameter and rises to 20–40% when the diameter is > 5 cm.

DIAGNOSIS

Misdiagnosis and delayed diagnosis can occur in up to 30% of cases. The differential diagnoses include renal colic, pancreatitis, diverticulitis and acute myocardial infarction.

- Ruptured AAA typically presents with severe abdominal and/or back pain which may radiate to the groin (thus mimicking renal colic). Patients may also present with syncope.
- Examination reveals a patient who looks unwell, with tachycardia, hypotension and an acutely tender abdomen (without guarding or rigidity). A tender, pulsatile abdominal mass is felt in approximately 50% of cases only. Absent femoral pulses and an aortic bruit may sometimes be detected.
- In the stable patient, CT scanning confirms the diagnosis of AAA, including the site, the extent and the presence or absence of rupture. Its disadvantage is the requirement for the patient to move to the radiology suite.
- In the unstable patient, the diagnosis must be made on history, examination and by use of ED ultrasound. Ultrasound is portable, safe, and increasingly available in the ED. A large number of studies suggest that in the hands of emergency doctors it is both sensitive and specific in diagnosing AAA.
- While allowing easy diagnosis of AAA, however, ultrasound cannot reliably diagnose rupture. Plain abdominal X-ray has a limited role, as only 60% of AAAs show significant aortic calcification and it cannot detect rupture.
- All patients suspected of AAA rupture require bloods for emergency cross-match (10 units) and estimation of haemoglobin, electrolytes, renal function, troponin and lipase. An ECG and chest X-ray should be performed if the patient is haemodynamically stable.

Management

- Management of **acute rupture** is rapid resuscitation while simultaneously organising immediate surgery. Patients should be monitored in an acute resuscitation area and 2 wide-bore intravenous cannulae inserted.
- Resuscitation involves oxygen, crystalloid fluids (such as normal saline) and early blood transfusion. Type O blood may

be required initially while awaiting full cross-matching. Large volumes of packed red blood cells, platelets and fresh frozen plasma may be required while arranging an operating theatre.

- The endpoint of fluid resuscitation is a systolic blood pressure of approximately 90 mmHg in a strategy termed 'hypotensive resuscitation'. Higher resuscitation blood pressures may increase bleeding and have been associated with worse outcomes in several studies.
- Incremental doses of IV morphine should be administered to control pain.
- 90% of patients with ruptured AAAs die without surgery although the mortality with surgery is still 50%. Surgical options include open repair of the rupture with insertion of a prosthetic graft or, more recently, percutaneous endoluminal repair and stenting. The endovascular approach has been proven to have a lower short-term mortality, but this advantage is lost over time due to increasing incidence of graft failure.
- The management of a **painful, non-ruptured AAA larger than 5 cm** is urgent surgical repair, as the risk of death from rupture outweighs that of elective repair (10%). Surgery is performed as soon as adequate CT imaging and rapid stabilisation of concurrent medical conditions have occurred.
- Suprarenal aneurysms have greater operative risk due to the need to re-implant the renal, coeliac and superior mesenteric arteries. Repair is commonly complicated by paraplegia, renal failure and mesenteric ischaemia.

Non-aortic abdominal aneurysms

Splenic artery aneurysms account for 60% of this group. They have a female predominance of 4:1 and are associated with portal hypertension and pregnancy. Rupture in pregnancy is associated with 50% maternal mortality, 95% fetal demise and delayed diagnosis.

Other sites of intra-abdominal aneurysms include hepatic, superior mesenteric and renal arteries.

Acute arterial insufficiency

OVERVIEW

Acute arterial insufficiency (AAI) is defined as sudden reduction in limb blood flow resulting in circulation inadequate to meet tissue metabolic demands. AAI is most commonly due to embolism or thrombosis associated with underlying atherosclerotic peripheral arterial disease.

The most common sources of emboli are the heart, aorta and larger arteries. Sources of cardiac emboli include atrial fibrillation, acute myocardial infarction, prosthetic valves and infective endocarditis. Thrombotic occlusion of synthetic bypass arterial grafts is more common than occlusion involving 'native' arteries. Thrombotic blockages are also associated with hypercoagulable states.

Common sites of occlusion include the femoral and popliteal arteries and, less commonly, the iliac, tibial and peroneal arteries of the leg. Upper limb AAI is relatively rare and usually due to emboli or aortic dissection.

DIAGNOSIS

Clinical presentation is related to the site of occlusion and the relative presence of collateral circulation.

Typically, the patient presents with acute onset of severe pain, paraesthesiae and coldness in the limb. Loss of motor function may supervene with ongoing ischaemia. **History** should seek to ascertain the onset and duration of symptoms plus any intercurrent medical diseases.

Physical signs include: loss of pulses distal to the occlusion, skin changes (including pallor, cyanosis or mottling), decreased skin temperature, loss of sensation and weakness. The presence of motor or sensory neurological signs implies prolonged ischaemia and a poorer prognosis for the limb. If AAI occurs in the presence of good collateral circulation, physical signs may be less florid.

Investigations should include arterial duplex (B mode and Doppler) ultrasound to confirm the diagnosis. CT angiography is sometimes required to establish the diagnosis and facilitate angioplasty. Full blood count, biochemistry, ECG and chest X-ray should be performed to ascertain likely causes and fitness for operating theatre.

MANAGEMENT

Treatment involves immediate anticoagulation with heparin to prevent clot progression, rapid stabilisation of any underlying medical conditions and emergency surgical revascularisation by thromboembolectomy (endovascular or open), angioplasty or arterial bypass grafting. Intra-arterial thrombolysis has been used in patients deemed not fit for surgery, but the mortality is higher compared with operative treatment.

Irreversible ischaemic changes occur within 4–6 hours and revascularisation is less effective after 8–12 hours.

Atheroembolism

Atheroembolism is a subset of AAI in which fibrin/platelet deposits embolise from proximal atherosclerotic lesions to distal-end arteries. It is associated with invasive arterial procedures such as cardiac catheterisation.

Patients develop signs of arterial insufficiency involving the extremities. Affected areas are painful, tender and may be either dusky or necrotic.

Treatment is unsatisfactory as anticoagulation, emergency surgery and thrombolysis all fail to reduce morbidity. Low-dose aspirin therapy should be started and vascular surgery review organised.

Chronic arterial insufficiency

The most common presentation is intermittent claudication associated with reduced pulses and trophic skin changes. Critical chronic arterial insufficiency is associated with ischaemic pain at rest and ankle systolic BP of less than 50 mmHg. Calculating an ankle/brachial index (ankle systolic BP divided by arm systolic BP) helps predict severity. A ratio of < 0.9 is abnormal and < 0.4 is indicative of severe disease.

The investigation of choice is arterial duplex ultrasound.

Chronic management revolves around cessation of smoking, regular exercise, aspirin, control of associated medical problems such as cardiac failure and a trial of alpha-blocking drugs.

Deep venous thrombosis

(See Chapter 11, 'Venous thromboembolic disease—deep venous thrombosis and pulmonary embolism.')

Editorial Comment

Never ignore marked or unrelieved pain as a possible indicator of a vascular complication—ischaemia, aneurysm, dissection, compartment syndrome—or the need for urgent referral.

Chapter 17
Orthopaedic principles—fractures and dislocations

John Raftos and Peter Locke

General principles

RESUSCITATION AND DETECTION OF OTHER INJURIES

Orthopaedic injuries often occur in multiply-injured patients. Resuscitation with identification and management of life-threatening injuries during the primary survey usually take precedence over the identification and management of orthopaedic injuries, which should be identified and managed during the secondary survey once the patient has been stabilised. Exceptions include:

- major pelvic fractures—may cause life-threatening haemorrhage which must be controlled in the primary survey
- femoral shaft fractures—may involve 1–2 L of blood loss and should be reduced and splinted during the primary survey.

ANALGESIA

(See also Chapter 13, 'Pain management in the emergency department.')
Most fractures and dislocations cause severe pain that requires urgent analgesia on presentation to the ED. Appropriate initial analgesic measures may include:

- inhaled nitrous oxide or methoxyflurane or intranasal fentanyl
- intravenous morphine (0.1 mg/kg for children, 2.5–5 mg aliquots for adults)
- oxycodone 5–10 mg orally
- compound oral analgesics (paracetamol plus codeine) may be used but their efficacy is not proven
- immobilisation with a plaster slab, traction splint, Zimmer splint, sling, etc
- regional anaesthesia (femoral nerve block for femoral shaft fracture).

DETECTION OF ASSOCIATED INJURIES

A thorough knowledge of anatomy is necessary to suspect and detect injuries to tendons, nerves, blood vessels and other viscera that are commonly associated with bony injuries.

EARLY REDUCTION OF FRACTURES

Some displaced fractures and dislocations should be reduced urgently to prevent serious permanent sequelae. These injuries (and their sequelae) include:

- traumatic hip dislocation (sciatic nerve injury, avascular necrosis, heterotopic calcification)
- true knee joint dislocation (popliteal artery injury with lower limb ischaemia, common peroneal nerve injury)
- supracondylar fractures of the elbow (median nerve, radial artery injury)
- elbow dislocation (ulnar nerve injury, heterotopic calcification)
- displaced pelvic fractures (ongoing haemorrhage)
- ankle fracture/dislocation (ischaemic necrosis of compressed skin, usually over one of the malleoli)
- shoulder dislocation (traction injury of the brachial plexus, axillary artery injury, recurrent dislocation).

EARLY REDUCTION OF DISLOCATIONS

Joint dislocation causes injury to the structures supporting the joint. Prolonged dislocation increases the likelihood of recurrent dislocation. Early reduction reduces the risk of recurrent dislocation and is effective analgesia. Most patients require little or no analgesia once the dislocation has been reduced, and their time in the ED is minimised with early reduction.

PROCEDURAL SEDATION FOR ED REDUCTION OF DISLOCATIONS AND FRACTURES

(See also Chapter 2, 'Securing the airway, ventilation and procedural sedation'.)

Performed by appropriately qualified ED specialists and registrars, procedural sedation is a safe technique for the reduction of most dislocations and the urgent reduction of some fractures in the ED.

- Ketamine is the preferred agent for use in children.
- A combination of propofol and fentanyl is ideal in adults because its short duration of action minimises the duration of altered consciousness and allows early discharge.
- Morphine plus midazolam is an adequate alternative in adults but has a longer duration of action.

Safe procedural sedation requires appropriate staffing with an airway-skilled doctor, other than the doctor who will perform the procedure, to perform the sedation and monitor the patient. ECG and oxygen saturation monitoring should be in place and advanced airway and resuscitation equipment should be at hand.

APPROPRIATE CONSULTATION AND REFERRAL

Each hospital has its own arrangements for referral of patients who need specialist orthopaedic assessment. If the patient needs orthopaedic assessment in the ED, then the orthopaedic registrar should be contacted. If outpatient orthopaedic referral is necessary, this is provided either at a hospital fracture clinic or in the rooms of the orthopaedic surgeon on call if there is no fracture clinic.

INJURIES OF THE HAND AND WRIST

(See also Chapter 18, 'Hand injuries and care'.)

The management of hand injuries is the domain of specialist hand surgeons. Fractures of any of the bones of the hand or carpus should generally be reviewed by a hand surgeon, as should any laceration of the hand or wrist with the potential for nerve or tendon injury, nail bed injuries, crush injuries, burns, hand infections and high-pressure injection injuries. Arrangements for referral to a hand surgery unit will vary from hospital to hospital and should be clearly laid out in the ED.

Upper limb injuries

CLAVICLE FRACTURE

Assessment

- Clavicle fracture is most commonly caused by falls onto the outstretched hand, less commonly by direct-force injury.
- Patients usually present with pain, tenderness and deformity and are reluctant to move the affected arm.
- Fractures of the medial and middle thirds usually heal without sequelae. Fractures of the outer third may be complicated by delayed or mal-union.
- Plain X-rays usually adequately demonstrate clavicle fractures.

Management

Orthopaedic registrar assessment in the ED is necessary for:

- angulated or displaced fractures
- fractures of the outer third which may need open reduction and internal fixation.

Management of undisplaced fractures of the medial and middle thirds is:

1. a triangular sling or proprietary shoulder support
2. simple analgesia
3. referral to the fracture clinic or orthopaedic surgeon's rooms.

ACROMIOCLAVICULAR (AC) SUBLUXATION/DISLOCATION

Assessment

- This is most commonly caused by a fall onto the tip of the shoulder or an impact on the tip of the shoulder during contact sport.
- **Subluxation** of the AC joint is associated with rupture of the acromioclavicular ligament and generally requires symptomatic treatment only.
- **Dislocation** of the AC joint is associated with rupture of the acromioclavicular ligament and the stronger coracoclavicular ligament, and may require open reduction and internal fixation, especially in sportspeople.
- Plain X-rays of the shoulder will show widening (subluxation) or displacement (dislocation) of the AC joint. Comparative X-rays of the normal side and weightbearing views may help with diagnosis.

Management

- Symptomatic management (triangular sling/proprietary shoulder support, ice, simple oral analgesia) is appropriate for **subluxation**.
- Patients with **dislocation** should be referred to the fracture clinic or orthopaedic surgeon for consideration of open reduction and internal fixation.

STERNOCLAVICULAR SUBLUXATION/DISLOCATION

Assessment

- Caused by:
  - — a direct blow to the sternum or medial clavicle *or*
  - — transmitted force from a blow to the posterolateral shoulder causing anterior dislocation of the clavicle, or to the anterolateral shoulder causing posterior dislocation.
- **Anterior dislocation** of the medial clavicle causes pain and localised deformity.
- **Posterior dislocation** of the medial clavicle has the potential to injure or compress the trachea and the major vessels and nerves that underlie the sternoclavicular joint, causing dyspnoea, chest pain, altered sensation in the arm or vascular abnormality in the arm.
- Plain X-rays are not sensitive for sternoclavicular dislocation. CT scan should be performed for diagnosis and to detect any injury or compression of intrathoracic structures.

Management

1. All patients with sternoclavicular dislocation should be seen by the orthopaedic registrar in the ED.
2. Subluxations and some anterior dislocations may be treated symptomatically.
3. Posterior dislocations and most anterior dislocations will require reduction under general anaesthesia.

ANTERIOR DISLOCATION OF THE GLENOHUMERAL (SHOULDER) JOINT

Assessment

- The mechanism of injury is a forced abduction and external rotation of the arm at the shoulder or a fall onto the hand forcing the humeral head anteriorly. It occurs most frequently during sport or in the surf in young people and in falls in older people.
- Every dislocation damages the rotator cuff and/or bony structures of the shoulder, and so recurrent dislocation is common. The incidence of recurrent dislocation after an initial dislocation is about 50% and increases after every subsequent dislocation, each of which tends to occur with decreasing force. The likelihood of recurrent dislocation is reduced by prompt reduction.
- The patient complains of pain in the shoulder and the arm is held immobile. Inspection usually reveals prominence of the tip of the shoulder and loss of the deltoid contour with an apparent hollow subacromially. Diagnosis may be difficult in obese individuals.
- Examine the patient for **common complications** of shoulder dislocation:
  - circumflex axillary nerve injury with loss of sensation over the deltoid and loss of deltoid function (usually masked by pain pre-reduction)—test for sensation in the 'nurse's cape' distribution over the deltoid
  - fracture of the humeral head or neck—inspect the humeral head and neck and the greater tuberosity carefully on X-ray
  - posterior cord brachial plexus injury with weakness of wrist extension through the radial nerve—test the function of the wrist and the hand, especially wrist extension
  - axillary artery injury—palpate the radial pulse.
- Plain X-rays will identify the great majority of shoulder dislocations. The humeral head usually lies in the subcoracoid position. Look for avulsion fracture of the greater tuberosity and

fracture of the humeral neck. Patients with greater tuberosity avulsion should have standard reduction. Patients with humeral neck fracture need orthopaedic consultation.

- CT scan may be necessary for the patient with a painful immobile shoulder and inconclusive X-rays.

Management

Some emergency doctors may opt to reduce recurrent shoulder dislocations without preliminary X-rays, but this cannot be regarded as standard practice.

1. Standard management for shoulder dislocation is prompt reduction in the ED. Reduction techniques that do not involve traction are preferred because they are said to reduce the likelihood of recurrent dislocation. Techniques include:
   - The Spaso (after Spaso Miljesic) technique. With the patient supine, the arm is lifted vertically with gentle traction and an assistant thumbs the humeral head while gentle external rotation is applied.
   - The Stimpson technique. The patient lies prone on a bed with traction applied with weights to the extended arm.
   - The Kocher manoeuvre. Counter-traction is provided by an assistant with a towel in the axilla. The operator applies axial traction using the flexed forearm as a fulcrum, followed by external rotation to 90°, and then adduction of the upper arm across the chest wall and internal rotation.
   - The Milch technique. With the patient supine on a bed, the arm is fully abducted and gentle external rotation is applied while an assistant thumbs the humeral head.
   - The Hippocratic method. With the patient supine on a bed, place the stockinged foot in the axilla for counter-traction, hold the arm at the wrist in both hands, and apply traction to the straight arm.
2. Reduction is usually heralded by a palpable 'clunk'.
3. Once reduction has been achieved:
   - Perform post-reduction X-rays to assess position and the possibility of bony injury.
   - Re-examine for neurovascular injury.
   - Immobilise the arm in a triangular sling/shoulder support.
   - Advise the patient to avoid abduction for at least 1 week.
   - Referral to the GP for follow-up is usually adequate if there is no evidence of associated fracture or neurovascular injury.

- Discuss referral to a specialist shoulder surgeon with patients with recurrent dislocation.

4 Successful reduction is generally a function of good technique and adequate sedation. The use of excessive force may result in humeral neck fracture, especially in older patients. If reduction is difficult, review the adequacy of sedation and/or seek orthopaedic assistance. Never apply excessive force.

POSTERIOR DISLOCATION OF THE GLENOHUMERAL (SHOULDER) JOINT

Assessment

- Posterior shoulder dislocation is uncommon (about 1% of all shoulder dislocations) and the diagnosis is often missed because the humeral head appears to be located on anteroposterior X-ray.
- The mechanism of injury is a forceful impact to the anterior aspect of the shoulder or tetanic muscle contraction during seizure or electric shock.
- The shoulder is painful and the patient is reluctant to move the arm, which is held adducted and internally rotated.
- The shoulder joint may appear located on the anteroposterior X-ray but careful inspection will show the 'light bulb sign' (the usually asymmetrical appearance of the humeral head becomes symmetrical because of internal rotation) or the humeral head overlapping the glenoid. The lateral X-ray will show the head of the humerus posterior to the glenoid.

Management

Reduction under procedural sedation in the ED is usually successful—axial traction is applied while the arm is abducted to 90° and then externally rotated.

HUMERAL HEAD AND NECK FRACTURES

Assessment

- The majority of fractures of the upper humerus occur in falls onto the outstretched hand in older patients.
- Fractures most commonly involve the surgical neck of the humerus but also involve the anatomical neck, the greater and lesser tuberosities and the articular surface, all either alone or in combination.
- The history is usually of a fall onto the outstretched hand causing pain, swelling and later bruising about the shoulder.

Bruising and/or reluctance to move the shoulder may be the only clinical features in older patients with dementia.
- X-rays of the shoulder are usually diagnostic. Look for associated shoulder joint dislocation, angulation, displacement, involvement of the articular surface and displacement of the greater tuberosity.

Management

Most patients with upper humerus fractures should be reviewed by the orthopaedic registrar in the ED to determine appropriate treatment:

- Surgical treatment with replacement hemiarthroplasty should be considered for adults with significant intra-articular involvement.
- Surgical treatment with closed reduction or open reduction and internal fixation should be considered for younger patients with significant displacement or angulation and for displaced avulsion fractures of the greater tuberosity.
- Epiphyseal fractures in younger patients often require closed reduction under general anaesthesia.
- Uncomplicated fractures of the neck of the humerus are treated conservatively in a triangular sling/shoulder support, or in a collar and cuff if there is impaction requiring gravitational reduction.
- Older patients may be significantly disabled by immobilisation of one arm. Social work involvement is necessary to make appropriate care arrangements while the disability persists. Overnight admission allows analgesia to be optimised and social arrangements to be made.

HUMERAL SHAFT FRACTURES

Assessment

- Humeral shaft fractures are caused by direct-force injuries, torsion or falls onto the outstretched hand.
- The patient presents with upper arm pain and is reluctant to move the arm, which is generally supported by the other hand.
- X-rays of the upper arm are usually diagnostic. Look for displacement, angulation and the presence of a 'butterfly' fragment.
- The radial nerve may be contused in the radial groove in fractures of the middle third of the humerus—always test extension of the wrist and fingers. The injury is usually a neuropraxia which will recover over 6 weeks to 6 months. Vascular injury is uncommon.

Management

The orthopaedic registrar should review all humeral shaft fractures in the ED.

Management includes:

1. Standard management of humeral shaft fractures is immobilisation in a 'hanging slab'. Apply ample padding, especially around the elbow, using an appropriate-width plaster slab. Start in the axilla and continue the slab under the flexed elbow, over the outer surface of the upper arm and well onto the shoulder. Wrap with a gauze bandage, and support in a sling or collar and cuff.
2. Some humeral shaft fractures will require open reduction and internal nail fixation. These may include those with a butterfly fragment and those associated with multiple injuries.
3. Supply appropriate analgesia and arrange review at the fracture clinic or orthopaedic surgeon's rooms.

SUPRACONDYLAR FRACTURES OF THE HUMERUS

Assessment

- Supracondylar fracture is most common in children, with peak incidence at 8 years, and is usually caused by a fall onto the outstretched hand.
- The patient presents with a painful, swollen elbow and is reluctant to use the arm, which is usually supported by the other hand.
- Assessment should include a full neurovascular examination of the hand, looking for **complications** of the fracture:
  - Brachial artery injury. The brachial artery may be compressed or, in severe cases, there may be intimal damage or rupture. Check the radial pulse and capillary refill in the fingers.
  - Median nerve injury. Check sensation in the radial palmar 3½ fingers and motor function in the abductor pollicis.
  - Increased tissue pressure/compartment syndrome. Haemorrhage and oedema around the fracture site may cause vascular compromise that is detected by regular vascular checks of the hand and forearm.
  - Volkmann's ischaemic contracture. A disabling ischaemic injury of the muscles and nerves of the forearm, this is caused by arterial injury or compartment syndrome following supracondylar fracture.

- X-rays will demonstrate a supracondylar fracture line. Look for displacement, angulation, comminution.

Management

- Urgent orthopaedic review is needed if there is evidence of vascular compromise.
- All supracondylar fractures should be reviewed by the orthopaedic registrar in the ED. Those with significant displacement or angulation will need closed reduction under general anaesthesia. Those with vascular compromise will need urgent reduction and vascular surgical assessment.
- Comminuted fractures in adults may require open reduction and internal fixation.
- Undisplaced fractures without significant swelling can be managed, after orthopaedic registrar review, with a collar and cuff, oral analgesia and referral to the fracture clinic or orthopaedic surgeon's rooms.

ELBOW DISLOCATION

Assessment

- Elbow dislocation occurs in both children and adults, usually as the result of a fall onto the outstretched hand. The radius usually dislocates posteriorly in response to forced hyper-extension.
- The patient presents with a painful, swollen elbow and is reluctant to use the arm which is usually supported by the other hand.
- Assessment should include a full neurovascular examination of the hand, looking for **complications** of the fracture:
  - Ulnar nerve injury. Check sensation in the ulnar palmar 2½ fingers and motor function in adduction and abduction of the fingers.
  - Brachial artery injury. The brachial artery may be compressed or, in severe cases, there may be intimal damage or rupture. Check the radial pulse and capillary refill in the fingers.
  - Median nerve injury. Check sensation in the radial palmar 3½ fingers and motor function in the abductor pollicis.
  - Increased tissue pressure/compartment syndrome. Haemorrhage and oedema around the fracture site may cause vascular compromise that is detected by regular vascular checks of the hand and forearm.

(*pto*)

- X-rays usually demonstrate the dislocation clearly. Intra-articular bone fragments are common and their origin is often unclear. Look for these carefully—they may inhibit reduction.

Management

1. Elbow dislocations are generally reduced in the ED under procedural sedation. Most will reduce with axial traction on the forearm, which is held in 30° flexion while the assistant thumbs the olecranon process. If this is not successful, then, with traction still applied, extend the elbow to unlock the coronoid process. An intra-articular bony fragment may prevent reduction—these patients will need open reduction.
2. Test range of elbow movement post-reduction—a full, smooth range suggests successful reduction; resistance to movement suggests intra-articular bone fragment or soft-tissue entrapment.
3. Post-reduction X-rays are performed to show alignment and the position of any intra-articular fragment.
4. Repeat the neurovascular examination post-reduction to ensure that none of the nerves has been entrapped in the reduction.
5. Support the reduced elbow in a long arm plaster back slab and refer to the fracture clinic/orthopaedic surgeon's rooms for review.

OLECRANON FRACTURES

Assessment

- These fractures are caused by either a fall onto the elbow or forcible contraction of the triceps.
- There is usually pain and swelling over the olecranon.
- X-rays clearly demonstrate the fracture in most cases. Look for displacement and the position of the fracture relative to the joint.

Management

- All olecranon fractures require orthopaedic registrar review in the ED.
- Management usually depends on the integrity of the extensor mechanism:
  - If the mechanism is intact and the fracture undisplaced, treatment consists of immobilisation in a long arm slab supported in a sling/shoulder support and review at the fracture clinic or orthopaedic surgeon's rooms.
  - If the extensor mechanism is disrupted, then open reduction and internal fixation is usually necessary.

PULLED ELBOW

Assessment

- Occurs in children aged 1–6 years when the radial head slips out from under the annular ligament as a result of axial traction when there is a sudden tug on the arm by either child or parent while the parent is holding the child's hand.
- The parent indicates that the child is not using the affected arm, which is usually held limply by the side or semi-flexed. There is often, but not always, tenderness over the radial head.
- X-rays are not necessary when the history is clear.

Management

- Reduction is achieved without anaesthetic. The operator, having gained the child's and parent's confidence, holds the elbow in one hand with the thumb over the radial head while the other hand fully supinates and then flexes the forearm. Reduction is usually palpable.
- The child does not usually begin to use the arm again immediately. Review about 15 minutes post-reduction usually shows that full movement has returned. No follow-up is necessary.

RADIAL HEAD AND NECK FRACTURE

Assessment

- These structures may be injured by direct force, but the most common mechanism of injury is a fall onto the outstretched hand.
- The patient presents with pain in the elbow and pain on movement. Supination and pronation are usually limited by pain. Firm palpation over the radial head reveals tenderness.
- Most of these fractures are undisplaced and do not require manipulation.
- The outstanding feature on X-ray is a positive 'fat pad sign', indicating the presence of an elbow joint effusion:
  - — visible posterior elbow-joint fat pad
  - — anterior bowing of the usually straight anterior fat pad
  - — a blood/fat level in the anterior fat pad.
- On X-rays, look for angulation in the normally smooth arc of the radial neck and intra-articular fracture of the radial head.

Management

- Undisplaced fractures of the radial head or neck are treated with triangular sling immobilisation and referral to the fracture clinic or orthopaedic surgeon's rooms.

- Angulated fractures of the radial neck and displaced intra-articular fractures of the radial head should be reviewed by the orthopaedic registrar in the ED and considered for open reduction and internal fixation.

RADIUS AND ULNA SHAFT FRACTURE

Assessment

- Isolated fracture of the shaft of one of the forearm bones is usually caused by direct-force injury. Fractures of both bones are much more common and are caused by transmitted forces from falls onto the outstretched hand. The position of the hand and arm at the time of the fall will determine the pattern of the fractures.
- The patient presents with pain, swelling, deformity and limitation of movement of the forearm.
- X-rays will demonstrate the pattern of the fracture. Both bones are usually broken or there is a pattern of fracture of one bone with dislocation of the other (Monteggia, Galeazzi fracture/dislocations), so views that include the whole of the forearm including the elbow and wrist joints are essential. Look for angulation, displacement and comminution.

Management

- All fractures of the shaft of the radius and/or ulna should be reviewed by the orthopaedic registrar in the ED.
- Management depends on patient age, the site of the fracture and the degree of angulation and displacement.
- A significant proportion of radial/ulnar shaft fractures will require either closed reduction under general anaesthesia or open reduction and internal fixation.

DISTAL RADIUS AND ULNA FRACTURE

Colles' fracture

Assessment

- Colles' fracture, first described by Abraham Colles in 1814, is defined as a fracture of the distal radius within 2.5 cm of the wrist joint with dorsal and radial angulation and dorsal displacement.
- It is caused by falls onto the outstretched hand and is commonest in older women.
- The patient presents with pain, swelling and deformity (often described as 'dinner fork' deformity) of the wrist after a fall. There is tenderness over the distal radius.

- X-rays show a transverse fracture of the distal radius. Look for angulation, displacement, comminution, intra-articular involvement.

Management

- Management depends on the nature of the fracture:
  - Fractures with minimal displacement and angulation are adequately treated by immobilisation with a short arm slab with the wrist in the neutral position.
  - Fractures that demonstrate features of instability (comminution, radial shortening, intra-articular involvement) may require open or closed reduction and internal fixation because they are at increased risk of mal-union.
  - Displaced and angulated Colles' fractures that are not unstable are managed with closed reduction and plaster immobilisation.
- Colles' fracture reduction is performed in the ED at some institutions. Procedural sedation and regional nerve block are the preferred anaesthetic options. Some institutions still use intravenous regional anaesthesia (Bier's block), which should be performed only by senior medical staff with a thorough understanding of its complications.
- **Complications of Colles' fracture** include:
  - mal- or non-union, especially with unstable fractures
  - median nerve compression
  - Sudeck's atrophy
  - rupture of the extensor pollicis longus tendon
  - residual wrist stiffness and pain
  - poor grip or function due to persisting dorsal angulation.

Editorial Comment

In any wrist injury (especially after a fall), look for/exclude **dislocated lunate**—pressure damage to median nerve—which needs urgent reduction and is often missed early.

Smith's fracture

Assessment

- Defined as a full-thickness fracture of the distal radius 1–2.5 cm from the wrist with volar displacement and angulation. Also known as a reversed Colles' fracture.

- It is caused by falls onto the outstretched hand with forced supination and by injuries that cause forced hyperflexion at the wrist (fall onto the back of the hand, handlebar injuries).
- The patient presents with pain, swelling and deformity (often described as 'garden spade' deformity) of the wrist after a fall. There is tenderness over the distal radius.
- X-rays show a transverse fracture of the distal radius. Look for angulation, displacement, comminution, intra-articular involvement.

Management

All Smith's fractures should be reviewed by the orthopaedic registrar in the ED, and most will require closed reduction.

Barton's fracture/dislocation

Assessment

- Barton's fracture/dislocation is an intra-articular fracture of the distal radius in which impingement of the carpus causes displacement of either the volar (more common) or the dorsal rim of the radius.
- X-ray shows an intra-articular fracture of the distal radius with either volar or dorsal displacement and angulation of the intra-articular rim of the radius, the carpus having been effectively driven into the distal radius.

Management

Closed reduction may be attempted but the carpus tends to hold the fragments apart, and so many of these fractures will require open reduction and internal fixation.

Scaphoid fracture

Assessment

- The scaphoid is the most frequently fractured carpal bone.
- Scaphoid fractures are usually the result of a fall onto the outstretched hand.
- About 70% of fractures involve the middle third ('waist') of the scaphoid, 10–20% involve the distal pole and 5–10% involve the proximal pole.
- The patient presents with pain and perhaps swelling of the wrist after a fall. Presentation may be delayed days or weeks after an apparent 'sprain' does not resolve. Examination reveals tenderness in the anatomical 'snuff box' and pain on axial compression of the thumb.

- X-rays (with scaphoid views) usually reveal a transverse fracture of the scaphoid but may be normal. If clinical suspicion is high and the X-rays are negative, there are several options:
  - Apply a scaphoid plaster and re-X-ray after 10–14 days
  - Perform a CT (or MRI) scan of the wrist
  - Perform a radionuclide bone scan of the wrist.

  The chosen option will depend on preference and availability of imaging.

Management

- All scaphoid fractures should be reviewed by the orthopaedic or hand surgery registrar in the ED to determine the need for internal fixation.
- Management is either immobilisation in a scaphoid plaster slab or open reduction and internal fixation. Fractures displaced by more than 1 mm are usually internally fixed. Some surgeons routinely internally fix proximal pole fractures because of their increased incidence of non-union and avascular necrosis.
- The main complications are:
  - avascular necrosis—occurs in 15–30% of scaphoid fractures, most commonly in proximal-pole fractures; the more proximal the fracture, the more likely is avascular necrosis
  - delayed and non-union—is most common in proximal-pole fractures
  - osteoarthritis—results from avascular necrosis, mal-union and non-union and leaves the patient disabled with a painful, stiff wrist.
- Delayed diagnosis and immobilisation of scaphoid fracture significantly increases the likelihood of avascular necrosis and non-union. Obtain further imaging (CT, MRI, bone scan) for patients with snuff box tenderness but normal initial X-ray.

Gamekeeper's/skier's thumb

(Also see a discussion of this topic in Chapter 18, 'Hand injuries and care'.)

Assessment

- This injury involves rupture of the ulnar collateral ligament of the thumb metacarpophalangeal (MCP) joint because of forced abduction and hyperextension of the thumb in motorcyclists, skiers and footballers.
- The patient presents with pain and swelling at the MCP joint and examination reveals laxity of the joint in abduction.

Management

Management is immobilisation in a thumb spica and referral to the fracture/hand clinic or orthopaedic/hand surgeon's rooms for consideration for surgical repair.

Fifth metacarpal fracture

(Also see a discussion of this topic in Chapter 18, 'Hand injuries and care'.)

Assessment

- The 'boxer's fracture' is a fracture of the neck of the fifth metacarpal from punching a person or a wall or occasionally from a fall directly onto the fifth metacarpal knuckle.
- X-rays reveal a fracture of the neck of the metacarpal, usually with volar angulation.
- Test for rotational deformity by asking the patient to flex the fingers. If there is significant ulnar or radial deviation of the flexed little finger, reduction is necessary.

Management

1. Reduction is best performed with a proximal digital block.
2. Immobilisation is best maintained with a gutter slab that holds the wrist slightly extended, the MCP joint in 70–90° flexion and the interphalangeal joints in extension (the 'position of safe immobilisation', POSI).

Punch injuries may also cause dislocation of the head of the fifth metacarpal, which often requires reduction under general anaesthesia and internal fixation.

METACARPAL AND PHALANGEAL FRACTURES

Assessment

- These fractures are usually caused by direct-force trauma.
- Examine for rotational deformity and associated injuries:
  - open fracture
  - tendon injury
  - digital nerve injury
  - nail bed injury.
- X-rays of the hand adequately demonstrate most metacarpal and phalangeal fractures. Look for angulation, displacement and tendon avulsion fractures.

Management

- Isolated, uncomplicated metacarpal fractures with minimal angulation and displacement can be safely treated with immobilisation in a volar slab in the position of safe immobilisation:
  - wrist slightly extended
  - the MCP joint in 70–90° flexion
  - the interphalangeal joints in extension.
- Refer to the fracture/hand clinic or orthopaedic/hand surgeon's rooms.
- Isolated, uncomplicated phalangeal fractures with minimal angulation and displacement can be safely treated with immobilisation by 'buddy-strapping' and referred to the fracture/hand clinic or orthopaedic/hand surgeon's rooms.
- Painful subungual haematoma should be treated by trephining the nail by gently pressing the tip of a red-hot paperclip onto the middle of the nail or drilling with a 21-gauge needle, over the haematoma.
- Angulated or displaced fractures, those with rotational deformity, open fractures and those complicated by tendon, nerve or nail bed injury need review in the ED by the orthopaedic or hand surgery registrar.

DISLOCATIONS OF THE INTERPHALANGEAL AND METACARPOPHALANGEAL JOINTS

Assessment

- Dislocations of the finger joints are usually caused by forced hyperextension and the dislocation is usually dorsal.
- Always X-ray deformed fingers before attempting reduction, because displaced fractures give a similar external appearance to dislocations.

Management

1. Most finger dislocations are easily reduced. Digital nerve block may be used, but many dislocations can be reduced without anaesthesia. The technique involves applying axial traction to the distal part while pressing with the thumb of the other hand over the base of the dislocated bone.
2. Failed reduction may occur when the head of the proximal bone is 'button-holed' through the volar plate, necessitating open reduction.

(pto)

3 Always obtain a post-reduction X-ray to exclude avulsion fractures.
4 Examine active movements of the finger post-reduction to detect rupture of the middle slip of the extensor tendon in distal interphalangeal dislocations.
5 Buddy-strap the reduced finger and encourage active movement.

MALLET FINGER

Assessment

- Mallet finger is caused by avulsion of the insertion of the extensor tendon mechanism from the dorsal base of the distal phalanx. It usually occurs in ball sports when the ball strikes the tip of the finger, forcing it into hyperflexion.
- The patient presents with pain and swelling at the distal interphalangeal joint and examination reveals weak or absent active extension.
- X-ray reveals a dorsal avulsion fragment. Look for the degree of separation and amount of joint-surface involvement.

Management

- Definitive management depends on the degree of separation and joint-surface involvement. The majority of patients are adequately treated with a mallet-finger splint (splinting the joint in mild hyperextension) for 6–10 weeks.
- Apply a mallet-finger splint and refer the patient for early review in the hand/orthopaedic clinic or the hand/orthopaedic surgeon's rooms.

BOUTONNIÈRE DEFORMITY

Assessment

- Boutonnière ('button-hole') deformity results from avulsion of the central slip of the extensor tendon from the base of the middle phalanx. The lateral bands then migrate towards the volar surface, causing flexion at the proximal interphalangeal joint and extension at the distal interphalangeal joint. The central slip disruption may be caused by laceration, dislocation of the interphalangeal joint or forced flexion of the extended finger.
- Most patients present with a tender, swollen proximal interphalangeal joint.
- X-rays may show an avulsion fragment adjacent to the dorsal base of the middle phalanx.

Management

All patients with boutonnière deformity should be referred urgently to the hand surgery/orthopaedic registrar for prompt surgical treatment.

DIGITAL NERVE INJURIES

Assessment

- All patients with any injury, especially lacerations, of the hand and fingers should be carefully examined for nerve injury before any anaesthetic agent is given.
- Sensory loss from digital nerve injury usually affects a quadrant of the finger.

Management

- Hand surgeons will usually attempt surgical repair of any digital nerve injury proximal to the distal interphalangeal joint. Any patient with digital sensory loss following a hand or finger injury should be referred to the hand surgery registrar for consideration of operative repair.
- Patients with lacerations should be treated with tetanus immunoprophylaxis and intravenous antibiotics pending hand surgery review.

TENDON INJURIES IN THE HAND

Assessment

- The majority of tendon injuries in the hand are associated with skin lacerations.
- Tendon injury must be suspected with any hand or finger laceration and its presence must be confirmed/excluded according to the following:
  - Test tendon function/finger movement.
  - Carefully inspect the wound for signs of tendon injury. Remember that many tendon injuries are not visible in the wound because the injury has occurred with the finger in a different posture.
  - If the laceration is in a position where tendon injury may have occurred and the laceration appears to extend past the deep fascia, tendon injury should be suspected.
  - Be wary of partial tendon laceration which will go on to rupture.

Management

Urgently refer all patients with actual or possible tendon laceration to the hand/orthopaedic registrar for formal exploration with a bloodless field in the operating theatre.

Pelvic fractures

Pelvic fractures occur in three broad settings:

1. As a result of simple falls from standing in older patients. These are usually undisplaced fractures of the pubic rami or acetabulum and usually do not require active treatment.
2. Avulsion fractures in adolescents and young adults.
3. As a result of major forces in young and old patients. Displaced pelvic fractures often cause life-threatening haemorrhage requiring urgent resuscitation and active definitive treatment.

PELVIC FRACTURES IN THE ELDERLY

Assessment

- These fractures occur as a result of falls from standing and include fractures of the pubic rami and undisplaced fractures of the acetabulum.
- The patient presents with hip pain, often localised to the groin in pubic ramus fractures, and is unwilling to bear weight.
- X-rays will often demonstrate undisplaced fractures of the pubic rami or acetabulum.
- CT imaging or radionuclide bone scan will detect occult fractures in patients who are unwilling to mobilise but have apparently normal X-rays.

Management

Management includes:

1. adequate analgesia
2. admission to hospital under the orthogeriatric or geriatric team
3. initial bed rest
4. prophylaxis against thromboembolic disease
5. early mobilisation
6. social work involvement to facilitate return to home
7. falls assessment.

PELVIC AVULSION FRACTURES

- Anterior superior iliac spine avulsion:
  - occurs in athletes and young people as a result of forceful contraction of the sartorius
  - is treated by rest from exercise for 2–6 weeks.
- Ischial tuberosity avulsion:
  - occurs in athletes as a result of forceful contraction of the hamstrings
  - may require lengthy rehabilitation and surgical treatment.

- Anterior inferior iliac spine avulsion:
  - occurs in athletes as a result of forceful contraction of the rectus femoris
  - is treated by rest from exercise for 2–6 weeks.
- Posterior iliac spine avulsion:
  - occurs in weightlifters
  - may require lengthy rehabilitation.

MAJOR PELVIC FRACTURES

Assessment

- These injuries occur as the result of major trauma:
  - falls from heights
  - motorcycle and motor vehicle crashes
  - crush injuries
  - industrial accidents.
- They may be complicated by:
  - life-threatening haemorrhage from arteries and venous plexuses within the pelvis and sacrum
  - bladder injuries
  - urethral injuries
  - gynaecological injuries
  - rectal injuries
  - neurological injury to the sacral nerves.
- A plain X-ray of the pelvis is a standard element of the primary survey for trauma management and will show most haemodynamically significant pelvic fractures. Look for continuity of the three circles (pelvic inlet, 2 obturator foramina), sacral fracture, sacroiliac dislocation. Major pelvic fractures usually involve double breaks in the pelvic ring; if one is identified, look for the second.
- CT scan gives accurate visualisation of pelvic and sacral fractures but should not be performed if the patient is haemodynamically unstable.

Management

Management of major pelvic fracture in the primary survey includes:

1. ABCs—identification and management of other life-threatening injuries
2. resuscitation—crystalloid or blood
3. analgesia with intravenous morphine
4. pelvic haemorrhage control:
   a. reduction and immobilisation in the ED—sheet tied around the pelvis, proprietary pelvic immobiliser

b urgent transfer to the angiography suite for radiological identification and embolisation of bleeding points

c transfer to the operating theatre once stable for closed reduction and application of external fixator immobilisation.

Lower limb injuries

FEMORAL NECK FRACTURES

Assessment

- These fractures are common in the elderly, most commonly caused by a simple fall from standing. They can occur with minimal or no apparent trauma in osteoporotic patients and as pathological fractures, especially with metastatic breast carcinoma.
- Most femoral neck fractures are clinically obvious. The patient is unable to stand or mobilise after a fall and there is characteristic shortening and external rotation of the affected limb. Be wary of the impacted fracture, in which the limb may appear normal and the patient may be able to bear weight, albeit with pain and a limp.
- X-rays will usually identify the femoral neck fracture. Look for position of the fracture, alignment, displacement, features of pathological fracture.
- When X-rays do not show an obvious fracture but there is pain or inability to mobilise, perform a CT scan or radionuclide bone scan to identify an occult fracture.

Management

- Patients with femoral neck fractures tend to be elderly with significant comorbidities. Many hospitals have joint orthopaedics/geriatrics (orthogeriatric) admission policies that provide thorough perioperative medical assessment and management. Ensure that all comorbidities are identified, assessed and optimised preoperatively by appropriate investigation and consultation.
- The management of femoral neck fracture is operative. The best mortality and morbidity outcomes are achieved with operation within 24 hours of injury.

HIP JOINT DISLOCATION

Hip dislocation occurs in two circumstances: traumatic and prosthetic.

Traumatic hip dislocation

Assessment

- Is a medical emergency because of risk of injury to the femoral head and sciatic nerve and requires urgent reduction.

- Usually caused by a high-velocity impact on the flexed, abducted knee as in motorcycle crashes and impact from the dashboard in high-speed motor vehicle crashes or in falls from significant heights.
- Is often associated with other injuries in the pelvis and knee with intra-abdominal and intrathoracic injuries.
- 80–90% of traumatic hip dislocations are posterior, 10% are anterior and the remainder are central.
- Major complications are:
  - avascular necrosis of the head of the femur
  - sciatic nerve injury
  - myositis ossificans.

  The likelihood of all of these complications is reduced by early reduction.
- The patient presents from a high-velocity impact with a shortened, internally rotated and adducted leg.
- Urgent assessment should include:
  - primary survey (ABCDE, resuscitation)
  - looking for injuries in other organ systems
  - examination of the knees and femoral shafts for associated injuries
  - assessment of sciatic nerve function—test dorsiflexion and plantarflexion at the ankle and sensation over the lateral border of the foot
  - palpation of the arterial pulses of the leg and foot.
- X-rays usually demonstrate the dislocation adequately. Always obtain X-rays of the pelvis, femur and knee joint. Look for associated pelvic, femoral, patellar or tibial fractures.

Management

Reduction may be performed in the ED under procedural sedation if the patient is otherwise stable. In unstable patients, the dislocation is reduced in the operating theatre after life-threatening injuries have been controlled.

Prosthetic hip dislocation

Assessment

Does not cause sciatic nerve or femoral head injury, but should still be reduced promptly to relieve pain.

Management

Usually reduced in the ED with procedural sedation. With the patient supine in bed, an assistant provides counter-traction to the pelvis while the operator stands on the bed and flexes the hip and knee to 90° and then applies vertical traction.

X-ray to confirm successful relocation and re-check sciatic nerve and vascular function.

FEMORAL SHAFT FRACTURES

Assessment

- The mechanism of injury usually involves significant force, as in motor vehicle crashes, falls, sporting accidents. Occurs most often in young adults. The fracture may be transverse, oblique or spiral.
- Clinically the thigh is swollen and tender and the leg may be angulated and/or shortened.
- X-rays of the whole of the femur and the hip and knee joints are needed.
- Complications include:
  - — blood loss of up to 2000 mL
  - — fat embolism
  - — vascular and nerve injury (uncommon).

Management

Urgent management should include:

1. primary survey (ABCDE, resuscitation)
2. looking for injuries in other organ systems
3. aggressive fluid resuscitation
4. urgent blood cross-match
5. consider femoral nerve block for analgesia
6. early reduction and immobilisation in a traction splint to reduce pain and haemorrhage.

Most femoral shaft fractures in adults are treated with open reduction and internal fixation. Children are usually treated in gallows traction.

DISTAL FEMORAL FRACTURES

Assessment

- Includes supracondylar and condylar fractures. Occur with major trauma in motor vehicle crashes and falls, and with minimal trauma in older and/or osteoporotic patients.
- Examination shows that the knee is swollen (with lipo-haemarthrosis in condylar fractures) and deformed with decreased range of movement.
- X-rays usually define these fractures well. Look for displacement, angulation and effusion and a blood/fat level in the knee joint.

Management

Give adequate intravenous analgesia and immobilise in a long leg plaster slab while awaiting urgent orthopaedic registrar review.

RUPTURE OF THE QUADRICEPS TENDON

Assessment

- Usually occurs in men from early middle age onwards when an axial force is applied to the leg with the knee fixed in flexion.
- The patient presents with pain around the knee after a fall and is unable to mobilise.
- Careful examination reveals a visible and palpable gap in the suprapatellar tendon immediately above the upper-pole patella.
- X-rays often show avulsion flakes from the superior border of the patella.
- Ultrasound confirms the diagnosis.

Management

Management is surgical repair of the tendon. Immobilise the knee in a Zimmer splint or long leg plaster slab and ask the orthopaedic registrar to see the patient in the ED.

PATELLAR FRACTURES

Assessment

- Caused by direct-force injury to the patella in falls from standing and from the dashboard in motor vehicle accidents or from sudden forceful contraction of the quadriceps.
- The patient presents with a painful knee after the accident. Knee joint effusion is often, but not always, present.
- X-rays should include anteroposterior, lateral and 'skyline' views. Undisplaced linear fractures may be difficult to see on plain X-ray. Obtain a CT scan of the knee when there is significant pain but no evident fracture on plain X-rays. Look for a knee joint effusion with a blood/fat level which is diagnostic evidence of a fracture.
- The orthopaedic registrar should review the patient in the ED.

Management

Management depends on patient age and the integrity of the quadriceps mechanism:

- If the mechanism is intact, management is usually with immobilisation in a Zimmer splint or long leg plaster.
- Open reduction and internal fixation is standard management if the mechanism is disrupted.

PATELLAR DISLOCATION

Assessment

- Patella dislocation most commonly occurs in adolescent females but is also common in young males, especially during sports. Dislocation is usually lateral and is caused by either a force applied to the medial patella or forceful contraction of the vastus lateralis with the knee flexed. Congenital predisposition is present in more than 50% of cases, with excessive external rotation at the hip joint being the most common precipitant. Recurrent dislocation is common.
- The diagnosis is usually apparent, with obvious lateral dislocation of the patella.
- Pre-reduction X-ray is not necessary when the diagnosis is clear.

Management

1. Reduction is often achieved without anaesthesia with the operator gently extending the knee fully while pressing on the lateral patella with the thumb. If the patient is reluctant to allow this, then procedural sedation should be used.
2. Post-reduction knee X-rays (anteroposterior, lateral, 'skyline') are performed to detect associated avulsion fractures.
3. The leg should be immobilised with the knee straight in a Zimmer splint for 3 weeks to allow the medial ligaments to heal. The patient is referred to the fracture clinic/orthopaedic surgeon's rooms and to a physiotherapist for strengthening of the vastus medialis.

TRUE DISLOCATION OF THE KNEE

Assessment

- True dislocation of the knee is a medical emergency because it is commonly associated with popliteal artery injury and the risk of amputation.
- The mechanism of injury often involves significant force as in high-speed motor vehicle crashes, pedestrian/car collisions and falls, but rotation on a planted foot during sport can cause dislocation, especially in heavy individuals.
- Associated injuries:
  - Up to 30% of knee dislocations are open.
  - Popliteal artery injury occurs in up to 79% of knee dislocations.
  - Common peroneal nerve injury with foot drop occurs in up to 40%.

  - Compartment syndrome occurs because of swelling around the knee joint and upper leg, and its presence increases the risk of nerve and muscle ischaemia and amputation.
- The risk of amputation because of arterial injury increases if reduction is delayed.
- 3 of the 4 major ligaments of the knee must be ruptured for the knee to dislocate.
  Examine for:
  - distal pulses, capillary refill, colour, temperature
  - common peroneal nerve injury—dorsiflexion of the foot and toes, sensation between the first and second toes dorsally
  - increased compartment pressure.
- Urgent X-rays confirm the diagnosis of knee dislocation.

Management

Management should include:

1. primary survey (ABCDE, resuscitation)
2. looking for injuries in other organ systems
3. urgent orthopaedic registrar review in the ED
4. prompt reduction in the ED using procedural sedation
5. post-reduction immobilisation in a long leg plaster slab
6. urgent CT angiography and vascular surgery consultation in all cases.

If reduction is delayed for more than 8 hours, the likelihood of distal amputation is about 80%.

TIBIAL PLATEAU FRACTURE

Assessment

- Classically described as 'bumper-bar fractures', these injuries are common in pedestrians struck by cars but also occur in falls from standing in the elderly and occasionally during sport. The causative force is usually applied to the knee laterally, driving the lateral femoral condyle into the lateral tibial plateau and opening the knee medially. The lateral tibial plateau is more frequently injured than the medial. Lateral tibial plateau fracture may be associated with medial collateral ligament (MCL) and anterior and posterior cruciate ligament (ACL, PCL) tears as the knee opens up from a laterally applied force.
- The patient complains of knee pain, usually has a knee joint effusion and is unable to bear weight.
- Tibial plateau fracture is easily missed on plain X-ray. Look for a knee joint effusion with a blood/fat level.

(*pto*)

- CT scan of the knee should be performed on any patient with knee pain and inability to mobilise and will detect tibial plateau fractures that are poorly delineated on plain X-rays.
- Examine for popliteal artery and common peroneal nerve injury.

Management

- Management depends on patient age and degree of displacement.
- Immobilise the knee in a Zimmer splint or long leg plaster slab and obtain orthopaedic registrar review in the ED.

ACUTE KNEE PAIN

The cruciate ligaments (anterior and posterior, ACL and PCL), collateral ligaments (medial and lateral, MCL and LCL) and the medial and lateral menisci are frequently injured during sport and in accidents in which linear and/or torsional forces are applied to the knee. Injuries to the ACL, PCL and the menisci, along with fractures of the distal femur, proximal tibia and patella, will usually cause acute knee effusion (lipo-haemarthrosis).

Acute inflammatory and infective monoarthropathies—gout, pseudogout and septic arthritis are the most common—often also present with acute painful knee joint effusion.

TRAUMATIC KNEE PAIN

Assessment

- All patients with acute knee injuries should have plain X-rays of the knee (anteroposterior, lateral and 'skyline') to demonstrate fractures:
  - tibial plateau fracture, femoral condyle fracture, patella fracture
  - avulsion fractures:
    - of the tibial spine in cruciate ligament injury
    - avulsion flakes from the upper-pole patella in quadriceps ligament rupture
    - avulsion flakes from the femoral condyles in MCL and LCL injuries
    - vertical avulsion flake from the proximal lateral tibia (Segond fracture, indicative of ACL tear).
- A careful history of the mechanism of the knee injury points to the probable derangement:
  - A linear force applied to the lateral knee will open the joint medially and compress the bones laterally, resulting in, with increasing amount of force:

- MCL tear—the most common knee ligament injury. Occurs most frequently in football tackles, skiing. There will be tenderness over the MCL above and/or below the medial joint line. Test for laxity to valgus strain—grade 3 injuries involve complete rupture, cause medial joint laxity and may require surgical repair. Grade 1 and 2 injuries are partial tears, there is no laxity and they usually heal without surgery.
- MCL tear plus medial meniscus tear—also occurs most commonly in football and skiing. As well as features of an MCL tear, there will be a knee joint effusion and tenderness over the medial meniscus at the medial joint line. Usually requires arthroscopic repair of the medial meniscus.
- MCL tear plus medial meniscus tear plus ACL tear—also occurs most commonly in football and skiing. As well as the features of MCL and medial meniscus injury, there will be laxity to an anterior stress. Usually requires arthroscopic ACL reconstruction.
- Lateral tibial plateau fracture plus MCL tear.

— PCL tear is usually caused by hyperextension of the knee, most commonly in football or skiing. There will be a knee joint effusion and laxity to posterior strain.

— Rotational forces, as in changing direction on a planted foot, cause meniscal tears and cruciate ligament injuries.

Examination of acute knee injury is often difficult because of pain and swelling but should always include the following.

1. Inspect for the presence and size of effusion. Compare with the other, normal knee; remember to milk the prepatellar bursa and test for patellar tap. Effusion suggests internal derangement and is unusual in isolated collateral ligament injuries.
2. Palpate for tenderness. Tenderness over the MCL and LCL above and below the joint line suggests collateral ligament injury. Tenderness in the joint line suggests internal derangement.
3. Test range of movement. A 'locked' knee is usually caused by acute or exacerbation of chronic meniscal tear.
4. Test for collateral ligament integrity. Laxity to valgus strain suggests MCL tear; laxity to varus strain suggests LCL tear.
5. Test for cruciate ligament integrity:
   — Anterior drawer sign. Supine on bed, hip at 45°, knee at 90°, sit on patient's foot and pull tibia forwards. Laxity suggests ACL tear.

(*pto*)

- Lachman test. Supine on bed, knee flexed to 20–30°, tibia lifted upwards. Laxity suggests ACL tear.
- Posterior drawer sign. Supine on bed, knee at 90°, sit on patient's foot and push tibia backwards. Laxity suggests PCL tear.

6 Test for meniscal injury:
- Apley grind test. Prone on bed, knee at 90°, apply axial force through leg and rotate.
- McMurray's test. Patient supine on bed, knee at 90°, thumb over joint line, rotate lower leg. Pain and palpable 'click' indicates meniscal injury.

Management

Initial management of knee ligament and meniscal injuries includes:

1. Give analgesia.
2. Consider aspirating a tense haemarthrosis for pain relief.
3. Immobilise in a Zimmer splint.
4. Refer to fracture clinic or orthopaedic surgeon's rooms for further assessment and management.

NON-TRAUMATIC KNEE PAIN

- All patients with knee pain, effusion and no history of injury should have plain X-rays of the knee along with screening blood tests (blood count, erythrocyte sedimentation rate, C-reactive protein, urate).
- Aspiration of knee effusion fluid for microscopy, culture and crystals should always be performed to exclude a diagnosis of septic arthritis.
- Septic arthritis requires admission to hospital for urgent surgical lavage and intravenous antibiotics.
- Acute gouty arthritis should be treated with oral prednisone 1 mg/kg up to 50 mg daily for 3–4 days and a non-steroidal anti-inflammatory agent.

TIBIA AND FIBULA SHAFT FRACTURES

Assessment

- Often seen in the younger age group during active adolescence and adulthood.
- Swelling and deformity are usually obvious.
- Open fractures are common.
- Usually require reduction under anaesthesia with external and/or internal immobilisation.

Management

Management includes:

1. analgesia, usually with intravenous morphine
2. orthopaedic registrar review in the ED
3. test for distal neurovascular compromise
4. urgent reduction of deformity in the ED with procedural sedation if there is evidence of distal vascular compromise
5. urgent attention to open injuries with lavage and antibiotics
6. immobilisation in a long leg plaster slab.

ISOLATED FIBULAR FRACTURES

Assessment

- These fractures are usually the result of direct-force trauma but may be associated with diastasis of the tibio-fibular ligament, especially if the fibular fracture is at the neck of the fibula.
- X-rays of the tibia and fibula should always include the knee and ankle joints. Look carefully for evidence of tibio-fibular diastasis if an apparently isolated fibular fracture is present.

Management

Isolated fibular fractures may be treated with either a firm bandage or a short leg plaster slab and referral to the fracture clinic or orthopaedic surgeon's rooms.

ANKLE LIGAMENT INJURIES

Assessment

- Common cause of presentation to EDs.
- Usually caused by trips where torsional force is applied at the ankle joint. Inversion injury is the most common.
- The lateral ligament of the ankle comprises:
  - anterior talofibular ligament
  - posterior talofibular ligament
  - calcaneofibular ligament.
- The medial (deltoid) ligament of the ankle consists of superficial and deep components.
- 75% of ankle injuries are ligament injuries without fracture, and 90% of these involve the lateral ligaments. 90% of lateral ligament injuries involve the anterior talofibular portion.
- The great majority of ankle ligament injuries are partial (grade 1 and 2) tears which will heal to full strength with conservative treatment. Full (grade 3) tears of more than two ligaments often result in persistent ankle instability and so will often require

surgical reconstruction. Assessment of instability is difficult at the acute presentation because of pain and swelling.

- The patient presents with a painful, often swollen, ankle.
- The decision to image the ankle depends on the independently validated Ottawa ankle rules: if there is pain in the malleoli and any one of
  - inability to bear weight both immediately and for 4 steps in the ED
  - bone tenderness over the distal 6 cm of the fibula or the tip of the lateral malleolus
  - bone tenderness over the distal 6 cm of the tibia or the tip of the medial malleolus

  plain anteroposterior and lateral X-rays of the ankle should be performed.

Management

For a patient with no evidence of fracture on ankle X-rays, management should include:

1. Adequate analgesia.
2. Explain that pain, bruising and swelling in ankle ligament injuries usually persists for 3–6 weeks and that sporting activity should be deferred for 4–12 weeks. Ankle strapping should be used for sport for up to 6 months after injury.
3. Apply a firm tubular bandage (e.g. Tubigrip).
4. Ice for 48 hours and elevate while sitting until swelling subsides.
5. Most patients will need crutches for the first few days.
6. Active weightbearing can be resumed when pain permits, usually in 3–5 days.
7. Arrange physiotherapy referral.
8. Arrange review by the general practitioner for assessment of instability after 1 week.

ANKLE DISLOCATION

Assessment

- This is a common injury and is usually associated with ankle fractures.
- The patient presents with pain, swelling and obvious deformity at the ankle joint.
- Distal neurovascular function is usually preserved, but the skin is stretched tightly over one of the malleoli and this may lead to ischaemic necrosis of the skin if reduction is delayed.

Management

Management should include:

1. Urgent reduction under procedural sedation in the ED, usually before X-rays have been performed. Most dislocations reduce easily with manual traction on the foot.
2. Immobilisation in a short leg plaster slab.
3. X-rays to reveal the associated fractures.
4. Urgent orthopaedic registrar review in the ED.
5. Associated fractures will usually require open reduction and internal fixation.

ANKLE FRACTURES

Assessment

- Ankle fractures are common and usually result from trips and over-balancing.
- Management depends on the integrity of the ankle mortise.
- Pott's classification is:
  - uni-malleolar—lateral or medial
  - bi-malleolar—lateral and medial
  - tri-malleolar—lateral, medial and posterior.
- The mortise is unstable if there is evidence of:
  - talar tilt or shift
  - displacement of any of the malleoli
  - bi-malleolar fracture
  - tri-malleolar fracture
  - uni-malleolar fracture with ligament injury at the opposite malleolus.
- Exclude talar dome injuries—often missed by X-ray.

Management

- Stable fractures in the anatomical position are usually treated conservatively in a short leg plaster slab with referral to the fracture clinic or orthopaedic surgeon's rooms.
- Unstable fractures are usually treated with open reduction and internal fixation.

The orthopaedic registrar should review all ankle fractures in the ED.

ACHILLES TENDON RUPTURE

Assessment

- Achilles tendon rupture is usually a sporting injury and occurs in adults from their 20s with forceful contraction of the posterior

compartment muscles, often when pushing off at tennis and squash, and in sprinters.
- The patient reports a sudden severe pain at the base of the leg. There is often an audible snap and the patient describes feeling as though he or she has been hit in the calf and is unable to walk or stand on the toes.
- The Thompson test is usually diagnostic. The patient either lies prone or kneels on a chair facing away, and the operator squeezes mid-calf—the foot plantarflexes with an intact Achilles tendon, but does not move when the tendon is ruptured.
- Ultrasound confirms the diagnosis, demonstrates partial rupture and differentiates between Achilles tendon rupture and calf muscle tears.

Management

Management is surgical repair of the ruptured tendon.

TALUS FRACTURES

Assessment

- Flake avulsion fractures are common with ligamentous injury of the ankle and foot and are usually treated as ligamentous injuries.
- Fractures of the neck and body of the talus require substantial force (falls from a height, compression of the foot against the firewall in high-speed motor vehicle crashes) and may lead to ischaemic necrosis of the talus.
- Most talus fractures will be visible on plain X-rays of the foot and ankle. CT scanning is indicated for patients with foot pain and swelling with apparently normal X-rays, e.g. talar dome fractures not visible.

Management

Patients with talar fractures should be reviewed by the orthopaedic registrar in the ED. Displaced fractures will require open reduction and internal fixation.

CALCANEUS FRACTURES

Assessment

- Calcaneus fractures are common, are usually the result of a fall from a height and are bilateral in up to 20% of cases.
- They may be a part of the complex of injuries caused by dissipation of energy from a fall onto the feet:
  — calcaneus fracture

- — ankle fractures
- — tibial plateau fracture
- — proximal femoral fracture
- — thoracolumbar vertebral fracture (with 10–20% of calcaneus fractures)
- — atlas and base-of-skull fractures.
- Assess all of the above areas for pain and tenderness and image any areas of concern.
- Plain X-rays will demonstrate most calcaneus fractures.
- Once a calcaneus fracture has been identified, obtain a CT scan of the calcaneus to demonstrate articular involvement, comminution, subluxation.

Management

- Calcaneus fractures should be reviewed by the orthopaedic registrar in the ED.
- Displaced and intra-articular fractures will need open reduction and internal fixation.
- Patients with bilateral fractures will need hospitalisation because they are unable to mobilise.

MAJOR FRACTURE/DISLOCATIONS IN THE FOOT

Subtarsal dislocation

Assessment

- Subtarsal dislocation occurs with major forces, as in falls from a height or compression of the foot against the firewall in high-speed motor vehicle crashes.
- May lead to avascular necrosis of the talus.
- Usually identified on plain X-rays.
- Requires CT imaging to identify associated fractures and articular involvement.

Management

- Urgent reduction is necessary if there are features of distal vascular compromise.
- Initial reduction may be performed under procedural sedation in the ED or under general anaesthesia in the operating theatre.

Chopart fracture/dislocation

Assessment

- The Chopart fracture/dislocation is essentially a dislocation of the midfoot on the hindfoot. It is an uncommon injury, caused by major forces as in falls from a height or compression of the foot against the firewall in high-speed motor vehicle crashes.

- There is fracture and dislocation about the talonavicular and calcaneocuboid joints.
- Plain X-rays may appear normal.
- CT imaging should be performed if there is pain and swelling of the foot with apparently normal X-rays. It will clearly identify the complex of injuries.

Management

- Urgent reduction is necessary if there are features of distal vascular compromise.
- The orthopaedic registrar should review all midfoot and hindfoot fractures in the ED.
- Management is by open reduction and internal fixation.

Lisfranc fracture/dislocation

Assessment

- The Lisfranc fracture/dislocation is essentially a dislocation of the forefoot on the midfoot. It is caused by major forces, as in a heavy weight falling on the foot or a trip off a kerb or step.
- The key to the injury is the articulation of the base of the second metatarsal with the midfoot, anchoring the forefoot and preventing lateral movement. Lisfranc fracture/dislocation occurs when lateral and rotational forces cause fracture of the base of the second metatarsal and disrupt Lisfranc's ligament, allowing lateral dislocation of the forefoot.
- X-rays of the foot may appear normal. Look carefully for fracture of the base of the second metatarsal and lateral displacement of the metatarsals.
- CT imaging should be performed if there is pain and swelling of the foot with apparently normal X-rays.

Management

- Urgent reduction is necessary if there are features of distal vascular compromise.
- The orthopaedic registrar should review all midfoot and hindfoot injuries in the ED.
- Management is usually by open reduction and internal fixation.

OTHER METATARSAL INJURIES

Fifth metatarsal fractures

Assessment

Fractures of the base of the fifth metatarsal are common. The two types of this fracture should be differentiated because their management differs. Both are caused by inversion injuries of the foot.

1. The 'Jones' fracture is a transverse fracture of the base of the fifth metatarsal and usually requires immobilisation in a boot or short leg plaster because of a tendency to non-union.
2. The 'pseudo-Jones' fracture is an oblique fracture of the base of the fifth metatarsal caused by avulsion of the insertion of peroneus brevis, usually heals well and is usually treated symptomatically in a firm bandage.

Management

Initial management includes:

1. a firm bandage or a short leg plaster slab
2. crutches
3. referral to the fracture clinic or orthopaedic surgeon's rooms.

Stress fractures

- The second and third metatarsals are prone to stress fracture because they have little mobility in the forefoot.
- The patient will complain of persistent forefoot pain without history of injury.
- There is often a history of recent increase in walking or running.
- X-rays are often normal.
- Radionuclide bone scan will demonstrate these fractures.
- Advise rest and refer to the fracture clinic or orthopaedic surgeon's rooms.

PHALANGEAL FRACTURES IN THE FOOT

Assessment

Toe fractures are common and are caused by direct injury. The big toe and the little toe are the most exposed and the most frequently injured.

Management

1. Fractures are usually minimally displaced and are best treated by buddy-strapping.
2. Painful subungual haematoma should be treated by trephining the nail by gently pressing the tip of a red-hot paperclip onto the middle of the nail.

(*pto*)

Open fractures of the toes require assessment in the ED by the orthopaedic registrar for lavage under general anaesthesia and intravenous antibiotics.

INTERPHALANGEAL AND METATARSOPHALANGEAL JOINT DISLOCATIONS

Assessment

- These are caused by direct injury and are usually easily reduced.
- X-ray all deformed toes before attempting reduction because of the possibility of fracture.

Management

1. Most toe dislocations are easily reduced. Digital nerve block may be used but many dislocations can be reduced without anaesthesia, depending on patient preference. The technique of reduction involves applying axial traction to the distal part while pressing with the thumb of the other hand over the base of the dislocated bone.
2. The relocated toe should be buddy-strapped, and the patient mobilises normally.

Open dislocations, fracture/dislocations and failed reductions should be reviewed by the orthopaedic registrar in the ED.

Editorial Comment

These patients commonly present to the ED.
Respect pain and swelling—suspect fracture.
Remember: (1) you are not a radiologist; (2) not all fractures are visible even on good films.
Ensure the patient understands the need for follow-up, confirmation of a diagnosis/formal X-ray report and the need for review if healing/pain/function is not to plan. Ignore this, and you could be sued.

Chapter 18
Hand injuries and care

Bill Croker and Iromi Samarasinghe

Hand injuries are common in emergency departments. Meticulous assessment and management is crucial because preservation of function is critical for livelihood and recreation.

Assessment

Document:

1. Handedness
2. Occupation
3. Special interests (guitar, piano, model making, etc)
4. Mechanism of injury (cutting, crushing, industrial, high-pressure injection, burn, bite)
5. Contamination
6. Time of injury
7. Specific symptoms (tingling, numbness, weakness)
8. Treatment so far
9. Immunisation status.

Examination

Document:

1. Position of hand—noting variation of finger positions from usual 'rest' posture
2. Location of injury
   - — name fingers (not number)
   - — palmar (volar) or dorsal surface
   - — radial or ulnar border
3. Perfusion
4. Nerve function (see below)
5. Tendon function (see below).

NERVE FUNCTION—SCREENING TESTS

Median nerve

- Motor: test abduction of the thumb from the plane of the palm while palpating the thenar eminence

- Sensory: volar surface—thumb, palm and radial 2½ fingers; dorsal surface—radial 2½ fingers distal to the proximal interphalangeal (PIP) joint.

Radial nerve

- Motor: wrist extension and extension of digits.
- Sensory: dorsal surface—radial 2½ fingers proximal to PIP joint and dorsum of hand.

Ulnar nerve

- Motor: adduction of fingers in extension (hold a piece of paper between the fingers).
- Sensory: ulnar 1½ fingers and hand on both volar and dorsal surfaces.

TENDON FUNCTION

Test each joint of the fingers and thumb in flexion and extension. This will detect complete laceration only. Warn the patient about the possibility of delayed rupture.

The exact posture of the injured part at the time of injury cannot be accurately known. Therefore, inspect the base of the wound through the full range of movement of the adjacent joints, watching for deficits in visible tendons. Testing flexor digitorum profundus (FDP) at the distal interphalangeal (DIP) joint requires the joint more proximal to be held in extension during flexion of the joint being tested. Testing flexor digitorum superficialis (FDS) at the PIP joint requires all fingers except the one being tested to be held in extension to neutralise the mass flexor effect of FDP at the PIP joint.

Treatment

INITIAL TREATMENT

1. Analgesia:
   - digital block (avoid adrenaline)
     Always check sensation prior to application of local anaesthetic.
   - wrist block
   - IV narcotics.
2. X-ray the injured part if there is a possibility of bony injury or foreign body.
3. Check tetanus status.
4. Carefully clean open injuries and remove debris.
5. Antibiotics if extensive injury or compound fracture.

6 Elevate (pillow-case sling from an IV pole if being admitted).
7 Keep fasted and commence IV fluids if surgery a possibility.
8 Splint injured finger, especially if protracted delay to specialist review.

SPLINTING

The hand is splinted in a position to minimise the risk of stiffness after treatment: wrist extended (40°); metacarpophalangeal (MCP) joints flexed (90°) and fingers fully extended. This position keeps the collateral ligaments of the fingers at their maximal length.

Splint only those joints that need to be included for a particular injury.

Explain to the patient the importance of moving any joint not enclosed in the splint, to minimise stiffness.

HAND THERAPY

Follow-up that involves a hand therapist ensures optimal outcome.

Soft-tissue injuries

LACERATIONS

These require careful inspection through full range of movement following local anaesthetic. Document any sensory changes prior to anaesthetic.

Sutures, if required, should be 5/0 non-absorbable and are removed after 5–7 days—longer if over extensor joints, in the elderly or in patients on steroids.

FINGERTIP INJURIES

While usually not large, these can be very painful.

Small skin loss without bone exposed

(Small skin loss = area smaller than a 5 cent piece.)

1 Anaesthesia.
2 Clean.
3 Apply 'wet' dressing (membrane) or chloramphenicol (Chloromycetin) ointment.
4 Change every 2–3 days until healed (dressing clinic, LMO or home).
5 Elevate (hand above elbow) to reduce pain and swelling for first 2–3 days.
6 Refer to the hand/plastic/orthopaedic team according to your hospital's practice for outpatient follow-up. (*pto*)

7. Active and passive mobilisation to avoid stiffness after first 2–3 days.
8. Analgesia.
9. Review for infection (increasing pain, spreading redness, fever—a late manifestation).

Larger defect or with bone exposed

Defects larger than 1 cm in diameter require skin graft. Refer to the hand/plastic/orthopaedic team according to your hospital's practice. Commence initial treatment.

FINGER LACERATIONS

Careful assessment for associated nerve and tendon injury. If present, refer as appropriate. Otherwise, suture as indicated.

PALMAR LACERATIONS

'No-man's land' is the zone from the midpalm to the PIP joint where the tendons of the flexor superficialis and profundus are enclosed together in tendon sheaths. Great care in assessment is necessary. Palmar skin is thick and difficult to suture. Anaesthesia is difficult to achieve with local infiltration for similar reasons.

Request senior review.

Nails

NAIL BED LACERATIONS

Meticulous repair is critical. It is not just cosmetic; poor technique results in a permanently split nail. Refer to the hand/plastic/orthopaedic team according to your hospital's practice for repair of laceration.

Preserve the nail; it can be used as a splint.

Commence initial treatment.

SUBUNGUAL HAEMATOMA

With NO injury to nail or surrounding nail margin

Crush injury. X-ray to exclude fracture. Drill through the nail in 2 or 3 spots with a 19-gauge needle spun between thumb and index finger to release blood.

Splint, analgesia, elevate for 48 hours.

Associated undisplaced fractures are considered 'open' and treated with oral antibiotics.

With injury to nail or surrounding nail margin

Or where the subungual haematoma is greater than 50%, there is risk of nail bed laceration. Refer for review by the hand/plastic/orthopaedic team.

AVULSION

Nails take 3 months to grow from nail bed to tip, delayed by a month if the bed is injured.

If the nail is avulsed there is a risk of nail bed laceration. Refer for review by the hand/plastic/orthopaedic team.

Tendons

LACERATIONS OF THE EXTENSOR SURFACE OVERLYING THE PIP JOINT

Otherwise innocuous-looking lacerations of the extensor surface of the PIP joint can transect the central slip of the extensor mechanism with preservation of extensor function initially. However, a boutonnière deformity will subsequently develop if the tendon has been cut.

Refer to the hand/plastic/orthopaedic team as per your hospital's practice for exploration and repair. Commence initial treatment.

MALLET FINGER

A mallet finger is an avulsion of the extensor tendon at its insertion into the distal phalanx. The patient is unable to fully extend their distal phalanx. It occurs when there is a sudden forced flexion of an extended finger (hit by cricket ball, basketball, etc).

Without fracture

Splint in gentle hyperextension for 6 weeks—commercially available splints recommended.

Refer to the hand/plastic/orthopaedic team according to your hospital's practice for outpatient management.

With fracture

If there is a fracture involving more than 30% of the articular surface, this will need to be meticulously repaired. Refer to the hand/plastic/orthopaedic team according to your hospital's practice. Commence initial treatment.

Nerve injuries

The digital nerves and arteries run in a bundle along the line joining the flexion creases of a flexed finger. Beyond the distal flexion crease, the nerve breaks up into terminal branches which are not practical to repair. Some sensation will return anyway.

Lacerations proximal to the DIP joint causing sensory loss require exploration. Refer to the hand/plastic/orthopaedic team according to your hospital's practice. Commence initial treatment.

Nerves regrow at a rate of up to 1 mm a day. After repair, no guarantee can be given about return of function, which takes several months even when repair is successful. Commitment to physiotherapy is required to optimise outcome.

Vascular injuries

The ulnar artery is the dominant artery of the hand.

1 Control brisk bleeding with direct pressure—gauze and gloved fingers—to prevent exsanguination.
2 If bleeding persists when pressure removed, apply an arterial tourniquet (blood-pressure cuff inflated to 50 mmHg above systolic pressure for no longer than 20 minutes) prior to exploration and definitive treatment. Tourniquets are very painful and carry the risk of tissue ischaemia if left inflated too long.
3 A history of pulsatile bleeding dictates exploration of the wound to tie off both ends of the artery, to prevent formation of a pseudoaneurysm.
4 Refer to the hand/plastic/orthopaedic team according to your hospital's practice.
5 Commence initial treatment.

Bony injuries

Also see a discussion of this topic in Chapter 17, 'Orthopaedic principles—fractures and dislocations.'

PHALANGES

Fractures with rotational deformities

1 Assess for the presence of any rotational deformation by getting the patient to touch their thenar eminence with all their fingers simultaneously. If the injured finger is twisted, then a rotational deformation is present.
2 Digital block.
3 Correct rotational deformation.
4 Buddy-strap finger (gauze between fingers to minimise rubbing).
5 Elevation, analgesia, active and passive movement of fingers to reduce stiffness.

6 Refer to the hand/plastic/orthopaedic team according to your hospital's practice for outpatient follow-up in about 1 week to ensure no delayed deformity.
7 If rotational deformation, or more than 10° of angulation, persists after reduction, refer to the hand/plastic/orthopaedic team according to your hospital's practice for accurate reduction and fixation.

Fractures without rotational deformities

If no rotational deformity is present, buddy-strap, elevate until acute pain settles and then use hand normally, provide analgesia and refer to LMO for review.

Any spiral fracture of digits or metacarpals is potentially unstable—refer to the hand/plastic/orthopaedic team according to your hospital's practice.

FRACTURES INVOLVING JOINT SURFACES

Commence initial treatment.

Refer to the hand/plastic/orthopaedic team according to your hospital's practice for accurate reduction and fixation.

DISLOCATIONS

Position of fingers needs to be accurately documented by X-ray or photo prior to reduction.

1 Digital block.
2 Reduce dislocation, usually by gentle traction. If unsuccessful, try increasing the deformation (i.e. if dorsal dislocation, apply hyperextension before traction).
3 Buddy-strap finger (gauze between fingers to minimise rubbing).
4 Elevation, analgesia, active and passive movement of fingers to reduce stiffness.
5 Refer to the hand/plastic/orthopaedic team according to your hospital's practice for outpatient follow-up in about 1 week to assess for instability and continued hand therapy.

COMPOUND FRACTURES

Commence initial treatment.

Refer to the hand/plastic/orthopaedic team according to your hospital's practice for washout, reduction and closure.

FRACTURE OF THE FIFTH METACARPAL NECK

Provided angulation of this common 'punching' injury is less than 45°, a simple volar back slab for 3–4 weeks will usually provide sufficient support. Refer to LMO for review to ensure fracture does not slip.

Otherwise, refer to the hand/plastic/orthopaedic team according to your hospital's practice for reduction.

CARPAL BONES

Scaphoid fractures

The scaphoid is the keystone of the carpus, and non-union following fracture results in chronic pain and instability. Early CT can clarify the diagnosis. Management is controversial; conservative management in a scaphoid cast or open reduction internal fixation (ORIF) should be deferred to the appropriate specialist team (see Chapter 17).

Emergency treatment is:

1. Apply scaphoid plaster of paris (POP) cast.
2. Elevate.
3. Refer to the hand/plastic/orthopaedic team according to your hospital's practice for outpatient follow-up in about 1 week.

Gamekeeper's thumb

Forced abduction of the thumb (as in skiing) results in rupture of the ulnar collateral ligament of the thumb.

Assess for tenderness over the ulnar border of the MCP joint. If present, treat with a scaphoid plaster and refer to the hand/plastic/orthopaedic team according to your hospital's practice for outpatient follow-up in about 1 week to reassess and for continued hand therapy.

Specific conditions

INFECTIONS

- Suspect foreign bodies.
- Pain on passive stretch suggests tendon sheath infection or compartment syndrome.
- If not septic and no suggestion of tendon sheath infection, foreign body or collection, commence oral antibiotics, splint, elevate and review in 24 hours (earlier if there is any sign of deterioration).
- If there is evidence of tenosynovitis, early referral for operative drainage of the tendon sheath under general anaesthetic is necessary. Refer to the hand/plastic/orthopaedic team according to your hospital's practice. Commence initial treatment, in particular early intravenous antibiotics.

Specific infections are discussed below. Refer to the hand/plastic/orthopaedic team according to your hospital's practice.

PARONYCHIA

Paronychia is infection of the tissues around the fingernail.

1. Digital block.
2. Soak the finger in warm water for about 10 minutes.
3. Blunt-dissect with fine scissors or number 11 scalpel under the skin fold to open the abscess.
4. Irrigate.
5. Pack.
6. Analgesia, elevate and review in 24 hours.
7. Antibiotics are only indicated if there is significant surrounding cellulitis. Oral cephalosporins are generally adequate, although non-multiresistant oxacillin-resistant *Staphylococcus aureus* (NORSA) strains, which are increasing in incidence, may respond to clindamycin. Refer to the Therapeutic Guidelines (www.ciap.health.nsw.gov.au/home.html).
8. Complications include subungual abscess, which requires nail to be removed.

Chronic paronychia

Usually occupational from prolonged exposure of hands to water; involves bacterial and candidal infection.

Treatment involves drying hands with 70% alcohol and applying a topical antifungal cream such as clotrimazole 1%. The nail is removed only if the infection is intractable. Refer to hand surgery for marsupialisation and wedge resection of nail.

PYOGENIC GRANULOMA

These are collections of granulation tissue developing around a foreign body such as suture material. Treatment is by curette or formal surgical excision with histological examination of excised tissue.

FELON

A felon is an abscess of the pulp of the distal phalanx, which requires drainage with digital nerve block to prevent complications. It usually presents with throbbing pain, swelling and tenderness without fluctuance.

- Apply digital nerve block and forearm tourniquet to provide a bloodless field.
- A central longitudinal incision avoiding crossing the flexion crease protects the digital neurovascular bundle and flexor tendon

sheath. Avoid incision of vertical pulp space fibres. Incision is made down to the bone avoiding FDP insertion.
- Delay to treatment may result in osteomyelitis, pulp necrosis or loss of pinch function.

HERPETIC WHITLOW

Herpetic whitlow is most commonly seen in healthcare workers. It presents as a vesicle around the nail or finger pad and is intensely painful.

Swabs may be taken for herpes zoster polymerase chain reaction (PCR).

Topical aciclovir is used with variable success. Unlike bacterial infections, incision and drainage is not indicated.

BITES

Bites have a high rate of infection.

If bite is **simple and superficial** (i.e. with no evidence of involvement of underlying structures) and seen in under 8 hours:
- irrigate copiously
- debride as necessary
- consider delayed primary closure
- elevate
- immobilise
- review at 24 hours to ensure no infection.

'Bites' or 'tooth penetration wounds' due to punching injuries should be X-rayed to ensure there are no tooth fragments in the wound. Oral flora inoculated into the MCP joint with clenched-fist injuries usually results in a septic joint effusion and requires operative drainage, splinting and elevation and broad-spectrum parenteral antibiotics (ceftriaxone + metronidazole; see Antibiotic Guidelines, www.ciap.health.nsw.gov.au/home.html).

For **all other injuries** (complex or deep lacerations, involvement of underlying structures or delayed presentation), refer to the hand/plastic/orthopaedic team according to your hospital's practice. Commence initial treatment.

CRUSH INJURIES

Crush injuries cause extensive soft-tissue damage, without necessarily causing any bony injury. Initial assessment may reveal minimal external evidence of injury. Contained bleeding and tissue oedema resulting from the crush injury can cause progressively increasing pressure resulting in tissue ischaemia—the compartment syndrome.

History should be extended to include mechanism of crush, duration of compression and areas included under the compressive forces.

Examine in particular for signs of the **compartment syndrome**: pain out of proportion to the injury, pain on passive stretch of the compartment, tense feel to the compartment and distal paraesthesia. Pulses are normal until very late in the evolution of the compartment syndrome.

Refer to the hand/plastic/orthopaedic team according to your hospital's practice for observation and possible fasciotomy. Commence initial treatment.

Treat associated injuries as appropriate (lacerations, fractures or dislocations, arterial injuries).

Strict elevation and hourly limb observations to detect early signs of compartment syndrome.

HIGH-PRESSURE INJECTION INJURIES

Industrial accidents involving injection (e.g. paint, grease, gas) into the hand are urgently referred to the hand/plastic/orthopaedic team according to your hospital's practice for observation and possible debridement of devitalised tissue or fasciotomy for decompression of ensuing compartment syndrome. Commence initial treatment.

BURNS

Burns of the hand represent a 'special area' injury and should be discussed with the regional burns injury unit. Commence initial treatment—adequate cooling (minimum of 20 minutes) at 15°C (range 8–25°C) within 3 hours of incident: generous analgesia.

Indications for referral to burns unit:

- Circumferential burns to hand or fingers
- Multiple digits or web spaces involved
- Burns involving joint surfaces
- Deep dermal burn or uncertain depth
- Electrical or chemical burn
- Crush injuries or other injuries or systemic illness
- Delayed healing, > 1 week.

If transfer to burns unit is recommended, the wound area should be wrapped in plastic cling wrap after cooling is completed. Hand burns that do not require transfer should have paraffin gauze dressing.

Superficial partial-thickness dorsal surface burns (classically scalds or fat burns) should be reviewed at 24 hours to ensure correct initial assessment and then can be treated with analgesia, elevation and daily dressings by LMO or dressing clinic.

HYDROFLUORIC ACID BURNS

Hydrofluoric acid is an industrial cleaning agent which causes liquefactive necrosis resulting in deep-tissue damage and intense pain, often without much external sign of injury.

Specific treatment is calcium, which can be administered by a variety of routes. Calcium gluconate 2.5% gel (made by mixing 10% calcium gluconate solution with 3 times the volume of KY gel) can be used topically. For finger burns, the gel can be placed in a latex glove and the affected hand inserted into it for up to 45 minutes. This can be repeated 6-hourly for 24 hours until pain eases.

Intra-arterial calcium gluconate is effective second-line therapy for more severe and extensive hand burns. Infusion of 10–20 mL of 10% calcium gluconate in 200 mL 5% dextrose over 4 hours via a radial artery catheter is more effective than intravenous administration and safer than local infiltration, which risks compartment syndrome due to the volumes required.

Refer to the hand/plastic/orthopaedic team, according to your hospital's practice, for treatment.

ELECTRICAL INJURIES

Initial assessment can be misleading, as the full extent of injury may not be apparent at first.

Perform a very careful neurovascular examination.

Refer to the hand/plastic/orthopaedic team according to your hospital's practice.

AMPUTATIONS

Indications for replantation or revascularisation include thumb amputations, amputation of multiple digits, individual amputations distal to insertion of FDS and cold ischaemia time less than 24 hours.

Refer to the hand/plastic/orthopaedic team according to your hospital's practice for consideration of replantation. Commence initial treatment.

Care of the amputated part

No amputated part should be discarded until a formal plan of replantation has been discussed with surgeon and patient.

1 Carefully and gently clean the part.
2 Wrap in sterile saline-soaked gauze.
3 Place in a sealed plastic bag in an ice-water bath at 4°C.
4 X-ray both the stump and the amputated part.

CARPAL TUNNEL SYNDROME

Compression neuropathy of the median nerve as it traverses the wrist deep to the flexor retinaculum can be chronic or acute (suppurative infection, burn, haemorrhage, postoperative) and idiopathic or secondary to increase in carpal tunnel contents (tenosynovitis, haematoma, oedema) or decrease in size of tunnel (arthritis, fracture or dislocation of the lunate).

Indications for decompression include acute carpal tunnel syndrome with rapid onset and progression of median nerve impairment, persistent symptoms despite conservative measures, impaired sensation in radial 2½ fingers or thenar muscle palsy.

1 Conduct a thorough neurovascular and functional assessment.
2 Splint and elevate.
3 Refer to the hand/plastic/orthopaedic team according to your hospital's practice for endoscopic release or open carpal tunnel release.

Editorial Comment

Hand/finger injuries are very common, but require extra knowledge and care to avoid major functional problems that may affect livelihood, etc.

Chapter 19

Urological emergencies

Phillip C Brenner and Ed Park

Balanitis

KEY PRESENTATION/CLINICAL FEATURES

- Infection of foreskin: bacterial or fungal.
- Associated with poor hygiene, diabetes.

MANAGEMENT

- Soap washes; soaking in antiseptic solution or antibiotic ointment (e.g. neomycin); topical antifungals.
- PO antibiotics are sometimes needed, and if whole of shaft involved then IV antibiotics.

COMPLICATIONS

Phimosis secondary to adhesions.

Common post-procedural problems

EXTRACORPOREAL SHOCK-WAVE LITHOTRIPSY (ESWL)

Key presentation/clinical features

Commonly, patients will present with pain and haematuria and will require narcotic analgesia and non-steroidal anti-inflammatory drugs (NSAIDs).

Investigations

- Urinalysis (UA) and midstream urine (MSU).
- Electrolytes, urea, creatinine (EUC), full blood count (FBC).
- X-ray of kidneys–ureters–bladder (KUB) is relevant to establish size of stone fragment passing down ureter or presence of steinstrasse (a series of stone fragments in a line).
- Measure diameter of largest fragment in millimetres.

Management

- Analgesia: intravenous (IV) opioids; indomethacin 100 mg 12-hourly per rectum (PR).
- Fever with temperatures > 38°C is an absolute indication for admission and indicates an infected, obstructed system requiring likely decompression by a double-J stent or nephrostomy.

- Anuria or raised creatinine due to bilateral disease or solitary kidney is similarly an emergency requiring admission.
- If patient is pain-free, discharge with indomethacin suppositories 100 mg 12-hourly PR (if no history of ulcer or other contraindication to NSAIDs) and oral opioids such as codeine phosphate 30 mg/paracetamol 500 mg combination tablets or oxycodone 5 mg 6-hourly PO.

TRANS-RECTAL ULTRASOUND PROSTATE BIOPSY (TRUS BIOPSY)

Key presentation/clinical features

This is performed in the office under ultrasound control or as a day-only procedure. The needle is passed trans-rectally and hence is prone to bacterial seeding and sepsis, which may be life-threatening.

Complications

- Sepsis: patients with any fever (temperature > 37.5°C) must be admitted for intravenous ampicillin and gentamicin (or ciprofloxacin if allergic to penicillin). Take blood and urine cultures and initiate resuscitation, and refer to ICU if there are signs of hypotension or anuria.
- Haematuria: only requires treatment if it precipitates retention or is massive. Use a 22 Fr three-way irrigation catheter.
- Retention: usually due to pre-existing prostatism. Pass a small (14 Fr or 12 Fr) Foley catheter. If this is not possible, use a small suprapubic stab catheter (12 Fr).

Epididymo-orchitis

KEY PRESENTATION/CLINICAL FEATURES

- Commonest cause of scrotal pain.
- Commonest in 19- to 35-year-olds:
  - < 35 years: usually gonorrhoea or chlamydia; in homosexuals, may be *Haemophilus*, coliforms
  - > 35 years: obstructive cause (urethral or prostate); infected urine extension via vas deferens to epididymis; coliforms from urinary tract infections (UTIs).
- Other causes are *Pseudomonas aeruginosa*, *Mycobacterium tuberculosis*, viral mumps, cryptococcal causes, amiodarone.
- There can be sudden pain, swelling to the epididymis/testis of < 6 weeks' duration; associated urethritis.
- Tender epididymis and/or testis.

DIFFERENTIAL DIAGNOSIS

- Testicular torsion
- Undisclosed trauma
- Fournier's gangrene.

INVESTIGATIONS

Bedside

Urinalysis.

Pathology

- MSU
- Urine chlamydia and gonorrhoea PCR
- Urethral swab: white cell count (WCC) > 5/mm^3 indicates urethritis.

Imaging

Colour Doppler ultrasound: reveals epididymal involvement, characteristic features; to assess flow into testicle.

MANAGEMENT

Supportive

- Bed rest
- Scrotal support

Specific

- Antibiotics
  - for suspected sexually transmitted disease (STD)
    - ceftriaxone 500 mg IV or with 2 mL of 1% lignocaine IM injection for 3 days
      plus
    - azithromycin 1 g PO as single dose
      plus
    - a further single dose of azithromycin 1 g PO in 1 week

    OR
    - doxycycline 100 mg 12-hourly for 14 days
  - for suspected non-STD
    - trimethoprim 300 mg daily for 14 days
      OR
    - cephalexin 500 mg 12-hourly for 14 days
      OR
    - amoxycillin + clavulanate 500 mg + 125 mg 12-hourly for 14 days.

If unwell (whether STD or non-STD suspected):

- gentamicin 4–6 mg/kg as single dose, then determine a maximum of 1–2 further doses based on renal function (see Antibiotic Guidelines 2010 for further details; www.ciap.health.nsw.gov.au/home.html)
  plus
- ampicillin or amoxycillin 2 g 6-hourly
  OR
- if patient is penicillin-hypersensitive, gentamicin alone is usually adequate
- if gentamicin is contraindicated, ceftriaxone as single agent 1 g once daily or cefotaxime 1 g 8-hourly.

- Discuss with urology if follow-up is needed, otherwise discharge with GP follow-up.

COMPLICATIONS

- Abscess formation
- Testicular infarction
- Chronic pain and infertility.

Pearls/Pitfalls/Controversies

- Involve urology with all presentations.
- Empirically treat all men for STD-related causes.

Fournier's gangrene

KEY PRESENTATION/CLINICAL FEATURES

- Necrotising fasciitis of scrotum, penis or vulva, usually from peri-anal infection or UTI extending from peri-urethral glands.
- Mixed aerobic/anaerobic microorganisms (anaerobic *Streptococcus*, Gram-negative rods, anaerobes, *Bacteroides fragilis, Escherichia coli*).
- Can progress very rapidly and dramatically.

HISTORY

- Risk: much more common in men; diabetes; obesity; immunocompromised individuals; alcohol abuse; chronic steroid use.
- Severe pain sometimes out of proportion to clinical findings.

EXAMINATION

- Patient is febrile, unwell, confused, signs of septic shock; can begin from anterior abdominal wall.
- Haemorrhagic, discoloured, necrotic, indurated, bulla formation in scrotal or perineal region.
- Crepitus.

INVESTIGATIONS

Bedside

Venous blood gas to assess lactate in septic patient (lactate > 4 mmol/L is associated with higher mortality).

Pathology

- FBC, EUC, glucose
- Blood cultures
- Wound swab if relevant.

Imaging

- Should not delay urgent surgery if diagnosis is very likely.
- CT can reveal air in fascial planes or deep-tissue involvement.

MANAGEMENT

- The first priority is urgent surgical/urological referral, as debridement is the specific management.
- Sepsis resuscitation:
  - antibiotics: meropenem 1 g 8-hourly IV + clindamycin 600 mg 8-hourly IV (see Antibiotic Guidelines, www.ciap.health.nsw.gov.au/home.html).
  - IV volume resuscitation with normal saline: can start with 10–20 mL/kg, then reassess.
  - as a guideline, aim of sepsis management is mean arterial pressure (MAP) > 65 mmHg, urinary output > 0.5 mL/kg/h, no confusion.
  - intubation for obtunded patient or inadequately ventilating patient
  - inotropes (noradrenaline, starting at 0.05 microg/kg/min) after adequate volume challenge (at least 2000–3000 mL) and ensure ongoing volume resuscitation occurs concurrently
- Supportive care:
  - analgesia
  - glucose control if hyperglycaemic in a diabetic patient (use half the recommended insulin dose in patients not usually on insulin (e.g. < 0.5 U to 0.5 U/kg/h).

- Hyperbaric oxygen therapy could be considered by the surgeons, if available, *after* surgical debridement.

COMPLICATIONS

Septic shock; multi-organ dysfunction.

Pearls/Pitfalls/Controversies

- Urgent surgical referral is required if this diagnosis is a possibility; maximise resuscitation early in the ED.
- Antibiotic treatment alone for Fournier's gangrene portends a 100% mortality rate.

Hydrocele

KEY PRESENTATION/CLINICAL FEATURES

- Fluid collection between the visceral and peritoneal layers of tunica vaginalis of the scrotum or along the spermatic cord.
- Causes are:
  - idiopathic—commonest
  - reactive collection secondary to infection; trauma; neoplasia (any inflammatory condition of the scrotum or its contents)
- Fluid trans-illuminates with torch and is usually painless.
- May be asymptomatic or have symptoms related to secondary cause.

INVESTIGATIONS

Depend on whether secondary cause is thought likely.

Imaging

Depends on suspected cause: scrotal ultrasound to confirm diagnosis or look for secondary causes.

MANAGEMENT

- Depends on cause.
- Indications to consider intervention for hydroceles include:
  - inability to distinguish from indirect inguinal hernia
  - failure of resolution after reasonable period of observation
  - unable to assess testis reliably
  - hydroceles secondary to disease (infection, tumour)
  - patient preference.

Paraphimosis

KEY PRESENTATION/CLINICAL FEATURES

- Inability to retract the pulled-back foreskin over the head of the penis in uncircumcised males, producing oedema and venous obstruction.
- May occur in elderly uncircumcised males who have the foreskin pulled back for catheterisation and it is then not retracted afterwards.
- Cannot occur in circumcised males.

INVESTIGATIONS

None are usually required.

MANAGEMENT

- Consider the need for procedural sedation before attempting retraction (penile nerve block using lignocaine *without adrenaline* is an alternative; inject around base of penis).
- Apply ice packs for 5+ minutes, then use lignocaine gel lubricant and gentle *continuous* traction (over minutes if needed), holding the shaft of the penis and slowly retracting the foreskin.
- If unsuccessful, involve urology for surgical correction.

COMPLICATIONS

- Venous obstruction leading to infarction, necrosis.
- Urethral obstruction secondary to swelling.

Pearls/Pitfalls/Controversies

- Always return the foreskin to its original position after examination/catheterisation of uncircumcised males.

Phimosis

KEY PRESENTATION/CLINICAL FEATURES

- Inability to pull the foreskin back from the head of penis; can produce secondary ballooning of foreskin, urine retention, balanitis
- Congenital or acquired (from recurrent balanitis and adhesions).

MANAGEMENT

- Congenital phimosis usually resolves with age.
- Urgent circumcision for acquired cases.

Priapism

- Low flow/veno-occlusive (commonest): painful, reduced venous outflow can lead to ischaemia, thrombosis from venous stasis; late erectile dysfunction occurs.
- High flow/arterial (rare): arterial laceration (can be trauma from direct injection), leading to uncontrolled inflow of arterial blood; long-term erectile dysfunction is unlikely.

KEY PRESENTATION/CLINICAL FEATURES

Causes

- Toxicological:
  - — cavernosus injection (prostaglandin E_1 or papaverine)
  - — psychotropics—phenothiazines (e.g. chlorpromazine), butyrophenones (e.g. haloperidol); selective serotonin reuptake inhibitors (SSRIs)
  - — rarely, sildenafil (Viagra), tadalafil (Cialis), vardenafil (Levitra); cocaine; anticoagulants; tetrahydrocannabinol (THC)
- Haematological: sickle-cell anaemia (in children too), leukaemia, myeloma, polycythaemia.
- Spinal trauma.
- Idiopathic.
- Trauma causing arterial laceration (high-flow).

HISTORY

- Low-flow priapism is painful.
- High-flow priapism painless, associated trauma.

EXAMINATION

- Look for trauma.
- Urine retention.
- Ask about penile implants.
- Low-flow form will usually have a soft glans; high-flow will have an engorged glans.

INVESTIGATIONS

Bedside

Consider intra-cavernous blood gas if unsure if low- or high-flow (high-flow will be arterial)—involve urologist first.

Pathology

Consider investigating possible underlying causes such as haematological malignancy or sickle-cell anaemia.

Imaging

Duplex ultrasound for high-flow; look for arterial laceration, then angiography can be used to embolise.

MANAGEMENT

Urgent involvement of urology.

Pharmacological

Trial pseudoephedrine 60 mg PO.

Needle aspiration

(Urologist should perform or supervise.)

- Aseptic technique
- Consider procedural sedation
- Local anaesthesia technique:
  - direct infiltration
  - penile nerve block (inject around base of penis; never use adrenaline-containing solutions).
- Insert 23-gauge butterfly needle laterally at 2 or 10 o'clock and at a 45° angle to the skin (not perpendicular to the skin, to avoid damage to the urethra and dorsal neurovascular bundle). Aspirate slowly (often ~30 mL aspirated); only one side needs to be aspirated, as shunts connect both sides.
- If retumescent, then agents such as
  - adrenaline (1 mL of 1:10000 [= 100 microg] diluted in 10 mL normal saline, giving 5 mL at a time)
  - ephedrine (30 mg diluted in 10 mL of normal saline, giving 1.5 mg at a time)

  can be injected directly, but a cardiac-monitored environment is needed and they should be avoided in patients who will have an increased risk of complications with these agents being absorbed systemically. Only consider use of these agents in consultation with a urologist.

COMPLICATIONS

- Penile ischaemia/necrosis
- Long-term erectile dysfunction.

Pearls/Pitfalls/Controversies

- Involve a urologist with all patients.
- Consider underlying causes and the need to look for them.
- Warn the patient about potential erectile dysfunction.

Prostate disease

PROSTATITIS

Clinical features

- Causes: *E. coli* is commonest.
- Increased urine frequency; urine retention; perineal or low back pain.
- Fever; tender, enlarged prostate.

Investigations

- Urinalysis
- MSU
- FBC, EUC; blood cultures if septic and unwell
- CT of pelvis with IV contrast can have characteristic findings.

Management

- Antibiotics as for UTI (see management of UTIs, below)
- Analgesia.

BENIGN PROSTATE HYPERTROPHY

Clinical features

- Prostatism: difficulty initiating urine stream, poor urine stream, inadequate emptying, post-void dribbling, nocturia.
- Very enlarged bladders can develop when there is a chronic degree of urine retention with bladder-wall stretching.
- Usually presents to the ED with urine retention or UTI.

Investigations

- Urinalysis ± MSU
- EUC, consider PSA (prostate-specific antigen—can be elevated in prostatitis), digital examination

Management

- For acute retention: see section on urine retention, below.
- Urologist follow-up is required.

Complications

- Chronic urine retention causing hypertrophied enlarged bladder and renal impairment.
- If patient presents post-TURP (trans-urethral resection of prostate), issues include:
  - bleeding
  - infection
  - post-TURP syndrome: hyponatraemia with confusion

(*pto*)

- impotence
- retrograde ejaculation.

PROSTATE CANCER

- Adenocarcinoma in > 95% of cases; peripheral gland involvement in 70%.
- Metastases: osteoblastic (not lytic) to the lumbosacral area, pelvis, spinal cord, ribs, thoracic spine, brain.
- Consider cord compression in these patients if they present with gait instability, urine retention or constipation, lower-limb weakness.

Renal/ureteric calculus

KEY PRESENTATION/CLINICAL FEATURES

- Typically occurs between 20 and 50 years of age, though can also occur in children; it is commoner in men (~3:1).
- Risk factors are dehydration, family history, inflammatory bowel disease, diseases associated with hypercalcaemia or hyperuricaemia, myeloproliferative disorders.

HISTORY

- Sudden, severe flank pain radiating to the groin or testis with nausea, vomiting.
- Patient is restless, unable to keep still and prefers to stand.
- Lower ureteric stones can present with ill-defined lower pain and an extreme desire to pass urine when the bladder is empty—i.e. may present with retention but without urine in bladder.

EXAMINATION

- Pallor, fever if infection present.
- Patient can be tachycardic, hypertensive from pain.
- There is usually a lack of abdominal tenderness; if found to be peritonitic on examination, look for differential diagnoses.

DIFFERENTIAL DIAGNOSIS

- Ruptured abdominal aortic aneurysm (AAA): around 40% can present with haematuria; suspect if it is a first presentation of flank pain in an older patient (> 60 years).
- Pyelonephritis, testicular torsion, ovarian torsion.
- Gastrointestinal causes: diverticulitis, retrocaecal appendix, pancreatitis, bowel obstruction.
- Herpes zoster in L1 nerve root.

- Musculoskeletal cause: radicular back pain from disc prolapse.
- Opioid-seeking patient.

INVESTIGATIONS

Bedside

- Urinalysis: 90% of cases have micro- or macroscopic haematuria—meaning that 10% have *negative* urinalysis results.
- In AAA, ultrasound study by accredited staff.

Pathology

- MSU
- FBC
- EUC, liver function tests (LFTs), lipase, beta-hCG
- Consider calcium and uric acid levels if there is recurrent calculus.

Imaging

- Stones are 90% radio-opaque (uric acid stones are radiolucent).
- CT KUB: sensitivity 97%, specificity 96%; reveals other diagnoses (e.g. AAA).
- Plain KUB: sensitivity about 58–62%. The ureter runs across the tips of the transverse processes of L2–L5, the upper and lower sacroiliac joint and next to the ischial spine; the ureteric orifice is medial, near the coccyx.
- Intravenous pyelogram (IVP): sensitivity approximately 96%; can reveal size and assess for renal function; use if CT KUB is not available.
- Renal ultrasound: sensitivity approximately 70%, but operator-dependent; stone size cannot be estimated.
- MRI: no radiation, therefore possible use in pregnant patients. (Note that the effects of magnetic exposure on the fetus in the 1st trimester are not known; a risk/benefit discussion with the radiologist and the patient is advised.) There may be a lack of availability; MRI can miss small stones and is an expensive technique.

MANAGEMENT

Supportive

- Analgesia with combination opioids and NSAIDs
  - opioids: faster-acting initial analgesia, e.g. morphine 2.5–5 mg; titrate to response; do not use pethidine
  - indomethacin 100 mg 12-hourly PR (check for contraindications).

- Intravenous fluids if patient is dehydrated or septic; note that use of greater than maintenance IV fluids to assist stone passage has no credible evidence to support the practice.
- Alpha$_1$-blockers (e.g. tamsulosin) reportedly can augment stone expulsion rate; consider if stone of a size likely to pass, uncomplicated and distally located; liaise with urology.

Specific

- Stone size and likelihood of being passed within 1 month:
  - < 5 mm will pass itself in 90% of cases
  - 4–6 mm, > 50% will pass
  - > 7 mm, 5% will pass.
- Stone location:
  - proximal ureter, 25% will pass
  - mid-ureter, 45% will pass
  - distal ureter, 70% will pass.
- Interventions include:
  - percutaneous radiological nephrostomy: drains obstructed kidney
  - ureteroscopic removal/stent
  - open surgery for large stones
  - extra-corporeal shockwave lithotripsy (ESWL)
- Renal calculi:
  - if < 2 cm can be treated with ESWL; larger renal calculi are best managed with percutaneous nephrolithotomy
- Ureteric calculi:
  - if in upper half of ureter, can be pushed back into kidney for ESWL
  - if in lower half of ureter, can be removed with ureteroscope.
- Advise admission if:
  - patient is septic (or has fever with temperatures > 37.5°C)
  - there is impaired renal function (creatinine > 0.2 mmol/L)
  - there is persisting pain
  - stone is > 5 mm
  - patient has a single kidney
  - there is extravasation of contrast from renal pelvis on imaging (rare); this indicates high-grade obstruction.
- Advise discharge if:
  - patient is pain-free and stone is < 5 mm
  - none of the above criteria for admission are present
  - can get patient to strain urine with fine sieve to see if stone is passed.

- Arrange follow-up with urologist—liaise locally regarding type of repeat imaging: either plain KUB or repeat CT KUB to ensure passage of stone.

COMPLICATIONS

- Obstructed kidney (can be painless): this is an emergency requiring urgent intervention
- Urosepsis
- Renal impairment
- Bleeding.

Pearls/Pitfalls/Controversies

- *Always consider AAA in patients with 'first-presentation' flank pain who are older than 60 years.*
- Assess scrotum for testicular torsion.
- Urgent intervention is needed for an obstructed kidney—either radiological or surgical drainage.

Testicular torsion

KEY PRESENTATION/CLINICAL FEATURES

- Peak incidence is in newborns and in puberty or a young teenager; 75% occur under the age of 20 years and it is rare after age 30—but can occur at any age, as the anatomical abnormality (enlarged tunica vaginalis preventing testicular anchoring—'bell-clapper deformity') that predisposes is present from birth.
- Presents with lymphatic and venous obstruction followed by arterial occlusion.
- Complete torsion is a 360° turn or greater; the more turns, the shorter the time to ischaemia.

HISTORY

- Sudden severe lower abdominal or scrotal pain in a previously well patient; often nausea, vomiting present.
- Some patients report previous short-lived (< 2 hours) episodes of the same type of pain.
- Can present without sudden onset of pain.

EXAMINATION

- Fever can occur uncommonly.
- Always assess testes in paediatric patients with abdominal pain or a distressed, crying infant.

- Look for a high-riding, abnormally lying, swollen, exquisitely tender testis (only with 360° torsion) with scrotal swelling.
- The presence of cremasteric reflex is an *unreliable sign* to exclude torsion.
- There may be minimal findings if torsion is < 360°.

DIFFERENTIAL DIAGNOSIS

- Epididymo-orchitis
- Torsion of testicular appendage
- Strangulated hernia
- Haematocele/hydrocele
- Henoch–Schönlein purpura (vasculitis)
- Idiopathic scrotal oedema.

INVESTIGATIONS

Surgical exploration when torsion is the most likely diagnosis.

Bedside

Urinalysis.

Imaging

Colour Doppler ultrasound:

- Compare blood flow with that on 'normal' side; if reduced, suspect torsion. An untwisted testis can have hyperaemia.
- Sensitivity is quoted to be as low as 82% up to 88.9% sensitive and 98.8% specific; the technique is operator-dependent. Note that *normal flow does not exclude torsion.*

MANAGEMENT

- Surgical exploration: if testis is viable, then orchidopexy should be performed; the other testicle should be fixed as well.
- If urological services are unavailable within a reasonable timeframe (< 6 hours), then perform manual untwisting (turn right testicle clockwise, left testicle anticlockwise) under procedural sedation. If successful, patient will have reduced or no pain. All patients still need urological assessment at the time of presentation.

COMPLICATIONS

The salvage rate depends on the number of turns and the time to surgery.

- Salvage rate is 100% if surgery is < 4 hours from onset; 80–90% if within 6 hours; 20–50% at 10–24 hours.

- Despite salvage, long-term damage such as reduced volume, sperm, motility can occur.

Pearls/Pitfalls/Controversies

- *Time-critical disease*: in a 'classic' presentation (sudden-onset pain and vomiting in a previously well asymptomatic patient of typical age with supportive clinical findings), the patient needs urgent transfer to the operating theatre.
- Ultrasound investigation should not delay clinical urological review in suspicious cases; *it does not exclude torsion ultimately* and all features of the patient's presentation need to be considered.
- When the duration of symptoms points to likely testicular infarction, the patient still needs urgent urological assessment.
- Can occur in previously repaired torsion (secondary to absorbable suture use, which is less commonly used).

TORSION OF TESTICULAR APPENDAGE

- Peak incidence 10–13 years of age; a common cause of scrotal pain at age 3–13 years.
- An embryological peduncle < 5 mm with no function can twist.
- The 'blue dot sign' is a tender blue spot on scrotum viewed with trans-illumination.
- Management is operative or, if certain of diagnosis, conservative. Always involve urology.

Urinary tract infections (UTIs)

Include: asymptomatic bacteriuria, urethritis, cystitis, pyelonephritis.

CAUSES

- > 90% of cases are caused by Enterobacteriaceae (e.g. *E. coli*) and *Enterococcus faecalis* (previously classified as *Streptococcus faecalis*).
- *Staphylococcus saprophyticus* (skin-commensal) is a cause of simple cystitis in young sexually active females.
- Consider non *E. coli* infection post-instrumentation or after prolonged recent hospital admission.

Risk factors

- Frequent sexual intercourse
- Previous UTI
- Pregnancy
- Foreign body in urinary tract (e.g. calculus, catheter)

(*pto*)

- Diabetes mellitus
- Anatomical/functional urinary abnormality
- Immunosuppressive state (e.g. HIV, transplantation, chemotherapy, corticosteroid use)

KEY PRESENTATION/CLINICAL FEATURES

Urethritis

History

Dysuria.

Examination

Urethral discharge.

Cystitis

History

- Dysuria, increased urine frequency
- Suprapubic pain

Examination

- Patient should look well.
- There may be suprapubic tenderness.
- Obviously blood-stained urine can be present.

Pyelonephritis

History

- Dysuria, increased urine frequency; sometimes lack of urinary symptoms
- Flank or lower back pain
- Nausea/vomiting

Examination

- Fever; assess whether patient looks well or unwell.
- Assess for features of systemic inflammatory response syndrome (SIRS): respiratory rate > 20/min or pCO_2 < 30 mmHg; heart rate > 90 bpm; temperature < 36°C or > 38°C; WCC < 4 or >12×10^9/L.
- Hypotension or relative hypotension in elderly patient (e.g. BP < 110 mmHg in 80-year-old).
- Flank tenderness or abdominal tenderness.

DIFFERENTIAL DIAGNOSIS

Pyuria

Previous recent antibiotics; renal calculi; non-specific urethritis in males; renal tract neoplasm; catheter; prostatitis; renal tuberculosis (TB).

Urethritis

Urethral trauma.

Cystitis

Vulvovaginitis.

Pyelonephritis

- Renal: calculus
- Gastrointestinal tract: appendicitis, diverticulitis, acute abdomen of any cause
- Gynaecological: ovarian cyst rupture, endometriosis
- Vascular: AAA rupture
- Musculoskeletal: radicular pain

INVESTIGATIONS

Regarding nitrites on urinalysis

- Only coliform bacteria reduce urinary nitrate to nitrite (*Enterococcus* spp and *S. saprophyticus* do not).
- Overall there can be a high false-negative rate (i.e. patient has UTI but no nitrites on urinalysis).

Urethritis

Bedside

Urinalysis.

Pathology

- Swab for STD culture
- MSU and chlamydia/gonorrhoea PCR

Cystitis

Bedside

- Urinalysis:
  - — leucocyte esterase test for WCC: reported 48–86% sensitive, 17–93% specific
  - — positive predictive value in symptomatic patients is 50%; negative predictive value is 92%. (Is a reasonable screening test if negative; however, in elderly individuals do not rely on it if UTI is considered a possible diagnosis.)
  - — if nitrites are positive, sensitivity for urinalysis increases.

Pathology

MSU:

- Significant bacteriuria is > 10^5 bacteria/mL (colony-forming units/mL); this indicates infection rather than contamination.

- Asymptomatic bacteriuria is the above amount grown, but no symptoms in patient.
- Symptomatic patient with bacterial count > 10^5 has a very high probability of infection.
- Asymptomatic patient with bacterial count > 10^5 and pregnant should be treated.
- Asymptomatic geriatric patient with significant bacteriuria is common in functionally impaired elderly people and should not be treated.

Pyelonephritis

Bedside

Urinalysis.

Pathology

- MSU
- FBC, EUC, beta-hCG in women ± LFTs; ± lipase
- Blood cultures

Imaging

- Consider if calculus or obstruction is suspected
- In ongoing fevers despite appropriate antibiotics
- Renal ultrasound can be performed as an outpatient in stable patients with a very likely diagnosis; assesses for abscess, hydronephrosis, anatomical abnormalities.
- CT KUB if calculus is suspected

MANAGEMENT

Urethritis

Fully treat if STD is suspected.

Cystitis

- Antibiotics
  - send urine for culture, but no need for any pathology or imaging in these patients
  - no need for consideration of IV antibiotics.
- Non-pregnant females:
  - trimethoprim 300 mg daily for 3 days
    OR
  - cephalexin 500 mg 12-hourly for 5 days
    OR
  - nitrofurantoin 100 mg 12-hourly for 5 days
    OR

— amoxycillin + clavulanate 500 mg + 125 mg 12-hourly for 5 days.

- Pregnant females (doses as above):
  — cephalexin (class A)
  OR
  — nitrofurantoin (class A)
  OR
  — amoxycillin + clavulanate (class B1).
- Males:
  — trimethoprim 300 mg daily for 14 days
  OR
  — cephalexin 500 mg 12-hourly for 14 days
  OR
  — amoxycillin + clavulanate 500 mg + 125 mg 12-hourly for 14 days.

Pyelonephritis

Supportive care

- If patient is unwell or has features of sepsis:
  — IV fluids
    - if severe sepsis, use 10–20 mL/kg normal saline
    - if ongoing significant hypotension, consider inotropes (noradrenaline 0.05 microg/kg/min) after at least 2000–3000 mL of fluid challenge and then ongoing fluid resuscitation with initiation of inotropes.

  — aim as a guideline in sepsis that MAP > 65 mmHg, urine output > 0.5 mL/kg/h
  — early IV antibiotics (within 1 hour).
- Analgesia.

Specific antibiotics

- If pyelonephritis mild with low-grade fever and no vomiting:
  — amoxycillin + clavulanate 875 mg + 125 mg 12-hourly for 10 days
  OR
  — cephalexin 500 mg 6-hourly for 10 days
  OR
  — trimethoprim 300 mg nocte for 10 days.
- If resistant to above or *Pseudomonas aeruginosa* is the cause:
  — norfloxacin 400 mg 12-hourly for 10 days
  OR
  — ciprofloxacin 500 mg 12-hourly for 10 days.

- If severe, use:
  - gentamicin 4–6 mg/kg for 1 dose, then determine dosing interval for maximum 1 or 2 doses based on renal function (see Antibiotic Guidelines 2010; www.ciap.health.nsw.gov.au/home.html for details of gentamicin doses)
    plus
  - amoxycillin or ampicillin 2 g 6-hourly IV.
- If patient is hypersensitive to penicillin, gentamicin alone is usually sufficient.
- If gentamicin is contraindicated, use as a *single* drug:
  - ceftriaxone 1 g daily IV
    OR
  - cefotaxime 1 g 8-hourly IV.
- The above regimens do not adequately cover for *P. aeruginosa* or enterococci.
- Change to PO administration when able; total duration of treatment should be 10–14 days, then send urine for culture 48 hours after finishing antibiotics.

COMPLICATIONS

- Septic shock
- Renal abscess
- Bacteraemia and seeding of other organs
- Secondary stone formation from certain bacteria: *Proteus* or *Klebsiella* (struvite/staghorn calculus).

Pearls/Pitfalls/Controversies

- In older patients, if suspecting UTI in differential diagnosis always send for MSU—do not rely on urinalysis.
- Tachycardia, postural BP drop or posturally related lightheadedness can be features of sepsis in a reasonably well-looking patient: these findings warrant longer observation or admission.
- Treat asymptomatic bacteriuria in a pregnant woman to reduce risk of infection and the increased risk of secondary miscarriage.

Urine retention

KEY PRESENTATION/CLINICAL FEATURES

Causes

- Obstruction: prostatomegaly; rectal constipation; blood clot; urethral stricture; post-TURP bladder neck stenosis; recent instrumentation.

- Neurogenic: spinal injury; cauda equina syndrome (*painless* retention).
- Toxicological (in younger patients): any drug with anti-cholinergic effects (e.g. antipsychotics, tricyclic antidepressants); alpha-adrenergics.
- Infection: UTI.
- Painful genital condition: herpes; trauma.

HISTORY

- Look for underlying cause.
- Sudden onset, preceding urinary symptoms, or worsening prostatism.

EXAMINATION

- Degree of bladder distension
- Rectal examination to assess constipation, prostate size, perianal sensation, tone.
- Always carry out a detailed neurological assessment to consider a neurological cause, including saddle sensation, tone.

DIFFERENTIAL DIAGNOSIS

- Pelvic haematoma will present as a suprapubic mass and retention, but the bladder is empty and no urine will be obtained from suprapubic puncture.
- Any cause of lower abdominal peritonitis will give the impression of retention, but bladder is empty from anuria. Irrigate 50 mL in and out of an indwelling urinary catheter (IDC) to confirm correct IDC position and emptiness of bladder.
- Lower abdominal mass, such as diverticular phlegmon, ruptured AAA or pelvic malignancy.

INVESTIGATIONS

Bedside

- Urinalysis for UTI.
- Bladder scanner if in doubt: normal bladder capacity is approx. 400 mL maximum; patients with a chronic degree of retention from prostate disease can have larger capacities, > 1 L.

Pathology

EUC, FBC, coagulation profile if patient is on anticoagulants.

Imaging

Urgently indicated if a neurogenic cause is being considered (MRI of spine).

MANAGEMENT

- Catheterisation options
  - IDC: try 16F then the less-flexible 18F; keep a firm hold on the shaft of the penis with slight traction upwards, perpendicular to the supine patient. Always note residual volume; rapid decompression of volume of > 1000 mL can cause bladder-wall bleeding.
  - Suprapubic catheter (SPC): liaise with urology before attempting insertion; should be done under ultrasound guidance; involve senior staff.
  - Only urology specialists should ever attempt introducer-based catheterisation.
- Patients can usually be considered for discharge with a leg bag and education with referral to a urologist/urology trial of void clinic.
  - Regarding trial of void (TOV):
    - measure pre- and post-void residual volumes, which should be < 150 mL.
- Clot-based retention:
  - Patients have frank haematuria and passing of clots, and usually a history of prostate or bladder cancer or a recent urological procedure.
  - Always assess if patient is on anticoagulation and assess the risk/benefit of reversing it if needed; consult appropriately.
  - Consult with urology.
  - Catheterisation should occur with a 3-way catheter (larger-diameter, stiffer catheters with a 60 mL balloon) placed using the same technique as for a normal IDC—avoid overly aggressive attempts. Irrigation helps dissolve or wash out clots.
  - Consult urology or urology ward about protocol for bladder irrigation.
- Investigate/manage any underlying condition.

COMPLICATIONS

- Transient loss of bladder tone occurs after significant retention; this can take 1–3 days to normalise, therefore the catheter should be left in for at least that long before TOV if patient has acute retention; in patients who have acute on chronic retention, the IDC should be left in situ until urology follow-up.

- Renal impairment
- UTI
- Post-obstructive polyuria:
  - occurs in patients who present with acute on chronic retention
  - requires admission under urology
  - give IV fluids as per urology, but as a guide the IV fluid rate needs to match the prior hour's urine output plus maintenance if NBM (nil by mouth)
  - EUC needs to be closely monitored.

Pearls/Pitfalls/Controversies

- Always do formal neurological assessment in patients with acute retention.

Urological trauma

KIDNEY

Key presentation/clinical features

- The kidney is the commonest organ injured, mostly through blunt trauma (< 15% is penetrating).
- Markers for significant injury include:
  - haemodynamically unstable patient
  - loin tenderness
  - macroscopic haematuria.

Differential diagnosis

For haematuria in trauma: lower urinary tract trauma (ureter, bladder, urethra).

Investigations

Bedside

Urinalysis

- *If microscopic haematuria:*
  - perform urgent imaging if there is:
    - hypotension at any time from trauma
    - suggestive injury (fall from > 3 m, flank bruising, direct blow, injury from deceleration > 60 km/h)
    - suggestive associated injury (fractured lumbar vertebrae; fractured lower ribs)
  - in blunt trauma with low suspicion of urological trauma, there is no need for imaging but urinalysis should be

repeated in 1–2 weeks to check for resolution; if there is ongoing haematuria, then consider CT KUB with IV contrast to assess for non-traumatic, pre-existing renal disease
  - in penetrating trauma, always perform imaging.
- *If macroscopic haematuria:*
  - always investigate
  - can be from any part of urinary tract.

Pathology

- FBC, EUC
- Blood group and hold

Imaging

- IV-contrast-enhanced CT KUB: assess the contralateral functioning kidney; delayed or absent function in affected kidney; contrast extravasation.
- IVP if CT is not available: assess contralateral kidney function and possible ureteric involvement.
- MRI: use if available in those with contrast allergy; results are as good as CT.
- A negative ultrasound does not exclude renal injury.

Management

Supportive care

- Trauma assessment to look for other injury
- Trauma resuscitation if required
- Analgesia
- Tetanus if a penetrating injury

Specific care

- Conservative
  - for stable patients with functioning kidney and minor extravasation.
- Surgical exploration acutely if:
  - unstable patient due to haemorrhage
  - major extravasation due to shattered or bisected kidney
  - renal peduncle disruption
  - continued subacute haemorrhage
  - urinoma with sepsis.

Complications

- Haemorrhagic shock
- Renal impairment
- Kidney loss

URETER

- Rare; in children trauma to the ureter an occur from deceleration injury.
- Usually penetrating and associated with more-severe injuries.
- Diagnosed on IV-contrast-enhanced CT KUB.
- Usually diagnosed at laparotomy for other injuries.

BLADDER

Key presentation/clinical features

- The majority of bladder injuries are associated with pelvic fracture; about 10% of pelvic fractures occur with bladder injury.
- Occasionally a stab wound or seat belt injury will rupture a full bladder.
- Most injuries are to the dome; blunt injuries can result in large lacerations.
- Suspect based on mechanism; displaced pelvic fractures.
- The patient may have difficulty voiding.
- Suprapubic bruising, tenderness, peritonism.
- Haematuria.

Differential diagnosis

Frank haematuria from kidney or ureter or urethra.

Investigations

Bedside

Urinalysis: macroscopic haematuria in the majority of cases.

Pathology

- EUC, FBC
- Blood group and hold

Imaging

- Retrograde cystogram: 350 mL of water-soluble contrast introduced into the bladder, then look for extravasation (indicates rupture), both during administration and after drainage.
- CT cystography: assess surrounding structures.
- Perform IV-contrast-enhanced CT KUB to assess the upper urinary tract.

Management

- Manage all aspects of the trauma patient—prioritise injuries and need for intervention.

- If no blood at meatus: gently pass a 16F or 18F catheter (IDC is preferred over SPC).
- If blood at meatus, a urethrogram must be performed first before catheterisation.
- Minor extraperitoneal rupture may be managed with catheter drainage alone.
- Bladder body injury can be managed with prolonged use of an IDC.
- Major extraperitoneal rupture, all intraperitoneal rupture and dome injuries must be explored and repaired.

URETHRAL TRAUMA

Key presentation

- Consider blunt (fall astride) injury or penetrating injury.
- Is more common than bladder trauma.
- The risk in males with anterior pelvic fractures including pubic symphysis diastasis increases with the number of pubic rami fractured and the degree of displacement (especially displaced superior pubic ramus fracture), and also if there is sacroiliac involvement with the pubic ramus fracture.
- In females, usually occurs only with major pubic symphysis diastasis; often with associated vaginal bleeding.
- No displaced pelvic ring fracture makes urethral injury very unlikely in the absence of direct trauma.

Clinical features

- Urine retention; frank haematuria; scrotal/penile 'butterfly bruising'; high-riding prostate.
- Some patients have no initial physical signs, then blood at meatus.

Investigations

Retrograde urethrogram to assess for complete tear.

Management

- If there is high clinical suspicion, displaced anterior pelvic fractures on X-ray or frank haematuria—consult urology urgently, and do not pass an IDC.
- For minor/incomplete injury: IDC is carefully placed under radiological control.
- For major injury: SPC and urethroplasty/re-anastomosis to repair.
- Penetrating urethral trauma is very unlikely if all the following are present: no meatal blood; normal urination or easy catheter insertion; normal urinalysis.

Complications

- Urine retention
- Strictures
- Haemorrhage

Pearls/Pitfalls/Controversies

- Always involve urology if there is high clinical suspicion of urethral trauma or displaced anterior pelvic fractures, before passing an IDC.
- Successful IDC insertion does not exclude small urethral perforation.

SCROTUM/TESTIS

Key presentation/clinical features

- In paediatric patients, consider non-accidental injury.
- Intratesticular bleeding can lead to intracapsular pressure rise and subsequent necrosis.

History

- Mechanism
- Pain

Examination

- Exclude other, more significant associated trauma
- Scrotal bruising and swelling
- Assess for testicle size, tenderness, lie
- Consider penile, bladder or pelvis trauma depending on mechanism

Injury patterns

- Scrotal wall haematoma
- Tunica vaginalis haematoma (haematocele)
- Intratesticular haematoma (or subcapsular)
- Testicular rupture

Investigations

Bedside

Urinalysis.

Imaging

Colour Doppler ultrasound: assess degree of injury. This technique can underestimate; a normal ultrasound does not rule out the need for exploration.

Management

- Supportive
  - ice bags, analgesia.
- Surgical exploration
  - if uncertain about the degree of trauma after clinical and ultrasound examination
  - for testicular injury/rupture/haematoma
  - if tunica albuginea disrupted
  - for large haematocele
  - for penetrating trauma.

Complications

Risk of orchidectomy with conservative management for significant injury.

Pearls/Pitfalls/Controversies

- Always involve urology.
- Clinical features cannot exclude rupture.

PENIS

Key presentation/clinical features

- Amputation often self-inflicted or patient was psychotic at the time.
- Fractured penis is traumatic rupture of the corpus cavernosum: the patient hears a loud snap like the breaking of a glass rod, associated with direct injury to the erect penis; it collapses immediately and develops a large swelling on the affected side. Rarely the urethra ruptures as well.

Investigations

Bedside

ECG and venous blood gas if toxicological features are associated.

Pathology

- FBC, blood group and hold if there is significant blood loss.
- Psychiatric- or toxicology-based pathology if indicated.

Imaging

Discuss with urologist.

Management

- Stop ongoing bleeding if present.

- Look for other injury/concomitant overdose if patient is in an abnormal mental state.
- Wrap severed penis if recovered in sterile saline-soaked gauze, place in sterile bag and then put on ice.
- Urgent urology referral ± psychiatric referral is required.
- Suspected fractured penis should be referred urgently to urology for urgent repair.

Complications

- After reattachment: stricture, urethral fistula, skin loss, impotence.
- After fractured penis: if no repair, 50% have impotence and traumatic curvature of the penis.

Pearls/Pitfalls/Controversies

- Manage underling mental health issues if present.

Varicocele

KEY PRESENTATION/CLINICAL FEATURES

- Dilation of the pampiniform plexus of the spermatic cord veins; commoner on left than on right.
- If isolated right-sided varicocele or painful varicocele, look for inferior vena cava obstruction.
- If asymptomatic or a dull ache is felt on standing, can produce testicular atrophy.
- There is an association with men who are infertile.

DIFFERENTIAL DIAGNOSIS

Other scrotal conditions such as epididymitis.

INVESTIGATIONS

Imaging

Ultrasound to assist diagnosis.

MANAGEMENT

- Analgesia; refer to urologist
- Conservative treatment
- Surgical repair

Chapter 20
Burns

Linda Dann

The skin is the largest organ in the body, approximating 15% of bodyweight and 4.9 square metres in an adult. It has a number of functions, which correspond to the rationale of management and the potential complications of burns:

- protection from the environment (infection)
- temperature control (hypothermia)
- fluid control (dehydration and fluid replacement)
- energy control (need for increased caloric intake in larger burns).

The majority of burns occur in the home and affect mainly young men and those at the extremes of age.

Types of burns

- Thermal (including scalds)
- Chemical
- Electrical
- Radiation

Specific other factors

- Eyes: chemicals, flash burns, molten metal
- Extremes of age (< 5 or > 65 years)
- Airway/lung injury—blast injury may be fatal if untreated
- Hands/feet/perineum
- Circumferential burns of limbs or torso
- Burns crossing joints (especially flexor surfaces)
- Deliberate abuse

Assessment of the burns patient

- History of the patient, including any chronic conditions that may affect wound healing such as steroid use, diabetes, etc. Check tetanus status.
- History of the events surrounding the injury, including:
  - time of injury (fluid requirements assessed from this time)

- location of event (in open air, in closed room, etc) to give an indication of concomitant injury including carbon monoxide or toxic fume inhalation, blast injury, trauma from fall, etc.

- Full examination to exclude other injury.
- Assessment of the depth and extent of the burn injury using standard protocols such as Wallace's rule of nines (see Quick Reference section) or the Lund and Browder chart (Fig 20.1).

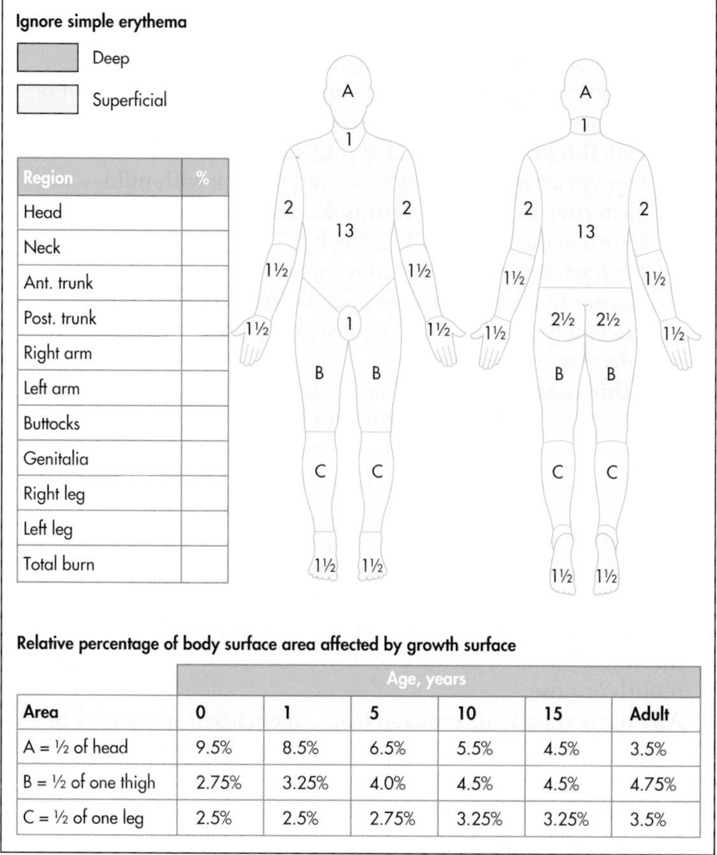

Region	%
Head	
Neck	
Ant. trunk	
Post. trunk	
Right arm	
Left arm	
Buttocks	
Genitalia	
Right leg	
Left leg	
Total burn	

Relative percentage of body surface area affected by growth surface

	Age, years					
Area	**0**	**1**	**5**	**10**	**15**	**Adult**
A = ½ of head	9.5%	8.5%	6.5%	5.5%	4.5%	3.5%
B = ½ of one thigh	2.75%	3.25%	4.0%	4.5%	4.5%	4.75%
C = ½ of one leg	2.5%	2.5%	2.75%	3.25%	3.25%	3.5%

Figure 20.1 Lund and Browder chart: estimation of extent of burn

Assessment of depth and extent of burn

EXTENT OF BURN

There are two methods of assessment of the extent of burns:

1. Wallace's rule of nines chart—varies with age, is good for quick assessment.
2. Lund and Browder chart—allows for age variation, is more accurate.

DEPTH OF BURN

The utilisation of terms such as first-, second- and third-degree has been largely replaced by:

- **Superficial.** Refers to epidermal reddening, e.g. sunburn. Extremely painful, no blistering, skin is red and heals spontaneously without scarring, usually within 1 week.
  Note: Superficial burns are not counted in assessing the extent of burn injury.
- **Partial-thickness.** Subdivided into superficial and deep:
  - *Superficial partial-thickness*—red or pink with mild blistering, as involves dermis. Extremely painful but heals spontaneously within 1–2 weeks.
  - *Deep partial-thickness*—may be initially red, then white. Harder to assess. Involves deep layers of dermis and is extremely painful. May require skin grafting to prevent infection and scarring.
- **Full-thickness.** Involves all layers of skin including blood vessels, nerve endings, hair follicles and the dermis. As a result, they are insensate, dry, white, translucent or even charred. All but the smallest (< 1 cm) will require skin grafting.

General management

- Remove the victim from the source of injury.
- Provide supplemental oxygen if there is any possibility of blast injury, smoke or toxic-fume inhalations, stridor, hoarseness of the voice, burns to the face or any evidence of soot around the mouth or nose.
- Any burned patient removed from an enclosed space may be assumed to have airway injuries even when no burns are evident.
- Adherent material should not be removed at this stage.
- Antibiotics are not required prophylactically—only if specific infection is demonstrated.

ANALGESIA

Superficial and partial-thickness burns are extremely painful.

- In minor or localised burns, application of cold water (for at least 30 minutes) and dressings alleviate pain.
- Simple oral analgesia may be required at home.
- Inability to control pain is an indication for admission, particularly in children.
- In more severe cases, initial management includes narcotic analgesia. Narcotics should be given intravenously and liberally, e.g. morphine 0.1 mg/kg initially, then titrated to response. Large doses are often required.

OTHER FACTORS

Airway/lung injury/inhalation injury

This may be caused by carbon monoxide or toxic fumes such as cyanide. Supplemental oxygen is required for all but minor burns and in all patients in whom there is actual or suspected inhalation injury (include patients with no evidence of burn but where there has been a fire in an enclosed space).

Intubation may be required early in patients with cyanosis, respiratory distress, stridor or hoarseness. Anticipate lung injury or swelling of the airway if facial burns are evident.

Circulation

Where possible, IV lines should be inserted through unburned skin. Fluid requirements may be high in extensive burns, at 2–4 mL/kg/% burn in the first 24 hours. Compartment syndrome or restriction of chest movement due to circumferential burns may require escharotomy as an emergency procedure.

Gastrointestinal tract

Gastric stasis or ileus can be assumed in all cases of > 20% burns. Except in minor burns, all patients should be nil orally until assessed regarding the need for urgent surgery.

Tetanus status

The usual protocols apply.

Fluid requirements

Significant fluid resuscitation after burns is required to maintain circulating volume and an adequate urine output. Volume losses can be anticipated and calculated from:

- patient weight
- extent of burn (body surface area—BSA)
- time from original burn injury.

There are a number of formulae available. The recommended fluid replacement and maintenance from the NSW Health burns transfer document are reproduced in Box 20.1.

Box 20.1 Recommended fluid replacement and maintenance in burns patients

Replacement

- In the first 24 hours after burn injury, 2–4 mL × kg × %burn BSA of Hartmann's solution.
- Give half of this amount in the first 8 hours and the remainder over 16 hours.

Maintenance

- Adult: replacement plus 2–3 L daily of maintenance fluid. Add potassium as required in maintenance for losses due to muscle/skin damage.
- Child < 30 kg: 4% dextrose + N/5 saline or 3.75% dextrose + N/4 saline according to weight

Urine output

- Adult: aim for 0.5–2 mL/kg/h
- Child: aim for 1 mL/kg/h if < 30 kg

NSW Severe Burn Injury Service. Burn transfer guidelines. NSW Department of Health; revised August 2004

Admission and transfer to specialised burns unit

Nowadays, patients aged 15–44 years have at least a 50% chance of surviving a 70% total BSA burn if treated in a specialist unit.

REFERRAL CRITERIA TO SPECIALISED BURNS UNIT

- Deep burns involving 10% or more of BSA in adults, or 5% BSA or more in children
- Burns involving the face, hands, feet, perineum, flexor joint surfaces
- Any inhalation injury
- Burns with associated injury, major pre-existing disease or suspected child abuse
- Significant chemical or electrical burns

ADMISSION CRITERIA TO GENERAL OR PLASTIC SURGERY UNIT

- Uncontrolled pain, particularly in small children
- Burns greater than 1–2% BSA full-thickness, or 15% BSA (adult) or 10% BSA (children) partial-thickness

Specific burns

THERMAL BURNS

Application of cool water (not ice) to minor burns for a minimum of 30 minutes may alleviate pain and reduce the severity of the injury. This is of no value if applied more than 3 hours after the injury.

If burns are extensive, there is a risk of hypothermia. Unburned areas should be kept warm with thermal blankets where possible.

Scalds are common in children—clothing soaked in hot liquid will cause further damage unless removed or cooled immediately. Adherent material should not be removed at home. Simple oral analgesia may be all that is required if small areas are involved.

Note: Accidental scalds usually have a scatter pattern with areas of unburned skin in between. A clear demarcation line may indicate deliberate abuse in children and in the aged.

CHEMICAL BURNS

Copious amounts of water for at least 20–30 minutes are required to effectively dilute chemicals in the first instance.

There is a risk of further injury from the dilute chemical run-off. Showers and removal of contaminated clothing may have occurred in the workplace.

Specific antidotes, if available, can be used after this initial treatment (see below, hydrofluoric acid).

The severity of chemical injury is related to a number of factors:

- pH of the agent
- concentration of the agent—some concentrated chemicals may produce heat when diluted, leading to thermal as well as chemical injury
- length of contact time
- volume of the agent
- physical form of the agent.

Acids generally produce coagulation necrosis by denaturing protein. This leads to the formation of eschar, which tends to prevent further penetration of the acid. Alkalis act both by denaturing protein and by fat saponification (liquefaction necrosis). As a result, there is no barrier to further penetration and the damage may be more severe.

Hydrofluoric acid (HF) is one of the strongest inorganic acids. Used mainly in industry (e.g. car detailing, glass etching), the commonest exposure is to the hands and fingers. HF penetrates deeply before dissociating to free hydrogen and fluoride ions. The hydrogen ions are corrosive. The fluoride ions (tissue chemical burn) combine with calcium and magnesium to form both insoluble and soluble salts. Systemic fluoride ion poisoning from severe HF burns can lead to hypocalcaemia, hypomagnesaemia, hyperkalaemia and sudden death. Symptoms of tissue destruction and necrosis may be delayed. Initial treatment utilises topical calcium gluconate gel. In severe cases, calcium gluconate may need to be injected subcutaneously or intravenously.

ELECTRICAL BURNS: LIGHTNING, HIGH-VOLTAGE AND DOMESTIC

Refer to Chapter 31, 'Electrical injuries'.

Prevention of infection

DRESSINGS

Necrotic tissue should be removed and the skin cleaned with a non-alcohol-based cleanser prior to the application of dressings.

Dressings alleviate the pain of irritated nerve endings by reducing exposure to air and clothing, resulting in a reduction in exposure to moisture and the risk of infection.

In small, superficial partial-thickness burns

For small, superficial partial-thickness burns, a variety of dressings have been suggested, including transparent dressings and Fixomul®, which do not require a daily change. Other closed 'burns' dressings, such as Vaseline® gauze or other dressings, require daily changes.

Silver sulfadiazine (SSD) cream is generally not recommended for outpatient care, as it may become a potential source of infection after 24–48 hours. Acticoat® is another silver-based product that has replaced SSD in many Australian burns units, but requires specialist application.

In deep partial-thickness and full-thickness burns

For deep partial-thickness and full-thickness burns, excision followed by split skin or full-thickness grafting may be required, unless skin substitutes are available.

Skin substitutes—characteristically the ideals are:

- is readily available
- acts as a barrier to moisture and microorganisms
- is robust, elastic and non-antigenic
- adheres to or integrates into the wound and minimises inflammation to promote healing.

Currently available skin substitutes are:

- biological skin replacements (allografts and xenografts) and bioengineered skin substitutes (autologous cultured and non-cultured skin products and biosynthetic skin substitutes)
- CellSpray, which involves spraying on a suspension of cells cultured from the patient's skin. The live skin cells rapidly proliferate to cover the burned area, and the risk of infection or scarring is reduced. Rejection is minimised as the cells are generated from the patient.

Specific other factors

Circumferential burns. Circulation may be distally compromised in peripheries due to eschar. Reduced chest-wall movement with hypoventilation is possible with circumferential burns to chest. Escharotomy may be required.

Note: Eschar is a result of full-thickness burn and is, therefore, insensate.

Flexor surfaces of joints. Early prevention of contractures is required. Compression garments may be applied in a burns unit.

Hands/feet/perineum. These are specialised skin areas with a high risk of circulatory compromise leading to the development of scars and subsequent deformity.

Child/aged abuse. Any suspicious burns, especially those with unusual appearance or in unusual places. The commonest burn injury in children is scalding.

Eyes. The eye is more resistant to acid than alkali. Copious washout, including eversion of the eyelids, is required to dilute the chemical prior to any specific antidote. Any solid particles must be removed from under the eyelids (especially powdered alkali), as this may otherwise lead to corneal scarring and opacification. pH should be checked to indicate that washout is adequate. Molten metal should be left to cool before removal by an ophthalmologist.

Flash burns. From arc welding, these are acute corneal burns that generally heal without sequelae within 24 hours. The onset of symptoms is delayed for several hours and they are extremely painful. Topical local anaesthetic may be required initially to examine the eye, but should not be used as treatment. Most do not require antibiotic treatment but pilocarpine drops can reduce pain, as can reduction of eye movement by application of eye pads.

Note: Be on the lookout for metallic foreign body overlooked on examination. Try not to pad both eyes if possible. Local anaesthetic puts patient at risk of being unaware of further foreign body. Sunglasses can help.

Extremes of age. In general, the larger the burn and the older the patient, the lower the chance of survival. A child has a relatively larger surface area in the most common burns, such as scalds around the head and face, increasing the risk of complications.

Airway/lung injury. If not immediately evident, blast injury, carbon monoxide or other toxic-chemical inhalation and burns to the upper airway are potentially fatal injuries if overlooked and untreated. A chest X-ray is required in any patient in whom airway injury is suspected.

Any other concerns can always be discussed with local burns unit medical staff.

Note: Burns must be regularly reassessed, as wound management varies according to the depth of the burn. This is often hard to accurately determine on presentation and is often initially underestimated. It becomes more obvious with time.

Online resources

Glattner R. Highlights of the 12th Annual Scientific Assembly of the American Academy of Emergency Medicine. San Antonio, Texas, Feb 2006.
www.medscape.com/viewarticle/528296_1

Chapter 21
Patient transport and retrieval

Neil Ballard

Transferring critically ill or injured patients between hospitals is a potentially dangerous business. Although these transfers occur commonly, care needs to be taken to ensure that they are performed appropriately and safely. The Australasian critical care specialty colleges have issued joint policy documents specifying minimum standards of care required in these circumstances, and these are essential reading for staff involved. (These documents are available on the website of the Australasian College of Emergency Medicine, www.acem.org.au.)

Although intrahospital transport is often thought to be routine, or not thought about at all, the issues raised below with regard to interhospital transport must be considered.

Indications for retrieval

Patients need retrieval or transport to another facility when their needs are beyond the scope of the facility that they are in. They may require a higher level of critical care, specialist surgical or medical services (e.g. neurosurgery or interventional cardiology) or investigations such as an MRI.

It is not unusual for critically ill patients to need transfer because no intensive care unit (ICU) beds are available. Time should be taken to ensure that this is the most appropriate course of action for a particular patient; if the patient is unstable or has a condition requiring urgent treatment and can be managed at the referring hospital, consideration should be given to moving another, more stable patient.

Why the patient is being transferred always needs to be borne in mind, for this will guide the urgency of the transfer. Once it becomes apparent that the condition of the patient is beyond the scope of care of the referring hospital, initiation of the transfer process should commence. In some circumstances this will mean activating a retrieval team even before the patient arrives at hospital, for example in the case of a multi-trauma patient and a small country hospital.

If the patient is being transferred for life-saving care (e.g. urgent neurosurgical decompression of an acute extradural haematoma), the patient needs to be packaged safely but quickly, taking time to do only procedures necessary for transfer. However, in other cases, such as a patient in septic shock being transferred for tertiary ICU care, time can be taken to optimise the patient's condition prior to transfer.

It is important to develop referral systems so that time is not wasted searching for a receiving hospital. These may be state-wide or regional systems, or simply agreements between small hospitals and larger centres. An essential component of such systems is the ability of a practitioner in a small facility to be able to find a receiving hospital and get clinical advice with little difficulty, preferably via a single phone call.

The retrieval team

Interhospital patient transport should be performed by staff with the skills, experience and training to deal with potential problems that may arise during the course of the mission. Within Australasia, there are a number of specialised medical retrieval services which generally follow the staffing model of an experienced critical care doctor (emergency medicine, anaesthetics or ICU) plus either a paramedic or a flight nurse. As well as interhospital transfer of critically ill and injured patients, these services may be involved in pre-hospital care.

If existing hospital staff are utilised in an interhospital transport, they need to be sufficiently experienced and skilled to make decisions and perform resuscitative measures in a potentially difficult environment, and they should be trained and familiar with the equipment that they use. The practice of sending an untrained junior doctor in the back of an ambulance with a critically ill patient can result in an adverse outcome for the patient, and a traumatic experience for the doctor involved.

Equipment

Monitors, syringe pumps and ventilators used in retrieval need to be light, robust and easy to use, with good battery life. Screens should be assessed for ability to be seen in variable light conditions (bright sunlight is particularly problematic) and at angles.

Airway, breathing and circulation equipment, plus appropriate medications and other necessary gear, should be kept in packs. These need to be checked regularly and staff involved in retrieval need to be familiar with the content and layout of these packs.

The retrieval environment

The hospital environment tends to be a familiar one: comfortable climate, controlled lighting, limited personal protection issues. However, interhospital transport of patients exposes both patient and staff to a number of different environments with various challenges.

Hot weather can result in dehydration and difficulty viewing monitors in bright sunlight. It can be difficult to assess a patient rugged up against the cold, or in the dark. Increasing altitude may result in hypoxia and cold. Interaction with unfamiliar staff of varying skills and experience at referring or receiving hospitals can present challenges, as can dealing with ambulance and other emergency services that one may come in contact with during interhospital patient transport. In such environments, the usual cues which alert one to deterioration in the patient's condition may be missed.

All of these elements impact on the patient, but also on the retrieval team. Lack of awareness of these hazards and precautions (e.g. food, fluids, good light sources) against them will result in fatigue and impaired decision making.

Retrieval vehicles

The vehicles generally used for interhospital patient transport are road ambulances, helicopters and fixed-wing aircraft. They have some similarities in that they all offer cramped and noisy workplaces and are thus difficult places in which to perform assessments and procedures. Lighting will be worse than in hospital, power for equipment may or may not be available and motion sickness may affect the patient or attendants.

- Road ambulances are commonly used for short-distance interhospital transfers (less than 100 km), but care must be taken to secure equipment properly.
- Helicopters tend to be used for medium-distance transfers (100–300 km), and often have the advantage of flying direct from referring to receiving hospital, but are more susceptible to bad weather than other modes of transport and are a particularly difficult environment in which to perform clinical assessment or procedures.
- Fixed-wing aircraft have a greater range and fewer weight constraints than helicopters, but transfers involve road-ambulance legs and more patient movements to and from stretchers, all with potential for mishap. Gravitational forces

on take-off and landing may result in marked haemodynamic instability (including cardiac arrest), particularly with hypovolaemic patients.

Fixed-wing aircraft used as air ambulances tend to be pressurised, but helicopters are not and so issues with hypoxia and gas expansion at altitude come into play. Gases expand by approximately 40% at an altitude of 8000 feet (2400 metres), and this may result in deleterious clinical effects if in a confined space. Pneumothoraces should be drained before transport.

An arterial partial pressure of oxygen (PaO_2) of 100 mmHg at sea level will fall to approximately 60 mmHg at 8000 feet if on the same fraction of inspired oxygen (FiO_2). This may make the difference between a patient being stable on high-flow oxygen via a non-rebreathing mask, and requiring intubation and ventilation. It may also result in medical attendants becoming hypoxic on minimal exertion during the mission, which may result in headaches, fatigue and impaired judgment.

The choice of retrieval vehicle should be made by a central tasking authority. This should take into account vehicle availability, weather, distance and clinical considerations.

Preparing a patient for retrieval

- The patient needs to be well packaged prior to interhospital transfer, always bearing in mind the clinical urgency of the case.
- It is difficult to do any procedures en route, so necessary procedures should be performed prior to departure, taking into account the likely or potential clinical course.
- If there is a concern about the airway, this should usually be secured by intubation prior to departure. The threshold for intubating a patient is lower than if they remain in a hospital environment.
- A minimum of two peripheral intravenous cannulae should be in place. Infusions should be rationalised to those necessary for transfer, and fluids should go through a pump (blood-giving) to ensure that they can run.
- Invasive blood pressure monitoring is more reliable than non-invasive readings, so an arterial line is preferable.
- Indwelling urinary catheters and gastric tubes are generally required. Awake patients should have an anti-emetic.
- Extreme care should be taken if moving an agitated or intoxicated patient. The risks of putting such patients in an

aircraft are considerable, so transfer should either be deferred or involve sedation or even general anaesthesia.

- Sufficient medications and infusions for the mission should be immediately available.
- Copies of notes and imaging should go with the patient.
- Accurate determination of the patient's weight is essential, as the movement of obese patients can be logistically challenging and beyond the capacity of usual means. Patient weight beyond 130 kg will generally require specialised transfer methods, as will extreme height or width.
- Be sure to keep the patient's family aware of what is going on and where the patient is going. Give them an honest idea of the likely clinical course.

In transit

With a well-prepared patient, the time in transit is generally spent keeping a close eye on the patient and dealing with problems should they arise. Occasionally, however, significant resuscitation will be necessary which makes for an 'interesting' journey.

Particular care should be taken any time the patient is transferred between stretchers, and during loading into and unloading from vehicles. These are danger times for inadvertent disconnections and even extubation, plus haemodynamically unstable patients can crash with even minor stimuli.

A clear and detailed record of the transfer should be kept.

Hand-over

Good hand-over is vital to ensure appropriate ongoing care of the patient. Hand-over at the receiving hospital should be to the most senior medical officer, and must also include the nursing staff who will be looking after the patient. Hand-over should follow a structured framework such as the ISBAR tool (Table 21.1—introduction, situation, background, assessment, recommendation), addressing clinical course and the immediate needs of the patient. Ventilation, monitoring and infusions should be transferred from the retrieval to hospital equipment in a systematic manner, ensuring the patient is appropriately monitored at all times. Be sure to pass on contact details of the patient's family. This is a vulnerable time for the patient.

The retrieval team is responsible for directing the coordinated hand-over and transfer of care. A patient retrieval hand-over procedure is outlined in Table 21.2.

Table 21.1 ISBAR clinical hand-over tool

I	**Introduction** Identify yourself, your role and location. Identify the patient
S	**Situation** State the patient's diagnosis/reason for admission and current problem.
B	**Background** What is the patient's history?
A	**Assessment** What are the most recent observations? What is your assessment?
R	**Recommendation** What do you want the person taking over care of the patient to do? When should this occur?

nswhealth.moodle.com.au/DOH/DETECT/content/00_worry/when_to_worry_06.htm

Pre-hospital care

Retrieval services may be involved in pre-hospital care of critically injured or difficult-to-access patents. Doctors in such services are generally specialists or advanced trainees in emergency medicine, anaesthetics or intensive care. The role of the doctor in such teams is to utilise critical-care skills in the field; for example rapid-sequence intubation, insertion of intercostal catheters or pre-hospital ultrasound scanning. The goal for medical pre-hospital teams is to provide these interventions in a safe and timely manner, accelerating rather than delaying the patient's journey to definitive care. The challenges of working in difficult environments often necessitate the development of protocols for such procedures with the aim to improve performance and safety. These protocols may include challenge–response checklists, which are common in aviation.

Editorial Comment

Every emergency department, especially those in smaller hospitals, must have an easily accessible document (e.g. on ED computer) that lists key phone numbers, checklists for doctors and nurses and how to organise transfers—the 'one phone call'—as well as who to call to have the matter escalated if the ED is overwhelmed or encountering a 'brick wall' at any receiving hospital. *Note:* Murphy's Law says—it will be at night, on the weekend and/or at holiday time, etc!

Table 21.2 Retrieval hand-over procedure

HAND-OVER: WHO, WHEN, WHERE, HOW	
Who	• The hand-over should be between the most senior hospital clinician responsible for the patient and the retrieval clinician
When	• The hand-over should take place at a predictable time—an estimated time of arrival for the retrieval team should be provided, with the expectation that the relevant team is **assembled at the designated time**. • The hand-over should occur **before the transfer of management** begins (unless urgent resuscitation is required). This ensures that all staff listen to the hand-over and then focus on the systematic transfer of patient care.
What	• At hand-over the following information is exchanged, along general ISBAR principles: — Presenting problem and relevant past history; use MIST/AMPLE — Initial and current management (including monitoring, infusions, ventilation) — Response to management and current condition (including current vital signs) — A problem list of perceived issues that need addressing within the next 60 minutes
How	1. Transfer to stretcher/bed • The hospital is responsible for ensuring that sufficient staff and equipment are available. The retrieval team is responsible for coordinating the move, as they are familiar with the retrieval equipment. 2. Transfer monitors • Monitoring should be transferred between the hospital monitors and retrieval bridge monitors one at a time. There should be no disruption to the continuity of monitoring. 3. Transfer therapies • Therapies should be transferred one at a time, at the direction of the retrieval team. *Ventilation:* — Hospital bed to retrieval stretcher = transfer ventilation last — Retrieval stretcher to hospital bed = transfer ventilation first; note when transferring from retrieval to hospital equipment, the retrieval team will prescribe initial ventilation parameters. *Drug infusions:* — One drug at a time, like-to-like, ensure no dead space *Specific therapies:* — i.e. intercostal drainage systems, external ventricular drains (EVDs), Sengstaken–Blakemore tubes, IV fluids *Routine therapies:* i.e. nasogastric tubes, urinary catheters, etc.

Modified from NSW Department of Health Retrieval Policy, 2011.

Online resources

ISBAR

nswhealth.moodle.com.au/DOH/DETECT/content/00_worry/when_to_worry_06.htm

Chapter 22
Mass-casualty incidents, chemical, biological and radiological hazard contingencies

Iromi Samarasinghe and Jeff Wassertheil

Aims and objectives

Incidents involving mass casualties are infrequent. However, they have the potential to overwhelm usual health resources with very little notice. It is therefore important that contingencies are developed, tested and ready for immediate implementation. Such contingencies outline the responsibilities for overall medical control, coordination and effective casualty management in major emergencies and disaster situations. They include the procedures for triage, first aid and resuscitation, some of which require modification when resource availability needs to be rationed.

Response plans must provide a framework for coordination of transporting injured or incident-affected individuals to appropriate treatment sites. Plans must incorporate procedures to enable the presence of medical, nursing and first-aid personnel, as well as other welfare personnel and psychological carers, to provide care at the scene of a mass-casualty incident (MCI).

At a hospital level, plans need to be developed, implemented, rehearsed and evaluated. This enables hospitals that are often full to manage a large number of patients in excess of usual workloads or capacities and, in certain circumstances, victims with special or specific management needs.

Incorporation of public health resources and interventions is integral to provide guidance and procedures where hygiene, sanitation, communicable disease or biological hazards potentially exist. Contingencies must provide an interface for concurrent activation of recovery plans. Access to appropriate and timely psychological support for victims and care providers is included in both early and ongoing recovery phases. The overall objective is to mitigate disasters by participation in event planning and medical and emergency service activation and training.

This chapter focuses on the health service response to an MCI, as it is not within the scope of this book to describe other emergency services frameworks.

Phases of a disaster

The phases of disaster management are prevention, preparedness, response and recovery.

PREVENTION

The prevention phase concentrates on strategies that minimise the severity of an incident. It aims to cushion the severity, reduce the effects, minimise adversity and contain the impact of a disaster. Prevention strategies also include incorporation of lessons learned from previous experiences. Legislation ensures plans are in readiness for such eventualities.

PREPAREDNESS

Effort in optimal preparedness promotes effective and optimal resource allocation and consumption. This phase occurs with an expectation that the plan will at some time need to be activated. Preparedness occurs from within and external to the health service.

Planning includes providers from both within and stakeholders from outside the health service that would be expected to respond in accordance with emergency management contingency plans. Local community stakeholders—such as the police, ambulance and the fire department—as well as public health and recovery agencies should be included in health service planning committees. Likewise, health service representation should be included in local council, shire or regional planning committees.

As highlighted under prevention, the recommendations from previous operational debriefings, adverse incidents or experience are woven into response plans.

Preparedness of medical services involves training and accreditation processes for each facility to work in conjunction with other agencies. Exercises to coordinate resources within and across agencies are aimed at improving the preparation phase.

RESPONSE

This involves the activation of a pre-determined and well-rehearsed emergency plan to respond to multicasualty external disasters resulting in the rapid mobilisation of personnel and other resources to manage the surge of patients.

RECOVERY

Recovery contingencies are implemented and provide for the short- and long-term recovery of the community (victims and helpers) affected by the disaster. This includes the health service staff and the repair and reinstatement of physical resources, consumables and services. A coordinated approach is required to rebuild the infrastructure and economic, social and emotional needs of the affected community.

Administrative and legislative mandates

A national legislative framework for emergency management provides for counter-disaster planning for response to and recovery from emergency situations that take place throughout Australia, and provides a blueprint for state or territory response plans.

MANAGEMENT STRUCTURE

National

At the Commonwealth level, Emergency Medicine Australia (EMA) is responsible for guidance and support of disaster-management procedures within each of the states and territories.

- EMA will fund any nationally coordinated response, especially any international deployments. A national response is triggered when an affected state is overwhelmed by a disaster and asks for assistance; when there is a political interest in the response involving international aspects, media or border regions; or when there is a terrorist threat and the National Counter Terrorism Committee is required to respond.
- The Commonwealth can also engage defence forces if a civilian disaster requires defence assistance. This commonly involves transportation, whether in the form of trucks for carrying equipment or aircraft for transporting casualties back to Australian shores. Highly trained medical teams may also be available if not engaged in areas of conflict.
- The Commonwealth can provide expertise in emergency management and assistance with political and media management.
- The Commonwealth can coordinate state assets such as aeromedical capability and medical teams. Although these medical teams are state-based and are designed for intrastate deployment, in the event that a state is overwhelmed other medical teams can be coordinated for interstate deployment.

- In addition, the Commonwealth can coordinate any foreign offers of help.
- COMDISPLAN has been established to coordinate the provision of Australian government assistance in the form of physical assets by funding the interstate deployment of medical teams and resources to the state in crisis.
- AUSTRAUMAPLAN allows the Commonwealth to become involved in a local incident if it is of national significance.
- OSMASSCASPLAN is a national overseas MCI response plan to deal with repatriation of Australian citizens, victims and nationals of other countries involved in an MCI in a foreign land.
- AUSASSISTPLAN involves Commonwealth funding, through the Department of Foreign Affairs and Trade (DFAT), for an MCI response in a foreign land. It differs from AusAid, which involves financial support from DFAT provided to a developing nation affected by a disaster.

State

Separate state emergency response plans, designed to provide long-term assistance to people and communities, are activated during the response phase of an incident to provide early commitment of resources. The principal role of the state Health Department is to deal with matters associated with the general health of the community and to provide health and medical services required as a result of a major emergency or disaster. Specific specialty plans for events such as shore retrieval, major burns management and terrorism and CBR (chemical, biological and radiation) incidents have been developed in order to harness a coordinated and cooperative multi-city response.

Very broadly, these state legislative frameworks provide for:

- disaster planning and response coordination of activities throughout the state to be enacted by the chief commissioner for police or nominated deputies
- roles and responsibilities of emergency services and support organisations for various types of emergencies or disasters
- the state Health Department to coordinate agencies involved in providing recovery actions in communities following major incidents and disasters.

The state Health Department ensures coordination of:

- provision of hospital and medical services
- provision of transport and hospitalisation for the injured or sick

- supply of medical and first-aid teams
- setting up of medical centres and casualty-clearing stations
- provision of disease control and other scientific and pathological services required
- health and scientific survey teams
- public health information, advice and warnings, to control and support agencies and for release to the affected communities.

The state Health Department has direct responsibilities as the control agency for:

- infectious disease outbreaks
- contaminated foodstuffs and water
- CBR substance releases.

It is also the support agency for all incidents, and provides advice to all combat and support agencies and to the general public in hazardous material, chemical, biological, radiological and nuclear incidents.

Accordingly, under these arrangements, the police and the various state or territory emergency service organisations develop the non-medical component of the state disaster emergency management plans. Under the various state emergency response arrangements, the Health Departments have statutory responsibility to provide the necessary planning and response required to deal with matters associated with the general health of the community and to provide medical and hospital services required as a result of a major emergency or disaster.

Individual local health districts will develop detailed plans specific to that local area. Local Emergency Management Committees, which include key stakeholders, ensure that the local community will be prepared and able to commit local resources.

An 'all hazards' approach to disaster planning ensures that contingencies are in place to respond to a variety of incidents involving a large number of victims. For instance, a disaster plan should be able to respond to a natural disaster such as a cyclone with some forewarning or a man-made disaster such as a terrorist attack which is a sudden-impact disaster without preparation time.

An 'all agencies' approach to disaster response helps to build a resilient community where all key stakeholders are prepared, trained and capable of responding to an MCI situation.

Medical response plans and agencies

A medical response plan (HEALTHPLAN) is a support plan for the state DISPLAN. It provides for a clinical-care organisational framework that outlines the roles and responsibilities of the various participating medical and healthcare responders, and provides the necessary integrated procedures for altering and mobilising medical and healthcare personnel, for establishing on-site medical control and for definitive treatment of casualties. The concept is that all arrangements and procedures made within the medical response can be applied from the smallest to the largest incident with a build-up of medical coordination and medical and health resources as necessary, following the general pattern of normal daily operational procedures wherever possible. This extends to contingency planning and has a presence at major events where potential public threat is perceived to exist.

The state DISPLAN is further divided into District and Local Emergency Response Committees, to ensure that an integrated effective response can be provided in times of emergency.

EMERGENCY SERVICE ORGANISATIONS

Also referred to as Combat Agencies, and include:

- police
- fire brigade
- rural fire service
- ambulance service
- state emergency service
- volunteer rescue associations.

EMERGENCY OPERATION CENTRES (EOCS)

EOCs will be activated when a major incident is declared and a coordinated support effort is required to assist with on-site medical care and transport of injured victims to appropriate hospitals for further treatment. For longer-term recovery assistance, EOCs are essential to coordinate the physical, medical, mental health and public health issues of victims and to assist with ongoing needs of communities. EOCs have representatives from all essential emergency service organisations. EOCs are activated at all levels of government, including receiving hospitals.

HEALTH SERVICE COMMAND AND CONTROL

This is determined by the state DISPLAN and is coordinated by the state HSFAC (Health Services Functional Area Coordinator) who controls the mobilisation of all healthcare personnel and resources to any emergency when the plan is activated. This includes:

- the mobilisation of resources to the incident site, and initiation of triage and treatment

- establishing 24-hour operational communications to initiate and instigate the necessary mobilisation of site medical commanders, medical response teams and notify casualty receiving hospitals in major emergencies
- the initial setting up of a casualty clearing station by the first ambulance team for triage and treatment on-site until a joint medical command post is established
- coordination of first aid with the ambulance service until the establishment of adequate medical response teams on-site
- coordination with Ambulance Command for transportation of casualties to appropriate hospitals
- coordination with HazMat and fire services for assistance with on-site decontamination of people exposed to toxic or microbiological hazards
- deploying the expertise of public health officers in emergencies where public health is threatened; all work within the framework of the Health Department public health sector for preventing and controlling outbreaks of communicable diseases, and for the preservation of acceptable standards for safe drinking water and foodstuffs.

HEALTH SERVICES FUNCTIONAL AREA COORDINATOR (HSFAC)

This senior medical advisor manages the internal administrative functions of the medical response plan and is responsible for activating a disaster response. All health personnel involved must be appropriately trained in emergency management and understand the command and control structure of disaster response. In some states the HSFAC is referred to as the Chief Health Officer.

Although specific contingencies and structures vary throughout Australia, the senior medical advisor generally manages the EOC when activated in support of the medical response system. The HSFAC also assists with the distribution of mass casualties to hospitals and, in times of major emergencies, will provide briefings via the Health Department to the appropriate minister and the media. The HSFAC is also responsible for coordinating resources by liaising with other agencies.

Pre-hospital medical coordination and disaster scene control

Although titles, role delineations, responsibilities, definitions and plans may vary among the states, the following principles are generic.

The descriptions below outline the events and actions that are required for proficient on-site disaster medicine management.

SITE MEDICAL CONTROL

The disaster-site medical procedures in place for establishing early medical control for the proper triage, treatment and transportation of casualties are initially provided by officers of the first responding ambulance vehicle. These officers carry out the roles of Casualty Collecting Officer (for assessment of numbers and types of casualties, to carry out a reconnaissance of the area and select an area suitable to set up a casualty collecting post, to report findings to Ambulance Control and to commence triage of casualties) and Transport Control Officer (to establish suitable access and turn-around for ambulance vehicles and to report this information to Ambulance Command for further incoming response vehicles).

As an ambulance commander arrives on-site, further assessments will be made and an Incident Command Centre established. All incoming medical responders report to the command post where tasks within the casualty clearing station (CCS) are allocated. Further medical assistance required on-site is requested through the chain of command via the site medical commander to avoid convergence and duplication of resources. A typical communication structure is outlined in Figure 22.1.

The medical services provided on-site will be limited initially, and will use the principle of doing as little as possible, as simply as possible, as quickly as possible and to as many as possible.

Life-saving procedures, such as airway management, immediate decompression of tension pneumothorax, arrest of haemorrhage, fracture stabilisation and relief of pain where necessary, may be the limit of medical assistance where medical resources are few. Effective triage prioritisation of casualties by a Triage Officer, usually an ambulance officer from the first responding team, is essential to determine number and type of casualty in the MCI. Early, accurate communication to the Incident Command Centre and further up the chain of command to the HSFAC will enable effective delivery of personnel and resources to the scene.

SITE MEDICAL COMMANDER

The site medical commander (SMC) directs medical aspects of treatment in the casualty clearing station. The medical commander coordinates medical teams on-site and is the top of the chain of command

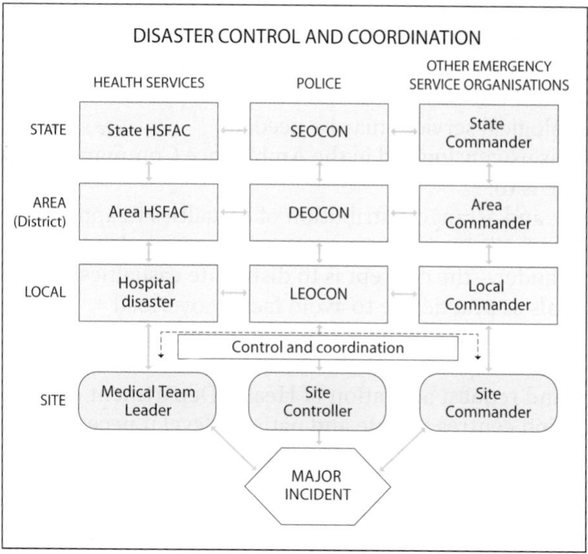

Figure 22.1 Linkage between emergency services organisations
DEOCON, LEOCON and SEOCON are the District, Local and State Emergency Operations Controllers, respectively

for medical response—all requests for resupply, resources and personnel pass through this officer. The medical commander determines the need for specialist teams, which include mental health and public health officers depending on the particular incident. As the SMC oversees several medical response teams, he/she does not get involved in medical care of individual patients.

The SMC is responsible for on-site medical coordination of all medical and health resources required, and for the command of all healthcare responders. The SMC is responsible for:

- in conjunction with the ambulance commander, establishing an effective medical controlled area (casualty clearing station) and effecting liaison with the police coordinator and other emergency services
- providing a frequent and accurate manifest to HSFAC and EOC detailing numbers and triage priorities of MCI victims following assessment of the casualty status
- assessing the on-site conditions with the ambulance commander and, if necessary, initiating the setting up of a second casualty

clearing station or designating area where transport of injured persons from the scene may safely incur significant delays
- assessing the requirement for relief of or for further medical teams at the scene, for further first-aid support and whether psychological services may be needed.

The SMC is usually located in the Ambulance Command Centre. The SMC's role is to:

- initiate and arrange distribution of casualties to appropriate hospital facilities, in conjunction with an ambulance commander—the concept is to distribute casualties to as many hospitals as practicable to avoid facility overload
- alert and mobilise medical teams and other medical and healthcare responders to the disaster scene
- liaise and request activation of Health Department emergency operation centres at state and national level if necessary, and provide situation reports at frequent intervals to EOC and to request further assistance
- instigate stand-down of the various medical and health responders as appropriate after consultation with the on-site ambulance commander and other emergency service authorities.

CASUALTY CLEARING STATION

This is initially established by the ambulance service and eventually managed by the medical response teams deployed to the scene. The primary requirement is that the casualty clearing station must be located in a safe place. When establishing a casualty clearing station, it should be a safe distance away from the 'hot zone', as sheltered as possible and of an adequate size to safely manage casualties delivered from the scene. It serves as a point for secondary triage by the medical response teams and for provision of essential treatments to safely package the casualties for transport to hospital for definitive care.

DISASTER MEDICAL RESPONSE TEAMS

Each team consists of 2 senior doctors and 4 resuscitation nurses, deployed from designated hospitals as determined by the state HSFAC. In Australia, all team members must be appropriately trained and accredited to work in the pre-hospital environment. All team members are registered on arrival at the site and need to be in appropriate pre-hospital uniforms, including regulation hats and footwear. Each team deployed to the incident site carries regulation disaster packs containing essential equipment.

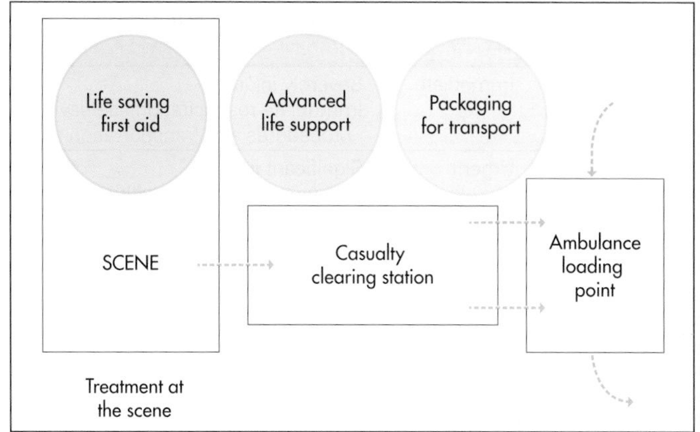

Figure 22.2 Schematic representation of a casualty clearing station

These teams provide treatment to injured victims based on disaster triage priorities (SMART triage, discussed below). Working in austere conditions with minimal resources, these teams provide essential treatment to allow safe passage of critically injured victims to hospitals for definitive care.

Disaster medical response teams have a critical role in minimising surge impact on hospitals by stabilising and sorting victims to allow them to be transported to hospitals outside the immediate network. Those not needing hospital or ED management can be referred to community-based resources either acutely or subacutely, in keeping with regional or municipal plans.

Triage

Triage generally implies direction of clinical resources to the most seriously ill or injured by a trieur or triage officer, in order to get the right casualty to the right place at the right time. In a mass-casualty situation, demand may be in excess of resource availability. It is neither ethical nor practical to classify clearly non-salvageable victims as top priorities.

TRIAGE SIEVE AND SORT

The triaging system in an MCI must be quick, simple, safe and reproducible. Triage performed by emergency personnel at the disaster site must be a 'quick look' and is referred to as *triage sieve*; this is followed

Table 22.1 Triage priorities and criteria for MCI victims

Priority	Colour	Description	Criteria
1	Red	Immediate	Severely injured Immediate resuscitation, life-saving procedures and transportation required
2	Yellow	Urgent	Significant injuries Intervention required within 4–6 hours
3	Green	Delayed	Casualty ambulant—'walking wounded' Has less-serious injuries, can await delayed treatment Uninjured psychologically-disturbed victims are included in this category
4	Blue	Expectant	Injuries so severe will require extensive medical care which will compromise the treatment of large numbers of other casualties
Dead	Black	Deceased	Medical officer is required to certify death on triage card Body becomes the responsibility of police/coroner's office Body not to be moved without police in attendance. Then body is stored in mortuary on/near incident site

by a more detailed reassessment in the treatment area of the casualty clearing station, referred to as *triage sort.* This process enables pre-hospital personnel to prioritise medical care and transport victims to definitive care in hospital in an organised and rational way.

Triage is a dynamic process that is repeated at each reassessment to ensure refinement of urgency stratification and to respond appropriately to the ongoing evolution of a casualty's injury complex and consequent physiology.

Sieve

This initial casualty assessment is based on the findings of a primary survey.

- If casualties are ambulant, they are initially regarded as walking wounded and are directed or escorted to a separate area of the casualty clearing station. These casualties are given a **priority 3** and will await delayed treatment and transport.
- If casualties are not ambulant, a triaging primary survey is performed. This looks at the airway, respiratory rate and

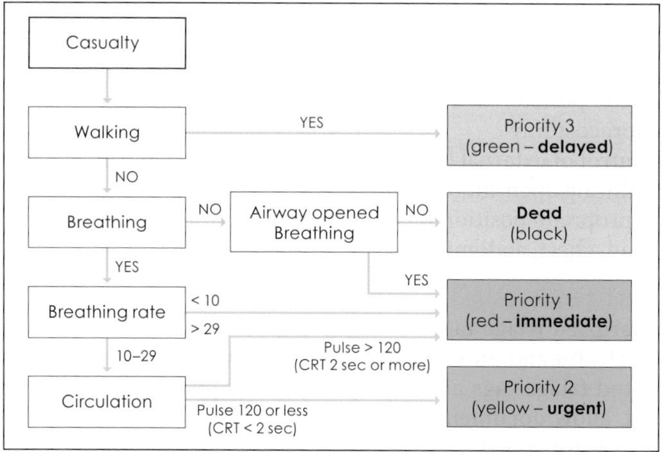

Figure 22.3 Triage sieve protocol

capillary refill time. If there is haemodynamic instability (see Figure 22.3), the casualty will be given a **priority 1** triage category to be moved to the casualty clearing station for commencement of immediate life-saving interventions.

- Non-ambulant casualties who are stable on primary ABC survey are given a **priority 2**. These second-priority patients may have significant injuries, but at the time of initial triage there is no evidence of airway compromise and they have normal respiratory and perfusion status assessments. These constitute most of the injuries that are time-critical on a pattern of blast injury. The implication of being stratified as a priority 2 patient is that treatment should be provided in a hospital within 4–6 hours.
- The operation of **priority 4** assignment is declared by the incident commander if the number of critically ill casualties far outweighs the resources available to treat at the scene or to transport to definitive care in hospitals. In normal circumstances these patients would be given a priority 1 for immediate intervention to treat life-threatening injuries, but in the resource-poor and austere conditions of an MCI the aim is to do the best for the most, and it may be deemed inappropriate to direct several personnel and much resources to provide treatment at the scene for a single victim in an MCI of great magnitude.

Treatment at the scene is limited to the institution of simple life-saving primary survey manoeuvres. These are:

- airway clearance by manual or other available methods
- decompression of a tension pneumothorax by needle thoracostomy
- control of external haemorrhage by compression bandage or splinting open-limb fractures
- appropriate positioning of unconscious patients or patients with head, chest, abdominal, pelvic or spinal injuries.

SMART tags

Standardised triage tags—SMART tags—are currently used across NSW Health and most other states and territories. These nationally accepted triage tags are waterproof, carry personal details of the victim, allow documentation of injuries, allow serial assessment of the Triage Revised Trauma Score (TRTS; see below) and can be used to document treatment instituted at the scene.

Priority 1 patients based on triage sieve assessment will be tagged with the red side of the SMART tag showing. These patients require immediate medical attention and are moved to the casualty clearing station as first priority, to commence treatment and transport to definitive care.

Priority 2 patients will have the yellow side of the SMART tag showing. The walking wounded, priority 3 patients, have the green side showing. If the casualty's triage priority changes, the SMART tag is easily changed to reflect this.

Those casualties that die at the scene have a separate black 'Deceased' SMART tag attached to them.

If use of priority 4 is declared at the MCI, the top left-hand corner of the red triage tag is folded over to show a blue patch. These casualties are critically ill and will require significant resources to treat.

In the event of an MCI involving a CBR agent, an alternative SMART tag is available which can be included in the plastic bag along with the standard triage tag.

Casualties must be re-triaged on the basis of response to simple first aid, injury pattern and likely prognosis. If critically injured or ill patients are unresponsive to these measures and unlikely to survive, they become second-priority casualties. This is sometimes known as reverse triage. In current MCI parlance, this is the priority 4/Blue/Expectant category. The incident commander must declare the operation of this triage category at the commencement of the emergency response, based on casualty numbers and availability of resources.

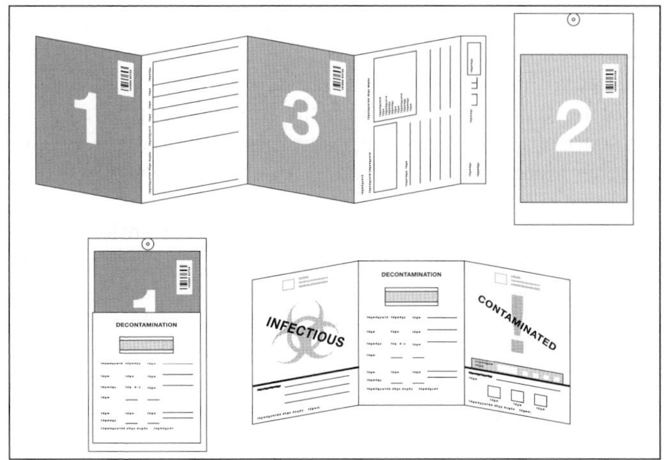

Figure 22.4 Triage cards—SMART tags (above) and CBR tags (below)

In this case the SMART tag's red priority 1 side will have the blue triangle folded down in the top left-hand corner. A doctor, preferably of 3 or more years' experience, or a senior nurse may be allocated to the care of extremely severely injured patients with a low probability of survival—the expectant category. Intensive efforts to resuscitate these patients may jeopardise the survival of large numbers of other casualties because of an excessive drain on resources. Supportive and palliative care only should be given until resources are available to commence more-vigorous resuscitation, if appropriate.

Sort

This triage method is the more formal risk stratification that identifies time-critical patients and assists in scheduling optimal allocation of available resources. It is commonly used by emergency medical personnel on admission of patients to casualty clearing stations or field hospitals.

This method of triage is based on the Revised Trauma Score (RTS) and is consistent with the Australasian Triage Scale and triage practices taught in emergency management of severe trauma (EMST), emergency life support (ELS), advanced paediatric life support (APLS) and major incident medical management and support (MIMMS) courses. It is a repeated process that is dependent on traditional ongoing patient observation.

Sort is generally implemented in the field utilising the RTS in order to rank physiological embarrassment and allocating an ordinal score. This assists with re-prioritisation or risk-stratification of casualties. Scores of 1–10 are associated with the Immediate (priority 1) category. A score of 11 identifies an Urgent (priority 2) patient. A score of 12 or higher identifies casualties that can wait for Delayed (priority 3) management (Figure 22.5).

Further refinement of triage can be assisted by attention to pattern of injuries or mechanism of injuries. However, in a trauma-related MCI, a considerable number of patients may be classified as time-critical on mechanism of injury alone (Table 22.2). Close observation of this latter group is necessary. Although these patients are of lesser priority owing to normal physiological parameters or the absence of an identified pattern of injury, they are victims of major trauma, have sustained major forces and are at risk of significant and occult internal injury.

TRIAGE REVISED TRAUMA SCORE (TRTS)

SYSTOLIC BP	CODED VALUE
> 89	4
76–89	3
50–75	2
1–49	1
0	0

RESPIRATORY RATE	CODED VALUE
10–29	4
> 29	3
6–9	2
1–5	1
0	0

GLASGOW COMA SCORE	CODED VALUE
13–15	4
9–12	3
6–8	2
4–5	1
3	0

Immediate priority 1	Urgent priority 2	Delayed priority 3
Score = 1–10	Score = 11	Score = 12

Figure 22.5 Triage Revised Trauma Score system to sort casualty priority

Table 22.2 Features suggestive of severe trauma or time-critical casualties

Pattern of injury	All penetrating injuries—head/neck/chest/abdomen/pelvis/axilla/groin
	Blunt injuries— • Patients with a significant injury to a single region: head/neck/chest/abdomen/axilla/groin • Patients with injuries involving 2 or more of the above body regions
	Specific injuries— • Limb amputations/limb-threatening injuries • Suspected spinal cord injury • Burns > 20% of body surface area or suspected respiratory tract involvement • Crush injuries where pressure is maintained for > 1 hour • Major compound fracture or open dislocation • Fracture to 2 or more proximal long bones • Fractured pelvis
Mechanism of injury	Car occupants involved in high-speed motor vehicle crash, e.g. impact speed > 60 km/h with major vehicle damage Pedestrians or cyclists hit by vehicles travelling at > 30 km/h Patients ejected from a vehicle Patients in a car that has rolled over Patients in a motor vehicle crash where there is a death of another or same vehicle occupant Patients who have fallen from a height > 3 metres Patients hit by an object that has fallen from > 3 metres Motorcyclists, cyclists Explosion victims Patients who are trapped and likely to remain so for > 30 minutes
Age and concurrent medical problems	Age > 55 years or < 5 years Pregnancy Significant underlying medical condition

Triage officers

It is preferable for the triage role to be undertaken by a senior doctor experienced and accredited in the sort and sieve methods of disaster triage.

FIRST-AID SERVICES

First-aid services can be provided by several different organisations. The common ones are St John Ambulance Australia and the Australian

Red Cross. These may be complemented by other first-aid providers such as the Australian Ski Patrol Association, the Royal Life Saving Society or Surf Life Saving Australia, depending on the circumstances. First-aid agencies are often activated by the ambulance service.

The principal role of first-aid organisations is to assist with minor injuries where the setting up of separate treatment centres is necessary to cope with walking wounded. First-aid teams generally work under the direction of a site medical commander or ambulance commander in casualty collecting stations or in field hospitals.

Communication

Good communication is essential to the effective functioning and coordination of an MCI operation. Breakdown in communication has been cited as one of the commonest failures of major-incident management. Various methods of communication are used in MCI management, including land-lines, mobile phones, megaphones and television broadcasts, but appropriate training in radio voice procedures is essential for those working in an MCI.

There are several advantages of radio communication through a specific network for the MCI, especially in remote areas and when mobile networks are jammed. All members of a medical response team are trained in NATO radio voice procedures, including use of standardised phrases (Table 22.3), phonetic alphabet (Table 22.4), clarity, brevity and accuracy.

Code Brown: hospital external disaster or emergency response plan

All public hospitals are required to have external disaster plans to cope with mass casualties directed to hospital facilities for treatment. In keeping with national standards for colour-coding emergency response plans, an external emergency, which includes disasters and MCIs, is referred to as a Code Brown.

Public hospitals are required to develop, implement and test contingencies for the reception of mass casualties. This is a requirement both of legislature and of the Australian Council on Healthcare Standards. During a health emergency, hospitals will have to convert quickly from their standard care capacity to surge capacity. This is achieved through re-prioritisation of healthcare needs to provide essential services to mass casualties. This would include cancellation of elective surgeries, early discharge of hospitalised patients and diversion of patients with minor complaints to alternative healthcare

Table 22.3 **NATO radio voice procedures**

Word/phrase	Meaning
THIS IS	When calling, say the call sign that you want followed by your call sign. For example: ALPHA THIS IS BRAVO.
OVER	I have finished speaking and it is your turn to reply.
OUT	I have finished talking to you.
RADIO CHECK	Can you hear me? If you can, then how well? Ideally it will be LOUD and CLEAR. If it isn't then describe it, such as WEAK BUT READABLE, etc. Reply in numerical/alphabetical order.
OK/ROGER	Use either word to show that you have received and understood the message. Note: 'COPY THAT' is just another, non-standard way of saying OK or ROGER but can be confusing if you really want them to copy it!
MESSAGE	I have a message for you—are you ready to receive it?
SEND	I am ready to receive your message.
MORE TO FOLLOW	The message isn't finished—but have you got it all so far?
SAY AGAIN	This can be SAY AGAIN ALL BEFORE or ALL AFTER or NUMBER or anything else that you didn't get down.
ACKNOWLEDGE	Please tell me that you have received the message. If you have, then respond as ROGER (or OK)—you do not have to read it all back.
WAIT	Give me 10 seconds to find a pencil or whatever.
WAIT OUT	I'll get back to you.
I SPELL	Say the word followed by I SPELL, then spell the word phonetically. If there is more than one word then say FIRST WORD—*say the word*—I SPELL … etc.

providers such as local GPs and medical centres. However, all public hospitals throughout the state are expected to maintain core functions during a Code Brown.

Some private hospitals participate in counter-disaster planning activities, especially if they are affiliated with or in close proximity to a large general hospital. Their external emergency response plans work side-by-side with the main receiving hospital, and a memorandum of understanding exists between the hospital management and the local health district or state HSFAC. They may be required to provide sheltered accommodation for casualties from an MCI or ongoing care of admitted patients being decanted from a local public hospital for it to receive casualties.

Table 22.4 NATO alphabet and numbers for radio communication in an MCI situation

Letter	Word	Letter	Word
A	Alpha	T	Tango
B	Bravo	U	Uniform
C	Charlie	V	Victor
D	Delta	W	Whisky
E	Echo	X	X-ray
F	Foxtrot	Y	Yankee
G	Golf	Z	Zulu
H	Hotel	**Numbers**	
I	India	1	Wun
J	Juliet	2	Too
K	Kilo	3	Th-ree
L	Lima	4	For-wer
M	Mike	5	Fi-yiv
N	November	6	Six
O	Oscar	7	Sev-en
P	Papa	8	Ate
Q	Quebec	9	Niner
R	Romeo	0	Zero
S	Sierra		

From the Advanced Life Support Group Australia (MIMMS), September 2003; updated November 2007.

Such plans may also include procedures for providing a trained and equipped medical team for casualty treatment at a disaster site. The provision of such medical teams may reduce the ED's effectiveness. The state HSFAC will give consideration to replacing or providing a team from another facility if the responding hospital is to continue to be a major casualty-receiving hospital. Some base hospitals in rural regions also have the capability to provide such teams, with smaller hospitals having a reduced capability.

Certain first-aid organisations such as St John Ambulance are also able to provide medical teams on request through the state HSFAC to the Commissioner of St John's Ambulance Australia. The Royal Flying Doctor Service (RFDS) of Australia has the capacity to provide medical teams for deployment to an MCI site within or outside its normal area of operation. The coordination of these resources is through the state HSFAC and the Chief Medical Controller of RFDS as well as the Director of the Aero Medical Retrieval Service.

PLANNING, EXERCISES AND REVIEW OF PLANS

All participating agencies integral to a medical DISPLAN response have subplans to ensure that effective response is available when required. Integrated medical response planning with other emergency services takes place at all levels, addressing various hazards that exist. The exercising and testing of plans takes place at frequent intervals and as necessary following planning reviews.

HEALTHCARE FACILITY EMERGENCY MANAGEMENT PLANS

The role of a healthcare facility in responding to external incidents will depend on the size and scope of healthcare services usually offered. Healthcare facilities that offer acute, subacute, long-term care and community outreach health care have a greater capacity to manage demand and overflows. The Code Brown plan of such large facilities will include arrangements for the reception of large numbers of casualties and will include designated treatment areas, security arrangements and the control of vehicular and pedestrian traffic to facilitate ambulance turnaround. Smaller hospitals can contribute by providing care to patients or casualties not requiring intensive resources or by assisting in decanting convalescing patients from other acute services, thus freeing resources to receive disaster victims.

Stages of response

In general, the phases of an external disaster emergency management plan are *alert*, *standby*, *activation* (declared or action), *stand down* and *recovery*.

Alert—*a disaster situation is possible*
- Begin preparations
- Develop contingency for potential escalation in required response

Standby—*a disaster situation is probable*
- Complete preparations
- Ensure readiness to receive casualties

Prepare to receive—*a disaster situation exists*
- Prepare to receive casualties

Stand down—*a disaster situation is contained*
- Cancellation of response
- Replacement of equipment
- All personnel resume normal duties

STAGES OF THE EXTERNAL EMERGENCY RESPONSE PLAN

Alert

A possible disaster may be advised by one of the emergency services, a media enquiry or a member of the public. Sometimes the alert is raised when ambulant victims present for treatment prior to any other notification. A chemical or biological exposure may be suspected when several patients present with similar symptoms or clinical syndromes over a short time.

All notifications or alerts should be validated. Each healthcare facility should have an incident response team (IRT) which can assess the situation and validate the alert. The IRT may be notified by the emergency department in the event of several casualties presenting to the ED, or by the area HSFAC. The IRT should consist of at least the hospital's disaster coordinator and incident commander. When the alert has been validated, the hospital incident commander, or similarly authorised person, will activate the external emergency response (EER) plan.

Occasionally, emergency services may need to be alerted by the health service after a number of patients have presented with a clinical syndrome suggestive of an exposure. Food poisoning and chemical exposures are examples of the latter.

Standby

Standby advises the health service of the presence of an external incident that may impact on hospital resources and services. During this phase, designated officers assess resources. Current staffing levels, any imminent shift changes and any extra staff that would be required in such a situation are noted. Bed availability is estimated.

An emergency operations centre (EOC) is established in the designated area. It is equipped with computers providing data relating to the Code Brown, and with adequate phone lines, radio communications and fax machines. The EOC is staffed by the hospital incident commander and the disaster coordinator as well as media relations officers and other essential executive officers. It becomes responsible for the management of all aspects of the external disaster as it affects the hospital. In addition to overseeing clinical operations in a Code Brown situation, the EOC manages planning, logistics and finance duties.

Staff must access action cards or documents and become familiar with their roles during the various stages of an EER. Staff not covered by specific action cards continue normal duties.

The operations chief will determine which staff are to be called in for duty and at what stage in the EER this should occur. If a protracted response is anticipated, staff may be required to come in several hours later. Notification is dependent on the nature of the incident. For example, for a Code Brown involving a chemical hazard it may be decided not to advise the senior surgical staff. In addition, the time of day may determine extent of notification within the healthcare facility. For example, an MCI occurring out of hours would be limited to the ED, ICU and operating theatres and might not include areas such as ambulatory care and other outpatient facilities which would not be staffed out of hours.

Activation (Prepare to receive)

Access to hospital beds

The following are principles to guide creation of bed capacity. It is desirable to accommodate all the disaster victims in one area or receiving ward. The following groups of patients are considered for discharge or transfer to less-acute facilities:

- electives with non-life-threatening conditions
- patients for routine investigation
- stable postnatal patients
- stable patients undergoing long-term treatment
- stable postoperative patients
- patients able to be accommodated by a 'hospital in the home' program.

Emergency department response

Aim

The aim of the ED is to rapidly assess and stabilise patients and then clear them from the department as soon as possible. If the external disaster is limited with no possibility of further casualties, a full patient assessment could be completed in the ED in keeping with usual practices. Most priority 1 casualties would require emergency operative management of open wounds and fractured limbs, and as such have no place in the ED on arrival from the scene. Other priority 1 casualties with blunt trauma would require ICU admission and the hospital's Code Brown plan should allow for direct or rapid admission of such patients to its ICU.

Call-in and notifications

Key clinical staff, clinical departments and management staff placed on standby are advised of the escalation. Clinical staff are initially summoned to the ED and prepared to receive casualties.

Triage officers

An appropriately trained senior medical officer would be allocated to perform secondary or tertiary triage on arriving casualties. The triage officer should be assisted by a clerical officer to document details on arrival. The triage officer should be in close communication with the ED team leader regarding numbers and acuity of casualties arriving from the scene. This is usually done via hand-held radio, as other modalities of communication can be unreliable in an MCI. There may be a need for more than one triage officer if the influx of casualties is high.

Resuscitation team leader

This role is allocated to an appropriately trained senior medical officer who may need to manage all the resuscitation rooms simultaneously. All available clinical support is directed to the critically ill casualties arriving from the scene. Close communication with both the surgical team leader and the ICU is essential for the safe and rapid disposition of these casualties.

Acute care team leader

A senior medical officer with appropriate training will oversee the care of patients with triage priority 2. Many of these patients may have significant occult injuries and may ideally need to be managed in resuscitation areas. Thorough clinical assessment and close monitoring is essential to avoid missing significant occult injuries.

Consulting space access

ED clinical staff should endeavour to discharge patients by expediting treatment, disposition, completion of clinical procedures and return of investigation results. Where possible, patients able to be managed in different environments, such as in general practice, could be directed to those services.

There is also an ongoing obligation to continue triage of non-disaster patients. It may be elected to simply use the Australasian Triage Scale with reverse triage of expectant cases designated as urgent.

Clinical records

Previously compiled standard clinical records containing medication charts, pathology and medical imaging request forms should be utilised for all MCI victims. Each MCI victim should be allocated an MCI medical record number for ease of tracking. The SMART triage tags should be retained within the clinical records.

Clinical zones

In order to coordinate clinical care, and depending on the size of the department and the anticipated workload, the ED can be divided into different zones with separate teams of clinical staff. Other clinical areas, such as outpatients, could be set up as satellite EDs to manage overflow ambulatory care patients.

Medical staff

During the standby stage of a Code Brown response, the emergency team leader should brief all medical and nursing staff on the expectations during the ensuing hours. It is preferable for ED doctors to be allocated to work in specific zones. Their roles should be clearly defined in their action cards. They should be appropriately dressed in personal protective equipment (PPE) and wear tabards showing their designation.

Additional medical officers may be requested through the EOC. It is imperative that staff follow their chain of command for all requests.

In trauma incidents, a surgeon should remain in the ED for immediate referrals and assessments. That surgeon is responsible for prioritising patients for theatre.

An anaesthetist will assist with urgent airway intervention, referrals and preoperative assessments as required.

Junior medical staff may be utilised to manage ambulatory patients in designated satellite areas. Similarly, medical and nursing students may be utilised appropriately in clinical areas.

Nursing staff

ED nursing staff roles generally parallel those of the medical staff, as treating teams are allocated to specific areas. Their role focuses on the nursing aspects of patient care and the management of the designated ED zones or other designated areas. Nurses receive and assess patients and assist with the examination and treatment of patients.

Senior nursing staff allocate nurses and clerical support staff to the designated areas and assist the triage officer in resource allocation.

Other

A particular focus is the availability of extra equipment, sterile stock and medications. All requests for re-supply must be escalated through the team leader to ensure that requests are not duplicated nor missed in the potentially chaotic working environment associated with a Code Brown response.

Box 22.1 Hospital-wide services necessary for external disaster plan

Departments and services contributing to Code Brown external disaster responses:

- Executive management
- Emergency department
- Intensive care unit and high-dependency unit
- Operating theatres and recovery units
- Receiving and non-receiving wards
- Outpatients department for managing ambulatory victims with minor injuries or psychological complaints
- Medical imaging
- Laboratory services
- Pharmacy services
- Supply and materials department
- Central sterilising supply department
- Environmental services
- Wardspersons and porters
- Linen and waste services
- Food services
- Engineering and facilities department
- Security
- Traffic control
- Mortuary services
- Social work department for management of worried-well victims and families of disaster victims
- Community relations and media management
- Volunteers

In-hospital responses

The detailed management of in-hospital responses and executive management issues are beyond the scope of this chapter.

Stand down

The cessation of the EER and return to usual operations is initiated by the hospital incident commander via the EOC. The response may conclude on advice from the disaster site or the area HSFAC. However, the response plan may require ongoing activation until pressure on the health service or hospital resources has subsided and normal activities can be resumed.

The stand-down mechanism may be total or progressive. Progressive stand-down can be initiated when certain areas are no longer required to function under response plan conditions.

Debriefing

There are two types of debriefing: operational debriefing and psychological debriefing. The latter has two components: immediate debriefing is a defusing of staff; formal counselling is offered for ongoing symptoms.

Operational debrief

A formal operational debrief, involving key participants and heads of departments, should be conducted within 1 week. This debriefing examines the incident and the organisational response. Reports are prepared for the external disaster committee. Recommendations in this report will form the basis of revisions to the healthcare facility's EER plan.

Defusing

Defusing is the immediate attention to the psychological needs of staff. This provides staff with an opportunity to express their feelings and thoughts about the episode.

Counselling

Counselling aims to assist staff with long-term distress suffered as a consequence of the disaster response. These services are generally provided by employee assistance programs or may be accessed through the various Health Departments.

Chemical, biological and radiological hazards

The approach to chemical, biological and radiological (CBR) exposures is similar in principle to multicasualty trauma incidents whether exposed victims are single casualties, several or within the context of mass casualties. The prime difference is the need to prevent contamination and/or infection of rescuers, healthcare providers and the community. The approach aims to provide optimum care while maintaining safety for other patients and staff. A second broad aim is to effectively decontaminate patients prior to entering the ED. It focuses on a sequence of actions and interventions that admits decontaminated casualties to EDs. A further aim is the expedient identification of causal agents that may enable specific treatment.

Acute recovery incorporates the restoration of areas used for decontamination to usual functions. It includes management of contaminated items for cleaning and inspection by hazard management or public health agencies. Where applicable, non-disposable medical equipment is cleaned and returned to regular use. Some contingency plans include specific equipment kits reserved for use in CBR incidents.

In the field, the sequence begins with identification of casualties and proceeds to isolation, decontamination, triage, treatment and transport to hospital. ED contingences are similar. However, treatment may need to commence before or concurrently with decontamination. The main risk for hospitals is the arrival of contaminated or infected individuals prior to recognition or advice of a CBR incident, with consequent contamination of the ED and, potentially, the whole healthcare facility.

FEATURES OF CBR AND NUCLEAR HAZARDS

CBR and nuclear substances potentially cause harm to human health. Incidents involving these substances often generate vapours, fumes, dusts and mists. Hazardous wastes can pollute waste streams, causing a threat to public health, safety or to the environment. They can also be invisible.

CBR hazards can be infectious, toxic, mutagenic, carcinogenic, teratogenic, explosive, flammable, corrosive, oxidising and radioactive and may cause immediate and/or long-term health effects. Exposure may result in poisoning, irritation, chemical burns, sensitisation, cancer, birth defects or organ disease of the skin, lungs, liver, kidneys and nervous system. The severity of the illness or disease depends on the nature of the substance and the dose absorbed.

Detailed information on all the hazards, their properties, effects and treatments is beyond the scope of this discussion. The following is provided as a broad overview.

MODE OF PRESENTATION

Education of all staff in recognising a contaminated or CBR-hazard-exposed person is necessary in order to minimise the risk of ED exposure and contamination. Self-presentation prior to notification by emergency services agencies is common in chemical incidents. Occasionally, emergency services may be unaware of the incident. In this situation the health service has a system-initiation function. In biological incidents, there is often a trickle followed by an epidemic flood of patients. Radiological incidents may involve burns, the consequences of initial radiation illness or the management of ongoing radioactivity.

An uninformed public, presentations of the worried well and an uncertainty or lack of knowledge by community-based doctors and healthcare providers compound ED impact. It has been estimated that the ratio of worried well to affected victims is 10:1.

CHEMICAL AGENTS

Nerve agents

Nerve agents are organophosphates. They block acetylcholine esterase inhibitors, causing a cholinergic crisis. Examples include Tabun (GA), sarin (GB) and VX.

Blistering agents

These irritate the epithelial surfaces by direct contact. The skin and mucosal surfaces are the target tissues. The mustard agents and lewisite are examples of this group.

Incapacitating agents

This group causes short-term disabling physical and/or mental effects by affecting higher cortical function. The group includes central nervous system depressants, stimulants and hallucinogens. To qualify for membership of this group, agents must be potent, last hours to days, not be potentially lethal at effective doses and have no long-term adverse sequelae. LSD (lysergic acid diethylamide) and 3-quinuclidinyl benzilate (BZ) are examples of incapacitating agents. BZ is an anticholinergic agent.

Blood agents—the cyanides

These agents impair cellular function by uncoupling oxidative phosphorylation.

Pulmonary/choking agents

Choking agents impair the respiratory system by irritating the respiratory tract mucosa and alveolar epithelium. These can produce a spectrum of illness from minor irritation to acute respiratory distress syndrome. Examples include chlorine and phosgene.

BIOLOGICAL HAZARDS

These are varied. Illness is usually of insidious onset. Because early symptoms may be non-specific, especially when patients may be prodromally unwell, early recognition can be difficult. Once the community is aware, workload is increased. Patient load will include those with non-specific symptoms, worried patients with usual clinical features of a non-exposure-related illness and those with unusual symptoms or clinical signs needing diagnostic refinement.

Patients exposed to microbiological agents may be recognised when a number of patients present with unusual similar symptoms or clinical signs. Alternatively an influx of patients with similar symptoms may present, with diagnostic refinement identifying a common broad illness such as pneumonia with isolation of an unusual causal agent.

Other dilemmas include when to immunise and when to definitively treat. These decisions must be made in conjunction with infectious-disease doctors and public health agencies. Rationalisation of available therapeutic substances is a logistical problem. The principles of managing this issue are no different to those of disaster triage and reverse triage. However, within this context, development of inclusion and exclusion criteria is more relevant.

The impact of the exposure on hospitals is likely to increase the workload of laboratory facilities in initial identification and ongoing examinations for isolation of infective agents or bacterial endotoxins and exotoxins.

RADIOLOGICAL HAZARDS

Two broad questions need to be asked when considering radiological exposure. Has the patient been irradiated? Is the patient radioactive? Irradiation alone can cause life-threatening illness. The latter additionally poses a risk to rescuers and ongoing careers.

All forms of ionising radiation can cause illness. Alpha particles generally have poor tissue penetration. They are of significance if ingested, inhaled or have contacted open wounds. Gamma rays penetrate tissues, directly affecting cells. Neutrons cause effects indirectly. Human tissue provides some resistance to beta particles, thus decreasing their impact and causing only tissue damage when they have penetrated cells. Bone marrow and gastrointestinal mucosa are the tissues at most risk. Injuries may be caused by a single radiation exposure, exposure to high levels of fallout and repeated exposures.

Acute radiation syndrome involves four phases: prodrome, latent period, manifest illness and death or recovery.

Prodrome

Initial symptoms often appear within 6 hours of exposure. Symptoms include nausea, vomiting, anorexia and general malaise. Treatment is largely symptomatic and supportive. A 48-hour lymphocyte count and chromosomal analysis of lymphocytes for dicentric fragments are predictors of likely bone marrow suppression and haemopoietic syndrome (see Figure 22.6).

Latent period

This phase is a variable symptom-free period of hours to weeks.

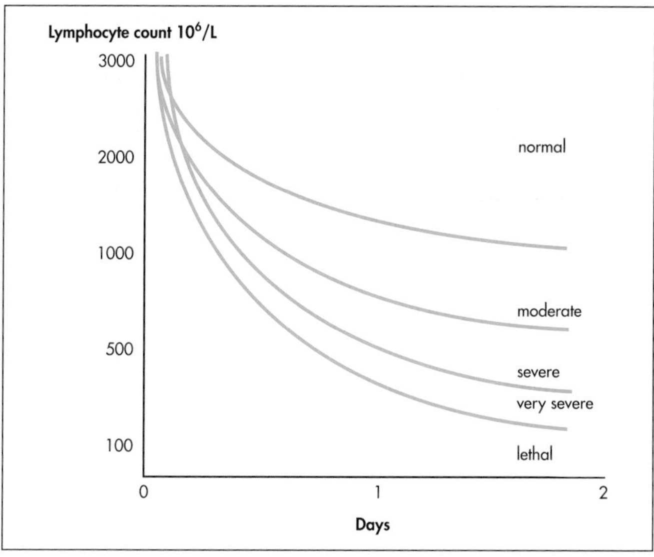

Figure 22.6 Lymphocyte count as a guide to severity of haemopoietic syndrome

Reproduced with permission from Emergency management practice manual 3: health aspects of chemical, biological and radiological hazards. Provisional edn. Australian emergency manuals series, part 3. Emergency Management Australia; 1999.

Manifest illness

In this, definitive radiation illness and its complications become evident. Four clinical syndromes are described: gastrointestinal, haemopoietic, vascular and cerebral.

- The symptoms of the gastrointestinal syndrome are similar to those of the prodrome phase with additional problems of diarrhoea, fever and gastrointestinal haemorrhage. Bowel perforation and septicaemia are complications of severe illness. Treatment is supportive with intravenous fluid resuscitation, dehydration and parenteral nutrition.
- The haemopoietic syndrome is the effect of bone-marrow suppression with increased susceptibility to infection, haemorrhage and occasionally anaemia. Treatment is generally supportive. Platelet transfusion may be necessary for thrombocytopenia-associated haemorrhage or if surgical intervention is required. Sepsis must be energetically treated. Wounds should be closed as soon as possible. Infected or

devitalised tissue should be excised. Early skin grafting of burns prevents opportunistic infection. Other blood products to enhance immunocompetence may be considered as clinically indicated.
- The vascular syndrome is due to vascular bed dilation and capillary leaking. Shock occurs as a result of volume loss and poor vascular resistance, due to stimulation of acute inflammation and release of vasoactive humoral mediators causing peripheral vasodilation.
- The cerebral syndrome comprises nausea, vomiting, cardiovascular instability, confusion, ataxia, seizure and loss of consciousness. There is a high mortality within 24–48 hours.

Recovery/death

Death or recovery over several weeks are sequelae of the illness.

GOALS OF EMERGENCY DEPARTMENT MANAGEMENT OF CBR EXPOSURE

The ED's goals are to:
- protect staff from toxic exposure
- rapidly assess and treat immediately life-threatening problems
- decontaminate
- determine the identity of the hazardous materials or chemical agents and provide specific treatment as indicated
- prevent cross-contamination of staff, visitors and other patients
- restore the clinical environment to normal functions following the incident.

Personal protective equipment (PPE)

The use of PPE by staff treating contaminated patients is the single most important line of defence against airborne agents. It prevents cross-contamination and provides a physical barrier and respiratory protection.

There are various safety standards of protective equipment. Hospitals generally require safety standard C equipment. The suggested contents of a level C PPE kit are outlined in Box 22.2.

Isolation areas

CBR plans must include the availability of an isolation area. In some instances, this may be a physical structure that has been developed in keeping with appropriate standards that have been incorporated into new or renovated facilities. In other circumstances, the isolation area may be makeshift or portable. Decontamination takes place within or immediately adjacent to the isolation area.

Box 22.2 Suggested contents of a level C PPE Kit

- Chemically-resistant splash suit with hood, storm flap and sealed seams
- Waterproof boots
- Butyl gloves—1 pair
- Nitrile gloves—6 pairs
- Full-face respirator with disposable filters—3
- Filter shower covers—3
- Chemically resistant tape—1 roll

Hot zone

The hot zone is an area of contamination. For practical purposes, this is an isolation area for dealing with contaminated casualties. In selecting an appropriate area for the hot zone, consideration needs to be given to wind direction, slope for run-off, access to water and drainage, ability to provide screening for privacy, traffic management and proximity to the ED.

Warm zone

The warm zone is a buffer area between hot and cold zones to minimise cross-contamination.

Cold zone

This is a clean, non-contaminated area.

Decontamination corridor

The decontamination corridor traverses the warm zone. The decontamination process is functionally a one-way sequence and process. Contaminated casualties enter the hot zone, pass through the decontamination process and exit into the cold zone, prior to definitive treatment within the ED.

Contaminated-area and hot-zone issues

Life-saving equipment required in this area will be out of service until decontaminated. All patient clothing and personal belongings are bagged and labelled. All items used and present in the hot zone must be decontaminated before reuse or, in the case of personal belongings, returned to owners. Specialist cleaning may be required.

Decontamination requires the availability of showering facilities. Screening is necessary for patient privacy. The area must be well ventilated. If necessary, ventilation may need to be enhanced using portable industrial exhaust fans.

In makeshift or portable situations, the contaminated hot zone, the uncontaminated cold zones and the ED should be easily identifiable and taped off to prevent accidental cross-contamination.

Contaminated waste and patient belongings are double-bagged, a red ('dirty') label is attached and the bag is placed in a yellow contaminated-waste bin. Extreme care should be taken with patient clothing and valuables. These must be clearly labelled, as they may be the only form of patient identification and may be required for forensic evidence.

Specimens that may cause cross-contamination through the normal means of transport must be transported in a safe manner. This may require specimens to be transported in labelled, sealed containers via a courier.

Decontamination

Decontamination aims to remove substance and stop ongoing exposure. Decontamination requires the removal of clothing and showering with copious amounts of water. If there is any doubt about contamination, then the person must be decontaminated. This also applies to emergency services personnel.

For safety reasons, only those staff designated as members of the decontamination team and wearing full PPE are permitted to decontaminate patients. If protective respiratory equipment is required, only staff trained in the equipment are to be deployed.

The following points serve as a guide to effective patient decontamination:

1 It is preferred that males and females be segregated.
2 The patient stands on a plastic sheet and removes clothing and personal belongings. These are wrapped in the sheet and placed in a bag. The bag is placed in a second bag. Identification and red 'contaminated' labels are attached.
3 Patients proceed to decontamination showers. Copious amounts of water and soap are used. Liquid, flour and disposable wipes and tissues may be required to remove thick liquid before showering.
4 Following decontamination, patients move through the warm zone or corridor to a 'clean area' or cold zone. The patient is dried and clothed in a standard examination gown. Once externally decontaminated, the patient has a green 'external decontamination' tag or armband applied and is moved to the triage area.

Editorial Comment

When a patient removes clothing, it should not be over their head. Consider cutting clothing off to avoid contamination of the face/airways.

Specific decontamination issues

- A contaminated appendage can be washed without wetting the whole body.
- Skin is washed down for 5 minutes with copious amounts of soap and water.
- Open wounds require gentle scrubbing or irrigation of wound for 5–10 minutes with lukewarm water.
- Eye exposures require irrigation of eyes with sterile normal saline for 15–30 minutes.
- Contaminated facial and nose hair and ear canals are to be gently irrigated, with frequent suctioning to ensure removal of contaminants.

Substance identification

Substance identification is necessary for correct decontamination and for providing medical treatment specific to the substance.

Chemical substances may be identified using:

- HazMat or product advice sheets
- computerised databases, e.g. Poisindex
- dangerous goods guide
- Poisons Information Centre—phone number 13 11 26 (Australia-wide).

A biological agent may have been identified and advised by the state public health agency. If a biological agent is suspected, identification strategies should be planned in conjunction with health service clinical microbiologists or infectious disease doctors. Forewarning of and close liaison with laboratory medicine is required.

Radiation hazard identification may have already been advised by the relevant public health and environment protection agencies. However, local nuclear medicine departments, especially those associated with radiotherapy treatment centres, may initially be of assistance. It is preferable that a radiation physicist assist with on-site assessment of patients and the local environment for radioactive contamination.

Staff roles

It is essential that all staff members are familiar with their roles in a chemical, biological or radiation incident/disaster. The roles are similar to those identified for response to traumatically injured mass casualties.

The triage nurse or officer remains 'clean', adjacent to the triage station.

The senior doctor in charge remains in the cold zone and allocates medical personnel to specific duties and areas, such as to isolation and decontamination. Doctors allocated to the hot zone must be familiar with the PPE, equipment and procedures for decontamination and treatment. The doctor in charge endeavours to determine substance identification and specific treatment.

The role of the nurse in charge of managing nursing and clerical resources parallels that of the senior doctor. A specific responsibility is to ensure that the decontamination area is screened off for patient privacy, clearly marked, signposted and isolated to prevent cross-contamination.

Decontamination teams

A decontamination unit consists of 2 teams, each with a minimum of 3 staff: doctor, nurse and patient services assistant. One team triages using either sieve or sort methods, and where appropriate clinically manages time-critical patients in need of emergency care. The second team concentrates on decontamination procedures.

Colour-coded role-specific action cards outlining team roles should be worn around the neck.

Men with full beards will not be able to obtain an accurate seal from the respirator and thus cannot participate in a medical decontamination team.

Clean-up and decontamination of hot zone equipment

Hot zone equipment may be separated into two groups, a chemical/disaster box and supplementary equipment, as outlined in Box 22.3.

Non-disposable hot zone equipment requires cleaning. Specialist cleaning may be necessary. These items should be doubled-bagged and labelled with a red 'contaminated' label.

Disposal of consumables, cleaning of equipment and restoration of decontamination areas to normal activities will vary among hospitals depending upon the set-up. Issues include:

- Chemical disposal of any contaminated waste water.
- Cleaning or disposal of contaminated clothing and contaminated disposable protective clothing.

Box 22.3 Suggested equipment lists for decontamination areas

Chemical disaster box equipment

- Personal protective equipment—disposable barrier suit, overshoes, nitrile gloves and respirator with disposable filter and air hose
- CBR procedure manual
- Liquid soap, flour, disposable wipes or tissues
- Clear bags for double-bagging of contaminated clothing and linen/ black pen to write on contents of bag (e.g. linen, patient clothing, disposable equipment)
- Plastic sheet
- Red CONTAMINATED tags and green DECONTAMINATED tags
- Red CONTAMINATED patient labels and green DECONTAMINATED patient labels
- Special specimen-carrying container for contaminated specimens
- Nozzle for hose
- Hazard signs and tape to identify isolation zone

Other equipment

- Hoses to connect to external outlets (depending on decontamination zone design)
- Dressing trolley for laying out resuscitation equipment
- Patient trolley(s)
- Portable oxygen and suction
- Transport resuscitation bag—adult and paediatric
- Defibrillator
- Portable BP cuff and sphygmomanometer
- Portable otoscope
- Towels, gowns to use after decontamination shower, warm blankets
- Clean trolleys for decontaminated patients
- Dirty linen skip

- Cleaning of the shower and hot zone areas. Cleaning staff may need access to PPE.
- Cleaning of contaminated equipment.
- ED staff may be able to clean equipment if this can be achieved safely. If not, specialist cleaning may be required.
- Disposable equipment will need to be replaced. This includes PPE equipment such as suits, gloves, overshoes and respirator hoods.
- Government agencies responsible for environment protection are notified if hazardous chemicals have entered the sewers or stormwater drainage system.
- Particulate matter removed from radiation exposure victims may need to be stored in lead-lined bags or sealed containers.

Staff decontamination

Staff should only remove and dispose of PPE and clothing when contaminated 'dirty' area clothing and linen has been double-bagged and trolleys and other equipment used in this area have been decontaminated.

Clinical and related wastes

The underlying principles for the treatment and disposal of clinical and related wastes are the health and safety of personnel and the public and the minimisation of overall environmental impact.

Clinical wastes include sharp items and human tissue wastes. Related wastes include cytotoxic, pharmaceutical, chemical and radioactive wastes. Ultimate disposal of wastes will depend on their nature and on national, state or local regulations governing the disposal of hazardous substances.

Wastes need to be segregated according to their category, bagged, packaged or containerised. Segregation practices need to facilitate the ongoing maintenance of safe waste movement and transport.

Plastic bags are used for the collection and storage of clinical and related wastes, other than sharps. They need to be of sufficient strength to safely contain the waste class they are designated to hold. They need to conform to colour coding and marking. If moist sterilisation is to be used for decontamination, bags must be suitable for that purpose. Bags may only be filled to a maximum of two-thirds of their capacity or to a maximum weight of 6 kg. This allows for secure final closure and unlikely tearing of the bag. Bags may only be secured with closure devices not having sharp protuberances such as staples or exposed wire ties.

Rigid-walled containers are used for collection of sharp items. Containers such as mobile garbage bins should be resistant to leakage, impact rupture and corrosion. These containers should be inspected after each use to ascertain that they are clean, intact and without leaks. Any containers should have interiors of smooth impervious construction to contain any spillage and to be able to be readily inspected, cleaned and sanitised. Rigid-walled containers must be appropriately colour-coded and securely closed, but not necessarily locked, during transport.

The key consideration for clinical and related wastes storage is their safe containment in a vermin-proof, clean and tidy area. Storage requirements will be dependent upon the volume and type of clinical and related wastes to be contained and the mode of waste treatment to be employed. Procedures will also be dictated by the logistics of waste treatment methods and the requirements of disposal facilities.

Waste segregation is maintained during the movement and handling of wastes. If waste is mixed or loses identification during movement, it must be treated at the highest level of contamination. Movement of wastes through patient care areas should be avoided. Industrial trolleys should be used to move clinical wastes contained in plastic bags or non-mobile rigid-walled containers.

Chemical exposure register

A chemical exposure register may be managed by the fire brigade or an appropriate HazMat management agency. However, hospital staff may be required to manage this.

All staff, including visiting emergency service personnel, and patients involved in contaminated areas must be listed on the register. The minimum details required in the register include name, hospital record number, designation and injuries sustained. Contact details of involved staff are recorded to ensure timely access if additional follow-up is required.

A tag stating the person has been exposed to a radiation, biological or chemical hazard and the substance involved is attached to the patient in the form of a wrist band. It is worn for a predetermined time, usually 48 hours in the case of a chemical exposure.

Online resources

South Australian Metropolitan Fire Service website
www.mfs.sa.gov.au

Victorian Metropolitan Fire Brigade website
www.mfb.sa.gov.au

Acknowledgements

Parts of this chapter were developed from the following documents:

NSW Health Medical Services Supporting Plan to NSW HEALTHPLAN, August 2010.

Canestra J, Jones S, Wassertheil J, Johnstone R (Frankston Hospital External Disaster Committee), eds. Respond Brown—external disaster plan. Victoria, Australia: Peninsula Health; 1999.

Jones S, Smith M, eds. Hazardous substance management. Victoria, Australia: Peninsula Health; 2000.

The section on radiation illness has been largely developed from: Holmes JL and Mark PD. Nuclear incident medical management. In: Emergency management practice manual 3: health aspects of chemical, biological and radiological hazards. Provisional edn. Australian emergency manuals series, part 3. Emergency Management Australia; 1999.

Tribute

I wish to acknowledge the life and contribution to emergency medicine of Associate Professor Jeff Wassertheil who passed away on 22 September 2008. He will remain a highly esteemed emergency medicine specialist, researcher, teacher, colleague and friend who, in spite of being in hospital, put the finishing touches into the previous MCI chapter of this book.

Gordian Fulde

Chapter 23
The seriously ill patient—tips and traps

Gordian W O Fulde

It is the purpose of every emergency department to assess, resuscitate, diagnose and treat, both definitively and symptomatically, the patients who walk or are wheeled in through the door.

The ultimate responsibility for this belongs to the medical officer. In order to cope when faced with a variable number of patients whose conditions vary in severity, an organised approach is essential.

There must be triage (sorting) and re-triage, especially if the department is busy. See Chapter 45, 'Advanced nursing roles'.

The emergency doctor should use a priority problem-oriented approach and make clear decisions. As the leader of the team of medical officers, nurses, clerical staff, radiographers, porters and the many others who are often needed to attend to a sick patient, this approach is imperative. The doctor must assess, resuscitate and manage the patient and the patient's relatives. As a rule, decision making is harder in the case of patients who are not critically ill. The majority of all admissions (60–70%) come from triage category 3. Such patients should be assessed and managed with emphasis on early symptomatic relief and reassurance.

A key to keeping control of a busy department is that the most senior medical and nursing staff must be aware of all patients (including those waiting in ambulances). This may involve, for example, after a resuscitation doing a 'flash' ward round to do a 'stocktake' and allocate priorities, make admission decisions, contact inpatient staff to come down or accept problems.

Emergency doctors must communicate well so that most parties, most of the time, have some idea what is happening or what they need to do. For example, with system problems, ensure you escalate 'up' early; that is, if beds are full and ambulances are waiting, ensure medical and nursing administration know (contacting them by mobile phone is best—they also want to know early).

Remember to ensure a safe and professional environment for patients and staff. Do not compromise this, as it is wrong and it will come back to bite you even though your motives were honourable.

Although it goes against human nature, ensure that difficulties are documented and submitted to the quality and risk system of your hospital. The system will respond, especially if serious or repeated problems are listed objectively. Emails to key people next working day also speed up action if critical issues are encountered. (See also Chapter 47, 'Administration, legal matters, governance and quality care in the ED'.)

In attending to the many problems encountered in an ED, rely on good clinical common sense in order to avoid pitfalls. At all times, play it safe. Be suspicious of any complication. Never be afraid to ask or 'google'. The patient must be managed in as close to an 'ideal' fashion as possible. Distractions such as work pressure or the many other difficulties faced in EDs (e.g. bed shortages) should play no major role in individual management. Of course, good written documentation is essential as evidence of what was done and why.

Warning—red lights—beware

For all of us there are red warning lights that alert us to potential pitfalls:

- **Re-presentations to the ED.** Think it through again; do not just accept the last diagnosis.
- **Patient sent in by another healthcare professional,** e.g. GP, community nurse. They are asking for your and the hospital's help.
- **If pain is severe and unrelieved, worry!** You have probably missed something. Continuing out-of-character pain is a very common feature of misdiagnosis—so re-think! At the very least, observe and ask.
- **Repeated questions or protests,** e.g. the patient, the patient's mother, anybody who keeps telling you 'they are sick' or 'this is not normal for the patient', are a key indicator of pathology going on.
- **Triage categories 3 and 4** are often quite sick (especially if old).
- **Check vital signs frequently yourself** (BP, pulse, respiratory rate, temperature, blood glucose level, coma scale, oximetry). They change quickly.
- **Unpleasant patients (with or without difficult relatives).** Never vary your standard approach and management. Document all. This also applies to VIPs and friends. Always be polite, not rushed, try to sit down, get eye contact and listen.
- **Hand-over patients.** Make sure you have the whole story and plan. In the USA this patient group features highly in court cases. Use the ISBAR tool (see Figure 21.1).

- **Poor history, poor examination.** History and examination are cornerstones of the diagnosis. If you are unable to get good facts, be very careful and conservative, and worry.
- **Investigations are never 100% accurate.** Even if a test is very expensive, do not worship it—it makes mistakes. Many tests confirm a diagnosis but do not fully exclude it. Look at the whole clinical picture. A multi-hundred-slice CT or multiple TESLAR MRI or even an X-ray does not necessarily mean you are expert enough (even in spite of pretty reconstructions) to definitively report. CT MRIs are finding new lesions that were not seen before and that may not be pathological.
- **Urgent treatment** (see Law 1, below). Sometimes you must treat on suspicion, *now!* For example, tension pneumothorax, bacterial meningitis, narcotic overdose, hypoglycaemia. Early pain control may also be needed.
- **Pain.** Always listen to the patient; go through all details of the pain (avoid leading questions!). This way you will probably get the diagnosis. Treat pain very early.
- **Abnormal results.** With so many tests now available, learn to scan for pivotal ones, i.e. those associated with time-critical bad outcomes. Ideally the lab should let you know by phone until all results go back to the orderer by smart-phone or such and alert you of an abnormal result via an alarm. An example of key abnormals is shown in Table 23.1.

Decision-making tips

In the ED, we are all seeing older, sicker, more-complicated patients. You must focus on:

- What made the patient come to hospital? What do they hope for?
- Are all the vital signs OK?
- Do I need extra help, extra information (old notes, GP, specialist advice)?
- Problems → plan of management.

An important question is: 'Does the patient need admission to hospital?' This is better approached from the other perspective: 'Is it safe or appropriate to send the patient home?' If the answer is to be 'yes', refer to the discharge checklist in Box 23.1.

The patient must be able to cope alone. Is there anyone to help? Can the patient take necessary medications, prepare and eat meals and go to the toilet? Also, can the patient survive any likely complication

Table 23.1 Critical results

General chemistry levels						
		Low critical values (= or <)		High critical values (= or >)		
Test (blood)	SI units	Paediatric (> 1 month to 16 years)	Adult	Neonate (up to 1 month)	Paediatric (> 1 month to 16 years)	Adult
Sodium	mmol/L	130	125		150	160
Potassium	mmol/L	2.8	2.8		6.0	6.0
Bicarbonate	mmol/L	16	10		35	40
Glucose plasma	mmol/L	2.5	2.5		15	25
Phosphate	mmol/L	0.4	0.4		2.8	2.8
Magnesium	mmol/L	0.5	0.5		2.0	2.0
Calcium (total)	mmol/L	1.6	1.6		3.2	3.2
Calcium (ionised)	mmol/L	0.8	0.8		1.6	1.6
pH		7.2	7.2		7.5	7.5
pCO_2	mmHg	–	–		–	70
pO_2	mmHg	40	40		–	–
Lactate	mmol/L	–	–		4.0	3.4
CarboxyHb	%	–	–		10	10
MetHb	%	–	–		10	10
Bilirubin	micromol/L			280		
Uric acid	mmol/L				0.400	
Urea	mmol/L				20	
Creatinine	micromol/L				100	

Haematology	
Platelet count	< 50 × 10^9/L
Absolute neutrophil count	< 1.0 × 10^9/L
Hb	< 80 g/L
WBC	< 2.0 × 10^9/L or > 30.0 × 10^9/L

Box 23.1 Discharge checklist—safe discharge, especially after-hours and for all elderly or disabled patients

1. Mobility—can the patient mobilise safely?

- Has the patient been observed to mobilise without assistance?
- If normally used, does the patient have a walking aid?
- Will the patient be able to sit in/get up from a chair?
- Will the patient be able to get into/up from bed?
- Will the patient be able to get from the transport vehicle into their residence (distance to front door, steps to negotiate)?

2. Social or family—is there adequate family or social support?

- Is someone available to take the patient home?
- Will someone be with the patient overnight if needed?

3. Nutrition, hygiene, comfort—can the patient attend to basic needs?

- Can the patient eat and swallow?
- Will the patient be able to shower/toilet without assistance (can they get clothes on and off)?
- Will the patient be able to prepare meals (can they open a can, is there food at home)?
- Is the patient pain free; does the patient have medications to take?

4. Cognitive function—is the patient likely to place himself or herself in a dangerous position?

- Can the patient be expected to avoid unnecessary personal risk (is there a history of wandering, leaving gas outlets open, etc)?
- Can the patient be expected to avoid self-harm, self-medicate?

5. Discharge instructions

- Letter
- Instructions understood
- Third party (GP, relative aware)

If NO has been answered for any of the above:

Determine whether the problem/potential problem can be adequately addressed (e.g. if the patient cannot walk from the car into their place of residence, ambulance transport may be organised) and document strategies below.

....

....

....

....

....

If NO has been selected for any of the above and appropriate management strategies can be identified, the patient should not be discharged at this time.

Patients choosing to discharge against medical advice must be asked to sign themselves out.

of the medical condition? The fact that the ED was excessively busy at the time and the hospital was full will not be at all useful as an excuse in a legal inquiry or a court case relating to the management of an individual who was inappropriately sent home. Always err on the side of safety and, if you are not sure what to do, get the most senior medical officer possible involved in the decision making. Always write details in the notes of what was decided, by whom and why.

Usually some follow-up, either by a local doctor, specialist or outpatients department, is indicated. This must be organised and noted in the patient's record.

Emergency department 'laws'

LAW 1: ALL PATIENTS ARE TRYING TO DIE BEFORE YOUR EYES

You must always think in terms of worst-case scenarios, e.g. cardiac infarcts, meningitis, subarachnoid haemorrhage, pulmonary embolism. This is even more vital where early specific treatment will cure and prevent death. It may seem dramatic, but if you treat or exclude these serious illnesses early, further management of the patient is often very straightforward. Remember, medicine is best geared to treat the serious illnesses and society expects us to get these right.

Once serious illness is excluded and explanations are given, the patient is often grateful and happy for follow-up by GP or specialist.

LAW 2: CALL FOR HELP EARLY!

The team approach for complicated emergencies, such as trauma and cardiac arrest, should be activated early, i.e. even before patients 'crash'. Early involvement of intensive specialists, those responsible for definitive care, is imperative. Never be reticent to ask for more help—a 'routine' case of acute pulmonary oedema is enough work for 2 doctors in the initial resuscitation phase. Always aim for the hypothetical optimum-care scenario, i.e. pretend that the patient is a loved relative.

If the patient is critical and unstable, call the arrest team or similar response team (e.g. medical emergency team) before it happens. The patient is much more likely to do better if you prevent the crash. See Table 23.2.

The patient who meets one or more of these criteria should be in a resuscitation area with adequate doctors and nurses. The 'drama' phase lasts only a few minutes and staff can return to their other patients as soon as you have control of ABCs.

Table 23.2 Calling for help criteria

Call for help for any patient who meets the following criteria

Change in	Physiology
Airway	Predicted difficult airway Unable to obtain
Breathing	All respiratory arrests Respiratory rate < 5 breaths/min Respiratory rate > 30 breaths/min O_2 saturation < 90%
Circulation	All cardiac arrests Pulse rate < 40 beats/min Pulse rate > 140 beats/min Systolic blood pressure < 90 mmHg
Neurology	Sudden fall in level of consciousness Fall in GCS ≥ 2 points Repeated or prolonged seizures Not-intubated GCS < 9
Other—any patient you are seriously worried about who does not fit the above criteria	For example: — Unable to obtain prompt assistance, resources — 'Difficulty speaking' — Agitation or delirium, violent — Any unexplained decrease in consciousness — Uncontrolled pain — Failure to respond to treatment

GCS, Glasgow Coma Scale score

Based on criteria set out in Parr MJ, Hadfield JH, Flabouris A et al. The medical emergency team: a twelve month analysis for activation immediate outcome and not-for-resuscitation orders. Resuscitation 2001;50:39–44.

Observation charts are now designed to highlight abnormal observations (e.g. Between the Flags). Do not ignore a deteriorating trend even if not abnormal yet.

LAW 3: BE FLEXIBLE

Many sick patients defy any discrete label or have a diagnosis backed up by clearly abnormal tests. Follow your clinical impression, keep looking and be prepared to be surprised and change your management direction. If in doubt, observe.

LAW 4: TREAT THE PATIENT, NOT JUST THE TESTS

Clinical impression (is this patient sick?) has been repeatedly shown to be highly accurate in picking up sick patients where scores, protocols, tests, etc have not clearly 'ruled in' a diagnosis (e.g. acute coronary syndrome). If in doubt, watch, observe, ask.

Do not feed the lawyers

- See above.
- Never openly criticise colleagues or management—you rarely have all the facts, let alone the other side's reasons. Clinical signs evolve and change.
- Respect the efforts of the healthcare workers. Do not talk shop (i.e. the imperfect world of healthcare and mistakes or problems) in public. It makes it worse for all. If there are problems, use the system/process to improve it, i.e. be constructive—there is always someone to discuss a problem with who can give advice on how to tackle it and achieve improvement. Also, positive feedback works well! Use it freely!
- Always find out early what the patient, relatives, GP, etc expect or want, especially if it is not clear what the problem is or why they came. You will make a lot of people happy with your service, even if you can only give an explanation of why you cannot meet their immediate perceived need. You also will save a lot of time and expense.
- To have a really good work environment, where the patient and you will do well, see Table 23.3.

INTERACTION WITH POLICE, LEGAL PROFESSIONALS, THE MEDIA

In the first instance, *say nothing*—until you have checked with someone more senior who knows what you are allowed to say, what the normal protocol is, e.g. whether the responding person should be the treating consultant, hospital medicolegal officer, hospital public relation officer, etc. An innocent comment taken out of context can cause no end of trouble.

The fun bits

Do these as much as you can:

- Teach—students, nurses, allied health and community (CPR); use aids such as photos and handouts and involve the learners.
- Engage in research—clinical audits, chart reviews (see benchmark article by EH Gilbert, SR Lowenstein et al. Chart reviews in emergency medicine research: where are the methods? Ann Emerg Med 1996;27(3):305–9).
- Mentor medical students, trainees, nurses—join up with other centres.

Table 23.3 **Emergency department 10 commandments**

1	IF IN DOUBT, ASK This includes asking medical, nursing, clerical and allied health staff
2	NO PATIENT IS TO BE DISCHARGED FROM THE EMERGENCY DEPARTMENT UNLESS THE EMERGENCY REGISTRAR/ CONSULTANT KNOWS ABOUT IT Especially if sent in by an LMO
3	BE SAFE: • universal protective measures • wash hands • safe shoes • safe sharps disposal • immunisations up-to-date • know 'needle-stick' protocol • know location of wall-mounted alarms • wear personal duress alarms • know hospital codes (see Figure 47.1)
4	IF YOU SUSPECT PROBLEMS, GET HELP EARLY
5	SEE PATIENTS IN THE TRIAGE ORDER THEY APPEAR ON THE EMERGENCY DEPARTMENT INFORMATION SYSTEM SCREEN and COMPLETE INFORMATION Print out discharge letter, instructions and results for the patient
6	ALWAYS CONSIDER ANALGESIA, GIVE ANALGESIA EARLY VIA THE MOST APPROPRIATE ROUTE (INTRAVENOUS UNLESS SPECIFICALLY CONTRAINDICATED)
7	WHILE ON DUTY IN THE DEPARTMENT, BEHAVE AS YOU WOULD LIKE A DOCTOR TREATING YOUR FAMILY TO BEHAVE
8	TREAT EVERYBODY EQUALLY: • socially • medically • be thorough and polite
9	WRITE NOTES GOOD ENOUGH TO USE IN A COURT APPEARANCE; DOCUMENT CLEARLY IN YOUR MEDICAL NOTES Include discharge instructions and whom notified
10	BE TIDY: • appearance • identification • names—yours legible, patient's on history and medication charts • do not leave X-rays out of packets and give back private X-rays, etc • keep consultation rooms clean • put used trays and sharps away • doctors, keep your office tidy • cot bed sides up when you leave the patient

- Simulation centres do course scenarios, and also have practice mannequins for anything from intubation to IVs (including intraosseous and LPs). Go and ask.
- Update yourself—ensure the department subscribes to journals, audio (*Emergency Medical Abstracts*, *Emergency Reports*, etc), journal club, podcasts, online resources, etc.
- Ensure that interesting articles are routinely circulated to staff; assist staff to attend conferences, courses, etc.
- Socialise—support departmental social and sporting events; everybody should attend some of the activities. Ensure they are well publicised and preferably that each group is represented. Get to know your fellow workers better—make the effort!

Chapter 24

Neurological emergencies

Donald S Pryor and Adam C F Chan

Coma or impaired consciousness

- Impaired consciousness is recognised and described by observation of response to sound, light, touch or painful stimulus. The Glasgow Coma Scale (GCS) gives a standard way of recording and monitoring the level of consciousness (see Chapter 15, 'Neurosurgical emergencies').
- Coma signifies diffuse disturbance of brain function, e.g. trauma, epilepsy, drugs, hypoxia, hypoglycaemia or metabolic abnormality, or it can be due to a brainstem lesion or brainstem compression.

HISTORY

Available information may be limited. Sources to contact include family, workplace, police, ambulance officers, family doctor, etc.

EXAMINATION

Look generally for signs of:

- head injury
- raised intracranial pressure (hypertension, bradycardia with dilated and non-reactive pupil is classical, see Chapter 15)
- drug overdoses—narcotics (needle track marks, pinpoint pupils)
- psychostimulants (dilated pupils, tachycardia, hypertension)
- tricyclic antidepressants (tachycardia, hypotension ± seizures)
- hypoxia (tachypnoea, cyanosis and abnormal pulse oximetry)
- hypercapnia (history of chronic airway limitation, oxygen given by ED or ambulance staff)
- metabolic causes—hypo/hyperglycaemia, sepsis, hepatic or renal failure, etc
- hypo/hyperthermia—measure temperature rectally; axillary or tympanic measurement is inaccurate in severe hypothermia or hyperthermia.

Look for specific CNS signs:

- Pupils: enlarged pupil with impaired response to light signifies a 3rd nerve lesion. This can alert to transtentorial herniation.

When bilateral, it suggests brainstem death. Small pupils occur with pontine lesions or opiate effect. Dilated pupils can be due to effect of psychostimulants.
- Eye movements: test by following a target or reflex with head turning (oculocephalic reflex). Failure of **conjugate** gaze to the side of the hemiplegia is common with a hemisphere lesion. When severe, the head and eyes stay deviated away from the hemiplegic side. **Dysconjugate** gaze is indicative of lesions of the 3rd, 4th and 6th cranial nerves or their nuclei or connections in the brain stem.
- Fundoscopy: look for papilloedema which usually indicates raised intracranial pressure. Pre-retinal haemorrhage, which may have a fluid level, suggests subarachnoid haemorrhage (SAH). Hypertensive or diabetic retinopathy may be present.
- Motor signs: look at posture and for absence of spontaneous movements.
- Tone—classically increased but, with acute CNS damage, decreased tone is usual.
- Tendon reflexes—classically increased but may be absent or reduced with an acute lesion.
- Plantar responses—classically extensor but may be absent with an acute lesion.

Note:

1. Decerebrate posturing may be confused with purposive movements.
2. Drug effects and hypoglycaemia may mimic focal neurological lesions.

INVESTIGATIONS

- Blood count, blood sugar level (BSL), electrolytes, urea and creatinine (EUC), liver function tests (LFTs) and calcium
- Serum paracetamol and urine drug screen
- Arterial blood gases (pH and pCO_2 level)
- Cerebral CT scans (first-line)
- Chest X-ray (CXR)
- If sepsis is suspected: blood and urine culture; lumbar puncture should only be performed if there are no contraindications (see 'Lumbar puncture', below)
- Urine analysis: catheterisation may be indicated to obtain urine for microscopy, drug screening, glucose and ketones; may be indicated for monitoring urinary output and nursing care reasons

MANAGEMENT

1. Ensure a patent airway and adequate oxygenation.
2. Establish venous access.
3. Treat hypo/hyperglycaemia.
4. Give naloxone 0.4 mg IV, up to 2 mg over 10 minutes for signs of narcotics overdose.
5. Give thiamine 100–200 mg IV for unknown cause of coma or signs of alcoholism/neglect.
6. Treat underlying conditions.
7. Monitor neurological signs and GCS half-hourly.
8. Maintain normal pulse, BP, temperature, hydration, monitor urine output and perform pressure care.
9. Raised intracranial pressure is usually an indication for immediate neurosurgical consultation. Treatment to gain time for definitive surgery may include:
   a. passive hyperventilation to a PCO_2 of 30–35 mmHg
   b. mannitol 20% (0.5–1.0 g/kg) by IV infusion over 20 minutes has an immediate effect which persists for hours
   c. in proven cerebral tumours, dexamethasone 12 mg IV—effect is not apparent for hours, but has the potential for long-term use.

SPECIFIC INVESTIGATIONS

Lumbar puncture (LP) only after cerebral CT scans (see 'Lumbar puncture', below).

Epilepsy

Fits are usually self-limiting and no urgent drug treatment is needed. However, prolonged or multiple fits require urgent treatment. Obtain history of:

- Epilepsy, antiepileptic drug and compliance
- Alcohol intake and timing of last drink
- Medications which may cause hyponatraemia
- Previous pseudoseizures—which are common and hard to recognise
- Malignancy and its treatment, which may cause hypercalcaemia
- Eclampsia in women of childbearing age.

During fits:

1. Immediate care should be directed to minimising injury from burns, cuts or falls.
2. Observe the features and duration of the fit: rigid (tonic) or jerking (clonic) or focal (arm, leg, face, eyes, lips, etc), responsiveness,

breathing, pallor, cyanosis, frothing, incontinence, eyes open or deviated, vocalisation, etc. Classification as *generalised* or *partial* will influence management.
3 Turn patient semi-prone and clear airway as soon as tonic phase and clonic movements cease.
4 Do not put anything between the teeth during a fit. Damage to the patient's teeth or the carer's fingers is more likely than any benefit.
5 Exclude hypoglycaemia early using bedside BSL testing.
6 Insert IV cannula and take blood.

INVESTIGATIONS

- Blood count, electrolytes, renal function, glucose and calcium
- Assay for antiepileptic drugs
- Cerebral CT scans

Consider other tests for less-common causes: HIV, syphilis.

PROLONGED FITTING OR FREQUENT FITTING (STATUS EPILEPTICUS)

Major generalised seizures lasting more than 30 minutes, or recurring rapidly without regaining consciousness in between, are life-threatening.

Treatment should be commenced after 5 minutes of continuous generalized seizure. This situation demands prompt airway management, high-flow oxygen, IV drug therapy, monitoring and support.

Treatment

1 Arrange transfer to a resuscitation area while commencing drug treatment. Establish IV access.
2 Give midazolam 2.5 mg IV with repeated bolus doses up to 15 mg (0.15–0.2 mg/kg for a child). IM administration can be used if venous access is delayed. Alternatives to midazolam are:
   — clonazepam 1–2 mg bolus IV (child 0.25–0.5 mg bolus)
   — diazepam 10–20 mg by slow IV aliquots of 5 mg, repeated if necessary (child 0.1–0.25 mg/kg).
3 Add phenytoin 15–20 mg/kg IV at no more than 50 mg/minute (if patient is not already taking phenytoin). For a child, administer 20 mg/kg IV at no more than 25 mg/minute. Monitor ECG and vital signs.
   OR
   Sodium valproate 10 mg/kg IV (child 15–30 mg/kg) up to 800 mg by slow IV injection followed by infusion of

1–2 mg/kg/h to a maximum of 2500 mg/day (or 40 mg/kg/day for a child).
OR
Other IV anticonvulsants, e.g. levetiracetam.

4. If seizures persist despite treatment, anaesthetise with thiopentone and muscle relaxant, provide ventilatory support and admit to intensive care unit.
5. Monitor temperature, oxygenation, acidosis, lactate, hydration, urine output, serum electrolytes and EEG.
6. Re-establish or adjust long-term oral anticonvulsants.

Cerebrovascular disease

Stroke is either cerebral infarction or haemorrhage. Infarction accounts for 80% of strokes. CT scans show haemorrhage immediately, but the signs of infarction are usually delayed for several hours. Transient ischaemic attack (TIA) is a focal ischaemic neurological deficit which usually lasts less than 1 hour.

INITIAL ASSESSMENT AND MANAGEMENT OF STROKE

Focus on:

- ensuring a clear airway, adequate oxygenation and circulation
- excluding stroke mimics, e.g. seizure, hypoglycaemia, sepsis, syncope, drug overdose, hypoxia, hyponatraemia and hemiplegic migraine
- documenting neurological deficits and level of consciousness
- identifying any cardiovascular abnormalities, e.g. atrial fibrillation (AF), signs of endocarditis, carotid bruit/dissection
- urgent cerebral CT scans to exclude haemorrhage or space-occupying lesions
- nil by mouth (NBM) until bedside swallow screen is performed
- aspirin as soon as haemorrhage is excluded and thrombolysis is not indicated
- regular monitoring of neurological status, blood glucose, blood pressure and hydration status.

Admit to stroke unit.

Thrombolytic therapy in stroke

- Thrombolysis is indicated for ischaemic stroke if the hospital is set up for this. Check for any contraindications such as recent surgery or anticoagulation. Follow the protocol to have the alteplase (rtPA) infusion commence as soon as possible within 4.5 hours of symptom onset. (*pto*)

- Alteplase 0.9 mg/kg up to a maximum dose of 90 mg. 10% of alteplase is given stat and 90% is given as IV infusion over 60 minutes. No antiplatelet or anticoagulation agents for 24 hours.

Common patterns of neurological impairment

- Hemisphere—hemiplegia with dysphasia or sensory inattention; embolism likely
- Internal capsule—pure motor hemiplegia; hypertensive lacunar infarction likely
- Brainstem—bilateral motor signs, sensory loss, vertigo/nystagmus, coma, ataxia, cranial nerve signs; vertebrobasilar system disease

Clinical diagnosis of pathophysiology

- Is it intracranial arterial occlusion due to atheroma, hypertension, and diabetes?
  or
- Neck vessel disease with embolism—carotid bruit?
  or
- Embolism from the heart—e.g. atrial fibrillation, prosthetic valve, infective endocarditis, recent myocardial infarction?

Investigations

- Perform urgent non-contrast CT scans, full blood count (FBC), electrolytes, creatinine, blood glucose level, coagulation studies, urinalysis, ECG and chest X-ray.
- Initial CT scans can be normal for ischaemic stroke, as infarction is best shown a few days after the onset. Early CT is used to exclude haemorrhage or brain tumour to allow the commencement of antiplatelet or thrombolytic agents.
- Magnetic resonance imaging (MRI) and magnetic resonance angiography can replace CT scans and carotid ultrasound when available. MRI shows infarction immediately after a stroke and can distinguish a new from an old infarct. Small lesions and brainstem lesions invisible in CT scans can be seen with MRI.
- Perform transthoracic echocardiography and carotid Doppler ultrasound studies. Transoesophageal echocardiography (TOE) may be needed to exclude cardiac embolism.

Stroke management checklist

- Oxygenation: maintain oxygen saturation at > 95%.
- Neurological status: hourly GCS and neurological observation for first 4 hours or until stabilised.

- Body temperature: control fever at < 37.5°C with paracetamol orally or rectally. Septic work-up if temperature > 38°C.
- Blood glucose: aim for 5–11 mmol/L. If BSL < 3 mmol/L, give 50% dextrose. If BSL > 11 mmol/L, cautious lowering of BSL can be commenced with SC insulin. Avoid hypoglycaemia.
- Blood pressure: established drug treatment for hypertension should be continued. Avoid new antihypertensive drug therapy during the first 24 hours, as it may worsen the ischaemia. However, treatment is indicated if systolic blood pressure (SBP) is >220 mmHg or diastolic blood pressure (DBP) is > 120 mmHg; but no more than a 10–20% reduction acutely.
- NBM and IV fluid to maintain hydration until swallow screen is performed.
- Urine output: bladder catheterisation may be needed to monitor urine output and assist nursing care of pressure areas.
- Deep-vein thrombosis (DVT) prophylaxis: subcutaneous low-molecular-weight heparin (LMWH) if not contraindicated.
- Antiplatelet therapy: start aspirin 300 mg stat then 150 mg daily.
- Anticoagulation: heparin or warfarin give no benefit in the initial management of acute ischaemic stroke due to increased risk of haemorrhagic transformation. Warfarin is protective in the long term with AF or other cardiac disease causing embolism.
- Positioning: coma position for impaired consciousness. Support for hemiparetic limbs, prevention of injury to the neglected side and general pressure care.
- Stroke unit: admission to a specialised stroke unit has proven benefits in reducing secondary complications and mortality.

TRANSIENT ISCHAEMIC ATTACK (TIA)

This is a neurological dysfunction resulting from focal brain or retinal ischaemia, usually lasting less than 60 minutes. It is often resolved by the time of ED presentation. Overall risk of stroke following TIA is around 8–10% at 1 week.

The diagnosis of TIA is intended to identify patients with platelet or cholesterol microemboli arising in neck vessel atheroma. Transient monocular visual loss is very suggestive of carotid artery stenosis.

The initial ED investigations for TIA should be the same as those given for stroke, above. Antiplatelet therapy can be commenced after cerebral haemorrhage is excluded by CT scan.

Hospital admission or specialised clinic referral may be needed to avoid any delay in stroke prevention measures.

INTRACEREBRAL HAEMORRHAGE

- Haemorrhage accounts for 10–15% of all strokes.
- Associated with high mortality—a 12-month survival rate of 30%.
- Bleeding due to anticoagulant therapy is common.
- Haemorrhage may be due to rupture of small vessels damaged by hypertension.
- With older age, amyloid angiopathy is common.
- Bleeding can be from arteriovenous malformation or aneurysm.
- Initial assessment and management are similar to ischaemic stroke, as listed above.
- Acute haemorrhage is easily recognised as a radiodense area in CT scans.
- Hypertensive intracerebral haemorrhage will usually be in the internal capsule/striatum or pons. Intracerebral haematoma from a berry aneurysm will arise from near the circle of Willis, and peripheral haematomas suggest amyloid angiopathy.
- MRI and contrast cerebral angiography may be needed to define suspected aneurysm or arteriovenous malformation (AVM).

Treatment

Treatment is as per the stroke management checklist given above, with the following modifications:

1. Cease all antiplatelet or warfarin therapy.
2. If patient is on warfarin use prothrombin complex concentrate, fresh frozen plasma (FFP) and vitamin K.
3. Institute antihypertensive treatment if SBP is > 180 mmHg or DBP is > 110 mmHg on 2 consecutive readings and after adequate analgesia. Lowering blood pressure acutely may compromise cerebral perfusion and must be done with caution.
4. Hydration: fluid restriction may be needed, as syndrome of inappropriate antidiuretic hormone secretion (SIADH) is common.
5. Consult neurosurgeon for possible surgical interventions. Surgical drainage may be life-saving for cerebellar haematoma.
6. Surgery may also be considered for presence of hydrocephalus, marked mass effect or haematoma associated with AVM or aneurysm.

Headache

The vast majority of headaches are benign and self-limiting. The goal of managing patients presenting to the ED with headache is to exclude potentially serious conditions and to relieve pain. Important diagnoses to be considered are:

- subarachnoid haemorrhage
- meningitis/encephalitis
- space-occupying lesions
- giant cell (temporal) arteritis
- acute narrow-angle glaucoma
- hypertensive encephalopathy.

MENINGITIS

Clinical features

- Headache with fever suggests meningitis, and there may be vomiting, photophobia, neck pain or stiffness, confusion, coma, irritability or fitting.
- Examine for neck stiffness and also purpura or hypotension in meningococcaemia; sources of infection, e.g. middle ear, sinusitis, cerebrospinal fluid (CSF) leak; or viral infection such as mumps or mononucleosis.
- Immune-deficiency states will totally change the bacteria likely to be responsible.

Investigations

- FBC, erythrocyte sedimentation rate (ESR), C-reactive protein (CRP), electrolytes, creatinine, blood glucose and CXR.
- Blood cultures.
- Nose, throat and ear swabs.
- Viral cultures, viral antibody titres.
- Cerebral CT scans must be obtained before a lumbar puncture (LP) is performed. Focal neurological signs, altered conscious state or features of raised intracranial pressure are all contraindications to LP if CT scans are not obtainable.
- An LP is needed to confirm the diagnosis and to identify and culture the organism.

Treatment

1. Give IV antibiotics as soon as the possibility of bacterial meningitis is realised. Do not wait for CT scans or LP. (Blood cultures or CSF polymerase chain reaction (PCR) may assist when antibiotic treatment has rendered the CSF negative to Gram stain and culture.)
2. Ceftriaxone 2 g IV every 12 hours (children 50 mg/kg/day).
3. Appropriate antibiotic for known organism/sensitivity, e.g.

benzylpenicillin 1.2–1.8 g every 4 hours (children 350 mg/kg/day) IV for *Meningococcus* or *Pneumococcus*.

4 Steroid therapy (IV dexamethasone 10 mg 6-hourly or 0.15 mg/kg) reduces neurological sequelae and mortality with known or suspected pneumococcal meningitis. Initial dose should be given prior to antibiotic therapy.
5 Treat disseminated intravascular coagulation, adrenal failure, SIADH and other complications.
6 Prophylaxis: it is recommended that household contacts of confirmed meningococcal and *Haemophilus influenzae* type b meningitis be given prophylactic antibiotics. Healthcare workers are not at increased risk for the disease and do not require prophylaxis unless they have had direct mucosal contact with the patient's secretions, as might occur during mouth-to-mouth resuscitation, endotracheal intubation or nasotracheal suctioning. The choices of prophylaxis can be rifampicin, ciprofloxacin or ceftriaxone.

LUMBAR PUNCTURE (LP)

Indications

The major role for LP in the emergency department is the diagnosis of infection or bleeding within the central nervous system (refer to Chapter 3, 'Resuscitation and emergency procedures').

Preparation

- Discuss the reasons, procedure and possible complications of the procedure with the patient or carer.
- Obtain verbal or written consent.

Complications

The most common complication is post-LP headache. It is caused by gravity-dependent traction on pain-sensitive intracranial structures due to low CSF pressure. The incidence of headache can be reduced by using a small-sizes LP needle (22-gauge) or pencil-point tip with a side hole (Sprotte needle). Bed rest has not been shown to improve the incidence of headache.

Other complications include:

- epidural haematoma
- local trauma to spinal cord or nerve roots
- infection such as discitis or epidural abscess.

Interpretation of CSF findings

- Normal CSF pressure is 5–20 cmH_2O when the patient is horizontal. High pressure may indicate the presence of space-occupying lesions or CSF outflow obstruction. Low pressure is associated with severe dehydration or CSF leak.
- Macroscopic appearance:
  - normal—clear and colourless
  - infection—cloudy
  - blood—pink or frank blood
  - old blood—yellow (xanthochromia).
- Laboratory testing:
  - urgent microscopy for cell count, differential and Gram stain
  - biochemistry: glucose and protein
  - xanthochromia if SAH is suspected
  - acid-fast bacillus and India ink stains if tuberculosis or *Cryptococcus* is suspected
  - cultures
  - antigen and PCR testing if antibiotic therapy was given prior to LP.

Table 24.1 Laboratory findings for CSF in meningitis

	Normal	Bacterial	Viral	Tuberculosis or fungal
White cell count/mL	< 5, and < 1 polymorphs	> 500 Polymorphs predominant	< 500 Monocytes predominant	< 500 Monocytes predominant
Glucose (mmol/L)	2.5–3.5	Low	Normal	Low
Protein (g/L)	0.18–0.45	High	Normal	High
Gram stain	–ve	+ve in 80%	–ve	–ve
Antigen	–ve	+ve in 80%	–ve	–ve

Additional considerations

- Pretreatment with antibiotics will diminish the yield of Gram stains and cultures but will not affect the CSF cell count.
- The initial CSF cell counts may show lymphocytosis in bacterial meningitis, and CSF may possibly be normal in culture-proven meningitis if LP is done in the early phase of the disease.
- The presence of a clot in one of the tubes or the clearing of CSF blood-staining from tubes 1–3 suggests traumatic LP. If traumatic tap is suspected, subtract 1 white cell for every 1000 red blood cells.

ENCEPHALITIS

Clinical features

- Headache and fever with neurological signs or fits suggests encephalitis.
- Impaired level of consciousness and delirium are common.
- There is overlap between meningitis and encephalitis.
- Encephalitis is mostly viral. Sometimes the specific virus can be identified from associated clinical features (e.g. mumps, rabies) or from laboratory tests, cultures and antibody titres, or from the epidemiology (e.g. Murray Valley encephalitis).
- Herpes simplex encephalitis demands early diagnosis as treatment is life-saving.
- Immunocompromised patients can present with parasitic or fungal as well as viral infections, e.g. toxoplasmosis, cytomegalovirus, progressive multifocal leuco-encephalopathy.

Investigations

- FBC, ESR, CRP, EUC, BSL and CXR
- Viral cultures and antibody titres
- Cerebral CT scans often show subtle changes, hypoattenuation in a temporal lobe and mass effect may be present
- Lumbar puncture—WCC 50–500/mL, mild elevation in protein, normal glucose; CSF sent for viral cultures, antibody titres and PCR for HSV and other viruses
- MRI is more sensitive and more specific than CT scans

Treatment

- Specific treatment is not available except for herpes simplex encephalitis which responds to aciclovir 10 mg/kg in IV infusions every 8 hours for 10 days. Each dose must be infused over not less than 1 hour.
- This drug should be commenced urgently on suspicion of herpes simplex encephalitis—i.e. clinical encephalitis with cells in the CSF.

SUBARACHNOID HAEMORRHAGE (SAH)

(See also Chapter 15, 'Neurosurgical emergencies'.)

Clinical features

- SAH should be considered in any new headache as the diagnosis is often missed. In particular, patients presenting with sudden onset of severe, 'worst ever' headache with or without neurological findings should be suspected of having a subarachnoid haemorrhage. Loss of consciousness and vomiting are common.

- Up to 50% of patients experience a 'warning bleed' associated with headache which settles spontaneously or with simple analgesia. Re-presentation with second bleed is usually catastrophic and associated with poor outcome. It is often due to a ruptured berry aneurysm and sometimes due to a vascular malformation.
- Hypertension, polycystic disease and aortic coarctation are associated with berry aneurysms. Monoamine oxidase therapy or illicit drug use may result in acute hypertension with SAH.
- On examination, look for meningism, altered level of consciousness, confusion or focal neurological signs (such as hemiparesis or dysphasia). Papilloedema may be present. Pre-retinal (subhyaloid) haemorrhage is virtually diagnostic. A cranial bruit may indicate an arteriovenous malformation. Absence of physical signs cannot exclude SAH.

Note: Migraine is not a likely diagnosis in a first-time severe headache.

Investigations

- Non-contrast cerebral CT scans in the first 24 hours will demonstrate subarachnoid blood in 90–95% of cases. Sensitivity of CT scans decreases with time: 80% positive at 3 days and 50% at 1 week.
- Lumbar puncture (LP) is necessary if there is clinical suspicion of SAH and CT scans do not provide a diagnosis. The diagnosis of SAH is dependent on the finding of red cells or xanthochromia in the CSF. Xanthochromia is due to breakdown products of haemoglobin in the CSF and is usually present within 6 hours of haemorrhage. Hence, LP can be delayed for 6–12 hours from the onset of symptoms to minimise false-negative findings.
- CT angiography has evolved as the preferred imaging modality for the cause of the haemorrhage. Digital subtraction or magnetic resonance angiography can be used as the next tier of investigation modality.
- Others: FBC, electrolytes, creatinine, BSL, ECG and CXR are relevant.
- SIADH, temporary hyperglycaemia and cardiac tachyarrhythmias may complicate the bleed.

Treatment

1. General supportive measures with airway protection, adequate oxygenation and blood-pressure control.
2. Relieve headache and restlessness. Use diazepam for sedation, narcotic analgesia for headache and antiemetics.
3. Maintain blood pressure in normal range by analgesia and sedation. Antihypertensive therapy should be used with caution.
4. Restrict fluids to 1200–1500 mL per day.
5. Antispasm drug treatment (nimodipine) oral or IV should be commenced within 48 hours of haemorrhage.
6. Monitor neurological signs.
7. Bed rest with head up by 30° in dark, quiet room.
8. Surgical clipping or coiling of the aneurysm or excision of or embolisation of an arteriovenous malformation remain the definitive treatments.

MIGRAINE

Clinical features

- The pathophysiology of migraine is complex and poorly understood. It is defined as idiopathic recurring headache disorder with attacks that last 4–72 hours.
- There is often presence of a family history and sometimes triggers such as food or menstruation. The headache may be preceded by a prodrome or aura of visual or other neurological symptoms.
- Typical characteristics include gradual onset, throbbing quality, unilateral location, nausea, vomiting, photophobia and prostration. Major but temporary neurological signs may result from migraine, causing diagnostic problems, e.g. aphasia, hemiplegia.
- Investigations will be normal and should be directed towards excluding other serious diseases as suggested by the clinical features—SAH, meningitis, etc.
- Although not life-threatening, migraine causes great suffering. When the diagnosis is secure, the goal is to relieve pain and other associated symptoms.

Treatment

1. Soluble aspirin 600–900 mg or paracetamol 1–1.5 g 4-hourly, up to 4 g/day.
2. Metoclopramide (10 mg orally or IV) has both antiemetic and direct analgesic effect.

3 Non-steroidal anti-inflammatory drugs (NSAIDs) can be an alternative: ibuprofen 400–800 mg orally or indomethacin 100 mg rectally.

If previous experience with these measures has failed:

4 Chlorpromazine: very effective treatment in 80% of patients who are unresponsive to oral analgesics. Preload patient with 1 L of normal saline, followed by chlorpromazine 12.5 mg given as a slow IV push over a few minutes. Further 12.5 mg boluses can be administered every 15–20 minutes, up to 37.5 mg if headache persists.
Hypotension should be treated with 500 mL boluses of normal saline and acute dystonia is treated with 2 mg of IV benztropine.

5 Sumatriptan is effective in 60–75% of cases. The recommended dose is 50–100 mg orally, 10–20 mg intranasally or 6 mg SC. Other triptans may be used: eletriptan 40–80 mg orally, naratriptan 2.5 mg orally, rizatriptan 10 mg wafer or zolmitriptan 2.5–5 mg orally.

If treatment with the above measures has also failed, consider:

6 Dihydroergotamine, a potent vasoconstrictor. The recommended dose is 0.5–1 mg SC or IM or IV with metoclopramide to minimise the gastrointestinal side effects. Note that ergot compounds are contraindicated with concomitant triptans.

Note: Narcotics are not advised.

GIANT CELL ARTERITIS (TEMPORAL ARTERITIS)

This disorder needs urgent diagnosis and steroid treatment, as delay may result in loss of vision. It occurs in older age (> 50 years), often female, and severe headache may be the only symptom. Jaw claudication and tenderness and swelling over the temporal artery may be present. The diagnosis is confirmed by a high ESR, temporal artery biopsy and response to steroids.

Treatment

If the clinical diagnosis is likely, commence steroid therapy immediately with prednisone 75 mg orally. Response within hours to the first dose of steroids can be diagnostic. Temporal artery biopsy and ESR help plan long-term treatment.

ACUTE NARROW-ANGLE GLAUCOMA

May present with unilateral headache and vomiting. Refer to Chapter 36, 'Ophthalmic emergencies'.

OTHER CAUSES OF HEAD PAIN

Very many other diseases of ears, eyes, nose, sinuses, teeth and temporomandibular joints may cause head pain.

Bell's palsy

HISTORY

This is an acute peripheral facial nerve palsy of unknown cause. There is rapid onset of unilateral facial weakness with reduced forehead and eyelid movements and sagging of the corner of the mouth.

Other features include ear pain, decreased tearing, hyperacusis and loss of taste on one side.

EXAMINATION

Conduct a neurological examination and look for vesicles or scabbing at or in the external ear canal (which indicates herpes zoster) or a mass in the parotid gland. Sparing of the forehead and eyelid muscles is suggestive of an upper motor neuron lesion because of bilateral innervation to this area.

TREATMENT

- Early treatment with oral prednisone 60–80 mg daily for 1 week, preferably within 3 days of symptom onset.
- Eye care with artificial tears or ointment or a patch to prevent drying and abrasion of the cornea.
- Antiviral agents have not been shown to have benefit in treating Bell's palsy in the absence of signs to suggest herpes zoster.

Paraplegia

Acute paraparesis or paraplegia is an emergency, as any delay in treatment may result in irreversible spinal cord damage. Mild or early cord lesions due to compression are most likely to benefit from prompt diagnosis and decompression and just such cases are more likely to be misdiagnosed.

CLINICAL FEATURES

Motor

- Weakness in the legs presents as difficulty walking. There is a pyramidal pattern of weakness (flexors and abductors more than and before extensors). Spasticity may be present.
- Tendon reflexes are increased with extensor plantar responses, but in an acute cord lesion upper motor neuron signs may be

absent. There may be flaccid paralysis with absent reflexes (spinal shock).
- Flexor spasms can be mistaken for voluntary movements.

Sensory
- Numbness or paraesthesias start in the feet regardless of the level of the lesion. Only when the damage has progressed will a distinct sensory level clearly indicate the segment of cord involved.
- In spinal cord disease, look for the highest abnormal signs. Minor abnormalities in the arms or a Horner's syndrome indicate that the disease is in the neck, when most of the deficit may still be in the legs.

Autonomic
- Careful interrogation is often necessary to reveal significant symptoms in early cord lesions.
- Constipation—insidious changes in bowel habit occur in subacute or chronic lesions.
- Urgency of micturition is often admitted only after leading questions. Retention of urine in severe lesions is revealed by a palpable bladder. The retained volume should be recorded if a catheter is passed. Retention with overflow (palpable bladder and large volume on catheterisation or ultrasound) should not be confused with simple incontinence.
- Erectile impotence may be revealed only on specific enquiry.

INVESTIGATIONS
- FBC, CRP, ESR, electrolytes, creatinine, LFTs, CXR and CT scan of cervical and thoracic spine.
- Urgent MRI of the whole spinal cord if there is any possibility of cord compression.
- Myelography is appropriate if MRI is not available.
- CT scans can show the lesion, particularly if the exact level is known, but MRI or myelography is needed to exclude a compressive lesion.

TREATMENT
- Emergency surgery to decompress the cord is the important measure to consider.
- Bladder care is also an urgent matter. Failure to relieve retention by catheter will damage the bladder. Leave an indwelling catheter draining.

(*pto*)

- Nursing and medical care is a specialised problem, and transfer to a special unit should be arranged without delay in acute or severe paraplegia.

Confusion

CLINICAL FEATURES

Document conscious state, behavioural and emotional disturbance, impairment of thought processes, disorientation, confabulation, delusions and hallucinations.

DIFFERENTIAL DIAGNOSIS

Exclude focal cerebral disorder—e.g. dysphasia.

Acute confusion

- Systemic infection—pneumonia, septicaemia
- Cerebral infection—meningitis, encephalitis, acquired immunodeficiency syndrome (AIDS dementia complex)
- Epilepsy—postictal, complex partial or absence status
- Metabolic—hypoglycaemia, uraemia, hepatic failure, hypercalcaemia
- Cerebral hypoxia—systemic hypoxia, hypotension, hyperviscosity
- Subarachnoid haemorrhage
- Cerebral tumour—including subdural haematoma
- Post-traumatic concussion
- Transient global amnesia
- Endocrine: hypothyroidism, hyperthyroidism, hyperglycaemia, hypoglycaemia, acute adrenocortical failure.
- Toxic—alcohol (Wernicke's, delirium tremens), barbiturates and sedatives, anxiolytics, antiparkinsonian drugs, illegal drugs
- Deficiency states—thiamine, vitamin B_{12}

Chronic confusion

- Dementia—Alzheimer's disease
- Vascular disease—multi-infarct dementia
- Cerebral tumour—including subdural haematoma
- Chronic encephalitis/meningitis—viral, syphilitic, AIDS
- Communicating hydrocephalus
- Metabolic—uraemia, hepatic, electrolyte disturbance
- Endocrine—hypothyroidism
- Toxic—drugs, alcohol, Korsakoff's psychosis
- Pseudodementia due to psychiatric disorder

Acute-on-chronic confusion

Usually an underlying dementia complicated by infection, drug toxicity or psychosocial disruption.

INVESTIGATIONS

1. Neurological and general physical examination
2. Exclude infection in lungs or meninges, hypoxia
3. FBC, ESR, CRP
4. Electrolytes, creatinine, blood glucose levels, LFTs, calcium, HIV, syphilis test (VDRL)
5. MSU, blood cultures
6. CXR, arterial blood gases/pH
7. Vitamin B_{12}, folate, thyroid function
8. Drug screen—urine and blood
9. Thiamine IV 100 mg
10. EEG
11. Cerebral CT scans or MRI

Chapter 25
Gastrointestinal emergencies

Greg McDonald and Christopher Wong

The aim of the emergency department assessment of patients with gastrointestinal (GI) tract emergencies is to rapidly identify and stabilise those patients requiring urgent surgical or procedural intervention. In pursuing this aim, the processes of assessment, investigations appropriate to the disease and management should be followed in an orderly and focused manner and must be performed simultaneously in the seriously ill.

Acute abdomen

An 'acute abdomen' may be defined as an acute intra-abdominal condition causing severe pain and often requiring urgent surgery. The causes may be:

- inflammatory, e.g. appendicitis, diverticulitis, cholecystitis, perforated viscus
- mechanical, e.g. incarcerated hernia, band adhesions, volvulus, intussusception
- vascular, e.g. aortic aneurysm, mesenteric infarction
- neoplastic, e.g. carcinoma colon
- congenital, e.g. malrotation, congenital atresia/stenosis, Meckel's diverticulum
- trauma.

ASSESSMENT

History

- Who is your patient? Age and sex are two important aetiological factors.
- Patients over the age of 65 years are twice as likely as younger patients to require surgical intervention.
- Consider gynaecological disorders, especially in women of childbearing age.
- Previous medical and surgical histories and a drug history will give important clues to diagnosis and need to be considered for operative fitness.

- When did the pain start? Acute onset of severe pain implies vascular events, perforated viscus or renal colic. Slower onset of pain tends to imply inflammatory causes.
- Where is the pain? Abdominal pain often localises to the site of the pathology. Has it moved? Initial visceral pain is usually diffuse and in the midline. As the disease progresses, somatic pain becomes more localised.
- What is the pain like? The colicky pain of bowel obstruction is typically episodic and gripping, with pain-free intervals. In the case of biliary and renal colic, there is constant pain which rises to a crescendo. Constant severe pain indicates advanced or serious illness.
- Which other symptoms accompany this illness? The onset of nausea and vomiting after the onset of pain suggests surgical illness. Constipation is non-specific, but absolute constipation (neither faeces nor flatus) indicates bowel obstruction. Diarrhoea, jaundice, haematuria, haematemesis or melaena suggest specific diagnoses.

Note: Only two-thirds of patients with acute surgical conditions have a classical history of illness. Children and the elderly are more likely to have atypical presentations.

Examination

General

Appearance: apprehensive and motionless with peritonitis, unsettled and agitated with colicky pain; pale and 'Hippocratic faeces' consistent with advanced disease.

Check temperature, hydration, pulse and blood pressure (with postural drop).

Abdomen

- Inspection—rigid, distended or scaphoid, visible peristalsis, operative scars.
- Palpation—diffuse or local tenderness, rebound, guarding.
  Note: 'Rebound' is not pathognomonic of peritonitis. It is falsely positive in up to one-quarter of patients, and subjective. Cough impulse and percussion tenderness are often more reliable.
- Percussion—local peritonism, air, fluid (shifting dullness), masses, organs.
  Note: Loss of liver dullness occurs with pneumoperitoneum.
- Auscultation—although not sensitive, you may hear peristaltic noises coinciding with colic in small-bowel obstruction; diffuse

increased bowel sounds in gastroenteritis; silent abdomen or occasional tinkling sounds in late bowel obstruction or diffuse peritonitis.

Special signs

- Murphy's sign in cholecystitis; Rovsing's, psoas and obturator signs in appendicitis; Cullen's (peri-umbilical) and Grey–Turner's (flank) signs of bruising in pancreatitis; costovertebral tenderness (renal punch) with pyelonephritis or perinephric abscess.
- Hernial orifices/scrotum and testes should never be forgotten.
- Rectal examination, as indicated, looking for blood (bright, melaena or occult), faecal loading, local tenderness, masses, prostatomegaly.
- Pelvic examination: incorrect and uncertain diagnoses occur much more frequently in women. A careful vaginal examination may help differentiate pelvic pathology. Ultrasonography when available is more accurate.
  Note: Cervical excitation is a 'classic' sign of ectopic pregnancy and pelvic inflammatory disease, but is a subjective sign.

Other systems

Exclude non-abdominal pathology causing abdominal pain, e.g. pneumonia, pulmonary embolus and myocardial infarction.

INVESTIGATIONS

Immediate

- Urine—urine analysis, microscopy and culture, pregnancy test (if appropriate)
- Blood—haemoglobin; haematocrit (packed cell volume, PCV); white cell count and differential; electrolytes, urea and creatinine (EUC); amylase/lipase (if appropriate); blood gases (if appropriate); group-and-hold serum/cross-match (if blood loss or operation likely)
- Stool—occult blood
- Organ imaging—abdominal X-ray, supine and erect; chest X-ray (CXR), erect

Semi-urgent (with appropriate indications)

- Blood—liver function tests (LFTs), coagulation studies
- Stool—smear and culture for colitis, enteritis
- Organ imaging—abdominal, ultrasound CT scan, angiography
- Endoscopy—proctosigmoidoscopy, panendoscopy

Value of investigations

Pregnancy should be considered in all women of childbearing years with acute abdominal pain, to exclude ectopic pregnancy in particular.

White cell count and other inflammatory markers (such as C-reactive protein) are non-specific unless elevated markedly (e.g. neutrophilia above 20×10^9/L). They are often late manifestations of significant pathology.

Serum lipase is the test of choice for pancreatitis. Serum amylase is frequently elevated in a variety of conditions. Levels greater than 3 times normal strongly suggest pancreatitis. Lipase is more sensitive and specific for pancreatitis.

Abdominal X-rays are an insensitive tool for diagnosing non-specific abdominal pain, but can be valuable in confirming specific and serious pathology. Bowel obstruction, paralytic ileus, and caecal and sigmoid volvulus have typical findings. A paucity of bowel gas may be the only clue to mesenteric infarction. Remember, check for calculi and for air in the biliary tree, and to look at the psoas shadows, the size and shape of solid organs. Avoid abdominal X-rays in pregnancy.

Erect chest X-ray will detect subdiaphragmatic free air, exclude pulmonary pathology and help preoperative assessment. Free air will be absent in about 20% of perforated peptic ulcers. Massive pneumoperitoneum suggests colonic perforation. The chest X-ray is the initial investigation for Boerhaave's syndrome (oesophageal rupture).

Abdominal ultrasound is the preferred imaging modality for women of child-bearing age and many paediatric diagnoses. It is usually indicated for right upper quadrant (RUQ) pain and cholelithiasis, obstructive uropathy, suspected abdominal aortic aneurysm and abdominal masses. It is the investigation of choice in paediatric intussusception, pyloric stenosis, appendicitis. Pelvic ultrasound is essential for the diagnosis of gynaecological and pregnancy-related diseases.

CT scanning: spiral non-contrast CT is the initial test of choice for renal colic. Contrast CT is useful in diagnosing many acute surgical conditions, e.g. acute pancreatitis, intra-abdominal sepsis, intra-abdominal trauma. It is increasingly used to confirm the preoperative diagnosis before laparotomy.

Proctosigmoidoscopy is a diagnostic tool in bright rectal bleeding, rectal mass and colitis, and is therapeutic in sigmoid volvulus.

Other specialised tests

Angiography may be both diagnostic and therapeutic in intestinal haemorrhage, mesenteric ischaemia and abdominal trauma.

Panendoscopy is indicated urgently in life-threatening upper GI tract bleeding and semi-electively in stable patients with suspected peptic ulcer or other inflammatory conditions of the upper GI tract.

MANAGEMENT

Surgical emergency

Indications for urgent intervention include leaking abdominal aortic aneurysm, perforated viscus, advanced peritonitis, mesenteric infarction and strangulated bowel.

Common indications for laparotomy

'Exploratory laparotomy' is now infrequently performed. After adequate resuscitation, most patients with an acute abdomen will undergo specific imaging prior to surgery. Where diagnosis is uncertain, exploratory laparoscopy may be useful.

Preoperative treatment

1 Airway/Breathing—correct hypoxaemia.
2 Circulation—intravenous access and appropriate blood tests; volume resuscitation; urinary catheter.
3 Analgesia is a high priority in moderate to severe pain. Titrated intravenous opiates are preferred. This will not mask or delay the diagnosis, and it will help clinical assessment by reducing distress and anxiety.
4 Antibiotic prophylaxis is required with diffuse peritonitis or if infective pathology is suspected. Ampicillin, gentamicin and metronidazole is the usual combination therapy, to cover coliforms, enterococci and anaerobes.
5 Other preparation—nasogastric tube; operative fitness (cardiorespiratory assessment); consent by surgeon.

Surgical admission

Some conditions for which admission to hospital for conservative treatment, observation and semi-elective operation is appropriate are discussed later.

Emergency department observation and disposition

Patients with mild or equivocal tenderness, minor or no laboratory abnormalities and whose condition settles can be discharged for follow-up in the community, after observation in the ED. Certain diagnoses, e.g. uncomplicated renal or biliary colic and peptic ulceration, are discharged in most cases for further investigations and referral.

Specific surgical conditions

ACUTE APPENDICITIS

This is the most common general surgical emergency. Most problems occur with extremes of age, < 5 and > 60 years, mostly due to atypical presentation and late diagnosis.

Assessment

- Classical history is vague periumbilical pain, anorexia, nausea, vomiting, pain migration to right iliac fossa, fever. However, this only occurs in about half of cases.
- Clinical features can be summarised by the Alvarado (MANTRELS) score and include:
  - M Migration of pain
  - A Anorexia
  - N Nausea/vomiting
  - T Tenderness at McBurney's point
  - R Rebound tenderness
  - E Elevated temperature
  - L Leucocytosis
  - S Shift to the left of white cell count.
- Rectal examination is no longer indicated in the diagnosis of appendicitis.
- Pelvic ultrasound is preferable to pelvic examination in excluding gynaecological pathologies.
- **Differential diagnoses:** mesenteric adenitis in children; diverticular disease/caecal carcinoma in adults; ovarian cyst, pelvic inflammatory disease, ectopic pregnancy.

Investigations

- If appendicitis is strongly suggested by clinical features, no investigations are required, other than for preoperative assessment.
- Ultrasound is preferred for evaluating right iliac fossa pain in children and fertile female patients if the diagnosis is uncertain.
- CT is more sensitive than ultrasound and may reveal alternative diagnoses; contrast is not needed with newer CT scanners.

Management

1 Surgery as soon as practical. Overnight delay in the stable patient does not significantly worsen outcome.
2 Suspected perforation/generalised peritonitis—urgent surgery.
3 Prophylactic antibiotics reduce infective complications. They should be given in the ED if peritonitis or abscess is suspected or if surgery will be delayed. Otherwise, antibiotics can be given at induction of anaesthesia.
4 Mass/phlegmon—intravenous antibiotics and fluids; nil by mouth; ultrasound/CT scan; operation at surgeon's discretion.

GALL BLADDER EMERGENCIES

Assessment

- 25% of women and 12% of men have gallstones.
- Past history of fat intolerance, belching and flatulence.
- RUQ pain becoming constant and severe.
- Mild fever and tachycardia; mild icterus in 10% of cases.
- Tender RUQ with positive Murphy's sign (sudden increased pain on inspiration).
- Palpable gallbladder in about one-third of cases.
- Complications include:
  — Empyema—toxic/shocked, high spiking temperatures; palpable tender mass as disease progresses
  — Local perforation—progressing fever, symptoms and signs. Local mass and peritonism
  — Free perforation—general peritonism
  — Cholangitis—secondary to obstruction (stone disease), instrumentation procedure (ERCP, cholecystectomy); ascending infection; fever/rigors (~90%); RUQ pain (~70%); jaundice (~60%).

Investigations

- Urine analysis—bilirubin; exclude renal pathology.
- White cell count—not reliable but WBC > 15,000/mL suggest more-severe disease or complication.
- LFTs—are non-specific but bilirubin > 60 mmol/L suggests common duct obstruction.
- Ultrasound demonstrates stones, debris within the gall bladder, wall thickening, masses or abscesses.
- Abdominal X-ray is not necessary but may be ordered to exclude other pathology and complications.

- Hepatobiliary iminodiacetic acid scan (HIDA) may be used if ultrasound is non-diagnostic, e.g. acalculous cholecystitis.
- Operative fitness assessment (e.g. ECG, CXR, haemoglobin (Hb), renal function).

Management

Uncomplicated biliary colic

Discharge home for outpatient investigation and referral if:

- pain resolves
- no significant local signs
- normal laboratory investigations.

Cholecystitis

1. Admit to hospital.
2. Nil by mouth and intravenous fluids.
3. Analgesia.
4. Antibiotics intravenously (ampicillin/gentamicin).
5. Endoscopic retrograde cholangiopancreatography (ERCP) is rarely indicated; but may be necessary with obstructing bile duct stone.
6. Cholecystectomy, depending on progression of conservative therapy.

Advanced/complicated disease

Examples of this are cholangitis, empyema, abscess, free perforation, septicaemia.

1. Rapid stabilisation and assessment as for 'surgical emergency'.
2. Antibiotics (ampicillin, gentamicin and metronidazole or equivalents).
3. ERCP for bile duct obstruction; urgent cholecystectomy or cholecystostomy for empyema and abscess.

DIVERTICULAR DISEASE

50% of people over 40 years of age have diverticular disease.

Assessment

- Previous symptoms—irregular bowel habit; diffuse, non-specific lower abdominal pain
- Diverticulitis—fever; altered bowel habit; left iliac fossa (LIF) pain and tenderness with or without local peritonism; LIF or pelvic mass
- Diverticular abscess—toxic; palpable mass
- Free perforation—generalised peritonitis
- Bleeding (see 'Lower GI tract bleeding', below)

Investigations

- Urine analysis and midstream urine (MSU), to exclude renal pathology
- White cell count
- Contrast CT scan is the imaging modality of choice to confirm the diagnosis and assess severity of disease
- Abdominal X-ray usually non-specific, but may reveal perforation, local or generalised ileus or large mass if CT scan is not readily available

Management

- Mild cases—stable vital signs; pain controlled, can tolerate oral fluids—may be managed as outpatients with oral antibiotics (e.g. amoxycillin + clavulanate).
- More severe cases: admit; nil by mouth; intravenous fluids; intravenous antibiotics (ampicillin/gentamicin/metronidazole).
- Complicated/severe disease—e.g. advancing peritonitis; CT findings—management as above; urgent surgical consultation.

Gastrointestinal bleeding

UPPER GI TRACT BLEEDING

Aetiology

- 50% peptic ulceration
- 5–15% erosive gastritis/oesophagitis/duodenitis
- 15% oesophageal varices
- 15% Mallory–Weiss syndrome
- 5% others (tumour, blood dyscrasias, etc)

Note: 30% of patients with known varices will bleed from other non-variceal causes.

Assessment

History

- Amount and nature of bleeding (haematemesis/melaena)
- Symptoms of occult bleeding
- Drug history—alcohol; non-steroidal anti-inflammatory drugs (NSAIDs); steroids
- Past GI tract disease/other conditions

Examination/immediate intervention

- Airway—intubation is indicated for airway protection in massive haemorrhage.
- Breathing—correct hypoxia.

- Circulation—assess for signs of shock.
  (*Note:* Initial haemoglobin may be near-normal in spite of massive blood loss.)
- Blood—for cross-match; haemoglobin; haematocrit; electrolytes; urea/creatinine; coagulation studies; liver function.
- General—evidence of chronic liver disease and hepatic encephalopathy; abdominal examination including rectal exam with or without proctoscopy; cardiorespiratory status.

Investigations

- Nasogastric tube insertion is rarely helpful; it may be performed for:
  - stable patients as a diagnostic tool
  - profuse haematemesis to empty stomach prior to endoscopy.
- Panendoscopy is the definitive investigation, and in many cases an effective immediate treatment of upper GI tract bleeding. Panendoscopy within 24 hours in stable patients reduces re-bleeding rates and shortens length of stay. Information regarding the aetiology, site and prognosis of the bleeding is gained. Urgent panendoscopy should be performed in cardiovascularly unstable patients and in those with profuse or persistent bleeding.

Management

1. Volume resuscitation with crystalloids and/or blood and/or clotting factors.
2. Close monitoring of vital signs, urine output and haemoglobin/haematocrit. Invasive monitoring in the ICU for patients who are cardiovascularly unstable, elderly or have cardiorespiratory disease.
3. For presumed non-variceal bleeding, commence proton-pump inhibitors (PPIs). PPIs reduce bleeding recurrence, reduce mortality and shorten length of stay for ulcer-related bleeding.
4. Urgent panendoscopy on high-risk patients with shock; blood requirements > 5 units; serious underlying disease; recurrent bleeding—especially if over 60 years of age. Endoscopy within 24 hours improves outcomes for all patients.

Non-variceal bleeding

- 80% of cases will settle spontaneously; 20% will require intervention for recurrent bleeding within 48 hours.
- Poor prognostic endoscopic findings in non-variceal bleeding are: gastric ulcer, especially lesser wall; posterior site in duodenum; visible vessel; sentinel clot or black spot in ulcer base.

Definitive treatment of non-variceal bleeding:

- endoscopic haemostasis
- surgery
- angiographic haemostasis (depending on availability).

Variceal bleeding

Poor prognostic factors include large blood requirements (> 4 units), active bleeding at endoscopy and Child's category C patients (advanced hepatic failure).

Further management:

1. Endoscopic banding or sclerosis is 90% effective in controlling variceal bleeding. Balloon compression prior and/or simultaneously aids sclerotherapy.
2. Vasoconstrictive drugs—e.g. octreotide, a somatostatin mimic—lowers azygous vein blood flow in patients with portal hypertension, decreasing bleeding. This is a useful adjunct when endoscopy is not readily available.
3. Sengstaken–Blakemore or Minnesota tube may be used as a temporary option for failed pharmacological or endoscopic treatment.
4. Angiographic embolisation.
5. Transjugular intrahepatic portosystemic shunt (TIPS).

LOWER GI TRACT BLEEDING

Causes of profuse, bright per rectal bleeding include: diverticular disease; polyps; angiodysplasia; carcinoma/colitis/solitary ulcer; haemorrhoids; Meckel's ulcer in children.

Note: Bright or maroon rectal bleeding is usually lower GI, but can occur with profuse upper GI tract bleed.

Assessment

History, examination and immediate intervention are as for upper GI tract bleeding. Elevated urea out of proportion to the creatinine can suggest an upper GI tract site of bleeding.

Investigations

Pathology work-up similar to upper GI bleed.

Management

1. Volume resuscitation.
2. Monitor vital signs, urine output, haemoglobin/haematocrit with or without central venous pressure (CVP).
3. Bleeding stops spontaneously in 75% of cases with conservative treatment.

4 Sigmoidoscopy/colonoscopy is usually done on a semi-elective basis if the patient remains haemodynamically stable.
5 If the patient remains unstable in spite of resuscitation, arrange urgent specialist referral for possible mesenteric angiogram or surgical treatment.
6 Radio-isotope scanning has a role in stable patients with uncertain sites of lower GI tract bleed.

Acute pancreatitis

the causes of acute pancreatitis are: gallstones (40–50%); alcohol (25–35%); idiopathic (20%); and others which include a variety of medications (5%).

ASSESSMENT

History

- Look for potentially reversible causes.
- Acute epigastric pain through to back, associated with nausea and vomiting.

Examination/initial intervention

- Airway
- Breathing—correct hypoxaemia
- Circulation—anticipate shock; fluid resuscitate as required.
- Blood—for lipase/amylase; haemoglobin/haematocrit; electrolytes; urea/creatinine; calcium; glucose; LFTs; blood gases; coagulation studies; group-and-hold
- Abdominal examination—temperature, jaundice; epigastric tenderness with or without mass; local/diffuse peritonism; Cullen's (periumbilical) and Grey–Turner's (flank) signs in haemorrhagic pancreatitis; paralytic ileus; subcutaneous fat necrosis
- Cardiorespiratory examination, especially to exclude complications (respiratory complications occur in 10–20% of cases)

Prognostic indicators

- Disease ranges from mild inflammation to severe extensive pancreatic necrosis (10–20%) and multi-organ failure, with mortality rates of > 20%.
- Assessment of severity is important for management and to predict outcomes.
- 3 known severity scores are performed 48–72 hours after

diagnosis. They may therefore not be useful in the ED setting, but can be used to observe progress after admission.

i Ranson's criteria:
   - Immediate—age > 55; hyperglycaemia; leucocytosis; lactase dehydrogenase (LDH); aspartate aminotransferase (AST)
   - Two days—drop in haemoglobin/haematocrit; shock; hypocalcaemia; hypoxia; azotaemia (elevated urea)
   - Score of 5 (at 48 hours) suggests serious illness

ii APACHE score

iii Balthazar staging on CT scanning

Investigations

- Amylase/lipase—levels more than 3 times normal confirm the diagnosis in the majority of cases. Lipase is more sensitive and specific, and is better than amylase in diagnosing chronic pancreatitis.
- Abdominal X-ray—does not need to be performed routinely, but can be used to exclude other diagnoses and complications. A 'sentinel loop' of localised small intestine may be present.
- Chest X-ray—raised left hemidiaphragm; pleural effusion; atelectasis; acute respiratory distress syndrome (ARDS).
- ECG to exclude myocardial infarct.
- Ultrasound should be performed to exclude gallstone pancreatitis. CT scanning with contrast may be performed within 72 hours to assess severity. It should be performed early when there is diagnostic uncertainty and in critically ill patients.

Management

1. Volume resuscitation.
2. Supplemental oxygen.
3. Monitor observations, urine output with or without CVP.
4. Nil by mouth; nasogastric tube for severe cases or if gastric dilation or ileus.
5. Analgesia—parenteral narcotics.
6. Insulin infusion if blood sugar level (BSL) > 15 mmol/L.
7. Observe for other complications—shock/acidosis; acute tubular necrosis; ARDS/disseminated intravascular coagulation (DIC); haemorrhagic pancreatitis; pancreatic abscess.
8. Early nutritional support—nasojejunal or parenteral.
9. Prophylactic antibiotics—for severe cases.

10 Early ERCP is necessary for gall-stone pancreatitis with an obstructing stone.
11 Laparotomy has up to 40% mortality. There are multiple options of invasive techniques to treat the complications of pancreatitis.

Gastro-oesophageal reflux disease (GORD)—oesophagitis

Remember: Indigestion is not a diagnosis; it is an excuse to stop thinking.

- In discussing GORD, it is crucial to consider an acute coronary syndrome. Improvement of 'indigestion' with antacids is not proof of upper GI tract pathology. 'Indigestion' is a common diagnosis in missed acute myocardial infarction (AMI). The mortality rate of missed AMI is around 30%.
- About 7% of the population reports daily heartburn. **Risk factors** for GORD include: obesity; alcohol; smoking; diabetes; pregnancy. **Exacerbating factors** are: chocolate/fatty and spicy foods; drugs, e.g. NSAIDs; cough medicines; bisphosphonates.
- The commonest **symptoms** of GORD are: heartburn; regurgitation; dysphagia (oesophageal stricture or spasm). Atypical symptoms relate to gastric reflux, which may be 'silent', e.g. cough/wheeze or hoarseness.
- GORD is the commonest non-cardiac cause of chest pain (~50% of cases).

ASSESSMENT

History

- Look for aetiological factors.
- Epigastric and/or chest pain, typically burning. Oesophageal spasm may occur without burning pain.
- Reflux, with or without cough/wheeze/hoarseness.
- Haematemesis/melaena.
- Cardiac risk factors and cardiac symptoms—could it be angina?
- Fatty food intolerance; belching; RUQ pain—could it be cholelithiasis?
- Weight loss; anorexia; jaundice—could it be upper GI tract malignancy?
- Malignancy/steroid use/HIV/immunosuppression—could it be infective oesophagitis?

EXAMINATION

- Airway; breathing; circulation.
- Abdominal examination—tenderness (epigastrium/RUQ); look for other causes of epigastric pain, e.g. liver, leaking abdominal aortic aneurysm. If suspicious of GI tract bleed, perform rectal exam for blood.

INVESTIGATIONS

- For uncomplicated GORD, none may be required. Do not forget an ECG. A trial of PPIs or H_2-receptor antagonists may give relief and suggest GORD, but does not rule out other diagnoses.
- Exclude other diseases: ECG/cardiac markers; CXR; LFTs; amylase/lipase; abdominal ultrasound.
- Assess complications of erosive oesophagitis, e.g. full blood count (FBC); iron studies.

MANAGEMENT

1. Lifestyle modification—weight loss; avoid precipitating foods/smoking; elevate head of bed about 20 cm; eat evening meal 3 hours prior to bed; smaller meals.
2. If uncomplicated GORD, commence treatment and refer to local doctor:
   a. antacids after meals and at night may control symptoms
   b. PPI or H_2-receptor antagonist.
3. Red flags include dysphagia/odynophagia; refractory symptoms after treatment; bleeding/anaemia; weight loss and aspiration. Consult a gastroenterologist.

Mesenteric ischaemia/infarction

Acute mesenteric ischaemia is a notoriously difficult illness to diagnose and treat. Reported mortality rates average about 70%. It is often diagnosed late because of non-specific initial symptoms and signs. By the time peritonism or advanced abdominal signs are present, extensive bowel infarction has usually occurred and the prognosis is grave. The bowel can tolerate about 4 hours of warm ischaemic time. Significant bowel necrosis occurs after 8–12 hours of ischaemia.

Mesenteric ischaemia is usually due to impaired circulation of the superior mesenteric artery (SMA): 50% is embolic, 25% thrombotic and 20% 'non-occlusive mesenteric ischaemia' (low-flow states). About 5% is due to mesenteric vein thrombosis.

ASSESSMENT

- Patients with SMA emboli will usually have a past history of atrial fibrillation or myocardial infarction.
- Patients with SMA thrombosis have evidence of other arteriovascular disease, and up to half will have experienced prior mesenteric angina.
- Low-flow mesenteric ischaemia occurs in patients with pre-existing hypotension, sepsis and vasoconstrictor infusions. The elderly and those on digoxin are particularly at risk.
- Mesenteric vein occlusion tends to occur in younger patients with hypercoagulable states and have a slower onset.
- Abdominal pain out of proportion to clinical findings is an important finding. The pain is typically acute-onset, severe, constant and generalised, sometimes colicky. It often responds poorly to analgesia. Many patients have vomiting and diarrhoea.
- Similar to other ischaemic pathologies, there are few initial physical signs. There is minimal, if any, tenderness. As the disease progresses, abdominal distension and GI tract bleeding may occur. Localised tenderness over infarcted bowel loops, diffuse peritonitis and systemic sepsis occur as the bowel becomes gangrenous and necrotic.

INVESTIGATIONS

- Most patients will have a series of screening pathology tests and abdominal and chest X-rays (see 'Acute abdomen') in the early stages in an attempt to find the diagnosis. By the time these non-specific investigations are significantly abnormal, the bowel is infarcting.
- Rising serial lactates suggest the diagnosis, but also occur late in the disease. Critically ill patients in septic shock need a work-up to assess severity and monitor resuscitation.
- The definitive investigation is an abdominal contrast CT angiogram. Whenever there is a reasonable index of suspicion of the diagnosis, this must be arranged urgently.

MANAGEMENT

1. Airway
2. Breathing—supplemental oxygen to correct hypoxaemia
3. Circulation—intravenous access; volume resuscitation as necessary; nil by mouth; urinary catheter
4. Analgesia—titrated intravenous opiates

(*pto*)

5. Antibiotics—ampicillin/gentamicin/metronidazole, or equivalent
6. Urgent surgical opinion/urgent radiological opinion (CT angiography can be curative, not just diagnostic)
7. Definitive treatment depends on the underlying cause and clinical situation
8. Advanced peritonitis from gangrenous bowel requires urgent laparotomy
9. Vasodilator and/or thrombolytic infusion can be administered at angiography
10. Specific embolectomy or thromboendarterectomy by a vascular surgeon may be necessary

Vomiting

Vomiting is a symptom, not a diagnosis. Most vomiting patients have benign, readily treated illnesses. Occasionally it is a symptom of a life-threatening problem. Management is directed at finding and treating the cause, assessing fluid deficits and controlling the symptoms.

ASSESSMENT

History

- Age—in infants and children consider pyloric stenosis, intussusception, viral gastroenteritis, reflux, sepsis and meningitis.
  Note: Children become dehydrated more quickly.
- Chest pain—acute coronary syndrome; Boerhaave's syndrome (uncommon).
- Abdomen:
  - Fever; viral prodrome; contacts with gastroenteritis or suspect foods; diarrhoea—infection, e.g. gastroenteritis or food poisoning
  - 'Heartburn'; epigastric discomfort; haematemesis/melaena—peptic ulcer disease; erosive oesophagitis; oesophageal varices; Mallory–Weiss tear
  - Abdominal pain—colicky suggesting bowel obstruction; RUQ suggesting biliary disease; RIF suggesting appendicitis; generalised and severe suggesting peritonitis
  - Previous abdominal surgery and colicky pain—adhesions and bowel obstruction
  - Jaundice; dark urine—biliary disease; hepatitis.

- Neurology:
  - Headache—migraine; meningitis or meningism; cerebrovascular event; sub-arachnoid haemorrhage
  - Vertigo/'dizziness'—labyrinthitis; vertebrobasilar disease or posterior fossa lesion.
- Vision—glaucoma.
- Pregnancy—in women of childbearing age.
- Diabetic or symptoms of diabetes—ketoacidosis.
- Drugs:
  - Medications—opiates; antibiotics; chemotherapy
  - Marijuana abuse—cyclical vomiting syndrome (repetitive hot showers is pathognomonic).

EXAMINATION

- Airway
- Breathing—ketotic
- Circulation—vital signs; peripheral perfusion; dehydration
- Disability—mental state; Glasgow Coma Scale (GCS); pupils
- Targeted examination guided by history

INVESTIGATIONS

- Investigations depend on the clinical context and the likely aetiology. They serve 2 purposes: establishing the underlying cause, and assessing complications of vomiting.
- Basic tests should include FBC; EUC; LFTs; BSL; urine analysis; beta-hCG in women of childbearing age.
- Disease-specific tests depend on the suspected diagnoses.

MANAGEMENT

1 Restore fluid deficits depending on degree of dehydration and EUC results.
2 If severe dehydration/shock, resuscitate with normal saline. Insert indwelling urinary catheter if persistent shock.
3 Otherwise, per oral/NG or IV rehydration, depending on the clinical context. (Children in particular respond well to oral and NG rehydration.)
4 Anti-emetics include:
   a dopamine antagonists—metoclopramide, prochlorperazine (beware acute dystonic reaction in young women and children)
   b serotonin antagonists—ondansetron.
5 Disease-specific interventions as indicated.

Constipation

As in vomiting, it is important to rule out serious underlying causes of constipation. It is the commonest GI tract complaint, affecting up to 25% of people at some time. 2% of the population have chronic or recurrent constipation.

Causes in children:
- functional (over 90% of cases, especially if > 1 year old)
- change in formula or to bottle-feeding in infants
- Hirschsprung's disease
- congenital anorectal or neurological diseases
- cystic fibrosis
- metabolic disorders.

Causes in adults:
- primary—functional (normal transit); slow transit; anorectal muscle incoordination
- secondary—
  - medications (up to 40% of cases), e.g. opioids, antidepressants, calcium-channel blockers, diuretics, iron, antihistamines, psychotropic agents
  - irritable bowel syndrome (IBS)
  - psychological conditions, e.g. anxiety, depression
  - anorectal structural abnormalities, e.g. anal fissure, haemorrhoids
  - endocrine and metabolic diseases, e.g. diabetes mellitus, hypercalcaemia, hypothyroidism
  - neurological, e.g. Parkinsonism, multiple sclerosis, spinal cord disease; autonomic neuropathy.

Note: Constipation is not a 'normal' part of ageing.

ASSESSMENT

History

- Frequency and quality of stool; effort of defecation; pain; incomplete evacuation; soiling; bleeding; nausea/vomiting; medications; urinary retention
- **'Red flags' in children**—delayed meconium; abdominal distension/vomiting; failure to thrive, recurrent pneumonia (cystic fibrosis); abnormal gait or lower limb tone; wheat intolerance (gluten enteropathy)
- **'Red flags' in adults**—age over 50 years; weight loss; rectal bleeding; family history of colon cancer

Examination

Examination is directed at finding underlying cause and confirming faecal loading.

- Airway; breathing; circulation
- Dehydration if vomiting; abdominal distension
- Abdominal examination—looking for obstruction, masses or hernia
- Anal inspection—congenital abnormality in children; anal fissure; haemorrhoids; rectal prolapse
- Rectal examination—to confirm faecal loading:
  - mandatory in an adult; may be replaced by plain abdominal X-ray in children if parents object or child distressed (level C evidence)
- Specific system examination to exclude secondary causes, e.g. neurological (altered anal tone, abnormal lower limb power/tone/reflexes)

INVESTIGATIONS

- None usually required if history of functional constipation in child.
- FBC; BSL; EUC; calcium; thyroid function; urine analysis in adults. Abdominal X-ray may be indicated to exclude obstruction and/or reveal extent of colonic loading.
- Sigmoidoscopy and/or colonoscopy (semi-elective) if 'red flags' in adult.
- Specific investigations or consultations if secondary cause suspected.

MANAGEMENT IN ADULTS

This is a possible protocol. Local preferences may apply.

1 Distal rectal vault only:
   a 1–2 Microlax enemas → wait 30–60 minutes
   b 1–2 bisacodyl enemas → wait 30–60 minutes
   c Fleet (phosphate) enema *OR* 20 mL lactulose in 100 mL water → retain for at least 10 minutes; may be repeated once
   d Manual disimpaction (with analgesia; sedation)
   e May need admission for repeat enemas.
2 Faecal matter above rectum:
   a Oral sorbitol (70%) 30 mL q2–3 hours
   plus
   b Fleet (phosphate) enema or lactulose enema as above → wait 4–6 hours

(*pto*)

c If no success (or oral sorbitol not available) → Glycoprep-C solution 1 sachet/litre orally per hour, up to 3 litres
OR
Movicol 8 sachets in 1 litre over 6 hours
OR
oral picosulphate 1–2 sachets in a glass of water (causes greater fluid and electrolyte shifts; use cautiously in the elderly due to dehydration; renal impairment; cardiac failure).

Admission may be required for observation, repeat enemas and/or oral agents.

Patients may be discharged if they have at least 1 significant documented bowel action, for follow-up by their doctor in 24 hours.

The discharge plan should include dietary advice, fluid intake, exercise, toileting pattern, aperients and review of causative medications.

Editorial Comment

Constipation is *not* a diagnosis, nor is it an excuse to stop thinking. Hospital EDs often have a very helpful protocol for this very common symptom (see Figure 25.1 overleaf). Be aware of red flags.

Hepatic failure—portosystemic encephalopathy

FULMINANT

- Acute hepatic failure, onset within 8 weeks
- Encephalopathy, jaundice, hepatic fetor, multiple-system complications (coagulopathy, immunosuppression, renal dysfunction)

Aetiology

- Viral hepatitis
- Paracetamol overdose/CCL4
- Drug reactions (e.g. isoniazid, methyldopa)

ACUTE-ON-CHRONIC

- Stigmata of chronic liver disease, jaundice, ascites, encephalopathy

Aetiology

- Alcoholic cirrhosis
- Chronic active hepatitis
- Post-necrotic
- Infiltrative
- Other

PRECIPITATING CAUSES OF ENCEPHALOPATHY

Fulminant

Encephalopathy from cerebral oedema is the hallmark of the disease. Coma has 80% mortality. Can be exacerbated by the conditions listed below.

Acute-on-chronic

- GI tract bleeding (especially upper)—elevated urea/creatinine ratio is suggestive; accounts for about 25% of cases
- Constipation
- Increased protein load
- Azotaemia/volume depletion—hepatorenal syndrome
- Hypokalaemia/alkalosis
- Hypoxaemia/hypoglycaemia
- Infection, including spontaneous bacterial peritonitis in ascites (usually coliforms or pneumococci)
- Ethanol, sedatives, opiates

ASSESSMENT

History

- Alcohol and drug history
- Rapidity of onset of symptoms
- GI tract bleeding

Examination/immediate intervention

- Airway
- Breathing—correct hypoxaemia
- Intravenous access
- Blood—for haemoglobin/haematocrit; coagulation studies; EUC; calcium/phosphate/magnesium; BSL; LFTs; arterial blood gases; viral serology, group-and-hold as necessary
- Dextrose—hypoglycaemia needs to be rapidly excluded and treated
- Encephalopathy—GCS; Mini Mental State; star chart (constructional apraxia); asterixis (flap)
- Further examination—fetor; evidence of chronic liver disease/ascites; liver/spleen/rectal examination; cause of likely decompensation, including rectal exam; complications (e.g. bleeding, cardiorespiratory, infectious disease, alcohol withdrawal)

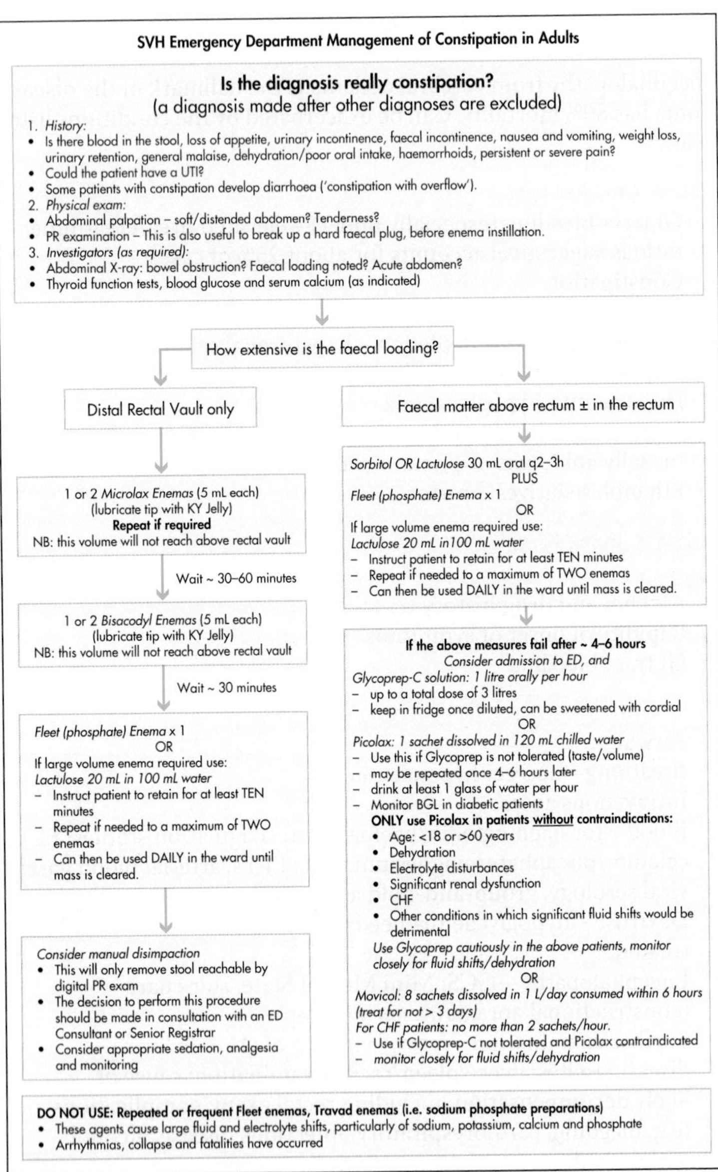

SVH Emergency Department Management of Constipation in Adults
Is the diagnosis really constipation?
(a diagnosis made after other diagnoses are excluded)
1. History:
• Is there blood in the stool, loss of appetite, urinary incontinence, faecal incontinence, nausea and vomiting, weight loss, urinary retention, general malaise, dehydration/poor oral intake, haemorrhoids, persistent or severe pain?
• Could the patient have a UTI?
• Some patients with constipation develop diarrhoea ('constipation with overflow').
2. Physical exam:
• Abdominal palpation – soft/distended abdomen? Tenderness?
• PR examination – This is also useful to break up a hard faecal plug, before enema instillation.
3. Investigators (as required):
• Abdominal X-ray: bowel obstruction? Faecal loading noted? Acute abdomen?
• Thyroid function tests, blood glucose and serum calcium (as indicated)
How extensive is the faecal loading?
Distal Rectal Vault only
1 or 2 Microlax Enemas (5 mL each)
(lubricate tip with KY Jelly)
Repeat if required
NB: this volume will not reach above rectal vault
Wait ~ 30–60 minutes
1 or 2 Bisacodyl Enemas (5 mL each)
(lubricate tip with KY Jelly)
NB: this volume will not reach above rectal vault
Wait ~ 30 minutes
Fleet (phosphate) Enema x 1
OR
If large volume enema required use:
Lactulose 20 mL in 100 mL water
– Instruct patient to retain for at least TEN minutes
– Repeat if needed to a maximum of TWO enemas
– Can then be used DAILY in the ward until mass is cleared.
Consider manual disimpaction
• This will only remove stool reachable by digital PR exam
• The decision to perform this procedure should be made in consultation with an ED Consultant or Senior Registrar
• Consider appropriate sedation, analgesia and monitoring
Faecal matter above rectum ± in the rectum
Sorbitol OR Lactulose 30 mL oral q2–3h
PLUS
Fleet (phosphate) Enema x 1
OR
If large volume enema required use:
Lactulose 20 mL in100 mL water
– Instruct patient to retain for at least TEN minutes
– Repeat if needed to a maximum of TWO enemas
– Can then be used DAILY in the ward until mass is cleared.
If the above measures fail after ~ 4–6 hours
Consider admission to ED, and
Glycoprep-C solution: 1 litre orally per hour
– up to a total dose of 3 litres
– keep in fridge once diluted, can be sweetened with cordial
OR
Picolax: 1 sachet dissolved in 120 mL chilled water
– Use this if Glycoprep is not tolerated (taste/volume)
– may be repeated once 4–6 hours later
– drink at least 1 glass of water per hour
– Monitor BGL in diabetic patients
ONLY use Picolax in patients without contraindications:
• Age: <18 or >60 years
• Dehydration
• Electrolyte disturbances
• Significant renal dysfunction
• CHF
• Other conditions in which significant fluid shifts would be detrimental
Use Glycoprep cautiously in the above patients, monitor closely for fluid shifts/dehydration
OR
Movicol: 8 sachets dissolved in 1 L/day consumed within 6 hours (treat for not > 3 days)
For CHF patients: no more than 2 sachets/hour.
– Use if Glycoprep-C not tolerated and Picolax contraindicated
– monitor closely for fluid shifts/dehydration
DO NOT USE: Repeated or frequent Fleet enemas, Travad enemas (i.e. sodium phosphate preparations)
• These agents cause large fluid and electrolyte shifts, particularly of sodium, potassium, calcium and phosphate
• Arrhythmias, collapse and fatalities have occurred

Figure 25.1 St Vincent's Hospital constipation management guidelines

DISCHARGE RECOMMENDATIONS:

FOLLOW UP: Patients should be advised to have follow up with GP the following day.
If unable to do this THEN have lactulose 20 mL orally bd PLUS a Glycerne suppository daily until reviewed by the GP.

Patients should pass at least one significant, documented bowel action prior to discharge.
Adequate fluid intake, higher fibre diet, exercise and other preventative measures (pear juice, prune juice) should be discussed.

Most patients can go home with:

- Lactulose 20 mL orally bd-tds
- Coloxyl with Senna 2 tablets orally bd

These should be titrated to at least one soft stool per day. Once this is achieved, the aperients can be weaned, i.e. first reduce Coloxyl with Senna to once daily then discontinue, followed by reduction in lactulose to once daily, then discontinue. Patients taking medications that cause constipation e.g. opiates, may need to be on long term laxatives.

For patients with significant faecal loading, faecal impaction or who have a PEG tube in situ, give

- Movicol 1 sachet dissolved in water bd-tds
- Coloxyl with Senna 2 tablets orally bd

Once the patient has at least one soft stool per day, replace Movicol with Lactulose and titrate as above.

Supplementary Information

Agent	Route	Category	Approximate time to effect	Side effects	$/dose in hospital
Microlax	Enema	Osmotic	Within 30 minutes	Slight burning sensation	0.66
Bisacodyl	Enema	Stimulant	Within 5 to 15 minutes	Anal burning, esp if not fully inserted	1.00
Lactulose	Oral liquid	Osmotic	Variable (hours)	Bloating, flatulence	0.20
Movicol	Oral liquid (125 mL)	Osmotic	30 to 180 minutes	Abdominal distension and pain, borborygmi and nausea, attributable to the expansion of the contents of the intestinal tract, can occur.	0.56
Glycoprep-C	Oral liquid (3000 mL)	Osmotic	30 to 60 minutes	Unpalatable (can be sweetened with cordial)	3.00
Picolax	Oral liquid (120 mL)	Osmotic	2 to 3 hours	↑ Na^+ ↓K^+, abdo discomfort, dehydration 2° poor intake Needs bacterial metabolism – effect reduced by broad spectrum antibiotics	1.14
Fleet	Enema (133 mL)	Osmotic	Within 2 to 5 min	↑ Na^+ ↑ $PO4^{2-}$ ↓Ca^{2+} dehydration	3.00
Coloxyl & Senna	Oral tablets	Stimulant	6 to 8 hours	Colic, cramps (dependence)	0.07

Drugs which can exacerbate constipation:

Opiates	Anticholinergics	TCAs	Ca Channel Blockers
Parkinson's therapies	Calcium supplements	Iron supplements	Diuretics
Antipsychotics	Anti-diarrhoeals	Sympathomimetics	Antihistamines

Adapted with permission: Austin & Repat Hospital, Victoria
Prepared by: S. Welch, Dr A Finckh, J. Gawthorne, J. Fagan.
Reviewed by: Dr C. Vickers
Date: 10/2005
Updated: 12/2009

Figure 25.1 continued

INVESTIGATIONS

- Septic work-up, including ascitic tap
- Arterial blood gases
- Serum ammonia (does not correlate well with severity of illness)
- Occult blood
- Chest X-ray
- ECG
- CT scan and EEG to assess encephalopathy/oedema and exclude other pathology
- Liver biopsy in some cases

Management

1. Treat precipitating causes, e.g. GI tract bleeding, constipation, volume depletion, electrolyte abnormality, infection.
2. Reduce protein absorption—oral lactulose (30–45 mL q8h); low-protein diet (20–40 g/day); oral antibiotics to treat gut flora such as neomycin or metronidazole may be used for patients intolerant of lactulose.
3. Other nutritional support, e.g. carbohydrates, zinc, magnesium.
4. Flumazenil may improve mental state by its actions on GABA receptors, but will not change long-term mortality.
5. Patients with potentially reversible coma will need endotracheal intubation and ICU transfer.
6. Consider reversal of portosystemic shunts in life-threatening encephalopathy not responding to treatment.
7. Liver transplant in selected patients.

Chapter 26
Endocrine emergencies

Anna Holdgate and Glenn Arendts

Emergencies in patients with diabetes

Diabetes is a disorder of glucose metabolism due to a relative (type 2) or absolute (type 1) insulin deficiency. With the rising rate of obesity in the community, diabetes is becoming increasingly common, and type 2 rather than type 1 diabetes is now often seen in young patients.

Diabetic patients may present to the emergency department with acute life-threatening derangements of glucose metabolism, with complications related to long-standing diabetes, or with unrelated health problems which require concurrent management of their diabetes.

DIABETIC KETOACIDOSIS (DKA)

Overview

DKA is due to insulin deficiency resulting in acidosis with ketosis, hyperglycaemia and fluid and electrolyte losses. It occurs in patients with type 1 (insulin-dependent) diabetes and may be the presenting problem in patients with previously undiagnosed diabetes. The principles in assessment and management of DKA are identifying and treating the precipitating cause, assessing the severity of the illness, correcting fluid and electrolyte disturbances and administering insulin.

Assessment

Patients with DKA commonly present with vomiting, polydipsia, polyuria, shortness of breath and abdominal pain. History and examination should be directed at identifying the precipitating event and assessing the degree of dehydration. Most commonly, DKA is precipitated in patients with type 1 diabetes by intercurrent infection, although other causes should be considered (see Box 26.1). It rarely occurs in patients with non-insulin-dependent diabetes.

A bedside venous blood sample will confirm the diagnosis by the presence of plasma ketones, acidosis (pH < 7.3 or bicarbonate < 15 mmol/L) and an elevated blood sugar level (BSL > 12 mmol/L). Urinary ketones will also be present.

Box 26.1 Precipitants of DKA

- First presentation of insulin-dependent diabetes
- Non-compliance/errors with insulin therapy
- Infection
  - — Urinary tract
  - — Respiratory tract
  - — Gastrointestinal
  - — Skin
- Other
  - — Steroid medication
  - — Myocardial infarction
  - — Pancreatitis
  - — Thyroid disease/surgery/pregnancy/trauma
  - — Alcohol abuse

Other important investigations include:

- Urea, electrolytes and creatinine (UEC)—potassium (K^+) abnormalities are common and creatinine may be elevated
- Full blood count (FBC)—elevated white cell count (WCC) suggests infection
- Midstream urine for microscopy and culture
- Blood culture if febrile
- Liver function tests; amylase and lipase if abdominal pain
- HbA_{1c} level—this indicates the level of blood sugar control over the past 3 months in long-standing diabetics
- ECG for silent myocardial infarction or arrhythmias
- Chest X-ray for respiratory infection

Management

Patients with DKA are often extremely ill and should be initially managed in an area of the ED with continuous ECG and oximetry monitoring, and regular blood pressure measurements. If there is a depressed level of consciousness, the patient requires supportive airway management and may need intubation. Ongoing regular measurement of BSL and serum K^+ should continue throughout treatment.

Fluid and electrolyte therapy

All patients with DKA are volume-depleted and require rehydration with intravenous fluids.

- Hypotension (systolic BP < 100 mmHg) should be treated with boluses of normal saline up to 2000 mL until BP has improved.
- In the normotensive patient, 1 L of normal saline should be given over the first hour, followed by another 1 L over the next 2 hours.

- Subsequent fluid therapy will be guided by clinical assessment of pulse rate and hydration status, but most patients will require 5–8 L of fluid over the first 24 hours.
- A dextrose-containing solution should be commenced once the BSL falls below 15 mmol/L, in addition to ongoing sodium requirements.

Potassium depletion is a feature of DKA, even in the presence of an initial elevated serum K^+. Serum potassium should be measured as soon as possible and is often available on the initial blood gas results. The administration of intravenous fluids and insulin will rapidly lower the measured K^+. If the initial K^+ is > 5.5 mmol/L, the level should be rechecked every 30–60 minutes as it will inevitably fall as a consequence of rehydration (and insulin treatment). Table 26.1 outlines the rate of potassium replacement. Monitoring of K^+ levels every 1–2 hours is essential during the initial phase of treatment.

Phosphate and magnesium levels are commonly low in DKA; however, there is no evidence to support the routine replacement of these electrolytes. Intravenous bicarbonate is of no proven benefit in patients with DKA, as the acidosis usually improves with rehydration and insulin therapy. Bicarbonate should not be given without consulting a critical-care specialist or endocrinologist.

The measured sodium level should be corrected for the elevated glucose, as the high BSL will artefactually dilute the sodium. The equation is:

$$\text{true sodium} = \text{measured sodium} + \frac{(\text{glucose} - 10)}{3}$$

Insulin therapy

Rehydration increases insulin sensitivity, and therefore insulin therapy should not precede fluid therapy. In children, many experts recommend that insulin therapy should be withheld for the first 1–2 hours of fluid resuscitation to avoid rapid falls in blood sugar. This should be discussed with a paediatric specialist early in the management.

In the initial phase, insulin should be delivered via continuous IV infusion. A second IV line is usually required for this purpose.

Table 26.1 Guide to potassium replacement in DKA

Serum K^+ (mmol/L)	Replacement therapy
> 5.5	Nil—repeat test in 1 hour
3.5–5.5	KCl 5–10 mmol/h
< 3.5	KCl 20 mmol/h, cardiac monitoring and central line

A common regimen is 50 units of Actrapid in 50 mL of normal saline via a syringe pump. The insulin infusion should commence at 0.05–0.1 units/kg/h (2–8 units/h), aiming for a fall in BSL of 2–4 mmol/h. The BSL should be measured hourly initially, and the insulin infusion adjusted according to the rate of fall.

The insulin infusion should continue until the urine is clear of ketones or the serum bicarbonate is greater than 20 mmol/L, regardless of the blood sugar level. Once the BSL falls below 15 mmol/L, rehydration should continue with a dextrose-containing solution. Subcutaneous insulin can be commenced once the patient has adequate oral intake and is no longer acidotic. The first SC dose must be given before the insulin infusion is ceased.

Other therapy

- Treatment of associated infection with appropriate antibiotics
- Subcutaneous heparin for thromboembolic prophylaxis
- A nasogastric tube may be necessary if there is persistent vomiting
- An indwelling catheter is often necessary to monitor urine output

Ongoing management

The aim of treatment is to correct fluid and electrolyte disturbances, lower the BSL to normal and control ketosis over 12–24 hours.

- Strict monitoring of BSL and serum K^+ every 1–2 hours initially is vital.
- Other electrolytes, especially sodium, should be checked at least twice daily.
- Regular reassessment of the patient's hydration status and acidosis is necessary to determine ongoing fluid management.
- The patient needs to remain closely monitored with hourly observations while the insulin infusion continues.

Cerebral oedema is a rare but life-threatening complication of DKA that is more common in children and usually occurs in the first 12 hours of therapy. Symptoms such as a falling level of consciousness, progressive headache, bradycardia and a rising blood pressure may indicate cerebral oedema and patients with any of these symptoms require urgent senior medical review.

Pearls and Pitfalls

- One of the commonest errors in managing DKA is failure to provide adequate potassium replacement. All patients with DKA are potassium-depleted and should have meticulous attention paid to potassium supplementation.

HYPEROSMOLAR HYPERGLYCAEMIC NON-KETOTIC STATE (HHNS)

Overview

This condition occurs primarily in older patients with non-insulin-dependent diabetes, although it has several clinical features in common with DKA. It is characterised by relative, rather than absolute, insulin deficiency leading to hyperglycaemia, hyperosmolarity and dehydration, with little or no acidosis or ketosis.

The goals of therapy are identification and treatment of the precipitating event, controlled correction of fluid and electrolyte abnormalities and correction of hyperglycaemia.

Assessment

HHNS often presents with non-specific signs such as confusion, vomiting and weight loss, developing over days to weeks in elderly patients with undiagnosed or poorly controlled diabetes. Polyuria and polydipsia are not universally present. There are many possible precipitating events, which are summarised in Box 26.2. These patients often have multiple comorbidities and may be on multiple medications.

Physical examination is focused on assessing the degree of dehydration and looking for evidence of a precipitating cause. The diagnosis is confirmed by the presence of severe hyperglycaemia (often > 50 mmol/L) and serum hyperosmolarity (> 350 mOsm/L), with minimal acidosis (pH > 7.3).

Box 26.2 Precipitants of HHNS

- Poor compliance
- Newly diagnosed diabetes
- Infection
  - Urinary tract
  - Respiratory
  - CNS
  - Skin
- Cardiovascular events
  - Acute myocardial infarction
  - Cerebrovascular accident/intracranial haemorrhage
  - Mesenteric ischaemia
- Other
  - Gastrointestinal haemorrhage
  - Pancreatitis
  - Renal failure
  - Diuretic therapy

Important early investigations include:

- UE—severe dehydration may be associated with hypernatraemia. The sodium level should be corrected for the BSL [true sodium = measured sodium + (glucose – 10)/3]. Potassium depletion and renal impairment are common
- Septic screen—urine, blood, skin swabs ± CSF for culture
- Chest X-ray—for evidence of infection and to evaluate heart size and presence of cardiac failure
- ECG—for evidence of myocardial infarction or atrial fibrillation
- CT of head—for cerebrovascular accident (CVA) or intracranial haemorrhage in patients with an altered level of consciousness

Management

These patients often have an altered level of consciousness and may have multiple comorbidities including heart and renal disease. Therefore they must be closely observed with full cardiorespiratory monitoring.

Fluid and electrolyte therapy

In the presence of shock (hypotension or poor tissue perfusion), **fluid therapy** should begin with 500 mL boluses of normal saline until blood pressure and tissue perfusion are restored. After correction of shock, fluid replacement should be performed relatively slowly. Although these patients are often profoundly dehydrated, this has usually occurred over a period of days to weeks and overly rapid replacement of fluid may lead to pulmonary or cerebral oedema.

- Most patients will have a fluid deficit of 8–12 L and this should be replaced over a 24–48 hour period.
- Fluid therapy should begin with 1 L of normal saline every 2–4 hours.
- If the corrected sodium is > 155 mmol/L or the sodium is rising, normal saline can be replaced by ½ saline/2.5% dextrose solution. The patient should be regularly assessed for clinical evidence of fluid overload, and may need central venous monitoring via a central line.

Potassium levels will fall rapidly once the patient is rehydrated and receiving insulin. Potassium replacement at 5–10 mmol/h should commence if the K^+ is < 5.0 mmol/L and urine output has been established. In the presence of oliguria and renal failure, K^+ replacement should be more cautious.

Insulin therapy

As for DKA, an IV insulin infusion should be commenced. Patients with HHNS are often insulin-sensitive and usually require 0.03–0.05 units/kg/h to achieve a fall in BSL of 3–5 mmol/h. As hyperglycaemia has developed over a long time period, it is appropriate to correct the BSL slowly, aiming for normalisation over 24 hours. This minimises the risk of cerebral oedema.

Other therapy

Precipitating illnesses should be actively sought and treated. Serious diagnoses such as mesenteric ischaemia must be considered. Thromboembolic prophylaxis with subcutaneous heparin is particularly important in HHNS due to the thrombogenic effect of profound dehydration, and the presence of serious comorbidities.

HYPOGLYCAEMIA

Causes

Hypoglycaemia most commonly occurs in diabetic patients on insulin or oral hypoglycaemic therapy. It can also occur in non-diabetics secondary to diseases such as sepsis, alcohol, hepatic failure, renal failure and insulin-producing tumours.

In diabetics, hypoglycaemia may be due to excess insulin or oral hypoglycaemic treatment, missed meals, physical exertion and alcohol. It may be the first presentation of renal impairment in patients on sulfonylureas.

Clinical features

Hypoglycaemia predominantly affects the brain and the autonomic nervous system.

- Neurological signs can vary widely and include agitation, aggressive or bizarre behaviour, coma, seizures, confusion, dysarthria and focal deficits such as hemiparesis (mimicking stroke).
- Autonomic features include sweating, tremor, blurred vision, vomiting and anxiety.
- The diagnosis is confirmed by BSL < 3 mmol/L on finger-prick sampling.

The diagnosis should be considered in all patients presenting with confusion, seizures or an altered level of consciousness.

Therapy

Hypoglycaemia is easily reversed with oral or intravenous glucose. Prolonged, untreated hypoglycaemia can lead to permanent brain dysfunction, so early diagnosis and treatment is essential.

- If the patient is still awake, oral glucose in the form of a sweet drink, biscuit or other sugary substance may be enough to restore BSL. If the patient is unable to swallow, 25 mL of 50% dextrose is given as an intravenous push through a large-bore IV cannula, followed by a 20 mL saline flush (to prevent phlebitis). If the patient does not recover within 2–3 minutes, or the BSL remains < 3 mmol/L, the dose can be repeated.
- If intravenous access is not possible, 1 mg of IM glucagon may temporarily reverse hypoglycaemia if the patient has normal hepatic function. This should be followed by oral or IV glucose.

Hypoglycaemia secondary to oral hypoglycaemic agents may be recurrent and prolonged, particularly in the presence of renal impairment. These patients require a dextrose infusion and observation in hospital until the BSL is stable.

Once the BSL is restored, assessment and treatment of the precipitating cause is essential.

Pearls and Pitfalls

- Always check the blood sugar level in any patient presenting with an altered level of consciousness, seizures or neurological signs. Hypoglycaemia is known as the 'great imitator' and may present in unexpected ways. Failure to diagnose this easily treated metabolic emergency can be disastrous.

THE 'HIGH-RISK' DIABETIC PATIENT

As well as the acute derangements of glucose metabolism outlined above, diabetic patients are at risk of other acute pathologies due to the long-term complications of their illness.

Infection

Diabetics are immunocompromised and thus are more prone to infection and are at greater risk of systemic sepsis than the general community. They may have significant infection in the absence of the usual clinical signs such as fever or elevated WCC. Therefore, diabetic patients with actual or potential infection warrant more extensive work-up than other patients, with a lower threshold for tissue and blood cultures, soft-tissue imaging and hospital admission.

In particular, soft-tissue infections are often polymicrobial and may invade into deeper structures such as muscle and bone. Specialist microbiology advice should be sought regarding antibiotic therapy.

Infarction

Macro- and microvascular disease seen in diabetic patients makes them more prone to acute vascular compromise in many organ systems, including the heart, brain, kidneys, gut and peripheral vasculature. Acute myocardial ischaemia may present atypically with minimal or absent chest pain, unexplained acute heart failure or non-specific vomiting. Abdominal pain in a diabetic patient has many potentially serious causes, including mesenteric ischaemia, myocardial infarction, leaking aortic aneurysm or renal infarction. Therefore these patients require thorough investigation which will usually include abdominal CT.

Other

Most patients with long-standing diabetes will have some impairment of renal function and are at relatively high risk of acute renal impairment, which may be precipitated by concurrent infection or any illness that leads to dehydration. Serum creatinine should be measured in any diabetic patient who presents with systemic illness.

Long-standing retinopathy may be acutely complicated by retinal haemorrhage, infarction or detachment, and any diabetic patient with acute eye symptoms should have urgent ophthalmology review.

THE DIABETIC PATIENT WITH UNRELATED ILLNESS

In addition to the specific conditions for which they are at higher risk, diabetics are subject to the same spectrum of illness and injury as the general population. Admission to hospital requires concurrent management of their diabetes as well as their acute illness, and this should begin in the ED. Poor glycaemic control in hospitalised diabetics increases the risk of death and infection and prolongs hospital stay. Acute illness will usually increase an individual's basal insulin requirements and most diabetics will require upward adjustment of insulin therapy in the early part of their hospital admission.

The BSL should optimally be maintained in the region of 5–8 mmol/L and there are several methods available to achieve this. Many hospitals have well-developed local protocols for managing diabetes, and these should be followed closely. For critically ill patients, particularly those with acute stroke, myocardial infarction and sepsis, blood sugar control is best achieved by continuous insulin infusion with close monitoring of finger-prick BSLs.

All patients with type 1 (insulin-deficient) diabetes who are not critically ill should continue to receive regular SC therapy with intermediate- and short-acting insulin, but will usually require higher doses.

Many type 2 diabetics will require a period of insulin therapy during hospitalisation, even if they are not usually managed with insulin. Basal insulin requirements should be provided with regular SC intermediate-acting insulin with additional short-acting insulin around meal times. This is preferable to 'sliding-scale' insulin therapy, as it provides more-stable glucose control.

Adrenal emergencies

HYPOADRENAL CRISIS (ACUTE ADRENOCORTICAL INSUFFICIENCY)

Presentation and clinical features

Hypoadrenal crisis develops in two clinical settings. Occasionally, the patient presents with acute haemorrhagic destruction of the adrenal glands due to sepsis, burns, trauma or anticoagulant therapy. More commonly, the crisis develops as an acute deterioration in patients with Addison's disease or other causes of chronic adrenal failure. This can be due to increased steroid requirements (e.g. infection), drug interactions that increase steroid metabolism, or non-compliance with maintenance steroid therapy.

The presenting symptoms are often non-specific and include lethargy, dizziness, nausea, diarrhoea and abdominal pain. However, in severe cases the patient presents with haemodynamic collapse—hypoadrenalism needs to be considered in any patient with unexplained shock.

Differential diagnosis

The differential diagnosis is very broad due to the non-specific presentations seen. Ascribing hypoadrenal symptoms to gastroenteritis or other intra-abdominal conditions is the most common misdiagnosis made.

Investigations

If acute hypoadrenalism is suspected, the following initial investigations may be helpful. Ideally these are done prior to starting treatment with steroids, unless the patient has frank shock and it is unsafe to delay treatment.

a UEC—the combination of a low bicarbonate level, hyponatraemia and hyperkalaemia is highly suggestive of hypoadrenal crisis. Renal failure may occur.

b BSL—hypoglycaemia
c Arterial blood gases (ABGs)—non-anion-gap metabolic acidosis.
d Ca^{2+}—hypercalcaemia.
e Random plasma cortisol level—a low level in the setting of acute stress is highly suggestive of adrenocortical insufficiency.
f Short corticotrophin test—this requires a baseline cortisol level, the administration of IV corticotrophin and then a repeat cortisol level 30–60 minutes later. This must occur prior to the administration of hydrocortisone (but not dexamethasone). In most cases of suspected insufficiency testing is possible, but if the patient is moribund and treatment cannot be delayed, omit this test.

Management

1. Fluids. The patient may present with haemodynamic collapse and require immediate resuscitation.
   - Hypotension should be treated initially with 1000 mL boluses of normal saline.
   - Hypoglycaemia, if present, should be treated initially with 25 mL of 50% dextrose IV.
   - Shock may be refractory to fluid resuscitation until hydrocortisone therapy is commenced. Even with adjuvant steroids, the patient may need vasopressor support in decompensated shock.
   - After resuscitation, further fluid requirements should be determined by assessment of the patient's hydration status. Normal saline should be used to replace any fluid deficit over the next 24–48 hours. If the patient has associated persistent hypoglycaemia, adding 50 g dextrose to each bag of normal saline given is preferable to using a dextrose-containing solution with a low sodium concentration.
   - Blood glucose, Na^+ and K^+ levels should be measured every 2–3 hours initially.
2. IV hydrocortisone (100 mg every 6 hours) should be given promptly.
3. Other important acute management issues include the treatment of any underlying precipitants, such as infection.

The majority of patients improve within 24 hours of commencing this treatment regimen. Oral combined glucocorticoid and mineralocorticoid therapy may then be commenced. Patient education after the acute treatment phase is over, concerning increasing their maintenance steroid requirements at times of stress or illness, is a vital part of management.

Pearls and Pitfalls

- In EDs, it is common to encounter cases of adrenal suppression due to chronic glucocorticoid therapy suppressing endogenous adrenocorticotrophic hormone (ACTH) production. When such patients become acutely unwell, they are at risk of developing a hypoadrenal syndrome, as their steroid requirements increase but they are unable to match this with increased production. To prevent this, any patient on continuous maintenance glucocorticoid therapy for the previous 6 weeks or more should have their dose augmented when they present to the ED with an acute stress. As a general rule, for any severe potentially life-threatening illness, give an additional 100 mg hydrocortisone over and above the patient's usual daily steroid dose. For less-severe illness, give 25–50 mg of additional hydrocortisone.

Thyroid emergencies

THYROTOXIC CRISIS ('THYROID STORM')

Presentation and clinical features

Patients at risk of thyrotoxic crisis usually have either undiagnosed or poorly treated hyperthyroidism. The precipitants of thyrotoxic crisis that should be looked for are shown in Box 26.3.

Box 26.3 Precipitants of thyrotoxic crisis

- Intercurrent illness or stress—infection, labour, major vascular events such as CVA
- Drugs—thyroxine overdose, amiodarone, iodinated dyes, salicylates, cessation of anti-thyroid drug therapy
- Trauma—multi-trauma, thyroid gland surgery, vigorous palpation of thyroid gland

Thyrotoxic crisis represents the extreme of hyperthyroidism, and the diagnosis is a clinical one. Three signs in particular help distinguish thyrotoxic crisis from uncomplicated hyperthyroidism:

a hyperpyrexia (temperature > 38°C)
b extreme tachycardia (heart rate usually 130–200 beats/min)
c CNS disturbance, ranging from restlessness and agitation to coma.

Vomiting and diarrhoea are common. Potentially life-threatening cardiac complications (arrhythmias, cardiac failure) occur in more than 50% of patients.

Differential diagnosis

- Sepsis
- Heat stroke
- Toxicological:
  - anticholinergic poisoning
  - sympathomimetic poisoning, e.g. amphetamines
  - neuroleptic malignant syndrome
  - serotonin syndrome
  - alcohol withdrawal

Investigations

No single test confirms the diagnosis of thyrotoxic crisis. Thyroid function tests (TFTs) confirm hyperthyroidism, but the levels of T_3 and T_4 in thyrotoxic crisis are usually no different from those in uncomplicated hyperthyroidism, and treatment should not be delayed for the TFT results. Hyperglycaemia, hypokalaemia, hypercalcaemia, abnormal liver function and leucocytosis occur commonly. CXR and ECG looking for specific cardiac complications should be performed.

Management

1. Supportive care. Patients with thyrotoxic crisis are usually extremely unwell and require continuous ECG, BP and temperature monitoring. Unstable arrhythmias and cardiac failure may be evident at presentation and require urgent treatment.

   These patients are hypermetabolic and have markedly increased oxygen, fluid, electrolyte and glucose requirements. High-flow oxygen by mask should be started. The patient can require 5–6 L of IV fluid in the first 24 hours, although less-aggressive fluid resuscitation may be necessary in the elderly or those with heart failure. Hyperpyrexia should be treated with external cooling methods, for example axillary and groin cold packs.
2. Beta-adrenergic blockers. These antagonise the peripheral end-organ effects of thyroid hormones and are the mainstay of emergency therapy. Oral (or nasogastric (NG)) propranolol commenced at 40 mg every 6 hours is the treatment of choice, although much higher doses may be required.

   Intravenous propranolol is not currently commercially available in Australia and, if the patient requires intravenous beta-blockade, esmolol is the best option due to its very short half-life. All beta-blockers can worsen cardiac failure and hypotension.

(*pto*)

3. Anti-thyroid treatment. Oral or NG propylthiouracil reduces the further synthesis of thyroid hormones and prevents the peripheral conversion of T_4 to the more active T_3. A loading dose of 400 mg followed by 200 mg every 6 hours is a typical regimen.
4. Corticosteroids improve survival in thyrotoxic crisis. Hydrocortisone 100 mg IV every 6 hours is an appropriate choice.

HYPOTHYROID CRISIS ('MYXOEDEMA COMA')

Presentation and clinical features

Myxoedema coma occurs most commonly following some precipitating event in a patient with unrecognised hypothyroidism (Box 26.4). The diagnosis is clinical and a high index of suspicion is required.

Box 26.4 Precipitants of hypothyroid crisis

- Intercurrent illness
  - Infection
  - GI tract bleed
  - CVA
- Drugs
  - CNS depressants
  - Beta-blockers
  - Cessation of thyroxine therapy
- Environmental
  - Extreme cold exposure

Myxoedema coma is the clinical extreme of hypothyroidism and is characterised by multi-organ failure due to reduced cellular metabolism. The cardinal features are:

a. decreased conscious state
b. hypoventilation progressing to respiratory failure
c. bradycardia and hypotension
d. hypothermia.

Increased total body water is common, leading to oedema, pleural and pericardial effusions, and hyponatraemia. Paralytic ileus and urinary retention may occur.

Differential diagnosis

- Environmental hypothermia
- Encephalopathies, e.g. hepatic, uraemic
- Cardiogenic shock
- Sepsis

Investigations

The diagnosis of myxoedema coma is clinical, although TFTs confirm hypothyroidism. A rapid free T_4 assay is often available and, if normal, excludes the diagnosis. Other important investigation abnormalities include:

a UEC—hyponatraemia, renal failure
b BSL—hypoglycaemia
c ABGs—elevated CO_2, hypoxia
d FBC—anaemia, low WCC
e ECG—bradycardia, prolonged QT interval
f CXR—pleural and pericardial effusions.

Hypothyroid crisis patients are commonly septic without exhibiting any of the usual clinical features of sepsis, and should have a septic screen as part of their initial work-up.

Management

1 Supportive care. These patients are profoundly unwell and require management in an area with full monitoring and resuscitation equipment.
   - Intubation and ventilation is often needed but requires special precautions due to hypothermia and gastric stasis.
   - Though oedematous, patients may have reduced intravascular volume; hypotension should initially be treated with 500 mL boluses of warmed IV normal saline.
   - Hypoglycaemia, if present, should be immediately corrected with 25 mL of 50% dextrose IV. Do not use hypotonic fluids; add dextrose to normal saline for maintenance if required.
   - Re-warming with warm blankets or a Bair Hugger is recommended provided it does not cause worsening hypotension from vasodilation.

2 Thyroid hormones. These are the mainstay of therapy in myxoedema coma. Controversy exists regarding the optimal dose, route and rate of thyroid hormone replacement. Initial IV therapy is preferred when ileus is suspected. Intravenous T_3 is the more readily bioavailable, and 10 microg can be given as a slow bolus every 4 hours initially. Oral T_3 or T_4 can be commenced once the ileus has resolved.

   As hypothyroid crisis usually develops slowly, rapid replacement of thyroid hormones may provoke serious complications such as cardiac ischaemia or arrhythmias. Providing supportive care is adequate, relatively low initial doses either IV or orally, titrated to clinical response, is prudent. (*pto*)

3 IV hydrocortisone 100 mg every 8 hours should be commenced, as myxoedema coma is often associated with adrenal dysfunction.
4 Hyponatraemia usually corrects with water restriction; but if severe and associated with altered conscious state, may require hypertonic (3%) saline.
5 Infection is common and should be covered with broad-spectrum antibiotic therapy.

Recovery time with treatment is highly variable, and improvement can occur anywhere from 24 hours to many days after commencing therapy.

Pearls and Pitfalls

- Up to 5% of female patients aged > 65 years encountered in the ED have unrecognised hypothyroidism. Even though very few of these patients will ever develop a hypothyroid crisis, it may be appropriate in the correct clinical context to assess for symptoms, signs and laboratory evidence of hypothyroidism in this at-risk population.

Editorial Comment

Be it an elderly female with increased confusion (hypothyroid) to a previously healthy, young patient (new-onset diabetes), remember to think *endocrine*, as illnesses are often initially subtle clinically but clear on simple blood tests.

Online resources

Diabetes mellitus, eTG complete (internet). Melbourne: Therapeutic Guidelines
www.tg.org.au

Chapter 27
Acid–base and electrolyte disorders

Derek Louey and Diane King

Electrolyte emergencies

(See Table 27.1 overleaf.)

Editorial Comment

Most electrolyte abnormalities, e.g. decreased level of consciousness from hyponatraemia, cannot be diagnosed by good clinical examination. Unless there is careful scrutiny of routine tests these will be missed, often with poorer outcomes.

CRITICAL OVERVIEW

Pathophysiology

- In health, serum electrolyte concentrations are usually tightly controlled over a wide range of inputs or losses by the endocrine and renal systems.
- Maintenance of electrolyte balance is achieved by altering oral intake, renal excretion or by the movement of water or electrolytes between fluid compartments.
- Serum electrolyte *concentrations* do not necessarily correlate with total body *stores*.

Derangement can occur as a result of overwhelming losses or gains, disordered homeostatic mechanisms or drug effects.

Obtaining samples

- Never decant excess blood between different specimen containers (because of preservative contamination)
- Never obtain specimens from a limb receiving IV fluids (because of dilution).
- Multiple needle entries, forceful aspiration or filling of containers, aerated collection and violently agitating samples increases the risk of haemolysis and spurious results.

Causes and mechanisms

There are various mechanisms affecting electrolyte balance.

- Disturbances result from:
  a Water/electrolyte losses or gains at extra-renal sites, i.e. enteral/gastrointestinal tract, parenteral/IV sites, skin
  b Compartmental shifts:
  intracellular fluid (ICF) ↔ extracellular fluid (ECF);
  vascular fluid ↔ interstitial fluid; ECF ↔ bone pool
  c Disordered renal homeostatic mechanisms (glomerular function/renal failure, tubular dysfunction/channelopathy) or abnormal endocrine control
  d Drugs exerting effects through any of the above mechanisms.
- Calcium, phosphate and magnesium abnormalities often co-exist.

The spectrum of likely causes differs between emergency department patients and hospitalised, postoperative or intensive-care patients (consult additional resources if there are other diagnostic considerations).

Clinical effects

- Electrolytes have varying roles in maintaining osmolar gradient and cell volume, governing the membrane potential of excitable tissue and regulating receptor signalling and enzyme function.
- The central nervous system (CNS), cardiovascular system (CVS), gastrointestinal motility (gastrointestinal tract) or neuromuscular system can be affected.
- Clinical effects can vary from mild and non-specific to severe and life-threatening.

Clinical impact is proportional to the *severity* and *acuity* of the derangement (and dictates the immediacy of treatment). If results are inconsistent with clinical information, repeat the test.

Rapid assessment

(See specific disorders.)

- Determine severity (see Table 27.1)
- Review volume status (dehydrated, hypovolaemic, oedematous)
- Review gastrointestinal (GI) intake and output (quantify oral intake including medications; vomiting; diarrhoea)
- Review parenteral fluids (total parenteral nutrition, TPN)
- Review skin losses (excessive sweating, extensive burns)
- Review medication history
- Review renal function and urine output
- Always compare with recent results to determine *chronicity* and *baseline values*
- Consider renal tubular or endocrine dysfunction—perform urine electrolytes

(*pto*)

Table 27.1 Electrolyte emergencies

Abnormality	Clinical indication	Treatment (only if clinical indication present)	Comments
Hyperkalaemia ($K^+ > 6.5$ mmol/L)	QRS widening; symptomatic arrhythmia	10–20 mmol calcium chloride or calcium gluconate IV over 5 minutes	Ca^{2+} temporarily stabilises membrane action potential (see text)
Hypokalaemia ($K^+ < 2.6$ mmol/L)	Arrhythmia	5–10 mmol potassium chloride IV bolus over 5 minutes	Continue monitoring during treatment
Hyponatraemia ($Na^+ < 110$ mmol/L)	Seizures or coma	1 mL/kg 3% hypertonic saline bolus over 5 minutes (repeat up to 2 times over 20 minutes)	Treatment may cause cerebral pontine myelinolysis and quadriplegia
Hypocalcaemia (total $Ca^{2+} < 2$ mmol/L)	Respiratory difficulties, hypotension, arrhythmias	5–10 mmol calcium chloride or calcium gluconate IV over 10 minutes	
Hypercalcaemia (total $Ca^{2+} > 3.5$ mmol/L)	Coma	Commence rapid rehydration with IV normal saline	Hydration optimises calciuresis (see text)
Hypophosphataemia ($PO_4^{3-} < 0.4$ mmol/L)	Arrhythmias	IV K_2HPO_4/KH_2PO_4 5–10 mmol/L over 60 minutes	Risk of dangerous hypocalcaemia with IV PO_4^{3-}
Hyperphosphataemia ($PO_4^{3-} < 2.25$ mmol/L]	Arrhythmias Respiratory failure	Saline rehydration Dialyse (if severe hypocalcaemia also)	
Hypomagnesaemia ($Mg^{2+} < 0.5$ mmol/L)	Arrhythmias	IV magnesium sulfate 10 mmol over 5 minutes	Rapid administration may cause flushing and hypotension
Hypermagnesaemia ($Mg^{2+} > 5$ mmol/L)	Arrhythmia Hypotension Respiratory failure	5–10 mmol CaCl or Calcium gluconate IV over 10 min	Ca^{2+} temporarily stabilises membrane action potential

- Consider specific endocrine tests if cause is not obvious (see chapters on adrenal failure, Addison's disease, hypoadrenalism, Conn's syndrome, parathyroid disorders, syndrome of inappropriate antidiuretic hormone (SIADH), diabetes insipidus)
- With multiple abnormalities—evaluate each abnormality individually and attempt to find a unifying explanation

Management

- Address the *cause,* not just the abnormality. More than one mechanism may be operating, e.g. poor oral intake + diuretics.
- Unless the abnormality is life-threatening, gradual correction (over 48 hours) is recommended.
- Resist the temptation to over-treat a stable abnormality in an asymptomatic patient where the management of the underlying condition has already been optimised.
- **Mild cases**—review and address causes, monitor abnormality.
- **Moderate cases**—as above, plus begin treatment and monitor response frequently.
- **Severe, life-threatening or resistant cases**—e.g. neurological (seizures, coma), CVS (hypotension, arrhythmia), respiratory muscle failure (hypoventilation, tetany). Get ICU opinion. Patients may need careful and vigilant management.
- Multiple biochemical abnormalities may be complex to manage. Seek expert assistance.
- Any replacement regimen for deficits needs to also account for ongoing losses.

(See Table 27.1.)

Disorders of acid–base balance

- Physiological significance: acid–base disorders risk interrupting/affecting enzymatic and hormonal function.
- Physiological control is *passive* (intracellular protein buffers, carbonic anhydrase buffer system) or *active* (CO_2 excretion via lungs, bicarbonate excretion via kidneys).

An acute derangement in acid–base balance invariably signifies a significant disease process. Most patients need admission or at least extended observation.

- Arterial blood gas (ABG) determination is essential to fully categorise the disturbance, e.g. acidosis/alkalosis; respiratory/metabolic; or mixed. Don't just look at pH (which may be near normal due to compensation).

- Clinical information and other lab tests will help determine the cause.

Treatment should generally be primarily directed at the *cause* of the disturbance and not simply by directly manipulating pH.

NORMAL VALUES

Normal values for pH, pCO_2 (partial pressure of carbon dioxide), PO_2 (partial pressure of oxygen) and HCO_3^- (bicarbonate level) in arterial blood are:

- pH 7.35–7.45
- pCO_2 35–45 mmHg ('respiratory acid')
- PO_2 100 mmHg
- HCO_3^- 24 mmol/L ('metabolic base')

DETERMINING THE ACID–BASE ABNORMALITY

(See Figure 27.1 overleaf.)

1. Check **pH**— if < 7.4 then patient is acidaemic; if > 7.4, patient is alkalaemic.
   - If acidaemic—is HCO_3^- < 24 (metabolic acidosis) or pCO_2 > 40 (respiratory acidosis), or both?
   - If alkalaemic—is HCO_3^- > 24 (metabolic alkalosis) or pCO_2 < 40 (respiratory alkalosis), or both?
2. Is the **respiratory compensation** for a metabolic abnormality incomplete or complete? (See 'Metabolic equations' in the 'Quick reference' section.)
   - If pCO_2 is lower than expected → concurrent respiratory alkalosis
   - If pCO_2 is higher than expected → concurrent respiratory acidosis.
3. Is the **metabolic compensation** for a respiratory abnormality acute/incomplete or chronic/complete? (See 'Metabolic equations and electrolytes' in the 'Quick reference' section.)
   - If HCO_3^- is lower than expected → concurrent metabolic acidosis
   - If HCO_3^- is higher than expected → concurrent metabolic alkalosis.

ABG interpretation may be difficult with a mixed respiratory and metabolic disturbance that results in near-normal pH, e.g. chronic respiratory acidosis with acute metabolic alkalosis. Use previously determined values to determine whether a new abnormality exists.

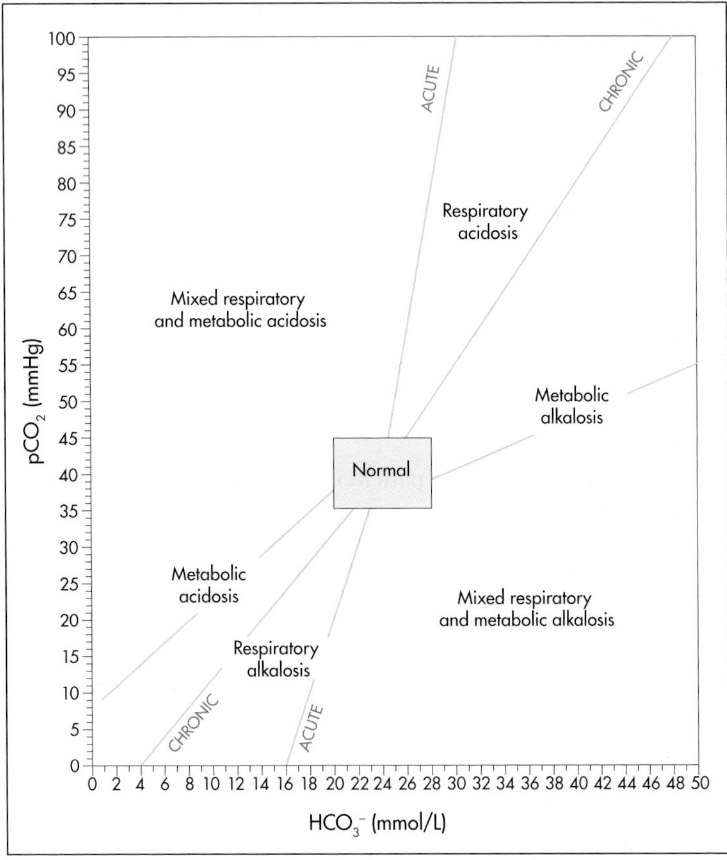

Figure 27.1 Acid–base nomogram

Anion gap

- Anion gap approximates the unmeasured anions (usually [protein$^-$], [SO_4^{2-}], [PO_4^{3-}]).
- It can be *estimated* as:

$$\text{Anion gap} = ([Na^+] + [K^+]) - ([Cl^-] + [HCO_3^-])$$

- Normal value for anion gap is 10–18.

The anion gap is important in *categorising* metabolic acidosis (see below).

Venous bicarbonate or total CO_2

- Normal values are venous bicarbonate 22–32 mmol/L and total CO_2 23–30 mmol/L.
- Some laboratories report total CO_2 in mmol/L. This largely approximates venous bicarbonate.

Cause of variances from normal

- ↓ indicates primary metabolic acidosis or primary respiratory alkalosis
- ↑ indicates primary metabolic alkalosis or primary respiratory acidosis

Clinical use

- Abnormal venous bicarbonate/total CO_2 indicates an acid–base disturbance—but note that normal values do not *exclude* an abnormality; this requires venous or arterial blood gas (VBG/ABG) values.
- In a patient with single pathology, venous bicarbonate may be used as a surrogate marker for pH to determine adequacy and progress of treatment, e.g. response to insulin in DKA, response to resuscitation in shock.
- Should not be used in multiple, concurrent acid–base abnormalities, e.g. chronic respiratory acidosis with acute metabolic acidosis.

Venous blood gas

- Normal values are pH 7.35, HCO_3^- 26 mmol/L, pCO_2 45 mmHg.
- There is evidence that venous pH, HCO_3^- and pCO_2 can be used to track changes in arterial values.
- Normal VBG values exclude acid–base abnormality.
- Quantification of abnormality is unreliable in the setting of shock.
- In a patient with isolated pathology and *not in shock*, VBG may be used to *monitor* acid–base status and hypoventilation instead of ABG.

Editorial Comment

The advantages of VBG over ABG are: easier to obtain, less painful and fewer complications. It should be used more often.

METABOLIC ACIDOSIS

(Mild: $[HCO_3^-]$ < 18 mmol/L; moderate: < 15 mmol/L; severe: < 12 mmol/L)

Metabolic acidosis is often associated with significant pathology. Aggressively search for cause, treat and monitor response (low venous HCO_3^- on serum electrolytes is the first clue).

Clinical effects are usually related to cause. Severe metabolic acidosis can contribute to circulatory collapse and diminished clotting function (important in shock and trauma).

Classification: distinguish *wide* (normochloraemic) from *normal* (hyperchloraemic) anion gap metabolic acidosis. (See above for notes on anion gap.)

Wide anion gap (normochloraemic) metabolic acidosis

Causes

Early sepsis, compensated hypovolaemic shock, inadequate fluid resuscitation and DKA are the most common ED causes of wide anion gap (AG) metabolic acidosis.

Other causes include renal failure, drug poisoning, thiamine deficiency, metformin (rare).

Assessment

- Rapidly assess the following:
  - Circulatory status (HR, BP, urine output)
  - Infection (fever)
  - Hyperglycaemia (bedside BSL, urinary ketones).
- Important lab tests:
  - Electrolytes
  - Anion gap
  - Renal function
  - Serum osmolarity
  - Serum ketones
  - BSL
  - WCC.

Management

1. Treat cause:
   - Hypovolaemia: fluids challenge until vital signs and urine output restored
   - Sepsis: fluids challenge, early administration of antibiotics
   - DKA: see Chapter 26
   - Renal failure: see below
   - Poisoning: obtain toxicology advice
2. Potassium deficit may be unmasked as the metabolic acidosis resolves. Begin replacement if patient is already hypokalaemic

or when adequate urine output is established (see section on hyperkalaemia, below)

Note: Do not treat a wide AG metabolic acidosis with bicarbonate infusion. Address the *cause.*

Normal anion gap (hyperchloraemic) metabolic acidosis

Causes

(Uncommon in the ED.)

- Bicarbonate loss from genitourinary system or GI tract, e.g. renal tubular acidosis, surgical fistula/stomal/drain losses, mineralocorticoid deficiency.
- Can be a complication of excessive infusion of normal saline.

Management

Get expert assistance.

- Sodium bicarbonate ($NaHCO_3$) IV, sodium bicarbonate/citrate PO
- If patient potassium-deficient: potassium citrate/bicarbonate PO, potassium acetate IV
- Total bicarbonate deficit (mmol) =
  $(24 - \text{existing } [HCO_3^-]) \times \frac{2}{3} \times \text{bodyweight (in kg)}$

METABOLIC ALKALOSIS

(Mild: $[HCO_3^-] > 25$ mmol/L; moderate: > 30 mmol/L; severe: > 35 mmol/L)

Clinical effects: in severe metabolic alkalosis, there is reduced oxygen delivery to the tissues (left shift of the oxyhaemoglobin (HbO_2) dis-association curve).

Causes

- Common: diuretic use, gastric losses (e.g. pyloric stenosis, bulimia nervosa)
- Less-common: mineralocorticoid excess (Conn's syndrome), diarrhoea from villous adenoma and laxatives

Perpetuating factors include dehydration, hypokalaemia.

Note: A wide anion gap in the setting of a metabolic alkalosis is suggestive of a concurrent metabolic acidosis.

Management

Note: Compensation for metabolic alkalosis is constrained by allowable limits of hypoventilation.

- If metabolic alkalosis is associated with volume loss and is non-oedematous, it is 'saline/chloride responsive' (urine $[Cl^-]$ < 25 mmol/L). Correct dehydration with normal saline.

- If oedematous: acetazolamide 250 mg 1–2 times/day.
- Potassium depletion needs to be corrected (see section on hypokalaemia, below).
- Stop any offending medications if possible.
- If the metabolic alkalosis is 'saline unresponsive' (urine [Cl^-] > 40 mmol/L), the patient may need hydrochloric acid (HCl) via central venous catheter (manage in ICU).

RESPIRATORY ACIDOSIS

(Mild: pCO_2 > 45 mmHg; moderate: > 55 mmHg; severe > 65 mmHg)
Clinical effects: in moderate to severe respiratory acidosis, somnolence then coma may occur due to decreased alveolar partial pressure of oxygen (PAO_2) (per alveolar gas equation).

Causes

- Any cause of respiratory depression or inadequate alveolar ventilation
- Acute cardiorespiratory illness (asthma/chronic obstructive airways disease, pulmonary oedema, pneumonia)
- CNS insults (opiates, benzodiazepines, acute space-occupying lesion)
- Trauma (head injury, flail chest, haemothorax/pneumothorax)

Management

- Treat cause.
- Mechanical ventilation (especially if drowsy/somnolent or severe head injury).

Note: Do not decrease FiO_2 (fraction of inspired oxygen) in an already hypoxic patient in an attempt to treat respiratory acidosis. Maintain an oxygen saturation (SpO_2) of at least 90–93% if CO_2 retention is of concern.

RESPIRATORY ALKALOSIS

Causes

- Uncommon but important causes include: sepsis, pulmonary embolism, salicylate poisoning (do not always assume anxiety).

Osmolarity, osmolar gap

PHYSIOLOGY

- Serum **osmolarity** is the serum concentration of substances to which a cell membrane is impermeable (normal values ~285 mOsm/L).

- It regulates movement of water between intra- and extra-cellular compartments and is controlled by antidiuretic hormone (ADH) and the thirst mechanism.
- Physiological plasma osmolarity (P_{osm}) can be *estimated* from the electrolyte results:

$$P_{osm} = 2 \times [Na^+] + [glucose] + [urea] \qquad \text{(all units are mmol/L)}$$

- P_{osm} can be *accurately measured* directly in the lab by freezing-point depression.
- The **osmolar gap** = measured osmolarity – estimated osmolarity.

CLINICAL EFFECTS OF DISTURBANCES

- If osmolarity is increased, this can lead to cellular dehydration; if decreased, oedema may occur.

Note: The degree of osmolar disturbance correlates with conscious state.

CAUSES OF DISTURBANCES

- **Raised:** free-water deficit, exogenous osmoles (e.g. alcohol, ethylene glycol, methanol, mannitol), excess endogenous osmoles (ketone bodies, lactate).
- **Lowered:** free-water excess, inadequate sodium replacement with isotonic losses.

Serum osmolarity can be used to distinguish true hyponatraemias from hyperosmolar and factitious hyponatraemia (see section on hyponatraemia, below.)

In the setting of acute poisoning and the *absence* of ketoacidosis, a raised osmolar gap suggests ingestion of osmolar-acting substances.

Urine osmolarity and other urine electrolytes

Urine electrolytes are useful in distinguishing extrarenal causes (e.g. excessive gains or losses) versus renal causes (e.g. tubular dysfunction or disturbed endocrine control).

- Urine electrolytes are ideally interpreted in the context of normal glomerular function, normovolaemia and cessation of offending drugs.
- Parallel changes (e.g. ↓ serum electrolyte, ↓ urine electrolyte) indicate an extrarenal cause with normal homeostatic response.
- Reciprocal changes (e.g. ↓ serum electrolyte, ↑ urine electrolyte) suggest primary renal or endocrine dysfunction or drug effect. For example, ↑ P_{osm} plus ↓ U_{osm} indicates SIADH; ↓ P_{K+} plus ↑ U_{K+} indicates mineralocorticoid excess.

Serum electrolytes and osmolarity can vary widely and therefore do not have specific reference ranges—they are interpreted together with concurrent serum levels.

Disorders of serum sodium

- Physiological significance: osmolar control of intracellular volume; the CNS is highly sensitive to imbalances in serum sodium.
- Physiological control: thirst mechanism, ADH at distal tubule and collecting duct.
- Major compartment: ECF (Na^+ is the most plentiful osmotically active cation).

Note: Water balance and water movement have a major impact on sodium concentration.

HYPONATRAEMIA

(Mild: $[Na^+] < 130$ mmol/L; moderate: < 120 mmol/L; severe: < 110 mmol/L)

Clinical effects

- Mild/chronic: patients are asymptomatic or have non-specific clinical features
- Moderate: confusion
- Life-threatening: cerebral oedema, seizure, coma (immediate treatment with hypertonic saline required)

Causes

(Causes are not usually due to pure sodium deficit.)

- Water excess—excessive water intake, too much 5% dextrose
- Sodium loss—diuretics, GI losses, excessive sweating (with replacement by salt-poor fluid)
- 'Oedematous states'—severe heart failure, liver cirrhosis, nephrotic syndrome
- Homeostatic failure—SIADH

Assessment

Verify with serum osmolarity:

- Low—true hyponatraemia (see below)
- Normal—normo-osmolar/factitious/pseudohyponatraemia (lipaemic specimen, hyperproteinaemic specimen)
- High—hyperosmolar hyponatraemia—DKA, hyper-osmolar hyperglycaemic syndrome (HHS), mannitol

Note: Beware of 'drip arm', where sample is taken from IV site with spurious concentrations of Na^+, K^+, Cl^-.

Table 27.2 Assessment of hyponatraemia

	Plasma osmolality (mmol/L)	U_{Na} (mmol/L)	U_{osm} (mmol/L)
Water intoxication Extrarenal sodium loss	Low	< 20	Low
SIADH (water retention) Mineralocorticoid deficiency	Low	> 40	High

U_{Na}, [Na^+] in urine; U_{osm}, urine osmolarity.

True hyponatraemia

Table 27.2 outlines possible diagnoses in hyponatraemia.

Potential causes of SIADH

- Acute illness
- Drugs—opiates, NSAIDs, various psychotropics, carbamazepine, cyclophosphamide, chemotherapeutics
- CNS and psychiatric conditions
- Neoplasia
- Acute and chronic pulmonary disease
- HIV

Management of hyponatraemia

- Hyper-osmolar hyponatraemia: address cause.
- Normo-osmolar hyponatraemia: repeat test with direct measurement method.
- If seizures or coma, *get help* (see Table 27.1).
- Moderately severe: 1 mL/kg/h 3% hypertonic saline. Monitor levels 2-hourly initially.
- If in shock or oliguric—bolus IV normal saline
- Once circulatory parameters are normal and urine output is > 0.5 mL/kg/h, apply fluid restriction to < 800 mL/day.
- Aim to increase Na^+ levels by 5–10 mmol/L/day.
  - Over-rapid correction may lead to central pontine myelinolysis and quadriparesis.
  - If [Na^+] rises too quickly despite careful fluid management, then obtain ICU opinion (may need desmopressin and 5% dextrose infusion to re-lower).
- In SIADH—also consider sodium tablets ± frusemide in difficult cases (seek expert assistance).
- In oedematous states—optimise medical management, consider vasopressin antagonists if persistent.

(*pto*)

Note: Continuing to administer excessive fluid (even normal saline) following initial resuscitation will continue to worsen hyponatraemia.

HYPERNATRAEMIA

(Mild: [Na^+] > 145 mmol/L; symptomatic >155 mmol/L)
Hypernatraemia is rare as long as there is a preserved thirst mechanism, normal ADH response and free access to water.

Clinical effects

- Mild or chronic cases: asymptomatic or non-specific clinical features.
- Severe cases: altered mental state (risk of central pontine myelinolysis, cerebral haemorrhage if acute).

Causes

- Inadequate water intake—institutionalised patients, altered mental state (common)
- Excess water loss—GI losses, osmotic diuresis
- Excessive sodium intake—salt poisoning
- Homeostatic failure—diabetes insipidus (DI); rare but important

Assessment

- Urine sodium, urine osmolarity (low in DI)
- Review drug history

Management

- Mild, well patient, able to drink: oral water rehydration
- If symptomatic or unable to drink: admit for IV fluid replacement and treat other comorbidities.
- If in shock or oliguric—bolus IV of normal saline
- Chronic hypernatraemia (duration > 24 hours):
  - give 60 mL/kg of ½ normal saline or 30 mL/kg of 5% dextrose over 24 hours to replenish water deficit.
  - Adjust rate to achieve a 10 mmol/L reduction over 24 hours. (Added K^+ will require a 25–50% increase in infusion rate.)
  - Additional fluid should be matched for other ongoing losses.
  - Avoid 5% dextrose if hyperglycaemic.
- Acute hypernatraemia (duration < 24 hours): give 6 mL/kg/h 2.5% dextrose. Aim for 2 mmol/L/h reduction.
- Repeat electrolytes frequently, 6- to 12-hourly depending on severity.
- Over-rapid correction may lead to cerebral oedema.
- In DI: give vasopressin or desmopressin (obtain assistance).

Disorders of serum potassium

- Physiological role of potassium: membrane potential of excitable tissue (especially cardiac muscle).
- Physiological control: renin–angiotensin–aldosterone at distal tubule.
- Major compartment: ICF (most plentiful cation).

HYPOKALAEMIA

(Mild: $[K^+] < 3.5$ mmol/L; moderate < 3.0 mmol/L; severe: < 2.4 mmol/L)

Clinical effects

- Moderate: muscle weakness (e.g. hypokalaemic period paralysis), ECG—shows flat T waves, U waves
- Severe: rhabdomyolysis, ventricular arrhythmia

Causes

- Potassium losses—vomiting, laxatives, diuretics, sweating, post obstructive diuresis
- Compartmental shifts—metabolic alkalosis, salbutamol, adrenaline, insulin
- Homeostatic failure—mineralocorticoid excess, renal tubular defects

Management

- Life-threatening (acute arrhythmia): *get help* (see Table 27.1); ultra-rapid IV potassium should be administered in ICU.
- Severe or nil by mouth ($[K^+] < 2.5$ mmol/L): give 10–20 mmol potassium chloride in 1 L of normal saline per hour. (A concentration > 40–60 mmol/L needs to be given by central line.) Initially monitor levels every 2 hours.
- Special cases: intravenous K_2HPO_4/KH_2PO_4 if concurrent hypophosphataemia, oral potassium bicarbonate ($KHCO_3$) or intravenous potassium acetate if concurrent normal AG metabolic acidosis (get expert assistance).
- Mild or moderate: potassium chloride slow-release tablets 600–1200 mg/day PO.
- Admit patient if hypokalaemia is severe, patient is symptomatic or has ongoing losses; otherwise outpatient review in 48 hours after initial treatment.
- In chronic depletion, total deficit can be 200–400 mmol.
- Successful treatment is dependent on addressing concurrent hypomagnesaemia (see section on hypomagnesaemia, below).

HYPERKALAEMIA

(Mild: [K^+] > 5 mmol/L; moderate: > 6.5 mmol/L; severe > 7.5 mmol/L)

Clinical effects

Severe: ventricular arrhythmia or bradyarrhythmia (do immediate ECG). ECG shows peaked T wave, ↓ QT → PR widening or BBB pattern → QRS prolongation → sine wave (arrows indicate worsening progression).

Causes

- Reduced potassium excretion—renal failure, angiotensin-converting enzyme (ACE) inhibitors, K^+-sparing diuretics
- Cellular injury—crush injury, rhabdomyolysis, haemolysis
- Temporary compartmental shifts—metabolic acidosis, beta-adrenergic blockers, digoxin toxicity
- Homeostatic failure—mineralocorticoid deficiency, renal tubular defects

Management

- Mild ([K^+] > 5 mmol/L): review cause ± rehydrate, Resonium 30 g PO/PR.
- Moderate ([K^+] > 6.5 mmol/L): 50% dextrose IV + 5–10 units Actrapid IV + 10 mg salbutamol nebulised, in addition to the above.
- Life-threatening (QRS widening, arrhythmia): *get help* (see Table 27.1); sodium bicarbonate ($NaHCO_3$) 1 mmol/kg over 30 minutes if there is concurrent metabolic acidosis; patient may need dialysis.

Most treatments only result in temporary transcellular shifts of potassium. Kaliuresis, dialysis or Resonium treatment will result in true elimination of potassium.

Note: Due to the complex interaction of parathyroid hormone (PTH) and calcitriol on the bones, calcium, phosphate and magnesium abnormalities often co-exist.

Disorders of calcium

- Physiological role of calcium: muscle contraction and blood clotting.
- Physiological control: PTH acting on bone pool, GI tract absorption and renal excretion (interacts with phosphate balance, calcitriol and magnesium balance).
- Major compartment: bone (some bound to serum albumin); in disease states, can be abnormally bound in the circulation, precipitate or be sequestered.

HYPOCALCAEMIA

(Symptomatic: total [Ca^{2+}] < 1.8 mmol/L; ionic [Ca^{2+}] < 0.7 mmol/L)

Clinical effects

- Mild: paraesthesia
- Moderate: tetany, ECG shows increased QT interval
- Severe: respiratory failure, torsade de pointes, hypotension, mental state changes

Causes

- Acute pancreatitis (precipitation)
- Massive transfusion (citrate sequestration)
- Tumour lysis syndrome (phosphate release)
- Acute renal failure
- Reduced PTH

Management

- If breathing difficulties, arrhythmias or hypotension: *get help* (see Table 27.1).
- Moderate/chronic: give 60–120 mL 10% calcium gluconate in 1 L 5% dextrose over 24 hours.
- Mild/chronic: treat the cause ± Caltrate (elemental calcium + vitamin D), calcitriol

HYPERCALCAEMIA

(Mild: total [Ca^{2+}] > 2.5 mmol/L; moderate: > 3.0 mmol/L; severe: > 3.5 mmol/L)

Clinical effects

- Acute or severe: changes in mental state/confusion (always consider this in cancer patients)
- Chronic: constipation and fatigue

Causes

- Malignancy/bone metastases (bone pool mobilisation)
- Thiazide diuretics (decreased renal excretion)
- Sarcoidosis (ectopic calcitriol production)
- Increased PTH

Management

(All therapies take time to work.)

- If comatose: *get help* (see Table 27.1).
- Correct dehydration until urine output is > 0.5 mL/kg/h.

- If hypercalcaemia is severe, commence saline calciuresis:
  - IV normal saline 1000 mL over 6 hours ± 20 mg frusemide over 2 hours; dialyse if unable to tolerate fluid loading and forced diuresis.
  - Alternatively, calcitonin 4 IU/kg with pamidronate 60–90 mg over 2 hours.
- Other treatments include prednisolone 20–40 mg/day (sarcoidosis, lymphoma), gallium arsenide/nitrate.
- If hypercalcaemia is mild or moderate—optimise hydration, address cause.

Disorders of phosphate

- Physiological role of phosphate: intracellular energy production
- Physiological control: calcitriol (interacts with calcium balance and PTH)
- Major compartments: ICF, bone.

HYPOPHOSPHATAEMIA

(Mild: $PO_4^{3-} < 0.8$ mmol/L; moderate: < 0.6 mmol/L; severe: < 0.4 mmol/L)

Clinical effects

- Usually due to chronic deficiency associated with reduced total body stores
- Moderate: mild weakness
- Severe: paraesthesia, mental state changes or arrhythmias, rhabdomyolysis (rare but may mask total body depletion)

Causes

- Decreased intake/absorption—chronic alcoholism, malnourishment (common), anorexia nervosa, antacid abuse
- Transcellular shifts—insulin (re-feeding syndrome, DKA treatment), post parathyroidectomy (hungry bone syndrome), respiratory alkalosis
- Homeostatic failure—increased PTH

Note: Beware of the refeeding syndrome in severe anorexia nervosa.

Management

- If arrhythmia: *get help* (see Table 27.1).
- Severe: intravenous K_2HPO_4/KH_2PO_4 40–80 mmol/L in 1 L normal saline over 24 hours.
- Moderate: PO elemental phosphorus 10–20 mmol/L 4 times daily.
- Mild and asymptomatic: resume normal diet.

HYPERPHOSPHATAEMIA

(Severity is related to the degree of hypocalcaemia.)

Clinical effects

Related to associated hypocalcaemia (see above).

Causes

- Transcellular shifts—acute tissue breakdown (rhabdomyolysis, haemolysis, tumour lysis), phosphate enemas
- Decreased excretion—severe renal failure, bisphosphonates, vitamin D excess
- Homeostatic failure—reduced PTH

Management

(All therapies take time to work.)

- If breathing difficulties, arrhythmias or hypotension: *get help* (see Table 27.1).
- Moderate/severe: commence urgent saline rehydration (but not in hypocalcaemia—consider dialysis).
- Chronic renal failure: seek advice.
- Mild: maintain hydration, address cause.

Disorders of magnesium

- Physiological significance of magnesium: membrane potential of excitable tissue (nerve, cardiac and skeletal muscle).
- Physiological control: nil (but can indirectly affect PTH and hence Ca^{2+}/ PO_4^{3-})—highly susceptible to major changes in intake or renal function.
- Major compartments: ECF (immediate), bone (large concentration but not rapidly mobilised).

HYPOMAGNESAEMIA

(Symptomatic: $[Mg^{2+}] < 0.5$ mmol/L)
Often associated with co-existing abnormalities, e.g. potassium, calcium, acid–base.

Clinical effects

- Moderate: ECG shows increased PR interval, increased QRS complex
- Severe: altered mental state, ventricular arrhythmias
- Other clinical effects related to associated abnormalities

Causes

Diuretics, chronic alcoholism, poor nutrition.

Management

- If arrhythmias: *get help* (see Table 27.1).
- Moderate: intravenous magnesium sulfate ($MgSO_4$) 20–60 mmol in 1 L normal saline over 24 hours.
- Mild: magnesium chloride ($MgCl_2$) 25–50 mmol over 24 hours

HYPERMAGNESAEMIA

(Mild: [Mg^{2+}] > 2 mmol/L; moderate > 3.5 mmol/L; severe > 5 mmol/L)

Clinical effects

- Mild: vomiting, flushing
- Moderate: hypotonia/reflexia, mental state changes, ECG shows increased QRS complex, peaked T waves
- Severe: respiratory muscle weakness, bradyarrhythmia, hypotension

Causes

Acute renal failure, iatrogenic (e.g. treatment of eclampsia).

Management

(All therapies take time to work.)

- If cardiorespiratory compromise: *get help* (see Table 27.1).
- Stop Mg^{2+} infusion, maintain urine output at > 0.5 mL/kg/h ± dialysis.

Rough correction factors for electrolyte abnormalities

See Table 27.3.

Acute renal failure

Acute renal failure is indicated by ANY of the following:

- ANY rise in serum creatinine (normal is < 120 micromol/L)
- Urine output < 30 mL/h

Box 27.1 lists life-threatening complications of renal failure.

Table 27.3 Approximate correction factors for electrolyte abnormalities*

Situation	Correction
Hyperglycaemia	True [Na^+] = measured [Na^+] + 0.3 × [glucose]
Metabolic acidosis	Reduce measured [K^+] by 0.5 for every ↓ pH of 0.1
Metabolic alkalosis	Increase measured [K^+] by 0.5 for every ↓ pH of 0.1
Hypoalbuminaemia	Add 0.1 total [Ca^{2+}] for every 4 g/dL decrease in albumin

* All measurements in mmol/L. Correction factors are rough guides only.

Box 27.1 Life-threatening complications of renal failure

- Severe hyperkalaemia (see section on hyperkalaemia)
- Acute pulmonary oedema
- Uraemic encephalopathy

EARLY ED ASSESSMENT AND MANAGEMENT

('Pre-renal, renal, post-renal'.)

1 Assess for and treat hyperkalaemia (see section on hyperkalaemia).
2 Restore renal perfusion: IV fluid bolus until urine output is > 40 mL/h or fluid overload develops.
3 Treat sepsis or UTI: urine dipstick, urine culture, IV antibiotics.
4 Relieve obstruction: IDC and measure hourly urine output ± urgent renal ultrasound to exclude ureteric obstruction ± urgent nephrostomy. Beware of post-obstructive diuresis resulting in hypovolaemia, hypokalaemia
5 Stop nephrotoxic drugs, e.g. NSAIDs, aminoglycosides, ACE inhibitors, frusemide.

PRE-RENAL (DEHYDRATION/HYPOVOLAEMIA) OR ESTABLISHED (ACUTE TUBULAR NECROSIS) RENAL FAILURE?

- Typically in pure dehydration, plasma urea:creatinine is > 20:1.
- 'Intra-renal' causes—check urine sediment for casts, protein and cells.

(See Table 27.4 overleaf.)

Box 27.2 (also overleaf) gives indications for haemodialysis.

HYPERLACTATAEMIA OR 'LACTIC ACIDOSIS'—CLINICAL USE, PROGNOSTICATION, DISPOSITION

- Normal value of lactate is < 2 mmol/L ('significant' is > 5 mmol/L).
- The body does not produce 'lactic acid'.

Note: Hyperlactataemia can occur with or without concurrent acidaemia.

Causes of raised lactate levels (often several mechanisms co-exist) are:

- Increased glycolytic activity, e.g. exercise, hypermetabolic states, critically ill patients
- Reduced metabolism, e.g. severe liver dysfunction

(*pto*)

Table 27.4 Pre-renal versus renal failure

Cause/mechanism	Pre-renal failure	Established renal failure (i.e. acute tubular necrosis)
Summary	Maximal water and sodium retention and maximally concentrated urine to maintain circulatory volume (U_{Na} ↓ but U_{urea}, U_{osm}, U_{creat} ↑↑↑)	Loss of concentrating power volume (U_{Na} ↑ and U_{urea}, U_{osm}, U_{creat} ↔)
$P_{urea}:P_{creat}$	20:1	10–15:1
U_{Na} (mmol/L)	< 20	> 40
U_{osm} (mOsm/L)	> 500	< 350
$U_{osm}:P_{osm}$	> 2:1	< 1:2
$U_{creat}:P_{creat}$	> 40:1	< 20:1
Fe_{Na}	< 1%	> 2%

$$Fe_{Na} = \frac{(U_{Na} / P_{Na})}{(U_{creat} / P_{creat})}$$

↓, decreases; ↑, increases; ↑↑↑, increases massively; ↔, remains unchanged; P_{creat}, plasma creatinine; P_{Na}, plasma sodium; P_{osm}, plasma osmolarity; P_{urea}, plasma urea; U_{creat}, urinary creatinine; U_{Na}, urinary sodium; U_{osm}, urinary osmolarity; U_{urea}, urinary urea.

Box 27.2 Indications for haemodialysis ('too much acid, water, potassium or poison')

- Severe metabolic acidosis
- Acute pulmonary oedema—fluids challenge does not re-establish urine output
- Hyperkalaemia not responding to medical treatment (see section on hyperkalaemia)
- Acute nephrotoxic exposures, e.g. lithium, methanol, ethylene glycol

- Poor tissue perfusion/oxygenation (type A lactic acidosis)—**important cause**
- Abnormal mitochondrial function (type B lactic acidosis)—e.g. metformin, thiamine deficiency.

Severity of abnormality generally correlates to short to mid-term morbidity and mortality (> 8–10 mmol/L predicts high mortality).

- Transiently high elevations can occur after prolonged exertion or seizures.
- Levels may be chronically elevated, e.g. in chronic liver failure.

- Serial measurements (and response to treatment) have a higher prognostic value than a single test.

The interpretation (as in all investigations) needs to consider other clinical data, i.e. other evidence of hypoperfusion, the disease process, its acuity and how readily it responds to treatment—e.g. haemorrhagic shock versus severe sepsis/multi-organ failure versus end-stage chronic liver failure.

Note: The main use of lactate level is to support a clinical suspicion of poor tissue perfusion or inadequate response to fluid/inotropic support. A normal lactate should not override clinical judgment.

Controversies in electrolyte management

- The practical value of the Stewart approach in assessing acid–base disturbances.
- Use of bicarbonate in severe wide AG metabolic acidosis with pH < 6.8.
- Iatrogenic factors in the pathogenesis of cerebral oedema in DKA.
- 5% dextrose, ½ normal saline or normal saline for hypernatraemia.
- The incidence of SIADH in hospitalised patients and implications for empirical fluid management.
- Use of diuretics to convert oliguric renal failure into non-oliguric renal failure.
- At what creatinine level to commence dialysis?

Online resources

UptoDate
www.uptodate.com/home/index.html

Chapter 28
Poisoning, overdosage, drugs and alcohol

Fiona Chow, Alex Wodak and Robert Graham

Editorial Comment

This is core knowledge required for many of the patients attending our emergency department.
Have the phone number of the Poison Information Hotline easily accessible in every ED:
13 11 26 (Australia nation-wide)
Use it! You can discuss the patient and their management (repeatedly if necessary), whether your enquiry is general or deals with an uncertain situation—history, presentation, unknown overdose agents.

Poisoning and overdosage

(Fiona Chow)

Poisonings and overdoses are common presentations in the ED. Most poisonings are deliberate or attempts to self-harm, though some are accidental. Non-accidental injury, negligence and the hazards of the environment also need to be considered. Poisonings can occur following drug ingestion by various routes of absorption, including oral, inhalational, parenteral, mucosal and transdermal, depending on the toxin involved.

ASSESSMENT

History

Important information:

- type(s) of toxin or drug
- quantity taken
- timing of the overdose
- single or repeated doses
- route—oral, inhalational, transdermal, mucosal, parenteral
- previous psychiatric history, including self-harm attempts
- collateral history from family, friends, ambulance staff—pill packets, drug paraphernalia, suicide note

- other medications prescribed, including herbal preparations and over-the-counter drugs
- past history—pre-morbid medical conditions

Circumstances associated with the overdose

(Deliberate, self-harm, accidental.)

- Examine the patient's psychosocial history.
- Direct questioning regarding suicidal ideation and intent and self-harm is essential.
- Good clinical practice involves psychiatric consultation prior to discharge in all cases of deliberate poisoning.
- In the case of an accidental overdose, consider the safety of the patient's environment, and continuing education. Factors such as accessibility of medicines or chemicals should also be considered (e.g. paediatric patient), and scrutiny of work practices may be pertinent.

INVESTIGATIONS

Investigations required depend on the circumstances of the individual case. Generally, the following pathology tests are required on admission:

- full blood count (FBC)
- electrolytes, urea and creatinine (EUC)
- blood sugar level (BSL)
- liver function tests (LFTs)
- paracetamol level.

Electrocardiography (ECG) should be performed routinely, as many poisonings can result in cardiovascular complications (such as arrhythmias and myocardial injury). Abnormalities such as sinus tachycardia, PR prolongation, widened QRS or QT prolongation or arrhythmia may be evident. Some poisonings require continuous cardiac monitoring (e.g. tricyclic antidepressants, digoxin, calcium-channel blockers and beta-blockers).

Depending on the clinical setting, other investigations would include:

- coagulation studies (paracetamol overdose, warfarin overdose)
- creatinine kinase ± urine myoglobin (rhabdomyolysis, ictal or post-ictal)
- specific drug levels (see Box 28.1)
- arterial/venous blood gas and co-oximetry (gas exchange, acid–base balance, carbon monoxide, amyl nitrite)

Box 28.1 Quantitative drug/toxic assays that may be measured in serum

- Carbamazepine
- Ethanol
- Digoxin
- Iron
- Lithium
- Paracetamol
- Phenytoin
- Salicylate
- Theophylline
- Valproate
- Co-oximetry (carboxyhaemoglobin, methaemoglobin)

- troponin
- calcium, magnesium, phosphate
- lactate
- urine drug screen
- beta-hCG if female
- chest X-ray (aspiration pneumonitis, pulmonary oedema, acute lung injury)
- abdominal X-ray (ileus; radio-opaque concretions, e.g. iron)
- computed tomography (CT) of brain (exclude other causes of clinical presentation, sequelae of poisoning).

PRINCIPLES OF MANAGEMENT

The key principles in the management of poisonings include:

- resuscitation
- risk management and prediction of toxic effects
- supportive care, investigation and monitoring
- decontamination and enhanced elimination
- specific treatments (e.g. antidotes)
- prevention of recurrence.

Resuscitation, stabilisation and supportive care

- All patients with an overdose should have intravenous access.
- Airway, breathing and circulation must be attended to, as poisoned patients may have decreased level of consciousness and thus an unprotected airway, respiratory depression or haemodynamic instability.
- Frequent reassessment of level of consciousness and vital signs is essential, as some poisonings can have delayed effects.

Decontamination

Decontamination is not essential for all poisoned patients. It will depend on the risk of toxicity versus the benefit of the decontamination procedure. The major modalities of decontamination are *external* and *gastrointestinal*.

External decontamination

Some toxins can be absorbed via dermal, mucosal and inhalational routes. In these cases clothes should be removed and the entire body washed with soap and water thoroughly in an attempt to minimise poisoning and to avoid exposure of treating staff to the toxin. The classic example is organophosphates. Another example is irrigation of an eye following a chemical burn.

Editorial Comment

When a patient removes clothing, it should not be over their head. Consider cutting clothes off to avoid contamination of the face/airways.

Gastrointestinal (GI) decontamination

- GI decontamination is associated with complications (see Box 28.2). Therefore, the key to GI decontamination involves assessing the risk of toxicity and hence the need for decontamination (risk–benefit analysis).
- If the overdose is associated with significant risk of toxicity, GI decontamination should be considered.
- It is unlikely to be of benefit if more than 2 hours after an overdose has elapsed. Exceptions to this are significant overdoses of slow-release preparations, drugs that have anticholinergic properties and drugs that experience secondary reabsorption via the enterohepatic circulation.
- No single modality is universally recommended for all overdoses.

Ipecac in the past was used to induce emesis, and traditionally was recommended for paediatric toxic ingestions. It is no longer routinely recommended. Studies have shown that it

Box 28.2 Potential complications of GI decontamination

- Aspiration pneumonitis
- Bowel perforation
- Bowel obstruction

does not alter patient outcomes and that its use can result in complications such as aspiration pneumonitis.

Gastric lavage has not been shown to be beneficial in the general management of the acutely poisoned patient. Complications include aspiration, hypoxia and GI perforation/trauma.

The efficacy of **activated charcoal** is time-dependent and therefore should be considered mainly in those presenting within 1 hour when the poisoning is assessed to be high-risk. The main complication of charcoal is pulmonary aspiration, especially in the obtunded patient. Toxins not well adsorbed by charcoal are listed in Table 28.1. Activated charcoal is also available with a cathartic (e.g. sorbitol). There is little evidence to suggest that the addition of a cathartic is superior to using activated charcoal alone.

Whole-bowel irrigation with agents such as polyethylene glycol is rarely used. It hastens the elimination of poorly absorbed or slow-release medications before they can be absorbed. Complications include vomiting, abdominal bloating and pain. Rarely, colonic or oesophageal perforation has been reported as well as GI bleeding (Mallory–Weiss tear) and pulmonary aspiration after vomiting. Occasions where it may be useful are:

- life-threatening ingestions of slow-release preparations
- life-threatening ingestions of enteric-coated preparations
- agents that do not bind to charcoal
- 'body packers and stuffers' (those who are acting as illicit drug 'mules').

Table 28.1 Drugs not well adsorbed by activated charcoal

Drug group	Examples
Alcohols	Ethanol, methanol, isopropyl alcohol, ethylene glycol
Metals	Lithium, iron, mercury, potassium, lead, arsenic
Acids and alkalis	
Hydrocarbons	Turpentine, kerosene, eucalyptus oil, benzene

Enhanced elimination

There are several forms of enhanced elimination that are more commonly used depending on the type of overdose. Again, assess the severity of the toxicity to determine whether employing these techniques will be beneficial.

Box 28.3 Situations when multiple doses of charcoal may reduce drug absorption

- The drug/s involved have significant reabsorption via the enterohepatic circulation.
- Stomach emptying is delayed (e.g. anticholinergic effects).
  Note: Ensure the presence of bowel sounds prior to repeating dose of charcoal, as ileus can occur due to anticholinergic effects
- The drug involved is *carbamazepine, dapsone, phenobarbitone, quinine* or *theophylline*.

Multiple doses of charcoal may decrease drug absorption in some cases (Box 28.3). This method of drug elimination works best when the drug involved is of small molecular weight, has a prolonged elimination time and a small volume of distribution. A suggested dosing regimen would be 25 g (adults) or 0.5 g/kg (children) every 2–4 hours. It is contraindicated if there is a bowel obstruction or decreased level of consciousness in a patient without a protected airway. Always check for the presence of bowel sounds before administering the next dose.

Urinary alkalinisation may be used for increasing elimination of weak acids. This can be achieved by intravenous administration of sodium bicarbonate. Give a bolus of 1 mmol/kg IV followed by an infusion (100 mmol of sodium bicarbonate in 1000 mL 5% dextrose in 0.9% normal saline over 4 hours). Adjust the rate to a urinary pH of > 7.5. Complications of bicarbonate therapy include fluid overload, alkalaemia, hypokalaemia and hypocalcaemia. The main indication is salicylate overdose.

Extracorporeal elimination includes haemodialysis and haemoperfusion. Dialysis is the most commonly used form of extracorporeal elimination. It can enhance elimination of various toxins (Box 28.4). Situations where dialysis may be considered are listed in Box 28.5.

Monitoring

Ongoing observation is often required to detect signs of toxicity (acute or delayed) or to monitor progress after treatment.

Examples include:

- continuous cardiorespiratory monitoring
  - ECG
  - blood pressure, heart rate
  - pulse oximetry, respiratory rate

Box 28.4 Drugs amenable to dialysis

- Carbamazepine
- Lithium
- Salicylates
- Theophylline
- Metformin
- Potassium
- Toxic alcohols (methanol, benzyl alcohol, diethylene alcohol, dipropylene glycol, ethylene glycol, propylene glycol, triethylene glycol)
- Valproate

Box 28.5 Indications for dialysis

- Failure to clinically improve despite full supportive and clinical treatment
- Inability to excrete or metabolise drug due to impaired route of elimination (e.g. renal failure, hepatic failure)
- Associated metabolic abnormalities that would be resolved with dialysis (e.g. metformin lactic acidosis)
- Acute renal failure caused by a potentially nephrotoxic drug
- Highly toxic poisoning or potentially lethal plasma concentration of the toxin/drug as determined by previous clinical reporting

- frequent reassessment of Glasgow Coma Scale (GCS) score
- core temperature (serotonin syndrome, hyperthermia, hypothermia)
- serial blood tests (some examples below)
  - drug levels (lithium, paracetamol)
  - LFTs (paracetamol)
  - prothrombin time (PT) or INR (paracetamol, warfarin)
  - BSL (hypoglycaemics, insulin)
  - methaemoglobin (amyl nitrite)
- urine output and urinary pH.

Supportive care

Listed below are several common toxic effects and corresponding management strategies.

Coma

- Reduced GCS is a common toxic effect of many drugs and poisons.
- Look for reversible causes and treat urgently—hypoglycaemia, opiate intoxication.
- Priority is focused on establishing a patent and protected airway.

- If coma was not a predicted outcome of the overdose, investigate for other causes. This may include a CT brain scan.

Seizures

- Benzodiazepines are first-line therapies for drug-related seizures.
- Barbiturates are second-line.
- Phenytoin is not indicated.
- If seizures are atypical (focal or partial), further investigation of the seizure is warranted.

Cardiovascular instability

- Management of hypotension involves intravenous access and fluids. Treat any associated arrhythmias.
- Inotropes and antidotes may be indicated to treat hypotension. Examples include calcium for calcium-channel blocker overdose, sodium bicarbonate for tricyclic antidepressant overdose, inotropes for beta-blocker overdose.

Hyperthermia

- Hyperthermia has life-threatening consequences such as multi-organ failure.
- Aggressive early treatment is essential.
- Cooled fluids, cooling blanket ± intubation, ventilation and paralysis are among the treatment options.
- Continuously monitor core temperature (rectal/bladder).

Metabolic and cognitive disturbances

- Screen for and treat conditions such as hypoxia, hypercarbia, glucose, acid–base and electrolyte abnormalities.
- Manage agitation and confusion initially with verbal reassurance. If unsuccessful, use benzodiazepines (first-line) or olanzapine to achieve gentle sedation. Key aims include safety of the patient (e.g. prevention of absconding) and safety of the staff.

Antidotes

For a list of antidotes, see the 'Quick reference' section, part 13.

Toxidromes and specific overdoses

The clinical presentation of some poisonings may be predictable based on the pharmacology of the drug/substance involved. Some classic toxidromes, with examples, are listed in Table 28.2.

Table 28.2 Some classic toxidromes

Toxidrome	Mnemonic/memory jogger	Clinical features	Examples
Anticholinergic	Mad as a hatter, red as a beet, hot as a hare, dry as a bone, blind as a bat	Delirium, flushing, hyperthermia, dry mouth and skin, dilated pupils, tachycardia, urinary retention, ileus	Tricyclic antidepressants, carbamazepine, antihistamines, phenothiazines, *Belladonna atropa*
Cholinergic—muscarinic effects	DUMBBELLS	**D**iaphoresis, **D**iarrhoea **U**rination **M**iosis **B**radycardia **B**ronchorrhoea, **B**ronchospasm **E**mesis **L**acrimation **L**ow BP **S**alivation	Organophosphates Carbamates
Cholinergic—nicotinic effects	'Days of the week' **M**onday **T**uesday **W**ednesday T**H**ursday **F**riday **S**aturday	**M**uscle cramps, **M**ydriasis **T**achycardia, **T**remor **W**eakness **H**ypertension **F**asciculations **S**ugar (hyperglycaemia)	Organophosphates Carbamates
Opiate		CNS and respiratory depression, miosis	Heroin, methadone, morphine, oxycodone, buprenorphine, fentanyl
Serotonergic		CNS, autonomic and musculoskeletal abnormalities	SSRIs, ecstasy, tramadol
Sympathomimetic	'Flight or fight' response	Tachycardia, hypertension, tachypnoea, agitation, hypervigilance, mydriasis	Cocaine, ecstasy, amphetamines

BENZODIAZEPINES

Overdoses of benzodiazepines are common and have a good prognosis with supportive treatment. CNS and respiratory depression are the main toxic effects. Flumazenil may confirm the diagnosis but is generally not used for treatment, unless reversing iatrogenic conscious sedation or if advanced airway management is unavailable. The half-life of flumazenil (about 1 hour) is much shorter than that of all benzodiazepines; repeat doses of flumazenil may be required to maintain effect.

Key points—benzodiazepines

- Care must be taken when using flumazenil in mixed overdoses, as some co-ingestants (e.g. tricyclic antidepressants) may be proconvulsant. The use of flumazenil in these situations may precipitate seizures and death.
- Other contraindications for flumazenil include known seizure disorder and benzodiazepine dependence.

OPIOIDS

This group of drugs includes those derived from opium as well as those that have opiate-like activity. Typical toxic effects are CNS and respiratory depression and miosis. Acute lung injury has been reported, typically occurring once ventilation has been restored following a period of respiratory depression. Other effects include mild hypotension (arteriolar and venous vasodilation).

Treatment of opioid toxicity is supportive, especially of the airway and ventilation, and sometimes involves the use of naloxone, either as bolus dose(s) or as an infusion. Several drugs in this group have atypical toxic effects (Table 28.3).

Table 28.3 Atypical opioids

Opioid	Atypical toxic effects of clinical significance
Tramadol	Serotonin syndrome, seizures
Dextropropoxyphene	Seizures, wide QRS arrhythmias (sodium-channel blockade), negative inotropic effects, hypotension
Methadone	Prolonged QT interval (possibly leading to torsades de pointes)
Pethidine	Seizures, serotonin syndrome
Fentanyl	Muscle rigidity (rapid injection)

Key points—opioids

- Check the duration of action of the opioid involved. Some are as short as several hours (fentanyl, heroin), and others as long as 24 hours (methadone and controlled-release forms of morphine and oxycodone). This may help to predict the likelihood of requiring a naloxone infusion and intensive care.
- Be mindful of more unusual routes of opioid administration such as transdermal patches (fentanyl).
- Naloxone can be life-saving. The treatment goal is adequate respiration as opposed to complete CNS recovery. Infusions can be used for intoxication with longer-acting opioids.
- The effects of naloxone are seen within minutes when administered intravenously. Duration of action is short (0.5 hours) in comparison to the majority of opioids. Close monitoring and observation is important after naloxone administration, as repeated dosing may be required.
- Naloxone can precipitate severe opioid withdrawal in the tolerant patient. Reverse respiratory depression with small increments in order to prevent severe withdrawal.
- Buprenorphine is a partial agonist. In overdose, naloxone can be used to reverse respiratory depression but a partial or complete lack of response may be seen.
- Children are at high risk of life-threatening opioid intoxication following ingestions.

PARACETAMOL

Paracetamol overdoses can be either single or staggered ingestions. There are 4 described stages of paracetamol poisoning (Table 28.4). Stage II marks the onset of liver injury. Renal failure is seen in 25–50% of those with hepatic dysfunction. Death is usually due to multi-organ failure, sepsis, haemorrhage, acute respiratory distress syndrome and/or cerebral oedema.

Key blood tests are paracetamol level and transaminases—aspartate aminotransferase (AST) and alanine aminotransferase (ALT). Prothrombin time (PT) and INR may also be indicated. Paracetamol levels are reported in various units (mg/L or micromol/L). When plotting the paracetamol level on the nomogram, always check that the units are corresponding to the correct axis. Failure to do so may have life-threatening consequences.

Paracetamol can be implicated in an accidental overdose. Remember to ask for quantities of paracetamol ingested in the patient

Table 28.4 Stages of paracetamol poisoning

Stage	Time to onset	Clinical features	Laboratory abnormalities
I	< 24 hours	Asymptomatic *OR* nausea, vomiting, malaise, diaphoresis	Normal LFTs; rarely metabolic acidosis (massive overdose)
II	Within 24–36 hours	Right upper quadrant pain/tenderness	ALT/AST ↑ (peaks by 72 hours)
III	72–96 hours	Jaundice, hepatic encephalopathy, coagulopathy, multi-organ failure, death	AST/ALT ↑↑, PT ↑, bilirubin ↑, glucose ↓, lactate ↑, pH ↓
IV	> 5 days	Recovery	Normalising of LFTs

↑, increase; ↑↑, large increase; ↓, decrease.

who has been self-medicating to achieve analgesia. Paracetamol is a common component of over-the-counter medications such as cold and flu preparations and migraine tablets.

Serious hepatotoxicity is less common in children than adults.

Charcoal can be given in those who present within 1 hour after potentially toxic ingestions.

Guidelines and treatment nomogram

A collaboration of clinical toxicologists in Australia and New Zealand resulted in new guidelines and a new treatment nomogram published in the *Medical Journal of Australia* in March 2008. The nomogram is shown in Figure 28.1 and the guidelines are summarised below.

Key points—paracetamol

- Presentation > 8 hours after ingestion increases the likelihood of hepatic failure and death.
- Presentation > 24 hours after ingestion with normal transaminases and an undetectable paracetamol level is associated with little risk of hepatotoxicity.
- *N*-acetylcysteine (NAC) commenced within 8 hours of ingestion is associated with 100% survival

Risk assessment:

The following are potentially hepatotoxic doses of paracetamol.

1 *Single ingestions*
   - — Adults and children > 6 years of age: > 150 mg/kg or 10 g (whichever is lower) over a period of < 8 hours
   - — Children aged 0–6 years: ≥ 200 mg/kg over a period of < 8 hours.

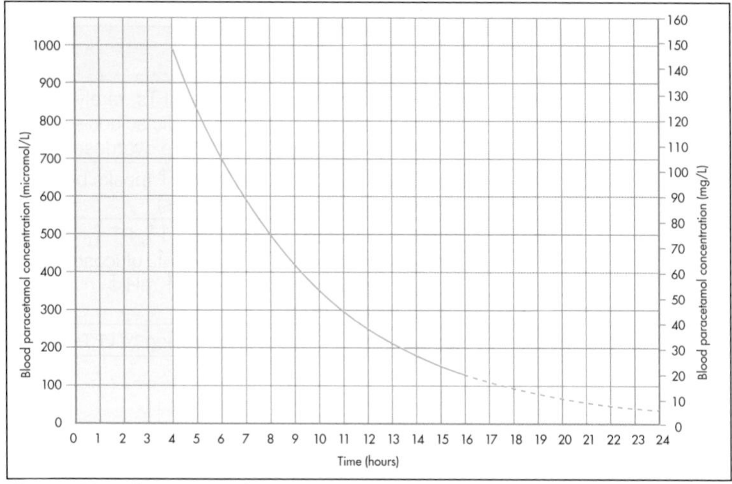

Figure 28.1 Paracetamol treatment nomogram
From Daly FFS, Fountain JS, Murray L et al. Guidelines for the management of paracetamol poisoning in Australia and New Zealand—explanation and elaboration. MJA 2008;188(5)296–302.

2 *Repeated supratherapeutic ingestions* (also given in Table 28.5, below)

— Adults and children > 6 years of age:
- > 150 mg/kg or 10 g (whichever is lower) over a single 24-hour period
- > 150 mg/kg or 6 g (whichever is lower) per 24-hour period over the preceding 48 hours
- > 100 mg/kg or 4 g/day (whichever is lower) in patients with predisposing risk factors (e.g. chronic alcohol use, use of enzyme-inducing drugs, prolonged fasting, dehydration, hepatitis)

— Children aged 0–6 years:
- ≥ 200 mg/kg over a single 24-hour period
- ≥ 150 mg/kg per 24-hour period for the preceding 48 hours
- ≥ 100 mg/kg per 24-hour period for the preceding 72 hours.

- **NAC should be *commenced immediately* if:**
  — Presentation is 8–24 hours after a known time of ingestion. The infusion can be ceased or continued once the paracetamol level and results of transaminases are analysed.

— Time of ingestion is unknown and paracetamol is detectable.
— There are signs of hepatic injury after any paracetamol overdose.

- Increases in AST and ALT levels are frequently the first laboratory sign of liver injury in paracetamol toxicity. Hepatotoxicity is defined as an AST or ALT > 1000 IU/L. King's College Criteria for paracetamol toxicity are predictors of poor prognosis. They are:
  — pH < 7.3 after adequate fluid resuscitation
  — creatinine > 300 micromol/L
  — prothrombin time > 100 seconds or INR > 6.5
  — grade III or IV encephalopathy.
- Early referral or consultation with liver transplantation services should be considered if any of the King's College Criteria are present, or there are worsening serial tests (↑ PT/INR or creatinine, ↓ pH and severe thrombocytopenia).

Management of acute single ingestions

Paracetamol levels measured > 4 hours post-ingestion can be plotted on a nomogram to determine risk of hepatotoxicity and indicate the need for NAC therapy.

Presentation within 8 hours

1. Measure the serum paracetamol (at 4–8 hours) and plot according to the nomogram. No other tests (e.g. LFTs, INR) are beneficial in making a risk assessment.
2. If the level is plotted above the treatment line, commence and complete NAC therapy. No further tests are required following completion of 20-hour NAC infusion. The patient is medically fit for discharge.
3. If the level is plotted below the treatment line, then no further medical treatment is required.

Presentation more than 8 hours after ingestion

1. NAC should be commenced immediately
2. Measure serum paracetamol level and ALT.
3. Treat according to results after plotting on nomogram:
   — If the paracetamol level plots *above* the treatment line, continue NAC.
   — If the paracetamol level plots *under* the treatment line and the ALT is *normal*, stop NAC. No further treatment is required.

(*pto*)

— If the paracetamol level plots *under* the treatment line and the ALT is *raised,* continue NAC infusion. Measure ALT after completion of NAC infusion.
  - If the ALT is *normal,* no further treatment is required.
  - If the ALT is *abnormal,* continue NAC (100 mg/kg over 16 hours) and recheck ALT/AST every 12–24 hours until falling.
  - If ALT/AST > 1000 IU/L check INR, renal function and platelet count every 12–24 hrs.

Management of staggered ingestions

A staggered overdose is one that occurs over a 24-hour period.

1 Check and plot the paracetamol level on the nomogram. Interpret the level as if the combined dose was taken at the time of the earliest ingestion.

2 Treat as per the guidelines under 'Management of acute single ingestions', i.e. within 8 hours post-ingestion pathway or more than 8 hours post-ingestion treatment pathway.

Repeated supratherapeutic ingestions

1 If the patient has ingested a potentially toxic dose (Table 28.5), measure serum paracetamol level and ALT.

2 If ALT is normal and paracetamol level < 12 micromol/L (20 mg/L), no further treatment is required.

3 If there is any other result, commence NAC and repeat paracetamol level and ALT at 8 hours.
   — If ALT is normal or static, no further treatment is required
   — If ALT is abnormal or worsening, continue NAC and check ALT and other bloods at 12-hour intervals.

Table 28.5 Repeated supratherapeutic doses that may be associated with hepatic injury

Adults and children aged > 6 years	Children aged < 6 years
> 150 mg/kg or 10 g (whichever is less) over a single 24-hour period	≥ 200 mg/kg over a single 24-hour period
> 150 mg/kg or 6 g (whichever is less) per 24-hour period over the preceding 48 hours	≥ 150 mg/kg per 24-hour period for the preceding 48 hours
> 100 mg/kg or 4 g/day (whichever is less) in patients with predisposing risk factors (e.g. chronic alcohol use, use of enzyme-inducing drugs, prolonged fasting, dehydration, hepatitis)	≥ 100 mg/kg per 24-hour period for the preceding 72 hours

Management of sustained-release paracetamol

1 If > 200 mg/kg or 10 g (whichever is lower) has been ingested, commence NAC.

2 Measure serum paracetamol level at 4 or more hours post-ingestion and then again 4 hours later if the first level was below the treatment line on the nomogram.
   — If both levels are below the line, NAC can be stopped.
   — If either level is above the line, continue NAC as per the guidelines under 'Management of acute single ingestions'.

Key points — *N*-acetylcysteine (NAC)

- NAC reduces the incidence of hepatotoxicity, hepatic failure and mortality in patients who present with normal liver function in the context of known ingestions.
- Adverse reactions include nausea and vomiting, anaphylactoid-type reactions—mainly cutaneous. Treatment of these reactions includes stopping the infusion, administering antihistamines and recommencing the infusion at a slower rate, then titrating back up. Bronchospasm, hypotension and angio-oedema have uncommonly been reported (< 2%).
- NAC has been shown to be useful even in late presentations with evidence of fulminant hepatic failure (decreases cerebral oedema, mortality). However, efficacy decreases the longer the delay beyond 8 hours post-ingestion.

ILLICIT DRUGS

The majority of these are best divided into *stimulants* versus *depressants* (Table 28.6 and Table 28.7). The others can be classed as *hallucinogens* (Box 28.6). *Amyl nitrite* is considered alone.

Stimulants

Cocaine and the amphetamines act via stimulation of the central and peripheral adrenergic receptors. They are sympathomimetic agents. The most common clinical effects of this group of drugs are outlined in Table 28.8. The most important clinical difference between cocaine and the amphetamines is that cocaine has a much shorter half-life and hence a shorter duration of action.

Cocaine

- Cocaine has additional properties to those above—it blocks sodium channels, is thrombogenic by promoting platelet aggregation and is vasospastic. It can also accelerate atherosclerosis.

Table 28.6 Stimulants

Drug name	Common street names
Cocaine	Coke
3,4-Methylenedioxy-*N*-methylamphetamine (MDMA)	Ecstasy
Methamphetamine	Ice, speed
para-Methoxyamphetamine (PMA) *para*-Methoxy-*N*-methylamphetamine (PMMA)	Red mitsubishi*, Dr Death, Killer
4-Methylthioamphetamine (4-MTA)	Flatliner
Synthetic cathinones, e.g. methylenedioxypyrovalerone (MDPV) or mephedrone (4-methylmethcathinone, 4-MMC)	Bath salts

* Not all pills with the red mitsubishi logo contain PMA.

Table 28.7 Depressants

Drug name	Common street names
Heroin	Smack, dope, hammer, gear
Gamma-hydroxybutyrate	G, GBH, fantasy, grievous bodily harm, liquid E
Ketamine	Special K, K, kit kat

Box 28.6 Hallucinogens and others

Hallucinogens	Others
• Cannabinoids LSD ('acid', 'blotter', 'dots')	• Amyl nitrite ('snappers', 'poppers', 'rushamines')

- Cocaine is more likely than amphetamines to cause seizures, arrhythmias and myocardial ischaemia. When combined with alcohol, cocaethylene can be produced which can enhance these cardiotoxic effects.
- Atypical chest pain is the norm for presentations of myocardial ischaemia, so a high index of suspicion must be maintained.
- Intake up to 4 days prior to presentation may be responsible for symptoms due to longer-lasting toxic metabolites.

Amphetamines

(MDMA, methamphetamine, PMA, PMMA, 4-MTA)

- These are more hallucinogenic due to their greater dopaminergic effect.

Table 28.8 **Clinical effects of cocaine and the amphetamines**

System	Clinical effect
CNS	Hallucinations (tactile, visual) Agitation Anxiety Psychosis Euphoria Seizures Tremor
Cardiovascular	Tachycardia Hypertension Chest pain (acute coronary syndrome) Arrhythmias (mainly cocaine)
Other	Hyperthermia Diaphoresis Tachypnoea Mydriasis Bruxism

- MDMA has been known to cause hyponatraemia and serotonin syndrome; therefore exercise caution in the delirious or post-ictal patient who has taken ecstasy.
- Hyponatraemia secondary to MDMA is thought to arise through several mechanisms—syndrome of inappropriate antidiuretic hormone (SIADH), water intoxication and loss of sodium in sweat (high ambient nightclub temperatures and dancing).
- Serotonin syndrome (Box 28.7) is diagnosed clinically according to features from three categories—autonomic, neuromuscular and central nervous system (CNS) abnormalities. It can be life-threatening. Management is supportive and, if patient is hyperthermic, early active cooling usually in association with intubation and paralysis is essential.
- The most common clinical presentation of 'ice' (methamphetamine) features aggression, paranoia, psychosis and agitation. The mainstay of treatment is sedation—options include benzodiazepines and antipsychotics (olanzapine, haloperidol). The route of administration of the sedatives will depend on the clinical state of the patient and the level of cooperation. Most cases are so severe that parenteral rapid sedation is the only management. In cases where intravenous access is problematic, intramuscular midazolam can be used. Sedation may need to be maintained until the effects of the amphetamine have ceased.

Box 28.7 Clinical features of serotonin syndrome

Autonomic dysfunction	Neuromuscular dysfunction	CNS dysfunction
Hyperthermia	Myoclonus	Confusion
Diaphoresis	Hyperreflexia	Disorientation
Sinus tachycardia	Muscle rigidity	Agitation
Hypertension	Tremor	Coma
Hypotension	Hyperactivity	Anxiety
Tachypnoea	Ataxia	Hypomania
Dilated pupils	Shivering	Lethargy
Unreactive pupils	Seizures	Insomnia
Flushed skin	Nystagmus	Hallucinations
Diarrhoea	Teeth chattering	Dizziness

- PMA and PMMA are more potent than MDMA but with a slower onset of action. Because of this, people tend to take more and consequently overdose. They are often sold as 'red mitsubishi' tablets or as ecstasy. They have been linked to deaths around the world, including Australia. Toxicity and death have been attributed to hyperthermia, rhabdomyolysis, seizures, disseminated intravascular coagulation (DIC), intracerebral haemorrhage or infarction, cardiac arrhythmias, electrolyte disturbances and multi-organ failure.
- 4-MTA has a mild stimulant effect, being less hallucinogenic and less euphoric compared with MDMA. It has been linked to multiple deaths in Europe though it is probably only lethal in excess or in combination with other drugs such as MDMA and cocaine.

Key points—stimulants

- Benzodiazepines are the treatment of choice for CNS and some cardiovascular (tachycardia, hypertension) effects of cocaine and amphetamine toxicity.
- Second-line therapies for hypertension include glyceryl trinitrate (GTN) or sodium nitroprusside infusions. Beta-blockers are contraindicated.
- Beta-blockers are contraindicated in the treatment of cocaine toxicity due to the potential for unopposed alpha stimulation. This can result in increased blood pressure, reduced coronary blood flow and reduced left ventricular (LV) function and reduced cardiac output.
- Management of chest pain in the context of cocaine or amphetamines is as with the usual work-up for acute coronary

syndromes. An ECG, chest X-ray and cardiac markers must be obtained and other causes for chest pain (e.g. dissection) should be ruled out. Aspirin, nitrates and diazepam should be given. The dose of diazepam is titrated to gentle sedation and the heart rate, aiming for settling of tachycardia (to reduce myocardial oxygen demand).
- Ventricular tachyarrhythmias due to cocaine toxicity should be initially treated with sodium bicarbonate.
- Do not assume that altered mental state or seizures are merely drug effects. Always exclude hyponatraemia as a cause and consider possible intracranial pathology.
- Aggressive early management of hyperthermia is crucial. Cooled fluids, cooling blanket and intubation, ventilation and paralysis (to prevent heat generation through shivering) are treatment options.
- Ecstasy may not be MDMA. It may contain any of the methamphetamines.

Depressants

Gamma-hydroxybutyrate (GHB) and analogues

This group of drugs consists of GHB, gamma-butyrolactone and 1,4-butanediol. They exhibit similar clinical effects. GHB was initially developed as an anaesthetic agent in the 1960s. It is a clear, colourless and reasonably tasteless drug with minimal 'hangover' effect which makes it palatable to the user and also accounts for it being implicated sometimes as a 'date rape' drug.

The most prominent clinical feature of toxicity is a rapid onset of coma, often to a GCS score as low as 3 (Box 28.8). Varying GCS over a short period of time can also occur. For example, a patient can oscillate from GCS 6 to 10 and then back to 6 in a period of 15–30 minutes. This phenomenon typically occurs as the drug effects are subsiding.

Due to the rapid onset and short duration of action, there is no role for decontamination. Treatment is supportive and care must be

Box 28.8 Clinical features of GHB intoxication

- Decreased GCS (often coma)
- Delirium
- Myoclonic jerking
- Hypoventilation
- Bradycardia
- Vomiting

taken with the intubated patient, as rapid recovery and violent arousal can result in self-extubation. Emergence delirium is often seen in the recovery phase.

Key points—GHB

- Patients have a good outcome with supportive care including intubation and ventilation.
- The drug has a short duration of action, with most patients recovering within 2–6 hours.
- GHB has an accumulative effect with repeated dosing and an additive effect with other CNS depressants such as alcohol and benzodiazepines. In these settings, recovery may be slower.
- Patients who are not improving or who have an atypical presentation should be further investigated (e.g. CT brain scan).

Ketamine

This is a dissociative anaesthetic agent. It is often swallowed, snorted or injected but can also be smoked. Users feel detached from their immediate surroundings, have 'out-of-body' experiences (flying, floating) and hallucinate. They do not respond to stimuli in their external surroundings. It is generally short-acting and fatalities are rare.

- Hypoventilation is uncommon.
- Effects can vary from appearing inebriated to being calm or agitated or violent. With larger doses, incoordination, inability to speak and confusion are common (see Box 28.9).
- Dystonic reactions, myoclonus, tremor and muscle rigidity can occur.
- Hypertension, tachycardia and bronchodilation are often seen.
- In overdose, coma occurs.
- Treatment options, depending on the clinical setting, include supportive care, sedation (benzodiazepines) and advanced airway management.

Hallucinogens

Cannabinoids

- Cannabinoids refers to active substances from *Cannabis sativa*. Cannabinol, cannabidiol and tetrahydrocannabinol (THC) are the major substances of this group. The principal psychoactive cannabinoid is delta-9-tetrahydrocannabinol.
- Marijuana is the name for a mixture of dried leaves and flowers of the plant.
- Hashish is the pressed resin. Hashish oil is the oil from hashish.

Box 28.9 Clinical effects of ketamine

- Euphoria, relaxation
- Feeling detached from one's body
- Distorted perception
- Confusion
- Anxiety, paranoia
- Slurred speech
- Blurred vision
- Lack of coordination
- ↑ Heart rate, blood pressure
- Nausea, vomiting
- ↓ Sensitivity to pain
- Inability to move
- Drowsiness
- Paralysis
- Muscle rigidity
- Hyperthermia
- Seizures
- Coma

- The concentration of THC varies from 1% in low-grade marijuana up to 50% in hashish oil.
- These substances may be smoked or ingested. Effects are apparent within minutes of smoking, and from 1–3 hours after ingestion.
- Clinical effects are listed in Table 28.9 overleaf.
- Serious toxicity is rare. The mainstay of treatment is supportive, with reassurance and benzodiazepines and/or occasionally antipsychotics (e.g. olanzapine) for gentle sedation in the agitated, paranoid or psychotic patient. Psychiatric symptoms are often due to underlying disorders.

Lysergic acid diethylamide (LSD)

- This is a synthetic hallucinogen which is able to alter and distort perception, thought and mood.
- It is sold as tablets, capsules, liquid, liquid-impregnated blotter paper or microdots, and is ingested. The onset of effects after ingestion is usually within 30–60 minutes, lasting approximately 10–12 hours.
- Auditory and visual hallucinations and size, shape and colour distortions may occur, as well as synaesthesia, a crossing-over of the senses often described as 'hearing colours' or 'seeing sounds'.

Table 28.9 Clinical effects of cannabinoids

System	Clinical effect
Psychological	Relaxation Sense of wellbeing Increased sensory awareness Slowing of time Panic
Cardiovascular	Tachycardia Postural hypotension
CNS	Reduced coordination Decreased muscle strength Sedation Dysarthria
Psychiatric	Dysphoria Panic reactions Psychosis
Gastrointestinal	Nausea, Vomiting (which can be cyclical and associated with excessive bathing activity)

- Users often experience many different emotions at once or swing between them.
- Potentially life-threatening complications include hyperthermia, coma, respiratory arrest, hypertension, tachycardia and coagulopathy, but have only been described in patients following a massive LSD overdose. Serotonin syndrome has been described with LSD use.

Key points—hallucinogens

- The most common presentation is of a 'bad trip'. Treatment involves providing a quiet room with minimal stimuli, reassurance and, if necessary, benzodiazepines.
- Trauma can also be a consequence of patients affected by hallucinogens.

Amyl nitrite

Amyl nitrite is a volatile nitrite and vasodilator. Nasal inhalation is the typical route of administration. Effects include facial flushing, lightheadedness, syncope, euphoria, sexual enhancement and disinhibition. It can cause methaemoglobinaemia, especially if ingested.

Table 28.10 Clinical effects of methaemoglobinaemia

Methaemoglobinaemia percentage	Clinical features
10–20%	Cyanosis
20–50%	Shortness of breath, dizziness, fatigue, headache
> 50%	Tachypnoea, lethargy, coma, seizures, death

Key points—methaemoglobinaemia

- Clinical features of methaemoglobinaemia are consistent with those of hypoxia (Table 28.10).
- Pulse oximetry typically reads around 85% and fails to improve with supplemental oxygen.
- Diagnosis relies on detection of the presence of methaemoglobinaemia on co-oximetry.
- Treat symptomatic patients with methylene blue 1–2 mg/kg IV over 5 minutes. Consider treating the asymptomatic patient with methaemoglobin levels of > 20%. Response should be apparent within 30–60 minutes. If not or dose is insufficient, the dose may be repeated.
- Monitor with serial methaemoglobin levels.

BETA-BLOCKERS

- Toxicity depends on which beta-blocker, the age of the patient, the presence of underlying respiratory or cardiac disease and co-ingestants (negative chronotropes).
- Of all the available beta-blockers, propranolol or sotalol toxicity are the most clinically significant and may be life-threatening.
- Clinical manifestations are usually apparent by 4 hours post-ingestion (Table 28.11) unless slow-release preparations were taken.
- ECG changes include:
  - rate decrease to approximately 60 bpm
  - PR prolongation (early indicator of toxicity)
  - QRS widening
  - QT prolongation.

Management

1. Continuous cardiac monitoring is essential and early invasive blood-pressure monitoring may also be required. Intubation and ventilation is likely for life-threatening overdoses.
2. Glucagon has always been the classic antidote, but other inotropes perform as well and are more easily available.

Table 28.11 Clinical features of beta-blocker overdose

System	Clinical features
Cardiovascular	Hypotension Bradycardia Arrhythmias
CNS	Delirium Coma Seizures
Respiratory	Bronchospasm Pulmonary oedema
Metabolic/endocrine	Hypoglycaemia Hyperglycaemia Hyperkalaemia

3 Treatment of bradycardia and hypotension includes atropine, adrenaline, isoprenaline and high-dose insulin (Box 28.10).
4 Give sodium bicarbonate for wide QRS and ventricular arrhythmias (as with tricyclic antidepressant overdose).
5 Remember that slow-release preparations exist.

Box 28.10 High-dose insulin in toxicity due to calcium-channel blockers or beta-blockers

- Rationale: insulin has an inotropic effect
- Use: cardiovascular collapse in calcium-channel blocker toxicity but can be considered for severe beta-blocker toxicity
- Dose:
  - glucose 25 g IV followed by insulin 1 U/kg IV
  - then glucose 25 g/h IV infusion and insulin 0.5 U/kg/h IV infusion
  - titrate to euglycaemia
  - watch potassium and glucose levels

CALCIUM-CHANNEL BLOCKERS

The centrally acting calcium-channel blockers (Box 28.11) are the most cardiotoxic in this group, and effects can be delayed (up to 16 hours) due to the sustained-release preparations available. Clinical features are outlined in Table 28.12.

Management

1 Activated charcoal can be administered in those that present up to 4 hours after an overdose of the sustained-release preparations.
2 Serial ECGs are recommended, even if initially normal.

Box 28.11 Types of calcium-channel blocker

Centrally acting	Peripherally acting
Verapamil Diltiazem	Amlodipine Felodipine Nifedipine Lercanidipine

Table 28.12 Clinical features of calcium-channel blocker overdose

System	Clinical features
Cardiovascular	Hypotension Bradycardia Any degree of heart block Cardiogenic shock Myocardial ischaemia Cardiac arrest
CNS	Confusion, drowsiness (due to hypotension, not the drug)
Metabolic/ endocrine	Hyperglycaemia Acidaemia

3 Early invasive blood-pressure monitoring and intubation for life-threatening overdoses (evident by hypotension despite fluid resuscitation) is recommended.
4 Atropine can be given initially for symptomatic bradycardia.
5 Hypotension should be managed aggressively, first with fluids, then with administration of calcium and next inotropes.
6 Give 60 mL of 10% calcium gluconate (0.6 mL/kg in children) or 20 mL of 10% calcium chloride (0.2 mL/kg in children) over 15 minutes. This may be repeated up to 3 times at 20-minute intervals. An infusion can be commenced, aiming for an ionic calcium level of 2 mmol/L.
7 High-dose insulin (Box 28.10) for haemodynamic instability following overdose.
8 Temporary pacing can be used, but needs to be ventricular to bypass the atrioventricular blockade. However, electrical capture is not always possible and, if it is successful, may not improve hypotension.

ORGANOPHOSPHATES AND CARBAMATES

- These are cholinesterase-inhibiting insecticides and pesticides.
- These compounds are well absorbed by inhalation, ingestion, even topical contact with mucous membranes or skin.
- External decontamination is warranted, aiming for prevention of contamination of staff as well as ongoing poisoning in cases of dermal exposure. Clothes should be removed by cutting off, avoiding contamination of face and airways, and bagged. Skin should be washed with water and soap. Treating staff should maintain caution when coming into contact with body fluids of these patients so as to avoid secondary poisoning.
- Poisoning results in a combination of excessive muscarinic and nicotinic activity (see Table 28.2).
- Red cell and plasma cholinesterase levels should be sent for. Red cell cholinesterase levels correspond to severity of toxicity whilst plasma cholinesterase levels indicate exposure to organophosphates.

Management

1. Indications for use of atropine include:
   - profuse diaphoresis
   - wheeze
   - cough
   - poor air entry
   - bradycardia
   - hypotension.
2. Secretions need to be controlled. The bronchorrhoea can lead to poor oxygenation, and non-cardiogenic pulmonary oedema has been described. In an adult give 1.2 mg of atropine (50 microg/kg in children) IV. Double the dose every 5 minutes until secretions are abolished, bradycardia resolved and air entry is improved (atropinisation). An infusion should then be commenced.
3. If atropine is required, pralidoxime should also be used. This reactivates anticholinesterases that have not yet formed irreversible bonds with the toxin ('ageing').

Delayed syndromes include an intermediate syndrome and also organophosphate-induced delayed neurotoxicity. The intermediate syndrome is characterised by neck flexion weakness, proximal weakness, loss of deep tendon reflexes, cranial nerve palsies and respiratory failure. It occurs in less than 40% of patients and appears 24–96 hours after acute exposure to organophosphates.

TRICYCLIC ANTIDEPRESSANTS (TCAs)

Examples: amitriptyline, clomipramine, dothiepin, doxepin, imipramine, nortriptyline, trimipramine.

TCAs are antihistaminic, anticholinergic and block sodium and potassium channels. They are also noradrenaline and serotonin re-uptake inhibitors and block gamma-aminobutyric acid (GABA) receptors. Overdoses are life-threatening, particularly at doses of > 10 mg/kg. Signs of toxicity (Table 28.13) are evident within 2 hours of ingestion and rapid deterioration can occur.

Early intervention with management of coma, hypotension, seizures and arrhythmias is life-saving. All patients must be cardiac monitored and observed for a minimum of 6 hours post-ingestion.

Table 28.13 Clinical signs of TCA toxicity

System	Clinical signs
CNS	Confusion Sedation Seizures
Cardiovascular	Sinus tachycardia Hypotension Arrhythmias

Key points—TCAs

- ECGs are essential. They should be repeated at intervals and the patient must have continuous cardiac monitoring.
- Intubate early if CNS depression, and hyperventilate.
- Seizures are treated with benzodiazepines.
- Hypotension can be managed with IV fluids, sodium bicarbonate and inotropes.
- Ventricular arrhythmias are treated first with repeated doses of IV sodium bicarbonate (100 mmol at 1- to 2-minute intervals). Defibrillation tends to be unsuccessful. Lignocaine is second-line drug therapy. Antiarrhythmics such as amiodarone and beta-blockers are contraindicated.
- Changes in the QRS interval (due to sodium-channel blockade) are predictive:
  — QRS > 100 ms predicts seizures, hypotension, coma
  — QRS > 160 ms predicts ventricular tachyarrhythmias
  — QRS interval of >100 ms is an indicator of toxicity.
- Early changes on the ECG are outlined in Box 28.12.

- Sodium bicarbonate should be given every 3–5 minutes until QRS narrows and hypotension improves.

Box 28.12 Early ECG changes in TCA toxicity

- PR prolongation
- QRS widening
- Large terminal R wave in aVR lead (especially ≥ 3 mm)
- QT prolongation

SELECTIVE SEROTONIN RE-UPTAKE INHIBITORS (SSRIs)

Examples: citalopram, escitalopram, fluoxetine, fluvoxamine, paroxetine, sertraline.

This is a common overdose and is usually benign.

Key points—SSRIs

- Nausea is common.
- Common early symptoms of a mild serotonin syndrome are: anxiety, mydriasis, sweating, tremor, clonus, tachycardia and hypertension.
- Seizures can occur.
- Rarely, serotonin syndrome can occur—especially if an SSRI is combined with other serotonergic agents (MAOIs, SNRIs, tramadol).
- Citalopram and escitalopram can cause QT prolongation.
- The toxic period is within 4–12 hours.

SELECTIVE SEROTONIN AND NORADRENALINE RE-UPTAKE INHIBITORS (SNRIs)

Examples: desvenlafaxine, venlafaxine.

These are serious overdoses with life-threatening CNS and cardiovascular toxicity.

Key points—SNRIs

- Common early symptoms are of a mild serotonin syndrome (see SSRIs, above).
- Seizures can occur; risk of seizures increases with dose.
- There may be a delay of up to 16 hours between overdose and symptoms.
- Serotonin syndrome can occur, especially if combined with other serotonergic agents (see SSRIs, above).

- Cardiovascular toxicity occurs with ingestions of > 7 g—hypotension, QRS/QT prolongation, cardiac arrhythmias.
- Patients should be monitored and observed for 16–24 hours.

MONOAMINE OXIDASE INHIBITORS (MAOIs)

Examples: phenelzine, tranylcypromine, selegiline, moclobemide.

Key points—MAOIs

- Moclobemide: minor toxicity regardless of dose—serotonin syndrome, QT prolongation.
- Phenelzine, tranylcypromine—potentially lethal, dose-dependent toxicity.
- MAOI adverse reactions:
  1. serotonin syndrome
  2. tyramine reaction (hypertensive crisis): occipital headache, hypertension, sweating, agitation, chest pain—post ingestion of tyramine- or dopamine-containing foods (e.g. aged cheese, salami, fava (broad) beans, beer, wine, pickled herring).
- Hypertension and tachycardia are usually managed with IV benzodiazepines or IV infusion of sodium nitroprusside or GTN, or IV boluses of phentolamine can be titrated to control severe hypertension.
- Watch for hyperthermia and treat aggressively.

QUETIAPINE

Quetiapine is an atypical antipsychotic which commonly causes sedation and tachycardia in the context of overdose. When combined with other sedating drugs (e.g. alcohol, benzodiazepines), the CNS depressive effects are additive.

- CNS effects: sedation, coma, delirium, occasionally seizures.
- Cardiovascular effects: hypotension, tachycardia (common), minor QT prolongation.
- Toxicity occurs within 4 hours and lasts up to 72 hours.
- Greater toxicity occurs with doses > 3 g.
- There is good prognosis with supportive and intensive care.

CARBAMAZEPINE

- Carbamazepine has anticholinergic effects, among other clinical signs (Table 28.14).
- Chronic overdose tends to cause headache, diplopia and ataxia.

Table 28.14 Clinical signs of acute carbamazepine toxicity

System	Clinical signs
CNS	Ataxia Nystagmus Dysarthria Decreased level of consciousness Seizures/status epilepticus
Cardiovascular	Sinus tachycardia Hypotension QRS prolongation

Management

1 Multiple doses of activated charcoal have a role in management.
2 Cardiac monitoring is recommended.
3 First-line treatment of seizures is benzodiazepines.

Drugs and alcohol

(Alex Wodak and Robert Graham)

Alcohol and drugs share the common property of affecting mood or thought (i.e. are psychoactive) in a pleasurable manner, and thus tend to be used repeatedly.

Problems resulting from alcohol and drug use can be classified as:

- *acute*—overdose, withdrawal
- *chronic*—organ damage, dependence.

After dealing with the presenting complaint, some attempt must always be made by the emergency medical officer to intervene effectively with the underlying cause of the presentation, i.e. the alcohol or drug use. An effective intervention could be as simple as an explanation or a referral.

ALCOHOL

- Use of > 60 g/day (males) or > 40 g/day (females) is considered hazardous.
  (*Remember:* 1 standard drink, e.g. 1 glass of wine, contains 10 g alcohol.)
- Over 5% of Australian men and 1% of Australian women drink hazardous quantities of alcohol.
- One in 6 medical admissions to Australian hospitals is directly attributable to alcohol, and another 1 in 6 patients drinks hazardously but admission is required for reasons unrelated to alcohol.

- Alcohol contributes to a substantial proportion of accident and emergency presentations.
- Studies show that ED staff grossly underestimate the proportion of intoxicated patients and, where recent alcohol use has been detected, the extent of intoxication is usually considerably underestimated.
- Alcohol can easily be measured in blood, breath or urine. Inexpensive portable machines are now available which will improve the rate and accuracy of diagnosis.
- The presence of high blood alcohol concentrations in an individual who appears to have no psychomotor impairment suggests the presence of tolerance to alcohol and thus regular consumption of large quantities.
- The most important aid to diagnosis is a high level of awareness.

Acute presentations

Overdose

- The signs of alcohol intoxication are well known, e.g. slurred speech, ataxia, clouded judgment, disinhibited behaviour.
- Alcohol intoxication can be fatal. The risk correlates roughly with the blood alcohol concentration (BAC). Any patient with a BAC of > 0.40 mg/100 mL should be regarded as high risk.
- Alcohol intoxication results in respiratory depression. Inhalation of vomitus is a serious potential hazard.
- Severely intoxicated individuals should be managed as other drug overdoses, i.e. carefully observed and nursed lying on the side. Emetics are dangerous and carthartics are unnecessary as alcohol is absorbed rapidly.
- The severity of CNS depression is increased by other sedatives such as benzodiazepines, barbiturates, antihistamines and opiates. Alcohol is commonly taken in combination with other drugs and often has an additive effect, which is not predictable. Alcohol ingestion often precedes the consumption of other drugs or acts of self-harm.

Alcohol Withdrawal Scale

The Alcohol Withdrawal Scale (AWS, see Figure 28.1, overleaf) is a widely used and simple instrument for measuring the signs of alcohol withdrawal. It has several virtues: the fact that it is a standardised instrument encourages a better quality of care, and the simplicity of the AWS makes it easy to use and encourages an earlier response. However, like all other instruments used in medicine, the AWS must

ALCOHOL WITHDRAWAL SCALE

MRN	SURNAME		
OTHER NAMES			
DOB	SEX	AMO	WARD/CLINIC

Please enter patient information or affix patient information label

Record AWS hourly for 4 hours, then at least 4/24 for 48 hours.

If total score is > 5 increase observations to hourly. If total score is > 6 notify medical officer.

DATE: / /	Time	Time	Time	Time	Time	Time	Time	Time	Time
Item 1 Perspiration									
Item 2 Tremor									
Item 3 Anxiety									
Item 4 Agitation									
Item 5 Temperature									
Item 6 Hallucinations									
Item 7 Orientation									
TOTAL SCORE									
Sedation/Type/Dose									

DATE: / /	Time	Time	Time	Time	Time	Time	Time	Time	Time
Item 1 Perspiration									
Item 2 Tremor									
Item 3 Anxiety									
Item 4 Agitation									
Item 5 Temperature									
Item 6 Hallucinations									
Item 7 Orientation									
TOTAL SCORE									
Type/Dose									

See over for explanations of items and scoring guide

Figure 28.2 Alcohol Withdrawal Scale

ITEM 1 PERSPIRATION	
No abnormal sweating	0
Moist skin	1
Localised beads of sweat on face, chest etc	2
Whole body wet from perspiration	3
Profuse maximal sweating—clothes and linen are wet	4

ITEM 2 TREMOR	
No tremor	0
Slight intentional tremor	1
Constant marked tremor of upper extremities	2
Constant marked tremor of extremities	3

ITEM 3 ANXIETY	
No apprehension or anxiety	0
Slight apprehension	1
Apprehension or understandable fear, e.g. of withdrawal symptoms	2
Anxiety occasionally accentuated to state of panic	3
Constant panic-like anxiety	4

ITEM 4 AGITATION	
No sign of agitation—resting normally	0
Slight restlessness, unable to sit or lie still, awake when others are asleep	1
Moves constantly, looks tense, wants to get out of bed	2
Constantly restless, getting out of bed for no obvious reason, returns to bed if taken	3
Maximal restlessness, aggressive, ignores requests to stay in bed	4

ITEM 5 TEMPERATURE	
Temperature of 37°C or less	0
Temperature of 37.1°C to 37.5°C	1
Temperature of 37.6° to 38°C	2
Temperature of 38.1°C to 38.5°C	3
Temperature greater than 38.5°C	4

ITEM 6 HALLUCINATIONS (Spontaneous sense of perceptions of sight, sound, taste or touch for which there is no external basis)	
No evidence of hallucinations	0
Distortions of real objects—aware these are not real if they are pointed out	1
Reports appearance of totally new objects or perception—aware these are not real if pointed out	2
Believes hallucination is real—remains orientated to place and person	3
Believes being in total non-existent environment, is preoccupied, unable to be reassured	4

ITEM 7 ORIENTATION	
Fully oriented in person, place and time	0
Oriented in person, unsure of place and time	1
Oriented in person, disorientated in place and time	2
Doubtful of personal orientation, disoriented in place and time, short periods of lucidity	3
Disoriented in place/time and person. No meaningful contact can be made	4

Alcohol withdrawal may be a life-threatening condition that requires medical intervention in clinical settings.

The alcohol withdrawal scale is designed to alert medical staff to the possibility that the patient may be developing alcohol withdrawal and may be in need of appropriate sedation.

be applied critically. The signs of alcohol withdrawal can be produced in many other conditions. Therefore, the diagnosis of alcohol withdrawal should always be reviewed and reconsidered in patients who do not respond quickly to treatment. It must be emphasised that the AWS is not a diagnostic tool, but one of measurement.

Alcohol withdrawal

- Withdrawal usually starts within 48 hours of abrupt cessation or decreased consumption of alcohol.
- In individuals who are used to high BACs and tolerant to alcohol, withdrawal symptoms may appear when the BAC has fallen but has not yet reached zero.
- Withdrawal is usually manifested by agitation, tremor and sweating. Confusion, anxiety and hallucinations are often present to a minor degree, but the patient can usually be 'brought back to reality' with prompt treatment.
- Hallucinations are usually tactile but less commonly visual. Auditory hallucinations can occur but usually suggest other diagnoses.
- The presence of severe confusion, tremulousness, anxiety and hallucinations, where the patient cannot be 'brought back to reality', constitutes delirium tremens (DTs). This is relatively uncommon.
- The risk of developing symptoms of alcohol withdrawal is poorly correlated with previous exposure to alcohol. Withdrawal symptoms following abrupt abstinence may not recur on future occasions.
- Alcohol withdrawal is exacerbated by physical illness, injury or surgery.
- Alcohol withdrawal is rarely a problem in the presence of advanced chronic liver disease, even if the patient has continued to drink alcohol until presentation. In such patients, other possibilities such as hepatic encephalopathy can mimic the symptoms and signs of withdrawal.

Persons withdrawing from alcohol are very sensitive to their environment. An uncaring or hostile reception by medical and nursing staff in a crowded and noisy ED often rapidly results in an aggressive and violent patient.

Management of acute presentations

- The key to management is manipulation of the environment. Emphasise peace and quiet, even lighting without sharp shadows, and most of all a caring attitude from staff. It is often difficult to obtain these conditions in EDs.

- Special detoxification centres are available in some centres for the management of persons intoxicated or going through alcohol withdrawal. If such a centre is not available or the patient has a medical or surgical problem requiring admission to hospital, the withdrawal can be attenuated by using a (cross-tolerant) sedative.
- **Diazepam.** This long-acting benzodiazepine is ideal for the management of withdrawal. The therapeutic index is high. The aim of management is to achieve patient comfort. The anticonvulsant properties of diazepam are also helpful.
  - Doses of 10–20 mg are given orally and repeated every 1–2 hours until the patient has been comfortably sedated. Smaller doses should be given in patients who have advanced chronic liver disease, with careful supervision as toxicity is more likely to result.
  - Frequent review is mandatory when the medication is being given every 2 hours. The diazepam is stopped once the patient is reasonably comfortable.
  - Diazepam can be given by slow IV injection under careful supervision if the patient is fasting, but this should generally be avoided.
  - Avoid discharging patients who are still receiving benzodiazepines. Review the diagnosis if the patient has not responded to 80 mg diazepam.
- **Haloperidol.** If alcohol withdrawal is severe (and not responding to benzodiazepines) or if delirium tremens is present, haloperidol is preferred. Doses of 2.5–5 mg can be given orally and repeated every 2–4 hours provided the patient is being closely supervised. Haloperidol can also be given parenterally. Doses can be increased if the patient is exceedingly restless.
- **Midazolam.** This can be used for the severely agitated patient in small IV boluses, 1–2 mg at a time, under close supervision when the above agents have still not worked adequately.
- **Phenothiazines.** These are not recommended for use in alcohol withdrawal (or delirium tremens) as they lower the seizure threshold.

Chronic presentations

Organ damage

Gastrointestinal bleeding is an emergency presentation frequently associated with excessive alcohol consumption.

Central nervous system

Fitting

- Occurs in 1–2% of episodes of alcohol withdrawal or delirium tremens. Caused by metabolic changes secondary to rebound hyperventilation following removal of alcohol, a CNS depressant.
- It is difficult to achieve therapeutic blood levels of phenytoin in patients who have suddenly stopped consuming alcohol.
- Diazepam is the best agent to control fitting in the ED.
- The first episode of fitting in an individual should always be investigated. Subsequent fits are only investigated if unusual features are present or if the seizure has occurred more than 48 hours after alcohol cessation.
- Long-term anticonvulsants to control fitting in patients who have uncontrollable alcohol consumption is often problematic. Phenytoin compliance is variable and patients will often fluctuate between phenytoin intoxication and zero blood levels.
- Subdural haematomas occur more frequently in patients drinking large quantities of alcohol because head injury, impaired coagulation and cerebral atrophy are common. They can present as epilepsy or as a space-occupying lesion. Early diagnosis is important, so a high degree of awareness is essential. Presentations are diverse but any unexplained drowsiness or lateralising signs should be investigated promptly.

Wernicke–Korsakoff syndrome

- The two conditions Wernicke's encephalopathy and Korsakoff's syndrome are now considered to be one entity.
- Episodes of Wernicke's encephalopathy are manifest by confusion, ophthalmoplegia, nystagmus and ataxia. Patients frequently present with only 1 or 2 of these signs. Treatment with parenteral thiamine is strongly recommended in all such cases.
- Thiamine is a cheap and safe preparation and should be administered generously to patients at risk of developing the Wernicke–Korsakoff syndrome. If untreated, this condition results in severe and irreversible brain damage requiring permanent institutionalisation. Prophylactic use of IV thiamine in at-risk patients is recommended.

Other

Other types of alcohol-related brain injury are common, rarely diagnosed and usually manifest with subtle impairment of decision making.

Metabolic problems

- Hypokalaemia is frequent and is usually due to poor nutrition, vomiting or diarrhoea. Hypomagnesaemia is also common. In the unwell patient with alcohol problems, it is prudent to correct such electrolyte abnormalities with intravenous replacement when IV access has already been established.
- Rarer metabolic problems resulting from alcohol include lactic acidosis, hypoglycaemia and renal failure secondary to myoglobinuria.

Trauma

Patients presenting with multiple injuries (including head injuries) are often severely intoxicated.

GI tract

Alcoholic hepatitis and pancreatitis (acute and/or chronic) often manifest in such patients and may have to be managed simultaneously.

Alcohol dependence

This is manifest by:

- narrowing of drinking repertoire—i.e. unable to vary type of beverage or quantity consumed according to the social occasion
- tolerance—i.e. increasing amounts of alcohol required to achieve the same degree of intoxication
- salience—i.e. alcohol seen to dominate the priorities in a patient's life
- compulsion to drink—i.e. patient plans the day so that steady supply of alcohol, often covert, is always available
- withdrawal symptoms—i.e. tremulousness, dysphoria, anorexia, nausea, vomiting, sweating (or some of these) usually occurring in the morning soon after waking
- relief of withdrawal symptoms—i.e. patient learns that withdrawal symptoms can be ameliorated by consuming alcohol and thus commences drinking earlier in the day as time passes
- reinstatement after abstinence—i.e. rapid development of dependence following prolonged abstinence and then relapse.

Note that the above criteria are essentially the same when considering the diagnosis of dependence for other drugs.

There is a wide spectrum of alcohol use disorders. Many patients in the ED are not dependent on alcohol but still have hazardous or harmful use. It is important to identify how severe the problem is, as the degree of severity affects management decisions.

Management of drinking problems

Diagnosis

- To achieve a high diagnostic rate, a high level of awareness of particular risk groups is essential.
- Males are more at risk than females, but this difference is becoming less.
- High-risk occupations include: employment in beverage industry, police force, armed forces, administrators, businessmen, employment away from family.
- The diagnostic rate will be improved by estimating BAC (or breath alcohol) as routine, especially in conditions such as trauma.
- A sound knowledge of alcohol-related medical conditions will increase the possibility of a correct diagnosis.
- Be alert for subtle signs, e.g. conjunctival injection, facial telangiectasia, Dupuytren's contracture, spider naevi.

Assessment and management

- Remember to ask every patient in a non-judgmental manner about alcohol consumption. Do not ask: 'Do you drink a lot?' Find out how many days a week a patient usually drinks, and how much of which beverage on each occasion.
- Assess the severity of alcohol dependence by asking about the presence of early-morning alcohol withdrawal symptoms (see above) or other indicators of alcohol dependence.
- Enquire systematically about medical or non-medical alcohol-related problems, including marital, employment, legal, financial and drink-driving complications.
- Recent research indicates that brief interventions by practitioners can be very effective, especially in individuals who have yet to develop well-established alcohol dependence or organ damage but are drinking hazardously.
- Establish a 'contract' with the patient and help to advise whether alcohol consumption should be reduced (and if so, how much) or whether abstinence is the desired goal.
- Discuss ways of achieving these ends.

- When a management plan has been established, arrange for long-term follow-up by the GP, social work department, community health centre, hospital clinic, Alcoholics Anonymous or SMART Recovery. A telephone service available in each state provides advice and contact details about specialist agencies and services available throughout Australia.

TOBACCO

Minimal intervention with smokers presenting to EDs for conditions unrelated to tobacco can achieve a modest but nonetheless significant reduction in smoking prevalence. All smokers should therefore receive advice to stop immediately, and to consult a GP or specialist agency if help is required in ceasing smoking. Smokers should be advised that mere reduction in tobacco consumption is pointless. Refer to the Quitline (13 7848).

Wherever possible, patients, relatives, visitors and staff must be discouraged from smoking for the comfort of the majority of the population who are non-smokers and, more importantly, because of the (now appreciated) hazards of passive smoking.

OPIOIDS

- Injecting drug users (IDUs) are a heterogeneous population. The conventional stereotype represents only one segment of this population.
- It is important to recognise that psychological as well as pharmacological factors maintain drug dependence.
- IDUs increasingly use a wide variety of psychoactive drugs. Cannabis, hallucinogens, cocaine, amphetamines, benzodiazepines, tobacco and alcohol are used as substitutes or adjuncts to opioids.
- Overdose is the major adverse pharmacological effect of opioids. Other problems result from microbiological (bacterial, viral, fungal and parasitic) and chemical contamination.
- The death rate is lower than generally recognised (approximately 1–2% per annum), while spontaneous remission is commoner than generally believed (approximately 40% per 10 years).

Acute presentations

Overdose

See 'Opioids' in the 'Poisoning and overdosage' section above.

Withdrawal

Opioid withdrawal is objectively milder than alcohol withdrawal and has been likened to a 'bad cold'. However, many experiencing heroin withdrawal complain about very distressing symptoms. Withdrawal can be recognised in patients who are often restless, have a tachycardia and sweat profusely. They may complain of diarrhoea or abdominal cramps, or a curious nasal snuffling may be apparent. The pupils are widely dilated. The most helpful objective signs are mydriasis and gooseflesh which can sometimes be seen fleetingly across the trunk and abdomen. Patients in opioid withdrawal should be referred to specialist detoxification centres (when available) unless a medical or surgical condition requires hospital admission.

Opiate withdrawal can be readily managed with sedation.

- Benzodiazepines can be effective; and clonidine, at a dose of 15 microg/kg/24 hours (in divided doses), is also used for this purpose. The medication is slowly reduced over 3–4 days.
- Alternatively, methadone can be given: usually 15–20 mg twice daily is sufficient, but slightly higher doses may sometimes be necessary. It is best to give methadone in divided doses for the first 1–2 days until the patient's opioid tolerance is known.
- In addition to the above, symptomatic treatment can be given for diarrhoea (e.g. loperamide) or abdominal pain (paracetamol or hyoscine).
- Sublingual buprenorphine is now regarded as the most effective drug for managing heroin withdrawal, but assessment of dose requires some experience. Delay initiation as long as possible, preferably until moderate withdrawal symptoms have developed.

Commencing the patient on methadone or buprenorphine can facilitate admission to a formal outpatient treatment program but does not oblige the patient to continue such treatment.

Organ damage

Local infections. Phlebitis, cellulitis or deep abscesses may develop from local injection sites. These can usually be adequately treated with antibiotics, but surgical intervention is sometimes required.

Systemic infections. Septicaemia, endocarditis, lung abscesses and brain abscesses are some of the serious and well-recognised systemic infections. The endocarditis is often right-sided and difficult to diagnose. Lung abscesses are often associated with endocarditis. The complications of HIV infections should also be considered in the differential diagnosis.

Hepatitis. This may be due to hepatitis B, C, D or sometimes hepatitis A virus. Admission to hospital may be required if the hepatitis is severe. Patients should be advised about the risk of spreading infection to others by needle or sexual contact. Advice should be given about alcohol consumption, diet and physical exercise, as the symptoms of hepatitis may be recurrent following overindulgence or participation in active physical exercise before the liver has recovered.

Patients with hepatitis B or C should be referred for long-term follow-up. Patients without evidence of hepatitis B should be encouraged to be vaccinated.

Diagnosis

Dependence is assessed by enquiring about drug use (number of injections per day, duration of drug use, expenditure on drug use) and psychological factors (which will be indicated by the damage to social development, e.g. relationships, employment).

The medical officer should be alert for drug-seeking behaviour, needle track marks or unexplained inconsistencies in the patient's history.

A history of the patient's drug use and drug dependence should be obtained and specific enquiry made about medical and non-medical opioid-related problems. Ask 'Have you ever injected drugs?' rather than 'Are you a drug user?'.

Management plan

All patients should be advised that help is readily available. The risks of needle sharing (hepatitis, HIV) should be discussed. A number of specialised agencies are available in major cities. Information about resources available for treatment can be obtained by contacting telephone information services (i.e. the Alcohol and Drug Information Service in NSW). Several larger hospitals have clinics for referral and community health centres usually have an alcohol or drug counsellor who can provide assistance.

Infection control procedures should be scrupulously followed because of the hazards of occupational exposure to agents such as HIV, hepatitis B or hepatitis C.

BENZODIAZEPINES

(Also see 'Benzodiazepines' in the 'Poisoning and overdosage' section above.)

A range of benzodiazepines is available with markedly different durations of action and some pharmacokinetic differences.

This group of drugs is relatively safe when used sparingly. Indiscriminate use is relatively rare but much more common in certain populations such as IDUs. Some elderly patients are very sensitive to even small doses.

Withdrawal

- The symptoms of benzodiazepine withdrawal may be somewhat similar to the original presenting complaint, e.g. insomnia, anxiety. Perceptual distortions are often present.
- Fitting can occur as part of benzodiazepine withdrawal. In severe cases, delirium can result without adequate treatment.
- Benzodiazepine withdrawal begins 5–7 days after stopping the medication. Onset may be earlier with shorter-acting drugs or later with longer-acting medication.
- Patients undergoing benzodiazepine withdrawal should always be referred for follow-up.

Organ damage

There is no significant organ damage associated with benzodiazepine use.

Dependence

To reduce benzodiazepine dependence, the dose and duration of treatment should be the minimum required to achieve the desired therapeutic effect. It should be noted that benzodiazepine users (when no clinical indication is seen to exist) should be referred for management. Usually it is possible to slowly reduce the dose over several weeks (with the agreement of the patient) by slowly reducing the dose of a longer-acting benzodiazepine (usually diazepam).

PRESCRIBED DRUGS

Emergency doctors should always be cautious about prescribing parenteral opioids to patients not known to the hospital, especially if the patient presents just before closing time and appears very familiar with drug names which are often slightly misspelt or mispronounced. Characteristic presentations are renal colic, backache, migraine or pancreatitis. Wherever possible, some objective evidence of the condition should be obtained, e.g. inspect freshly voided urine (passed under supervision) for the presence of microscopic haematuria in renal colic. Take-away doses of parenteral opioids should not be provided unless there is a good indication, e.g. disseminated malignancy or authentic letter from a medical practitioner. Avoid the prescribing of pethidine, which is responsible for the most difficult cases of iatrogenic dependence.

There is an increasing trade in and use of prescribed opioids, especially oxycodone in the form of Oxycontin, which can be inhaled (after vaporisation) or injected. Illicit use of methadone and buprenorphine may also present with resulting pathologies and/or drug-seeking behaviour.

COCAINE

(Also see 'Cocaine' in 'Poisoning and overdosage' above.)
Cocaine use has been increasing in Australia for some years but is still mainly confined to Sydney and is still much lower than in most other Western countries.

Overdose

- Psychosis is a common presentation. This should be treated with benzodiazepines. Aggressive behaviour is common.
- Seizures—again, benzodiazepines are recommended. Caution should be used when intubating as cocaine causes sensitisation of the bronchial tree.
- Arrhythmias, myocardial ischaemia, cerebral ischaemia may occur.

Withdrawal

Some individuals report a rebound, self-limiting period of mild depression following cessation of cocaine use. It is uncertain whether this represents a true withdrawal phenomenon.

Chronic use

Organ damage

- Snorting of cocaine is associated with the development of nasal septal necrosis.
- 'Free-basing' of cocaine is a method of inhaling cocaine following treatment of the salt (cocaine hydrochloride) with volatile solvents. Pulmonary damage can occur following inhalation of cocaine (as free base).
- IV administration is associated with problems similar to the complications of heroin IV self-administration.

Management

Cocaine users who present with psychosis should be scheduled to remain and treated until they have returned to their normal state. Drug and alcohol counsellors are of assistance. Telephone information and counselling services provide information on specialised agencies.

ECSTASY

(Also see 'Amphetamines—MDMA' in 'Poisoning and overdosage' section above.)

MDMA is a drug which has both amphetamine and mild hallucinogenic properties. Use of MDMA increased rapidly in many countries around the world in the 1990s, although the drug had first been synthesised many decades earlier. Side-effects are uncommon but deaths have been attributed to MDMA. There is controversy about the degree of risk, but deaths are rare compared with the very large estimated number of episodes of use. There is also concern based on animal studies of possible nerve and brain damage. However, it is often difficult to ascertain the extent of risk of illicit drugs because of the uncertainty about the nature of the drugs actually taken. The short-term risks of MDMA may be reduced by ensuring that people who are taking the drug do not become dehydrated.

GAMMA-HYDROXYBUTYRATE (GHB)

(Also see 'Gamma-hydroxybutyrate (GHB)' in 'Poisoning and overdosage' section above.)

In the last few years, GHB has become popular in many Western countries. GHB releases dopamine in the brain, causing effects ranging from relaxation to sleep at low doses.

Disorientation, nausea, muscle spasms, vomiting, convulsions and deep coma have been described following use of the drug. As with other illegal drugs, the dose taken is always uncertain. Deaths following the use of GHB have been reported and admission to intensive care is not uncommon among those who require treatment from ED of major hospitals. The risks are higher when combined with other drugs, especially alcohol.

TRENDS

The use of legal and illegal drugs is volatile. Overall, alcohol consumption has been declining in Australia since the early 1980s, although binge-drinking among young people is increasing. Tobacco consumption has been declining slowly for some decades. Cannabis consumption has been increasing for decades in Australia but consumption has fluctuated somewhat in recent years. Amphetamine consumption has been increasing in Australia for more than a decade. The number of people injecting heroin in Australia has been increasing rapidly for decades but declined during the heroin shortage that began in late 2000 and continued during 2001. Cocaine and amphetamine use increased as heroin availability declined. Recently, heroin availability and use have increased.

Other modern recreational drugs are discussed earlier in this chapter in the section 'Poisoning and overdosage'.

Online resources

Australian Drug Information Network
www.adin.com.au

Chapter 29

Drowning

Paul M Middleton

Epidemiology

Globally, drowning caused the deaths of 175,000 children and adolescents in 2004, and is the leading cause of overall deaths in children younger than 15 years in countries such as China and Bangladesh. The disparity between wealthy and poor countries is vast, with boys from low-income countries in the Western Pacific 10 times more likely to drown than those in high-income countries in the region, and girls 14 times more likely to drown than their high-income counterparts.

In 2011 a record 315 people drowned in Australian waterways, surpassing the average of 311 between the years 1995 and 2000. Men were almost 3½ times as likely as women to drown, and rivers and creeks were the site of the largest number of deaths in 2010–2011, partly driven by 38 deaths in the Queensland floods.

Children aged between 0 and 14 years were the most common age group to drown in swimming pools, with 28 deaths in children under 5 years, 57% of whom fell or wandered into water. Indigenous Australians are 4 times more likely to drown than other Australians, and alcohol or drug use was implicated in 17% of drownings in Australia.

Editorial Comment

There are fewer events as distressing to parents, family and ED staff as a child drowning. Recognise this early. Mobilise resources for support. If set up for it, having the parent(s) present with a dedicated staff member during resuscitation can be very beneficial in both the short and the long term. It has been shown also to improve staff satisfaction.

Pathophysiology

The concepts of 'wet' and 'dry' drowning, based on the presumption that a variable degree of laryngospasm occurs which, in some patients, prevents any aspiration of water or other substances into the airway, bronchial tree and lungs, have been discarded at the World Congress on Drowning.

The International Liaison Committee on Resuscitation (ILCOR) advisory statement on drowning describes an involuntary period of laryngospasm secondary to the presence of liquid in the oropharynx or larynx. It has been described that most patients aspirate less than 4 mL/kg of fluid and that approximately 10–20% of individuals maintain tight laryngospasm until cardiac arrest occurs and inspiratory efforts have ceased. This has been confirmed by autopsy studies, with 10% of patients showing no aspiration and approximately 20% of patients presenting with normal chest radiographs. Other sources suggest that drowning probably never occurs without aspiration to some degree.

What appears clear is that initial voluntary breath-holding precedes a variable degree of aspiration of water, followed eventually by apnoea, with the common pathway in all drowning being profound hypoxia associated with acidosis and hypercapnia. This hypoxia leads not only to unconsciousness, loss of airway reflexes and aspiration, but also to the cardiovascular effects of drowning. These include extreme bradycardia, ventricular fibrillation and asystole, which are often exacerbated by hypothermia in cold waters. Hypothermia is common in child victims of drowning due to their large surface area to body mass ratio and, although hypothermia has been associated with a poor prognosis after drowning as it is related to the duration of submersion, it has also been associated with a better prognosis, particularly in children, presumably due to a protective effect on cerebral organ function with the rapid onset of low temperatures. There have been several cases reported of survival of both children and adults following submersion in cold water for up to 66 minutes.

Following early survival, lethal hypoxia may still develop. However, in these later instances the hypoxia is due to the effects of surfactant disruption and abnormal function, atelectasis and intrapulmonary shunting. This profound secondary hypoxia may itself lead to respiratory failure and cardiac arrest.

In some groups of patients, aspiration of sand, silt, stagnant water, sewage and vomitus may result in bronchial occlusion, bronchospasm, inflammatory damage to alveolar capillary membranes, abscess formation and pneumonia. Late, atypical pneumonias may be caused by less-common pathogens such as *Aeromonas*, *Pseudallescheria* and *Burkholderia*.

Precipitating events

Drowning is sometimes precipitated by an injury or a medical condition. Loss of consciousness for whatever reason may result in drowning, particularly concussion, stroke or cardiac arrhythmia; this last cause may be underestimated in older adults with ischaemic heart disease, but also in younger patients with unrecognised prolonged QT syndromes. Concussion may be associated with motor vehicle crashes or diving, as are serious trauma including cervical spine injuries. It is also important to recognise the role of intentional injury, homicide, suicide and child abuse.

Outcome

The commonest cause of death in hospitalised drowning patients is post-hypoxic encephalopathy. Other common causes of death are acute respiratory distress syndrome (ARDS), multi-organ dysfunction syndrome (MODS) or sepsis syndrome.

Generally speaking, judging prognosis after a drowning incident is difficult, but there are recognised associations with particular outcomes. Pointers towards poor prognosis include:

- prolonged submersion
- delayed or no basic life support (BLS)
- requirement for basic life support (BLS)/advanced life support (ALS) in the emergency department
- unreactive pupils
- acute resuscitation efforts lasting longer than 25 minutes.

Individuals with any of these features have been reported to survive without disability, although the chances of successful resuscitation to a favourable neurological outcome are usually slim. Importantly, age has no independent association with outcome.

Examination

Examination should follow a systematic course, as described by ABCDE. Treatment should follow the same schema and should be delivered in systems immediately when any abnormality is identified.

Drowning victims may be classified into one of four groups, based on presenting physical examination:

1 asymptomatic
2 symptomatic
   — airway compromise—partial or complete requiring prior intervention

  - breathing—hypoxic, dyspnoeic, tachypnoeic, decreased oxygen saturation
  - circulation—bradycardia, tachycardia, hypotension
  - dysfunction—decreased level of consciousness, localising signs, other neurological deficit, anxiety
  - exposure and environment—hypothermia, metabolic acidosis

3 cardiopulmonary arrest
  - apnoea
  - asystole (55%), ventricular tachycardia/fibrillation (29%), bradycardia pulseless electrical activity (PEA) (16%)

4 obviously dead
  - normothermic with asystole
  - apnoea
  - rigor mortis
  - dependent lividity
  - no apparent CNS function.

INVESTIGATIONS

Investigations performed depend on the presenting condition and the potential for the investigations to change management. Routine blood tests that do not have the potential to change management are a waste of time and resources. In symptomatic patients, appropriate investigations may be:

- chest X-ray
- cervical spine X-ray
- 12-lead ECG
- core temperature
- pulse oximetry
- arterial blood gases (substantial deficits in gas exchange may exist in drowning patients; continuing monitoring of ventilation and metabolic status may be accomplished with serial venous blood gases)
- blood glucose
- full blood count
- urea and electrolytes including creatinine
- coagulation screen
- other investigations as suggested by history, e.g. troponin.

Later investigations may include computed tomography (CT) of the head and neck.

Management (ABCDE)

Key to the management of drowning patients, as with other critically ill or injured patients, is assessment and intervention in systems defined by ABCDE. This system of management fundamentally relies at its core on the maximisation of perfusion, ensuring the delivery of oxygenated blood to the brain and other vital organs.

Pre-hospital management differs very little from ED management in that the priorities are identical; however, as with most critically ill or injured patients, minimising any delay and striving for rapid transport with essential life-saving interventions being performed are the keys to optimum survival. It has been suggested in the USA that as life-savers are able to respond in a much shorter timeframe than ambulance services, they should receive extended training in advanced airway manoeuvres such as laryngeal mask airway (LMA) placement; however, in Australia lifesavers are often trained to a substantial degree in resuscitation, including the use of airway adjunct and bag–valve–mask devices.

The ILCOR and Australian Resuscitation Council guidelines on the management of cardiac arrest strongly suggest that drowning victims be given up to 5 rescue breaths before the commencement of chest compressions, in contradistinction to other cardiac arrest aetiologies where immediate chest compressions are prioritised. This is because cardiac arrest in drowning is clearly associated with hypoxia, and rescue breathing should contribute to the relief of this hypoxia.

If no resuscitative efforts have been initiated, and there is apnoea or no cardiac output, commence cardiopulmonary resuscitation (CPR) with a compression ratio of 30:2, first administering 5 rescue breaths in an attempt to achieve 2 effective ventilations; early defibrillation should be performed where appropriate; correction of any likely causative factors undertaken, which in this case would clearly include hypoxia and hypothermia; and regular IV adrenaline (epinephrine) administered every 3–4 minutes.

AIRWAY

The airway should be checked for foreign material and suction performed under direct vision. A *look, listen* and *feel* process will allow assessment of airway patency and respiratory effort. Basic airway manoeuvres such as a jaw thrust will be useful, whereas chin lift and head tilt should be reserved for patients with a clear history of non-trauma.

Clearance and maintenance of a patent airway, preferably by the most definitive means available, are of primary importance,

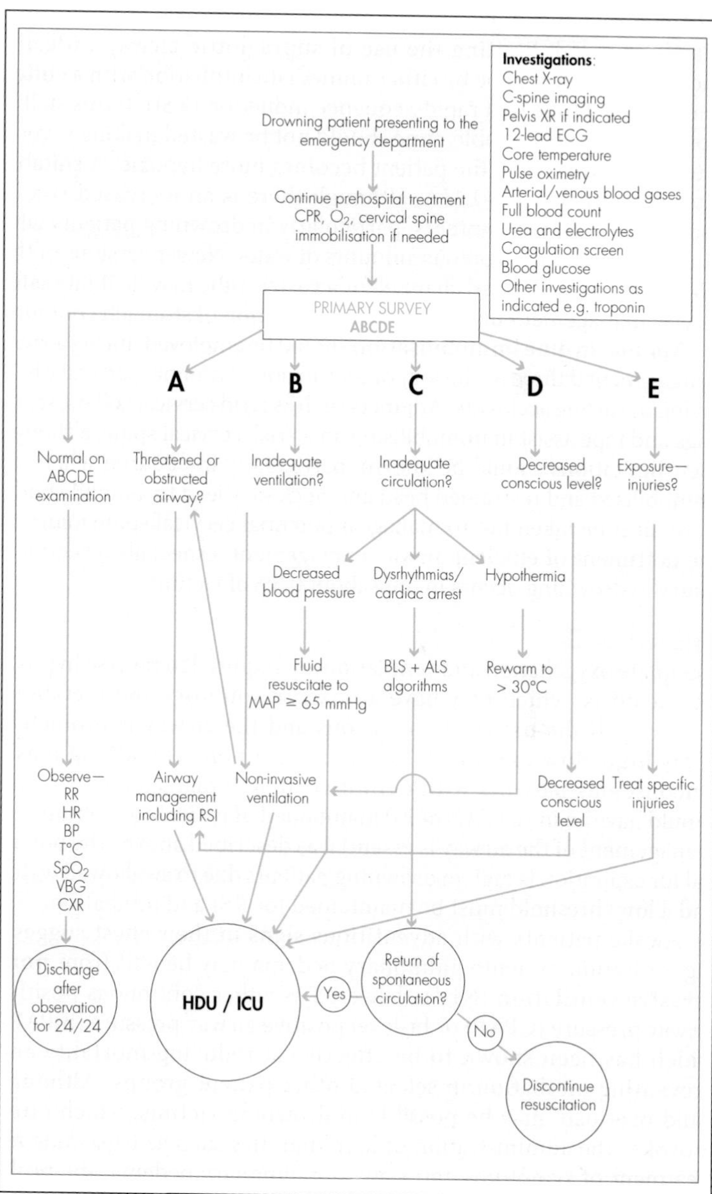

Figure 29.1 Drowning algorithm

particularly since high positive end-expiratory pressures (PEEPs) may be needed, limiting the use of supraglottic airways. Ideally, therefore, this would be by either immediate intubation with a cuffed endotracheal tube or a rapid-sequence induction (RSI). If this skill is not immediately available, time should not be wasted making several attempts at this while the patient becomes more hypoxic. A suitable alternative may be an LMA, although there is an increased risk of aspiration of gastric contents, particularly in drowning patients who may have swallowed copious amounts of water. Newer versions of the LMA with an embedded channel for a gastric tube may facilitate safer airway management utilising suction aspiration of stomach contents.

Manual in-line immobilisation should be employed during airway management if there is a history or a suspicion of trauma, particularly in diving or surfing accidents. Adjuncts such as rigid cervical collars, sandbags and tape assist in immobilising an at-risk cervical spine, although their limitations should be known, particularly in children where an immobilised and restrained head and neck may lead to a mobile body. Care must be taken not to manage a potential cervical spine injury to the detriment of efficient airway management, especially as cervical injury in drowning occurs in only about 0.5% of victims.

BREATHING

Adequate oxygenation and ventilation are required to reverse hypoxia and acidosis, which may have a mixed respiratory and metabolic aetiology. If the patient is conscious and the airway is protected, apply **high-flow oxygen** at 15 L/min via a non-rebreathing mask. Unconscious patients with definitive airway management in situ should have an initial FiO_2 of 1.0 maintained. If patients are obtunded, management of the airway is essential as described above. The potential for aspiration is high in drowning patients due to swallowed water, and a low threshold must be maintained for RSI and intubation.

Awake patients with adventitious signs in their chest suggesting aspiration or acute pulmonary oedema may benefit from **non-invasive ventilation** (NIV), delivered as either continuous positive airway pressure (CPAP) or bi-level positive airway pressure (BiPAP), which has been shown to be effective at reducing mortality and preventing intubation in selected other patient groups. Although 'fluid overload' may be possible in drowning victims, which often provokes the administration of loop diuretics such as frusemide for treatment of symptoms and signs of pulmonary oedema, the probable cause is more likely to be hypoxia- and acidosis-induced acute myocardial dysfunction with fluid maldistribution, and therefore NIV and potentially high-dose nitrate infusion may be the most appropriate treatment.

Conscious patients should be **monitored** by means of continuous pulse oximetry and, ideally, side-stream end-tidal CO_2 ($EtCO_2$) monitoring, which may give evidence of hypoventilation. Nasal-prong $EtCO_2$ monitoring equipment is not common; however, it has been shown to be efficacious in monitoring patients at risk for compromised ventilation. Ventilated patients should routinely have $EtCO_2$ monitored and ventilation titrated to allow maximum cerebral perfusion; in the presence of head injury, maintenance of $EtCO_2$ at 35 mmHg is appropriate.

Indications for RSI and intubation may be:

- altered level of consciousness and inability to protect airway or handle secretions
- high alveolar–arterial (A–a) gradient—a PaO_2 of 60–80 mmHg or more on 15 L/min oxygen by non-rebreathing mask
  Note: It is essential to estimate alveolar oxygen concentration to effectively use arterial blood gases (ABGs).
- worsening respiratory failure as demonstrated by clinical deterioration, increased work of breathing or drowsiness, together with worsening hypercapnia.

Note: Venous blood gases (VBGs) are often used for monitoring in the ED, with $PvCO_2$ being approximately 5 mmHg higher than $PaCO_2$; however, a trend of increasing $PvCO_2$ in serial samples has the most value in discriminating patients with respiratory failure. Measurement of serial ABGs should be utilised in intubated and ventilated drowning patients, preferably from an indwelling arterial catheter, in order to monitor the alveolar–arterial oxygen gradient.

Intubated patients should have an orogastric tube inserted to treat intragastric swallowed fluid and air. Have a high index of suspicion for tension pneumothorax if there is hypotension resistant to fluid resuscitation, particularly in the setting of potentially serious trauma associated with drowning. Small pneumothoraces may be managed by observation; however, if patients are intubated and ventilated, positive pressures may turn a simple pneumothorax into a tension pneumothorax, and placement of intercostal catheters may be an early necessity.

CIRCULATION

Patients in cardiac arrest following drowning who require BLS or ALS and are not hypothermic have a poor prognosis. Routine BLS should be implemented, with the caveat mentioned earlier that up to 5 rescue breaths should be delivered prior to commencing chest compressions.

Cardiac arrhythmias are secondary to hypoxia, acid–base disturbance and hypothermia, rather than to electrolyte disturbances caused by fluid aspiration, and any type of cardiac arrhythmia may be observed, particularly bradycardia and atrial fibrillation which are statistically the most common abnormalities. If the patient is hypothermic with a core temperature less than 30°C, only 3 attempts at defibrillation should be made, then BLS continued without further attempts until the temperature is above this threshold. Adrenaline and other intravenous drugs should be withheld until the core temperature is above 30°C.

Venous access should be urgently obtained with a large-bore cannula, and cardiac arrhythmias should be treated according to ALS algorithms. Boluses of crystalloid or colloid fluid are useful in maintaining perfusion of vital organs, although importantly attempts should not be made to attain 'normal' blood pressures, particularly in the presence of potential serious trauma or covert blood loss. A mean BP of 65–70 mmHg will be sufficient to maintain cerebral and renal perfusion in a supine patient. Patients may display hypotension and BP instability after prolonged periods of immersion, due to the effects of the hydrostatic pressure of the water on the body.

Rewarming is essential (see the 'Hypothermia' section in Chapter 32): wet clothing should be removed, the skin should be dried and the patient should be wrapped in warm blankets with aluminium foil or a space blanket outside this. Intravenous fluids should be warmed to 40°C; ventilator circuits should contain a humidifier/warmer to ensure ventilatory gases are also close to body temperature. Children lose heat quickly due to the large surface area to body mass ratio, and therefore careful management of temperature is mandatory.

A **low threshold for intraosseous cannulation** should be maintained, especially in cardiac arrest or critical condition post drowning; this may be achieved in adults as well as in children. Care should be taken with central venous cannulation as the hypothermic myocardium may be sensitive and prone to dysrhythmias. Resuscitation should not be ceased until the core temperature is above 30°C, and there are still no signs of life or organised cardiac function.

DISABILITY

Cerebral function is best preserved by prompt and effective management of airway, breathing and circulation. Neurological observations and sequential recording of Glasgow Coma Scale (GCS) scores monitors trends.

EXPOSURE AND EVERYTHING ELSE

Drowning patients need to be fully exposed to assess for injuries and potential related or causative factors. Remove all wet clothing and dry the patient, then promptly cover with blankets, followed by a space blanket as previously described to retain heat and to start or continue the process of rewarming. Core temperature should be recorded, and an indwelling temperature probe and a urinary catheter should be inserted during this part of the examination.

A log-roll should be performed to ensure that there are no missed injuries, bearing in mind that in unconscious patients, particularly those retrieved from inland waterways, beaches, etc, there is a higher risk of concomitant spinal injury, and taking particular care of airway adjuncts that have already been inserted. This means that manual in-line immobilisation (MILS) should be maintained until subsequent imaging, ideally a CT scan of the entire spine, is performed and interpreted by an appropriately trained clinician. Log-rolling should be performed using a controlled spinal technique, ideally a '3 under, 3 over' method that prevents pelvic tilting and lateral flexion of the spine.

Appropriate imaging should be performed at this stage, including a chest X-ray, and a pelvic X-ray if serious trauma is suspected as part of a mechanism of injury prior to drowning.

Online resources

2010 American Heart Association Guidelines for Cardiopulmonary Resuscitation and Emergency Cardiovascular Care Science. Part 5: Adult Basic Life Support
http://circ.ahajournals.org/content/122/18_suppl_3/S685.full

Drowning (Shepherd SM, Martin J, Norris R et al.)
www.emedicine.com/emerg/TOPIC744.HTM

International Life Saving Federation—World Drowning Report 2007
http://ilsf.org/sites/ilsf.org/files/filefield/world-drowning-report-final-sept-27-2007.pdf

Royal Life Saving Society Australia. National Drowning Report 2012
www.royallifesaving.com.au/__data/assets/pdf_file/0006/4002/2012-Drowning-Report.pdf

World Congress on Drowning 2002, Final recommendations
www.cslsa.org/events/ArchiveAttachments/Spr03Minutes/AttachmentG2.pdf

World Health Organization. Children and drowning
www.who.int/violence_injury_prevention/child/injury/world_report/Drowning_english.pdf

Chapter 30
Envenomation

Shane Curran and Thomas McDonagh

Introduction

Australia is home to many venomous creatures. Australian animals that are important in causing envenoming in humans include snakes, spiders, octopuses, fish and other marine creatures. The distribution of venomous creatures is wide, and each region has its own pattern of envenomation. Local knowledge is very important and local expert knowledge can be invaluable.

Resources that are available to you include the local emergency doctor or the on-call toxinologist, who can be contacted via the Poisons Information Centre (nationwide tel. **13 11 26**). They are available to discuss management of patients with possible or definite envenomation.

Snakebite

Australia is home to a number of the most venomous snakes in the world. Snake venom is a complex mixture of substances. Australian snakes produce venoms that have a range of clinical effects, including neurotoxic (presenting as progressive paralysis), myotoxic (causing rhabdomyolysis and subsequent renal failure) and coagulopathic (causing severe coagulation disturbances) (Table 30.1).

Snakebite is a medical emergency. Patients presenting following possible snakebite should receive urgent assessment and management. Patients who have significant envenomation may initially appear well.

Potential early life threats include paralysis and respiratory failure or haemorrhage due to coagulopathy. Look for evidence of ptosis, diplopia, dysarthria or dysphagia, or haemorrhage from skin, gums, needle puncture sites, gastrointestinal tract or intracranial.

The majority of snakebites will not result in significant envenoming, and so will not require antivenom. This is because many snakebites are 'dry bites' where no venom is injected. The amount of venom injected by a snake depends on snake maturity, fang length, venom yield, snake temperament, the number of bites and the time since the

Table 30.1 Clinical effects of Australian snake venom

	Defibrination coagulopathy	Anticoagulation	Paralysis	Myolysis	Renal failure
	Low fibrinogen Raised FDP/XDP	Normal fibrinogen Normal FDP/XDP			ATN
Brown snake	+++				+
Tiger snake	+++		++ Presynaptic	+++	+
Taipan	+++		+++ Presynaptic	+++	+++
Mulga snake (king brown)		++	++	+++	+
Sea snake				+++	
Death adder		+	Postsynaptic		
Red-bellied black snake	Venom is low in potency and small in volume—no major complications				

ATN, acute tubular necrosis; FDP/XDP, fibrin degradation products.

snake's last meal. Overall, fewer than 1 in 4 patients with a snakebite requires antivenom.

Editorial Comment

Check up-to-date guidelines as to antivenom use and doses, as this is constantly changing—for example, in many cases less is now given due to current research and evidence.

FIRST AID: THE PRESSURE–IMMOBILISATION TECHNIQUE

Snake venom spreads via the lymphatics, and its spread is increased by muscle contraction or activity. The pressure–immobilisation method of first aid prevents spread of the venom via the lymphatics and can prevent clinical envenomation. See Table 30.2 for when to use the technique.

- It involves applying a firm broad bandage, commencing at the site of the bite and then applying the bandage over the entire limb, extending both proximally and distally. The pressure is the same as that used for a sprained ankle. A splint (it is possible to use a stick) is then applied to the limb, to immobilise the limb and reduce muscle contraction. The patient is then kept as still as possible and transported to hospital.
- The pressure–immobilisation technique can prevent clinical envenomation if applied early and correctly. Both the limb and the patient should be immobilised. The bandages are kept in place until facilities are available to treat clinical envenomation in a hospital with a supply of antivenom.
- It is important not to wash the site of the bite, as it may contain traces of venom that are important for identifying the snake type.
- If a patient arrives following a possible snakebite and has had no first aid but is well and there are no signs of envenoming, there is no need to apply the pressure–immobilisation technique.
- If deterioration occurs when the bandages are removed, the bandages should be reapplied.
- The pressure–immobilisation first aid is not removed until the patient has been assessed and there is no clinical or laboratory evidence of envenoming or, in the envenomed patient, the antivenom has been commenced. The bandage can be removed halfway through the antivenom infusion.

Table 30.2 Use of the pressure–immobilisation technique of first aid

Pressure–immobilisation is recommended for:	Do not use pressure–immobilisation first aid for:
All Australian venomous snake bites, including sea snake bites	
Funnel web-spider bites	Redback spider bites Other spider bites, including mouse spiders, white-tailed spiders
Bee, wasp and ant stings in allergic individuals	Bee and wasp stings in non-allergic individuals
Blue-ringed octopus bites Cone snail (cone shell) stings	Bluebottle jellyfish stings Box jellyfish and other jellyfish stings Stonefish and other fish stings
	Bites or stings by scorpions, centipedes, beetles

Adapted with permission of the Australian Venom Research Unit.

VENOM DETECTION KIT

The venom detection kit (VDK) developed by Commonwealth Serum Laboratories (CSL) is important in the management of the patient with snakebite. The VDK can detect minute amounts of snake venom if present, and is used to determine what family of snake that venom came from.

- The VDK does not indicate that a patient has been envenomed. It also does not determine whether a patient should be given antivenom
- The VDK *does* indicate which antivenom to use, once the decision to give antivenom has been made.

The decision to give antivenom is a clinical decision based on symptoms, signs and pathology testing.

- A swab of the bite site is best, as this is where venom is present in the highest quantities. A small window can be cut in the bandages overlying the bite site. When the swab has been taken, the bandage is reapplied.
- Urine is the second best for venom detection, as Australian snake venoms are excreted in the urine. False-positive results are higher in urine testing with the VDK, so care is needed in interpretation in the non-envenomed patient. A positive urine result is not an indication for antivenom.
- Blood or serum is not used.

The venom detection kit is used by trained laboratory staff and takes at least 20 minutes to complete.

ANTIVENOM

- Antivenom exists for all major terrestrial snake types in Australia, and a multi-valent antivenom is available for sea snakes.
- Antivenom is the definitive treatment for a patient with systemic envenomation. The administration of antivenom can reverse the clinical effects of envenomation. The treatment of envenomation following snakebite involves the administration of adequate quantities of the appropriate antivenom.
- Antivenom is produced by CSL from antibodies harvested from horses that have been injected with subclinical doses of snake-venom toxins. As the antibodies are obtained from horse serum there is the risk of anaphylaxis, allergic reaction or delayed serum sickness. Prior to administration, therefore, preparations should be made to treat a possible anaphylactic reaction. Currently, premedication with adrenaline is not recommended.
- Monovalent antivenom is indicated if the type of snake is known, when the VDK determines the type of antivenom to be given, or in geographical areas where the occurrence of snakes is limited to specific snake types. Monovalent antivenom is preferred as it is less expensive, is a smaller load of foreign protein and has fewer side-effects.
- Polyvalent antivenom contains antibodies to the venom of all groups of land snakes. It consists of a large volume and is expensive. It is used when treatment with antivenom is indicated, the snake type is unknown and the VDK procedure is negative or will take too long to perform. It may be used when a patient presents with significant envenoming on arrival so that the determination of snake type with the VDK will take too long.
- In certain areas a mixture of monovalent antivenoms, based on the local prevalence of snake types, may replace polyvalent antivenom.
- The dose of antivenom is dependent on the dose of venom injected by the snake, *not* patient size, so children require the same amount of antivenom as adults do.
- Antivenom is always given intravenously and multiple ampoules may be necessary. The antivenom is diluted 1:10 in saline or Hartmann's solution. The volume of fluid (but not the dose of antivenom) may need to be modified in children.

- Premedication with adrenaline, antihistamines or steroids is not recommended.

LABORATORY TESTING

Laboratory tests are vital to assessing the patient possibly bitten by a snake, as patients may remain asymptomatic for some time. A patient with suspected snake bite needs to be managed in a hospital with laboratory facilities and this may require patient transfer.

Patients with possible snakebite should have **blood** taken for:

- coagulation—activated partial thromboplastin time (APTT), prothrombin time (PT), fibrinogen level, D-dimer/fibrinogen degradation products (XDP), platelet count
- creatine kinase
- renal function
- electrolytes.

Urine should be tested for myoglobin and blood.

If there is no access to a laboratory, a whole-blood clotting time can be performed to determine the presence of coagulopathy. To perform a whole-blood clotting time, 5–10 mL of blood are placed in a clean plain-glass test tube and allowed to stand. The time to clotting is measured and is normally less than 10 minutes. A time prolonged more than 20 minutes indicates coagulopathy.

Laboratory tests may be normal initially and need to be repeated. If all tests are normal, then the first-aid bandages should be removed and pathology tests repeated after 1 hour. As onset of coagulopathy may be delayed, blood tests should be repeated at 6 hours.

SIGNS AND SYMPTOMS

- Local signs of snakebite may vary from obvious bite marks, with local pain and swelling, to a trivial puncture or scratch. The absence of bite marks does not exclude significant snakebite, as no visible bite mark is quite common.
- General symptoms may be non-specific, such as nausea, headache, abdominal pain and collapse.
- Specific symptoms may include muscle pain, bleeding sites and muscle weakness.

In an emergency, it may be possible to determine the snake from the clinical and laboratory effects. It is advisable to seek expert advice prior to administering antivenom.

DISPOSITION

- Admit and observe all cases of possible snakebite. Patients should be checked frequently for signs of envenomation, and blood tests should be repeated, even if normal initially. Urine should be tested again for blood and myoglobin. The patient should be observed for early signs of paralysis, e.g. ptosis, diplopia and dysarthria, as small muscles are paralysed first.
- Patients who receive multiple doses of antivenom should also be given doses of steroids to prevent serum sickness.
- All patients with brown snake bite should be admitted for 24 hours.

Pearls and Pitfalls

- Not all patients bitten by snakes will suffer envenomation. Antivenom is not indicated in all cases—each case needs to be assessed individually.
- The patient with bite marks may not be envenomed. The patient with no bite mark and no symptoms may be envenomed.
- Early symptoms suggest severe envenoming.
- First aid should not be discontinued if antivenom and treatment facilities are not immediately available.
- The patient should be managed in a hospital with antivenom and laboratory facilities. This may require transfer of the patient, leaving the pressure–immobilisation first aid in situ.
- The VDK does not confirm or exclude envenoming. The VDK is used to determine which of the snake groups is responsible, so which antivenom is used.
- In the envenomed patient, multiple ampoules of antivenom are often necessary.
- Exotic snakes are kept in zoos and game parks and also illegally by collectors, so bites from non-Australian snakes can occur.

Spider bites

REDBACK SPIDER (*Latrodectus hasseltii*)

Redback spiders are common throughout Australia. They are common in urban areas, in and around houses, gardens, sheds, rubbish piles and discarded objects. It is the female spider that is responsible for envenoming. The bite of the redback can become very painful but envenoming is not normally life-threatening.

- Only one-fifth of bites will result in significant envenoming. Only people with significant envenoming receive antivenom.

- The redback bite is usually felt as an initial mild sting, with no signs of a bite at the site. Between 10 and 60 minutes later, the bite site may become painful. The pain can become severe and extend to the regional lymph nodes. Following this, pain may extend to the whole limb and the abdomen, and headache may occur. There may be nausea, vomiting, malaise and hypertension. An area of sweating may develop surrounding the bite site. The patient may be sweating profusely and this may be generalised or localised to the bite site, or in an area remote from the bite.
- Redback spider bite has been mistaken for acute surgical abdomen in children or myocardial infarction in adults.
- The triad of local pain, sweating and piloerection around the bite site increasing in the hour after a bite is diagnostic.
- Profuse sweating and pain in both arms or both legs following a bite is characteristic of systemic envenoming.
- If there is clear evidence of envenoming, then redback antivenom is given. The decision to treat is a clinical one; there are no tests to assist in the diagnosis.
  - Redback antivenom is given by IV or IM injection. There appears to be no clinical benefit of IV over IM administration. It can be repeated in 1 hour, if there is incomplete reduction of symptoms, or if symptoms return. No premedication is required, but facilities to treat anaphylaxis should be at hand.
  - Redback antivenom can be useful for relief of symptoms up to days after the initial bite. The need for multiple doses is not uncommon. Advice should be sought if multiple doses of antivenom are needed.

FUNNEL-WEB SPIDER (*Atrax* spp.)

There are at least 40 species of funnel-web spiders, but only one is known to cause death in humans. It is the Sydney funnel-web (*Atrax robustus*), which has a restricted range that includes the Sydney, Gosford and Wollongong regions. Other types are found over a wider range along the eastern seaboard of Australia.

- Following a bite from the Sydney funnel-web, death can occur within 1 hour. The effects are a bite that is usually painful, followed by perioral tingling, fasciculation of the tongue, profuse sweating, lacrimation and salivation, then skeletal muscle fasciculation and spasms. Hypertension and tachycardia usually occur and there may be rapid onset of pulmonary oedema.

- First aid is with the pressure–immobilisation technique. Definitive treatment is with Sydney funnel-web antivenom. Multiple vials of antivenom, usually 2–4, may be required. Resuscitation with airway control and ventilation may be necessary. Atropine may help reduce secretions.
- All Sydney funnel-web spider bites should be admitted for close observation.

The Sydney funnel-web spider appears similar to a number of non-venomous big black spiders (e.g. mouse spiders, trapdoor spiders). It is therefore important to have an approach to the management of the patient who presents with a *big black spider* bite if you practise within the distribution of Sydney funnel-web spiders. The unknown *big black spider* bite in these areas should be managed with pressure–immobilisation first aid, transport to a facility with antivenom and close observation for signs of envenoming.

WHITE-TAILED SPIDER (*Lampona cylindrata*)

The white-tailed spider is a common hunting spider that is often found in houses. Definite bites from this spider may cause some local pain and inflammation, but are usually only mild or moderate. The evidence linking the white-tailed spider to necrotic ulcers is limited, and research has failed to show that its venom causes significant skin damage.

- The patient who presents with a white-tailed spider bite usually only requires reassurance.
- There is an extensive list of causes of skin ulcers or necrotic skin lesions. Patients presenting with these may need referral to their GP or dermatologist.

NECROTIC ARACHNIDISM

Many spiders can cause a bite that may be painful and mildly inflamed locally. In some patients the skin may ulcerate. These small ulcers usually heal without specific treatment.

The development of lesions that ulcerate and develop necrosis is usually only tenuously linked to a spider bite. Patients with skin lesions often presume it was a spider bite, even though no spider has been sighted.

A number of overseas spiders not found in Australia, such as the recluse and fiddleback spiders, are implicated in causing necrotic skin ulceration and systemic illness.

There is little evidence to suggest that any single species of Australian spider is the cause of necrotic skin damage. In many cases, the cause of the tissue damage is a secondary bacterial infection.

Management includes adequate debridement of the wound, microbiological specimens and antibiotics if required. They may need investigation for other causes.

Marine envenomation

BOX JELLYFISH OR SEA WASP (*Chironex fleckeri*)

The box jellyfish is one of the most venomous creatures in the world. It is found in the tropical waters of northern Australia, and is most commonly encountered in the summer months.

- The venom of the box jellyfish contains cardiotoxic, neurotoxic and dermatotoxic compounds. Its tentacles contain stinging cells called nematocysts that contain the venom, and a spring-loaded harpoon. On contact with a victim the nematocyst releases the coiled harpoon, which pierces the skin and releases the stored venom. Victims may further discharge nematocysts as they attempt to remove the tentacles that still contain intact stinging cells.
- Clinically, there is severe localised pain, and local skin changes range from painful erythema to full-thickness skin necrosis. Typically, there are linear red welts that may go on to blister and ulcerate. Confusion, agitation and collapse with respiratory or cardiac arrest can occur.
- Rarely, envenomation may be very rapid and death can occur in 5 minutes, probably due to direct cardiotoxicity. Immediate and prolonged CPR is indicated in the event of cardiovascular collapse.
- The extent of envenoming is dependent on the area of skin suffering tentacle contact. An area of tentacle contact of 10% of the total body surface area is potentially lethal. One metre of tentacle-to-skin contact in a child, or several metres in the adult, can result in severe envenoming.
- Immediate first aid is vital. First, do not try to remove the tentacles. Any undischarged nematocysts can be inactivated by applying large volumes of household vinegar (dilute acetic acid). A pressure bandage is not applied as it can increase toxin load.
- Antivenom is available and is given by IV injection. IM injection of antivenom is no longer recommended as it will not be effective in the case of cardiovascular collapse. Early administration of antivenom may result in reduced pain and reduces skin necrosis and scarring.
- Severe envenoming is rare and most box jellyfish stings require only first aid.

IRUKANDJI (*Carukia barnesi*)

The irukandji is a small jellyfish, about 2 cm in diameter, found in the coastal waters of northern Australia.

- The sting of the irukandji is moderately painful, with little skin damage, but within 30 minutes onset of systemic envenoming may occur, with severe abdominal and back pain, nausea and vomiting, and muscle or joint pain. Sweating and agitation occur, and the patient is hypertensive and tachycardic. Symptoms are thought to be due to catecholamine release.
- The best form of first aid is application of vinegar.
- Treatment includes analgesia, and antihypertensive treatment may be required, in which case alpha-blocking drugs (phentolamine) may be used.
- No antivenom is available to treat irukandji envenomation.

PORTUGUESE MAN-O'-WAR OR BLUEBOTTLE (*Physalia* spp.)

The Portuguese man-o'-war, or bluebottle, occurs throughout Australian coastal waters, where it is often found washed up on beaches. It has a typical bright blue appearance, an air-filled flotation sac and long tentacles.

- The bluebottle causes a painful sting with localised discrete wheals and surrounding erythema. A line of redness with raised wheals or blisters is typical. Systemic symptoms are uncommon, but comprise nausea, vomiting, headache and abdominal pains. Deaths have not been reported following bluebottle sting in Australia.
- First aid involves washing the sting site with sea water, and removing the tentacles with forceps. Vinegar is not recommended.
- Treatment consists of hot-water immersion at 45° for 20 minutes. Analgesia is indicated, as is local anaesthesia.

BLUE-RINGED OCTOPUS (*Hapalochlaena* spp.)

The blue-ringed octopus is found in coastal waters around Australia. They are small, only a few centimetres in size, and exhibit electric-blue rings when aroused.

- A bite from the blue-ringed octopus may be painless and difficult to see, and so may go unnoticed. The bites usually occur when the octopus is handled. The victim, often a child, will usually report playing with a small octopus in or around a coastal rock pool.

- The saliva of the blue-ringed octopus contains a potent neurotoxin, tetrodotoxin, which causes a rapidly progressive flaccid paralysis, followed by respiratory failure and hypotension.
- First aid involves applying a pressure–immobilisation bandage.
- There is no antivenom, and treatment is based on maintaining supportive measures. Respiratory support with ventilation may be required for a few days, until the effects of the toxin wear off.

SEA SNAKES

Sea snakes are found predominantly in the tropical waters of northern Australia. There are more than 30 species found in Australian waters. They are inquisitive and rarely aggressive. All are potentially dangerous to humans, but very few sea snake bites of significance occur. Bites may occur when a sea snake is being handled or removed from the nets of a fishing trawler.

- Sea snake venoms contain postsynaptic neurotoxins and myolysins. Victims may therefore develop paralysis, with ptosis and diplopia, or muscle pain, weakness and myoglobinuria and hyperkalaemia, and renal failure may occur secondary to muscle breakdown. Coagulopathy is not a feature of sea snake bite.
- Treatment is with the pressure–immobilisation technique of first aid.
- Sea snake antivenom is available and is used for neutralising venoms of all species of sea snakes. Sea snake venoms are not reliably detected by the VDK.

STONEFISH

The stonefish is responsible for a painful sting that usually occurs when waders step on the fish in shallow waters around reefs and rock pools. They are well camouflaged and their spines may pierce the sole of a wader's shoe.

- When the fish is stepped on, the spines inject venom, which causes instant and severe pain. Local swelling, which may be marked, follows. Dizziness, nausea, hypotension and pulmonary oedema may rarely occur.
- As some components of the venom are denatured by heat, first aid involves immersing the limb in hot water. The water should not be hot enough to cause a scald.
- Analgesics are usually required. Local or regional anaesthesia may help in providing analgesia.

- Antivenom is available if there is significant envenoming, and is indicated if there is severe local pain. The number of ampoules given relates to the number of puncture wounds from the venomous spines.
- A remnant of the spine may remain embedded in the foot and removal is necessary. Imaging with X-ray or ultrasound may be indicated.
- The role of prophylactic antibiotics is unclear. However, wound irrigation, debridement and removal of foreign debris is paramount.
- Secondary infection is the major complication and may be from marine or aquatic organisms.

Pearl

- Treat all painful penetrating marine injuries with hot-water immersion. Use water at 45° and first immerse an unaffected limb to check that the temperature is tolerated, especially when anaesthetics are used.

Tick bites

- Ticks most commonly cause a local skin reaction, consisting of irritation and pruritus as the tick attaches and sucks blood from the host. Multiple bites may cause a rash.
- There are many species of tick and the most dangerous are those that cause paralysis, belonging to the *Ixodes* group. The *Ixodes* paralysis tick is found along eastern coastal strip of Australia.
  - Paralysis occurs due to a neuromuscular-junction toxin that occurs in the saliva of the *Ixodes* ticks. The toxin causes a progressive flaccid paralysis. Paralysis may take a few days to develop.
  - Tick paralysis is rare, and usually occurs in children less than 3 years old and presents as an ataxic gait with drowsiness, malaise and unsteadiness or leg weakness. The weakness may progress slowly, and even up to 48 hours after removal of the ticks.
- A thorough search should be conducted to find ticks, which may be multiple, including scalp, ear canals, axillae, natal cleft and genitals. Ticks are removed by using tweezers on either side of the embedded mouthparts. Care is taken not to squeeze the body of the tick, or more toxin can be injected. Care is also taken

not to break off the mouthparts that may remain embedded in the skin.
- Paralysis is treated with appropriate supportive care. Tick antivenom is no longer available.
- A local reaction to the tick bite that may last a number of weeks is common, especially if the tick has been incompletely removed.

Centipedes and scorpions

None of the species of centipedes or scorpions found in Australia are dangerous to humans. In other parts of the world they may be responsible for life-threatening envenomation.

Scorpions sting with their tail, not with their paired pincers. They may cause a painful bite, but the pain does not usually last long. Systemic symptoms are unusual and are not usually severe.

Additional resources

- Many hospitals have their own policies for management of potential bites.
- Many smaller hospitals have a clinical relationship with a larger hospital, and a local or regional emergency doctor will be available on the end of a phone. (Use them!)

Pearls and Pitfalls

- The most common pitfall is not relying on the history that is provided to you or underestimating the potential for envenomation.
- Unexplained coagulopathy, muscle pain or weakness should include envenomation as a differential diagnosis.
- Children with unexplained irritability, pain or sweating or boys with unexplained groin pain should have redback spider bites as part of the differential diagnosis.
- Gloves and forceps are used to remove marine tentacles from patients, as undischarged nematocysts can injure the first aider.
- Failure to apply, or removal of, a pressure–immobilisation bandage in snake or funnel-web envenomation may cause worsening symptoms; a pressure bandage should be applied and left in situ until no longer necessary.
- The decision to administer antivenom when clinically indicated should not be delayed.
- Adequate antivenom should be used as indicated on either clinical or laboratory grounds. (continues overleaf)

- Being bitten does not automatically indicate the need for antivenom administration. Many definite bites do not result in envenoming.
- A positive result for a VDK does not indicate the need for antivenom administration. There may be venom on the skin without systemic envenoming.
- The VDK tells us which antivenom to give, but not whether we should give it. The decision to give antivenom is based on clinical and laboratory findings of envenomation.
- Toxinologists who are on call do not regard any question as silly if it relates to a patient or presentation you do not fully understand. They are available through the Poisons Information Centre, **tel. 13 11 26**, Australia-wide.
- Ask for advice, and ask early. There are no stupid questions, only stupid people who don't ask questions.

Online resources

Australian Venom Research Unit
www.avru.org/general/general_main.html

Clinical Toxinology Resources
www.toxinology.com

Emergency Therapeutic Guidelines, toxinology
http://proxy9.use.hcn.com.au

Chapter 31
Electrical injuries

Gordian W O Fulde and Christopher J Mobbs

Overview

In Australia, people come to emergency departments as the result of an electrical injury, including by lightning. Some 15–20% are aged 0–14 years.

Each year there are preventable deaths attributable to electrical injury (> 90% are male). Many deaths from lightning strikes (mostly male) could have been avoided.

Electrical injuries are more common in males, and mostly occur in the young adult and adult years. The most common locations for injury are, in order, the home (often children < 6 years old) and the workplace.

The **source of an electrical injury** may be divided into 3 broad subgroups, with important differences in assessment and management of patients relevant to each. For example, cardiac arrest, as provoked by an electrical current, will more commonly be asystole from a lightning strike and ventricular fibrillation (VF) from a household AC current. The three subgroups, therefore are:

1. Lightning injury
2. High-voltage (> 1000 V) electrical injury
3. Low-voltage (< 1000 V) electrical injury.

Low-voltage electrical injury may be further sub-divided into patients *with* or *without* cardiac and/or respiratory arrest.

PATHOPHYSIOLOGY

Electricity may cause injury via 3 broad mechanisms:

1. Electricity causing direct tissue damage, altering cell membrane resting potential and eliciting muscle tetany, cardiac arrests and arrhythmias (thus better results from prolonged CPR).
2. Conversion of electrical energy into thermal energy (heat), causing tissue destruction and coagulative necrosis.
3. Traumatic injury resulting from falls or violent muscle contractions.

The site of either direct tissue or thermal energy damage depends on the pathway of current flow. Skin wound inspection alone will miss and underdiagnose damage to deep and distant structures.

PHYSICS

Electricity is the flow of electrons from higher to lower potential. Direct current (DC), from sources such as car batteries or defibrillators, flows in one direction. Domestic alternating current (AC) switches to and fro at 50–60 cycles per second (Hertz), as this confers advantages in terms of current generation and transmission. Ironically, human muscular tissue is sensitive to frequencies in this range, with tetany of peripheral muscles and VF arrest of cardiac muscles a risk during contact with household electricity. Domestic voltage in Australia is 230 V.

Lightning contains around 10×10^6 volts and a current of 10,000–200,000 amperes. However, as the result of the incredibly brief time (microseconds to milliseconds) involved in a lightning strike, the final amount of current is much less than expected.

It is the electrical current that is important in terms of human morbidity and mortality, and thus basic electrical injury potential rests with two laws:

- Ohm's law:

$$\text{Resistance (ohms)} = \frac{\text{Voltage (volts)}}{\text{Current (amperes)}}$$

- Joule's law:

$$\text{Heat generated} = \text{Current}^2 \propto \text{Resistance}$$

So, while dry, thick, calloused skin may be more resistant to injury by virtue of its very high resistance (up to 100,000 ohms) the resistance of moist skin is only 1000 ohms. It is therefore of vital importance to preach **good electrical safety**, especially in the home and workplace, and especially relating to moisture and electrical appliances and the installation of circuit-breakers.

Similarly, it is the role of all health professionals to educate the public about **safety during electrical storms**. Those who enjoy outdoor recreation, such as golfers and hikers, are the major group of people affected by lightning strike. Solo people who are struck make up 70% of the recorded mortality. Most fatalities (about 70%) are recorded between midday and 6pm. Deaths occur 5 times more frequently in the country than in urban areas. The summer storm season is associated with the highest mortality rate. The annual mortality rate is decreasing in all recording countries.

Three major predictors of mortality are: cardiac arrest at the time of injury, cranial burns (5× increased) and leg burns.

In order to **avoid lightning** there are some simple measures which should be followed:

- Stay indoors during a storm, or seek shelter in a building or car (not a convertible).
- Avoid contact with any metal such as golf clubs, umbrellas, tent poles, gates, roofs or hair clips.
- Do not stand next to or under the tallest object in sight, such as a tree, pole or haystack.
- Avoid being in a group—split up so that someone can call for help if necessary; give CPR (fixed dilated pupils can be an electrical brain injury which responds to CPR).
- Do not stand with your feet apart, as this increases your stride potential and can result in major burns.
- If caught alone, the correct procedure is to curl up on the ground, preferably in a ditch, well away from higher objects.
- It is important to note that, contrary to popular belief, lightning does strike twice or more in the same spot.

Wide-band magnetic direction finders are increasingly used to warn of incoming lightning storms. Lightning injuries can be markedly decreased by taking measures to prevent oneself becoming a conductor, and by not being near an obvious one. Piloerection during an electrical storm can mean that a lightning strike is imminent, and immediate evasive measures along the lines of those described above should be taken.

Low- and high-voltage electrical injury

- The type and amount of current can be inferred from the nature of the source. Electricians and other tradespeople may be able to give accurate information as to strength of power source and current type. However, within appliances, conversions from the more dangerous AC to DC, and to a different voltage, are possible.
- Entry and exit wounds may be visible, but their absence does not rule out serious injury and they may give no indication as to severity of underlying organ damage. The current between any such wounds does not necessarily travel in straight lines.
- Electrical flash burns, often seen in tradespeople, may occur where a short-circuit causes an explosion, e.g. on a switchboard. It is likely that patients have had very little actual current pass

through them, and dermal and corneal burns and sequelae of any blunt trauma may dominate the clinical picture.
- If a patient was 'frozen' to the circuit, due to muscle tetany with AC, a life-threatening injury may have occurred, with multi-organ and limb damage.
- Significant electrical injury resembles more closely a crush injury than a burn. Necrosis of deep soft tissues and organs has both immediate (e.g. cardiac arrest) and long-term (e.g. rhabdomyolysis and renal failure) adverse sequelae. Tissues and organs distant to the site of electrical injury may be affected, as large- and small-vessel arterial and venous thrombosis occurs.
- Infants and young children are prone to sustaining oral electrical injuries from electrical appliances. Mucous membranes have less resistance than skin and the current is therefore higher. These injuries may lead to eventual scarring and deformity of the face in later years. If the current travels close to the eyes, cataracts may form.
- Injuries, burns and complications are frequently under-diagnosed and poorly documented. Because litigation can ensue, good clinical recording is mandatory—as with all instances of burns and trauma in the ED. Diagrams are essential, photography desirable.

MANAGEMENT

Pre-hospital

The most important initial consideration is the safety of the rescuer and other bystanders. No more electrocutions should be allowed to occur. All wires and appliances should be considered live, as should any patients still in contact with them. Power should be shut down and/or the victim should be removed from the current with a non-conductive substance—for example a rubber car mat. Any water or moisture should be regarded as electrically live and the potential source of more electrical injury.

An electrocuted patient must then continue to be treated along standard life support guidelines. Nowadays, with automated and semi-automated external defibrillators (AEDs/SAEDs) available in many public areas, these devices should be utilised as rapidly as is safely possible, as early defibrillation from VF gives the greatest chance of survival. CPR has higher success rates with electrical injuries.

Hospital

- The standard approach to an *unconscious or critically ill patient* must always be employed. This includes neck immobilisation where necessary and exclusion of other causes of altered conscious state such as hypoglycaemia, overdose, cerebrovascular accident or trauma. This approach is particularly important in view of the fact that the prime treatment modality for the electrically injured is support of systems while waiting for recovery, and attempting to avoid complications.
- The majority of survivors presenting to the ED after an electrical injury are relatively well. A high level of suspicion for secondary traumatic injuries needs to be maintained, however, if there is a possibility of a fall, having been thrown or a violent muscle contraction. Emergency doctors should think of 'worst-case scenarios', as electrical injuries can affect multiple systems and may well be covert. It is essential to keep an open mind as to causation, and to carefully explore the possibility of serious concomitant disease.
- A thorough ABC reassessment and then a meticulous whole-body examination (primary then secondary surveys) with aggressive early management of any injuries must occur. Fractures may be present; fasciotomies of digits and limbs may need to be done in the ED. An ECG should be performed.
- A good urine flow (1 mL/kg/h) in the face of myoglobinuria (urine dipstick positive for blood) or shock is essential, as with standard treatment of rhabdomyolysis. Urinary alkalinisation and use of mannitol and/or frusemide may be indicated and late renal failure with acidosis must be anticipated.
- A check of tetanus immunisation status is mandatory.
- Cardiac monitoring and admission for observation is indicated in high-voltage (> 1000 V) injury, following seizures or loss of consciousness, raised cardiac markers and with ECG changes including arrhythmias. Arrhythmias will usually settle spontaneously and without sinister sequelae. Admission may also be required as dictated by traumatic injury, exacerbation of pre-existing chronic illness or in the elderly.
- Thus patients with 'low-voltage' injuries not meeting the adverse criteria detailed above may be discharged home with simple analgesia as required, following a normal ECG. No blood tests are necessary. An exception to this rule is in the case of

the pregnant female; the fetus, situated within amniotic fluid within a hyperaemic uterus, is at great risk, even with apparently 'minor' exposures having no noticeable effect on the mother. An urgent obstetric ultrasound and consultation should be sought.

- Adequate follow-up, both physical and psychological, must be arranged, as a high proportion of patients have some long-term effects following a significant electrical injury. Neurological damage has an especially poor prognosis. Electrical burns should be referred to a specialist burns centre.
- Many electrical injuries may involve workers' compensation or insurance claims, so good documentation is useful.

Lightning injuries

PHYSICS

Lightning occurs when particles moving up and down during a thunderstorm create static electricity. A massive negative charge builds up on the underside of a cloud until the charge difference between it and the positively charged ground is enough to cause electrical discharge. This lightning strike may last between 1 and 100 milliseconds. It differs from 'high-voltage' electrocution in additional ways—the energy level is many tens of millions of volts, it is a direct current (DC), it may cause a shock wave and may demonstrate the 'flashover' phenomenon, where the current passes over and around, rather than through, the patient.

Lightning is also associated with asystolic cardiac arrest, rather than ventricular fibrillation. Good CPR rather than early defibrillation is of paramount importance as, although return to sinus rhythm may spontaneously occur, there is a risk of secondary hypoxic arrest if resuscitation is delayed.

Some 30% of victims who are struck die, and up to 75% can have serious complications.

MECHANISMS OF STRIKE

1 **Direct strike**
   a Current passes through patient.
   b Current passes over surface of patient (flashover), often via wet clothes, which can explode or burn.
2 **Side flash**
   The patient becomes part of the main conductor. This occurs for example when standing under a tree which is struck by lightning. The current can pass as in a direct strike.

3 **Direct contact**
The patient is in physical contact with the main conductor.

4 **Stride potential**
This arises when current from a lightning strike travels along the ground near a person who has his/her legs separated. The current takes the path of lesser resistance up a leg, across the body and down the other leg, rather than along the high-resistance ground. This process is associated with a significant mortality.

PATHOPHYSIOLOGY

As the injuries sustained are both multisystemic and multifactorial in aetiology (from diverse sources such as electricity, heat, blunt trauma and anoxia), the clinical possibilities are vast. Certain injuries and their sequelae are typical or may even be diagnostic (see Table 31.1).

- Cardiac—asystolic arrest
- Neurological—loss of consciousness, paraplegia, hemiplegia, amnesia, seizure, tinnitus, autonomic nervous system dysfunction including fixed dilated pupils
- Vascular—keraunoparalysis; vascular spasm with absent pulses, mottled limbs. Usually resolves over a period of hours
- Skin—'Lichtenberg flowers'; may look severe but fade within hours
- Severe burns with their sequelae of renal failure, anaemia and tissue damage are very uncommon.

Table 31.1 Special injuries often associated with lightning

Skin	Burns—feathering or flowers (transient, not burns but electrocution showers) Superficial (often in patterns of sweatlines, or wet exploded clothing) Deep entry and exit wounds; imprints of metal buttons, belt clips, ignited clothing
Ear	Tympanic membrane rupture, barotrauma
Eye	Onset of cataracts, eye trauma and disruption of anatomy
Heart	Asystole, ventricular fibrillation, arrhythmias, infarct (rare), transient hypotension or hypotension
Limbs	Trauma; keraunoparalysis, a temporary neurovascular dysfunction in the majority of serious strikes, usually resolves in hours but permanent sequelae are possible
Central nervous system	Seizures, mental state similar to that after electroconvulsive therapy Amnesia (very common), psychological sequelae

As a generalisation, patients who survive the initial strike will usually have no major problems. Clinical expertise, including a high index of suspicion, must be used to rule out potential complications to the eyes, ears, heart and nervous system.

MANAGEMENT

Pre-hospital

- Rescuer safety is vital. A very special aspect of lightning victims is that they require aggressive resuscitation even in the light of asystole, apparent fixed dilated pupils or pulseless limbs, for the reasons detailed above.
- This is also the reason for a group caught by a storm splitting up—CPR can be administered to the victim by those not affected.
- A particular pitfall to avoid is withholding CPR to the victim of a lightning strike in the mistaken assumption that they remain charged by electricity.
- Paradoxically to usual disaster responses, if several people are struck by lightning at once, the care must go to the sickest (arrested) first, as the walking and talking wounded will survive whereas the arrested patient has only a brief opportunity to be salvaged.
- The diagnosis itself may be challenging, as the strike may be unwitnessed. Again, a high index of suspicion must be maintained and clues such as multiple unconscious people, exploded clothes and Lichtenberg flowers may point to the cause.

Hospital

- Patients may arrive arrested, unconscious, amnesic, as a trauma patient or as one that has very few clinical problems.
- A standard approach, e.g. advanced cardiac life support (ACLS), advanced trauma life support (ATLS), is indicated with simultaneous assessment and management systematically by an organised team.
- The clinical picture dictates the management. It is essential that other possible causes and concomitant illness be sought and excluded as part of the patient's management.
- As always, the ABCs are secured. Lightning-strike patients rarely need fluid loading. Hypothermia due to exposure is common. If there is any loss of consciousness, arrhythmia or rise in cardiac markers, cardiac monitoring for 24 hours is indicated. MRI is

useful for subtle lesions of the brain and spinal cord. Usually the surviving victim needs mainly supportive treatment.

- Special attention should be paid to the ear and eye examinations, for tympanic rupture and corneal defects respectively. Other ocular pathology will also need to be excluded, most easily when the patient is alert and able to cooperate with full eye examination. Basal visual acuity should be recorded if possible.
- Disposition is guided by the same considerations that govern other electrical injuries. A period of observation in hospital is warranted for changes in neurological or cardiological status and for other organ-specific pathology.

TASERs and electrical weapons

- Modern law enforcement deploys TASERs (Thomas A Swift Electric Rifles), and emergency departments see and assess these patients based on understanding that their use is a valid alternative to lethal force (guns).
- The literature supports the assertion that when used appropriately (adequate training) and with an exposure of < 15 seconds, these weapons do not cause fatalities or cardiac arrhythmias. Certain subgroups of people—those taking stimulants such as crystal methamphetamine, cocaine, hallucinogens, LSD, phencyclidine etc, and older patients with comorbidities—have been associated with arrhythmia and mortality.
- As with any electrical injury, secondary traumatic injuries from falls, etc must be looked for.
- The weapon's technology is based on DC, high voltage with low current (amperes). Two barbed metal hooks attached to wires are shot at the person by compressed gas. The hooks embedded in the skin deliver the electrical current, causing muscle contraction (tetany) to immobilise the person. Police TASERs have video recording inbuilt.
- At times EDs are requested to help remove the barbs; also at times the barbs can be embedded in special tissues, e.g. face, eyelids, etc. Normal injury and wound care applies.
- The literature supports the approach that if a TASER victim has no injuries and is asymptomatic they do not require admission, clinical observation or comprehensive laboratory or diagnostic work-up.

Pearls and Pitfalls

- Do not become a victim of electrical injury—ensure self and bystander safety before attending patient.
- Early CPR is potentially life-saving.
- The victim of lightning strike does not remain electrically charged.
- Even apparently 'harmless' electrical injury may have fatal consequences for the intra-uterine fetus.
- Asymptomatic patients following a 'low-voltage' electrical injury may be safely discharged from the ED following a normal ECG.
- Preach prevention, especially to golfers.

Online resources

E-medicine article, Electrical injuries in emergency medicine (Cushing TA, Wright RK, April 2013)
http://emedicine.medscape.com/article/770179-overview

UpToDate; search on 'electrical injuries'
www.uptodate.com

Chapter 32
Hypothermia and hyperthermia

David Lewis-Driver

Although Canadians write more about hypothermia and Saudis write more about hyperthermia, in fact neither condition is rare in Australia. Heat waves and fun-runs occur every year in every Australian city; at the opposite end of the spectrum, hypothermia is a regular accompaniment to injury and disease throughout the year, and can occur in summer—for example when nursing-home patients are left scantily clothed under an air conditioner to cool them. It is important, too, to remember that the average multiple-trauma patient in any country will become hypothermic unless specific preventive steps are taken.

Physiology

Temperature control requires a functioning hypothalamic centre, adequate cardiovascular function to be able to dissipate or conserve heat, adequate muscle bulk to generate heat, intact skin and sweat glands and sufficient common sense and mobility to escape the heat or cold. All of these may be affected by disease, trauma or environmental factors.

In both hyperthermia and hypothermia, skin circulation is a problem. Overheating cold skin induces vasodilation, which feels good but may overwhelm the pumping capacity of a cold heart, resulting in 're-warming shock'. Ice on hot skin induces vasoconstriction, which may limit heat transfer.

Hypothermia

This condition is defined as a core temperature of < 35°C. It is classified as shown in Table 32.1.

Table 32.1 Classification of hypothermia

Temperature (°C)	Grade	Signs
35–32	Mild	Shivering/apathy
32–28	Moderate	Confusion, ↓ heart rate, ↓ blood pressure
< 28	Severe	Cardiovascular failure

PHYSIOLOGY

The body responds to a fall in temperature by attempting to seek warmth and by shivering. If these efforts fail because of environmental factors or drugs, injury or disease and the temperature continues to fall, an initial rise in respiration, heart rate and blood pressure is followed by a gradual slowing of all body systems, with death due to cardiovascular failure. Central nervous system (CNS) slowing results in apathy and confusion, and cardiovascular system slowing proceeds to death in asystole, unless an irritable heart is jolted into ventricular fibrillation (VF).

In general, slow warming and gentle handling are appropriate. Vigorous attempts at external re-warming can result in skin burns or death from 're-warming shock', an ill-understood phenomenon that can best be considered as shunting of needed blood to the surface while the core is still too cold to cope with the demand. Core temperature lags behind surface temperature during re-warming, and healthy volunteers start to feel better when re-warmed while their core temperature is still falling due to continued cold penetration. An 'undressing phenomenon' is also well described, where failure of skin vasoconstriction as a terminal event allows return of skin circulation and leads to a sensation of warmth so that victims are found to have undressed themselves as a last act before death.

DIAGNOSIS AND DIFFERENTIAL DIAGNOSIS

If temperature is not a routine observation on every patient, ensure it is taken in those patients who are potential hypothermia candidates, as outlined in Box 32.1.

If the temperature is < 36°C on a standard instrument, use a low-reading thermometer. The tympanic thermometers commonly used in EDs will generally read down to 26°C and are thus adequate to suggest the diagnosis. However, they are not accurate enough to guide treatment. Use an electronic probe—rectal in an awake patient and oesophageal in an intubated patient.

INVESTIGATIONS AND MANAGEMENT

Mild hypothermia (35–32°C)

1. **Stop further heat loss.** The most powerful way to prevent heat loss in any ED patient is to stem conduction and radiation loss—i.e. remove wet clothes and provide a blanket or space blanket. This is also called passive external re-warming, because prevention of heat loss allows the patient's own metabolism to raise body temperature.

Box 32.1 Conditions associated with hypothermia

Conditions associated with accidental hypothermia

- Trauma that limits protective mechanisms, e.g. neck of femur (NOF)
- Overdose
- Alcoholism

Conditions that may cause hypothermia

- Sepsis
- Myxoedema or adrenal insufficiency
- Parkinsonism (failure to shiver)
- Wernicke's encephalopathy
- Drugs, e.g. phenothiazines, beta-blockers, clozapine, sedatives
- Hypoglycaemia; diabetic ketoacidosis (affects the body's 'thermostat')
- Pancreatitis
- Myocardial infarction or other cause of low cardiac output
- Malnutrition/anorexia
- Burns; extensive skin rashes (excessive heat loss)

Conditions that hypothermia may be mistaken for

- Cerebrovascular accident (CVA)
- Dementia; confusion in the elderly; delirium
- Hypoglycaemia
- Myocardial ischaemia
- Drunk and disorderly patient
- Myxoedema

2. **Treat the underlying cause** (Box 32.1).
3. **Monitor temperature.** A rise of > 0.5°C per hour is acceptable, but do not exceed a rise of 2°C per hour with a Bair Hugger (see below).
4. **Apply a Bair Hugger**, if available. This method of active external warming using hot air is commonly available and is unlikely to cause re-warming shock or burns. Active warming, however, is not vital unless the patient is incapable of generating heat because of systemic disease or a condition (e.g. CVA) that has reset the temperature centre. If a Bair Hugger is used, do not exceed a rise of 2°C per hour. It is probably better to leave the arms exposed, because the main risk is that sequestered cold blood will be restored to the circulating pool by skin vasodilation, causing an afterdrop in the core temperature. This risk is less from the trunk than the limbs.
5. **Give oxygen and monitor oxygen saturation.** If the saturation monitor will not read because of vasoconstriction, warm the finger or even do a digital block to overcome vasospasm.

6 **Set up IV access and take blood** for:

- Blood sugar level (BSL). Physiologically, hypothermia causes first a rise in BSL due to catecholamine-induced glycogenolysis, then reduced insulin secretion. Finally (below 30°C), insulin stops working. However, there is a strong association with hypoglycaemia in alcoholics, and elderly or malnourished patients may have exhausted glycogen stores by the increased metabolism of shivering. Treat hypoglycaemia but not hyperglycaemia. If re-warming does not correct hyperglycaemia, exclude haemorrhagic pancreatitis (a complication of hypothermia) or diabetic ketoacidosis (a cause of hypothermia).
- Urea and electrolytes. Fluid shifts and renal dysfunction mean that sodium and potassium can go in either direction. Minor changes in the initial results do not require treatment and can simply be observed during re-warming. Significant changes should be treated and may be a clue to the underlying cause of the hypothermia.
- Lipase. Pancreatitis is both a cause and a result of hypothermia.
- Full blood count (FBC). Expect the haematocrit to be high (due to cold diuresis—an attempt to compensate for central fluid overload due to peripheral vasoconstriction) and the white cell count (WCC) and platelets to be normal or low (due to sequestration). A normal Hb/Hct (haemoglobin/haematocrit) may indicate anaemia and a normal WCC does not rule out infection. Thus the main reason for doing the tests is that a high WCC increases suspicion of an underlying disease process.
- Troponin. Patients who become hypothermic during surgery have a higher incidence of myocardial events. Sub-endocardial infarctions have been found at autopsy in the absence of ECG changes. In elderly patients, repeat troponin after re-warming.
- Creatine kinase (CK). May be a clue to rhabdomyolysis in overdose or injury.
- Not coagulation screens. Hypothermic patients bleed more after surgery and trauma, and this is generally attributed to failure of one or more of the enzymes in the coagulation cascade and qualitative platelet dysfunction. However, coagulation screens will generally be normal because these

tests are done in the lab at room temperature. Re-warming is the best treatment. It is not generally possible either to get the lab to re-do the tests at the patient's temperature or to make fresh frozen plasma (FFP) work while the patient is still cold.

7 **Give fluid.**
  - 500–1000 mL of dextrose/saline or normal saline (warmed!).
  - Hartmann's solution is contraindicated because the cold liver cannot metabolise the lactate.
  - Assume that the patient is dehydrated due to 3rd space shifts and cold diuresis. Some fluid is required to compensate for the return of skin flow during re-warming, but when the patient is warmer the 3rd space fluid will return.
  - Elderly patients require cautious fluid replacement but younger patients can have the full litre fairly quickly.

8 **Do an ECG.** Hypothermia increases conduction times and often causes a slow atrial fibrillation which reverses with re-warming. The classical ECG change is the appearance of a J wave between the QRS complex and the T wave. Some computerised ECG programs interpret this wave incorrectly as myocardial infarction.

9 **Institute cardiac monitoring.** VF is the terminal event in a significant number of hypothermia deaths, and is commonly thought to be provoked by jostling or rescue or treatment procedures. It is unlikely above 29°C, however.

10 **Monitor blood pressure (BP).** If it drops, turn off the Bair Hugger if it is being used (re-warming shock due to skin vasodilation).

11 **Take an ABG** (arterial blood gas) and use the result, which is uncorrected for temperature. Expect hypoxia (due to ventilation/perfusion defects plus shift in oxyhaemoglobin curve plus increased haematocrit) and a lactic acidosis due to shivering. Below 32°C a respiratory acidosis due to slowed respiration will be added. Try to keep the uncorrected pH close to normal, but only by warming and ventilation. Bicarbonate (HCO_3^-) level is not indicated.

12 **Measure urine output.** Use an indwelling catheter (IDC) if required. None of heart rate (HR), BP or urine output will be *reliable* indicators of hydration status, but urine output will be the best of the three.

13 **Keep nil by mouth** until 35°C is reached (poor gut motility).

14 **Consider central venous pressure (CVP).** This may be the only way to measure fluid replacement requirements in the elderly, but the risk of coagulopathy is a strong disincentive. If a CVP catheter is introduced, it should stop well above the right atrium to avoid an arrhythmia in the irritable heart.
15 **Do a chest X-ray (CXR).** Cold induces bronchorrhoea and reduces ciliary activity and resistance to infection, making bronchopneumonia more likely.
16 **Give thiamine to alcoholic or malnourished patients**, because of the association between Wernicke's encephalopathy and hypothermia.
17 Confirm that the patient can protect the airway, cooperate with treatment, maintain a satisfactory partial oxygen pressure (pO_2) on oxygen, and has a fairly stable HR, BP and cardiac rhythm. If not, proceed to the more aggressive measures in the next section.

Moderate hypothermia (32–28°C)

Treatment should not be based on temperature alone, particularly since core temperature may not initially reflect the re-warming that has been commenced. BP, HR, oxygen saturations and ability to protect the airway all influence treatment decisions. Because VF is a frequent complication in this temperature range, patients with frequent ventricular ectopic beats (VEBs) merit vigorous re-warming.

In addition to the measures above, most moderately hypothermic patients will need:

1 **Intubation.** The patient will be hypoventilating and having problems dealing with copious bronchial secretions.
   - Use standard drugs and dosages. Pharmacokinetics and pharmacodynamics are altered by hypothermia, but there is no specific information to guide dosing. Below 30°C, most drugs do not work at all, and 'cold' intubation may be required. At higher temperatures, if the drugs work, they will generally have a longer half-life.
   - Insert a heat–moisture exchanger into the circuit. 70% of respiratory heat loss goes into humidifying expired air. Most EDs do not have mechanisms for heating inspired air, and this additional effort brings marginal benefit.

2 **Nasogastric tube (NGT).** Cold reduces gastric motility and distension is likely.
3 **Active external re-warming.** If a Bair Hugger is not available, put hands and feet in warm water or use radiant heat or

hot-water bottles. Be careful of burning poorly vascularised and insensitive skin.

Severe hypothermia (< 28°C)

1 Most of these patients will need active core re-warming and ICU admission. Heated gastric lavage and/or bladder irrigation through the NGT and IDC are non-invasive but not as effective as peritoneal lavage (one or two catheters) or thoracic lavage (two catheters). The most effective re-warming procedure is extracorporeal rewarming using cardiopulmonary bypass or haemodialysis machines.
2 Give broad-spectrum antibiotic prophylaxis because of the high incidence of sepsis due to impaired resistance.

If there is no cardiac output

Death from hypothermia will be preceded by slow HR and respirations, so more care than usual in seeking signs of life is indicated. Unfortunately, the muscular rigidity associated with severe hypothermia is similar to rigor mortis, so the clinical diagnosis of death is difficult without an ECG. But there are also cases of cold asystolic people recovering or being resuscitated, so the axiom 'no one is dead until they are warm and dead' creates a dilemma in the ED, particularly if CPR has been started pre-hospital.

Some guidelines are:

- Temperature < 15°C or potassium > 12 mmol/L is unsalvageable.
- 32°C is a reasonable level to achieve. Once it has been reached, if resuscitation has not already been successful, it probably will not be.
- With temperatures < 32°C, if cardiopulmonary bypass is available, use it. If it is not available, use warmed fluids through two intercostal catheters while CPR continues. VF may not respond to either drugs or defibrillation if temperature is < 32°C.

PRE-HOSPITAL CARE

Shivering is a very effective method of heat production, so simply rescuing and drying the patient is a good start. A warm carbohydrate drink provides core re-warming and energy for more shivering. Warm blankets stop shivering but are now considered to do no harm and they make the patient feel better.

Jostling a severely hypothermic patient (including unnecessary CPR) may precipitate VF. This makes the decision about whether to commence CPR very difficult. If the victim has no pulse or respirations, bag them with oxygen for a few minutes. This may improve output enough for a carotid pulse to be detected. (Wait at least 60 seconds before declaring it absent.) If there is still no pulse, CPR will not make things any worse. Start CPR unless:

- it will endanger rescuers by evacuation delays
- there are obvious lethal injuries
- airway is blocked with ice
- chest is too rigid to be compressed.

Hyperthermia

Hyperthermia is technically different to fever. It is an increased body temperature due to failure of the temperature regulation systems. Unlike hypothermia, it is not possible to say that the diagnosis is defined by temperature. However, it is reasonable to say that below 40°C urgent treatment is unlikely to be needed. Above 42°C, cellular damage is likely whatever the cause—fever or hyperthermia.

DEFINITIONS

In **fever**, the body's temperature regulation is reset to a new level. Resetting the temperature control with antipyretics may help.

Heat stress is a sense of discomfort in a hot environment.

Heat exhaustion is thirst, weakness, dizziness, etc, plus a normal or mildly elevated temperature due to water or salt depletion.

Heat stroke is a medical emergency; described below.

HEAT STROKE

This is defined as collapse plus CNS abnormalities plus temperature > 40°C occurring once temperature regulation is overwhelmed. In athletes it occurs despite sweating (exertional heat stroke), but in sedentary elderly or frail people (classical heat stroke) it usually occurs after sweating stops. There is a risk of multi-organ failure from the combination of hyperthermia and an exaggerated acute-phase response. Once this response has started, temperature correction may not be enough to avert death.

Key clinical features are:

- CNS disturbances, including altered behaviour, delirium, convulsions
- dry skin (when sweating eventually fails)
- hypotension
- muscle rigidity, rhabdomyolysis
- coagulopathy, petechiae
- renal failure.

Diagnosis

Diagnosis is easy if a patient has been exercising in hot conditions, but the presentation may be more subtle. Refer to Table 32.2 for a list of situations that predispose to hyperthermia.

Table 32.2 Conditions predisposing to hyperthermia

Condition	Reason
Advanced age	Impaired adaptation/mobility
Infancy	Immature sweating
Cardiac disease/drugs	Unable to increase cardiac output
Dehydration/diuretics	Less circulating fluid
Anticholinergics/skin disease	Reduced sweating
High humidity	Reduced evaporative cooling
Hyperthyroidism/stimulant drugs	Increased heat production

As with hypothermia, surface temperature may not reflect core temperature. Tympanic infrared thermometers are technically capable of detecting high temperatures, but results may be unreliable due to technique. As with hypothermia, the diagnosis should be confirmed with a rectal probe if suspected.

Differential diagnosis

Temperature of > 40°C plus CNS dysfunction equals heat stroke unless an alternative diagnosis is evident. The most obvious alternative diagnosis is a febrile illness, particularly CNS infection. A more detailed list of differential diagnoses is found in Box 32.2.

Box 32.2 Differential diagnosis of heat stroke

- Meningitis/encephalitis
- Cerebral malaria
- Thyroid storm
- Anticholinergic poisoning
- Delirium tremens
- Neuroleptic malignant syndrome

Investigations

- FBE—WCC usually high
- BSL—usually high but give glucose if low
- Electrolytes
- Liver function tests (LFTs)
- CK to check for rhabdomyolysis

- Urine analysis to check for myoglobinuria
- Coagulation studies
- ECG
- CXR to check for aspiration, acute respiratory distress syndrome (ARDS)
- ABG

Management

Heat stroke is a medical emergency. If the diagnosis is suspected, commence treatment immediately.

1. **Cool the patient.** Remove clothing as far as modesty permits, place a fan at each end of the bed, and continuously spray the patient with water at room temperature (or warmer) using a misting device. This evaporative cooling is the most effective cooling mechanism. If the temptation to use ice is irresistible, try to confine it to strategic areas (groin and axilla). Aim to reduce the temperature to 39°C within 30 minutes. Stop cooling when 39°C is reached.
2. **Give oxygen.**
3. **Intubate** if hypoxic or unable to protect the airway.
4. **Give normal saline.** Marathon runners can have 1 L stat and 1 L in the first hour. Other patients should have half this. If BP and urine output are not restored, use CVP to monitor further replacement. Pulmonary oedema is a risk because of renal failure and cardiovascular compromise.
5. **Insert an IDC.** Monitor urine output. If myoglobinuria is present, alkalinise the urine with HCO_3^- and give mannitol.
6. Consider sedation. Use a benzodiazepine to sedate the patient if agitated or confused and to control seizures.
7. Do not use aspirin or paracetamol. In theory they will not work: aspirin will exacerbate bleeding and paracetamol will require metabolising by a deranged liver. In fact, pyrogenic cytokines have been implicated in heat stress, but there have been no controlled trials of antipyretics.
8. Consider chlorpromazine 25 mg IV injection if shivering is impeding cooling, but do not use it routinely because it may lower BP and impair sweating.
9. Use FFP and platelets if bleeding is a problem. Disseminated intravascular coagulation (DIC) may be present, but treatment with heparin is controversial. Coagulation defects should correct with time and cooling.

If symptoms and blood abnormalities do not correct with cooling, ICU admission will be required. Heat stroke has a significant mortality rate.

Pre-hospital considerations

Cooling, rest and fluids are the cornerstones of pre-hospital care. Fans and evaporative cooling are preferred for the frail elderly. Fun-runners and athletes can be put into an ice-slurry bath. Despite inducing vasoconstriction and shivering, this is effective and has been shown to be safe in young people.

MALIGNANT HYPERTHERMIA

This is a rare complication of anaesthesia that usually occurs soon after anaesthesia, but may be delayed up to 11 hours. Most anaesthetic agents (including suxamethonium/succinylcholine) can cause it. Temperature is 41–45°C. Treatment is similar to heat stroke but with the addition of dantrolene 2–3 mg/kg/day.

NEUROLEPTIC MALIGNANT SYNDROME

This is an idiosyncratic reaction occurring in about 0.2% of patients given neuroleptics. Haloperidol is the commonest offender. Dopamine receptor blockade leads to skeletal muscle spasticity (generating heat) and impaired hypothalamic regulation (interfering with response). The patient has a temperature of > 41°C plus muscle rigidity plus altered consciousness plus autonomic instability. Treatment is as for heat stroke. Both dantrolene and bromocriptine are thought to be helpful, although there have been no controlled trials.

Pearls and Pitfalls

- Rapid re-warming may be dangerous. 0.5–2°C per hour is enough.
- Bair Huggers are safe and effective, but generally not essential if the temperature is above 32°C.
- If the oxygen saturation monitor will not read because the finger is too cold, a digital block may help.
- Hypothermia interferes with the coagulation cascade, but coagulation tests will be normal when the blood is warmed in the lab. There is no need to order the test.
- The classic triad of heat stroke is hyperthermia plus neurological abnormalities plus dry skin.
- Aspirin and paracetamol will not lower the temperature in heat stroke.

Controversies

Will intubation precipitate ventricular fibrillation in the cold heart? There are isolated reports, but a multicentre study that collected 117 intubated hypothermic patients (Ann Emerg Med 1987;16:1042–55) showed no problems.

Online resources

Cardiac arrest in accidental hypothermia
http://circ.ahajournals.org/content/122/18_suppl_3/S829.full#sec-102
Cardiac arrest in avalanche victims
http://circ.ahajournals.org/content/122/18_suppl_3/S829.full#sec-108
Practical recommendations for heatstroke management
http://ccforum.com/content/11/3/R54

Chapter 33
Childhood emergencies

Gary J Browne, Nicholas Cheng and Bruce Fasher

The child in the emergency department presents a challenge to the busy emergency doctor, particularly in a setting where both adults and children are being treated and the general culture is not a paediatric one. Children are different in that they are dependent, developing and growing rapidly (see Table 33.4, later in the chapter). They also differ in their spectrum of disease and response to illness. The most common reasons children present to Australian EDs are:

- respiratory conditions (bronchiolitis, asthma, croup and other respiratory infections)
- gastroenteritis
- other febrile illnesses (viral and bacterial)
- trauma (the most common cause of death in children).

When faced with a paediatric case, keep in mind that you are managing both the child and the family. Parents/carers may perceive their children to be sicker than the staff assesses them to be. In many instances they may prove to be right! It is crucial for a successful consultation to listen to the parents and get a clear understanding of their concerns. At the same time, do not be dismissive of the child; involve him/her in your history taking as a prelude to examination. Parental anxiety and coping skills also need to be assessed and any social disadvantage noted. The relationship between the parent and the child should also be noted.

In all childhood emergencies, take a careful history and examine the whole child. A child can deteriorate rapidly. This must be anticipated. If there is any doubt about a child's condition, a paediatrician should be involved and, if a paediatric unit is not available on site, transfer to a paediatric hospital considered.

PAEDIATRIC PARAMETERS

In dealing with a sick child it is important to recognise how physiological parameters change with age and the impact that this may have on the interpretation of observations and management.

Respiratory and cardiovascular

Table 33.1 Normal respiratory rate and cardiovascular values

Age	Normal respiratory values (breaths/min)*	Normal cardiovascular values (beats/min)**
Infants	40	160
Preschool	30	140
School age	20	120

* Endotracheal tube size = (Age in years ÷ 4) + 4
** Blood volume = 80 mL/kg; systolic blood pressure = 80 mmHg + (Age in years × 2)

Weight

In ideal circumstances, a child should be weighed and the weight, height and head circumference plotted on appropriate growth charts. In emergencies, weight can be estimated using either a Breslow tape or simple formulae:

$$<10 \text{ years old: weight} = (\text{age in years} + 4) \times 2$$

$$10 \text{ years or over: weight} = 3 \times \text{age in years}$$

Immunisation in childhood

The ED offers an excellent chance to give catch-up immunisations. The recommended schedule (see Table 33.2) changes frequently and is listed in the current *Australian Immunisation Handbook* (readily available from the Commonwealth Department of Health and Aged Care, tel. 1800 671 811, or from the website http://immunise.health.gov.au/handbook.htm.). There are few contraindications.

Resuscitation

In the emergency situation, a child's condition can deteriorate very rapidly. This is due to:

- the dynamic and unpredictable responses a child can have to stress
- physiological limitations, e.g. hypoglycaemia is poorly tolerated
- anatomical differences, e.g. small airways and fatiguable respiratory muscles
- developmental differences, e.g. neonates and small children have immature immune systems
- ability or inability to communicate
- immature psychological responses, affecting communications and cooperation
- illness responses, e.g. meningitis may not produce neck stiffness.

Table 33.2 NSW immunisation schedule

Age	Disease	Vaccine
Childhood vaccines		
Birth (maternity units)	Hepatitis B	H-B-VAX II (babies before 8 days of age)
2 months (all vaccines may be given as early as 6 weeks)	Diphtheria, tetanus, pertussis (DTP) *Haemophilus influenzae* type B (Hib) Hepatitis B Polio	Infanrix hexa
	Pneumococcal	Prevenar 13
	Rotavirus	Rotarix
4 months	Diphtheria, tetanus, pertussis (DTP) *Haemophilus influenzae* type B (Hib) Hepatitis B Polio	Infanrix hexa
	Pneumococcal	Prevenar 13
	Rotavirus	Rotarix
6 months	Diphtheria, tetanus, pertussis (DTP) *Haemophilus influenzae* type B (Hib) Hepatitis B Polio	Infanrix hexa
	Pneumococcal	Prevenar 13
12 months*	Measles, mumps, rubella (MMR)	Priorix
	Haemophilus influenzae type B (Hib)	Hiberix
	Meningococcal C	Meningitec
18 months	Varicella (chickenpox)	Varilrix
4 years* (all vaccines may be given as early as 3½ years)	Diphtheria, tetanus, pertussis, polio	Infanrix IPV
	Measles, mumps, rubella (MMR)	Priorix

Continues overleaf

Table 33.2 NSW immunisation schedule continued

Age	Disease	Vaccine
Adolescent vaccines (school-based program)		
Year 7	Human papillomavirus	Gardasil
	Diphtheria, tetanus, pertussis (DTP)	Boostrix
	Hepatitis B (catch-up only)	H-B VAX II
	Varicella (catch-up only)	Varilrix
Year 9	Human papillomavirus (males only)	Gardasil
Adult vaccines		
All 6 months and over (with medical conditions predisposing to severe influenza#)	Influenza	Influenza
Aboriginal—15 years and over		
Pregnant women		
65 years and over		
All—65 years and over	Pneumococcal	Pneumovax 23
Aboriginal—50 years and over		
Aboriginal—15–49 years with medical risk factors†		

* Refer to the *Australian Immunisation Handbook* (10th edition) for the vaccination of children with underlying medical conditions.
\# Refer to the *Australian Immunisation Handbook* (10th ed), pp.252–4.
† Refer to the *Australian Immunisation Handbook* (10th ed), pp. 330–3.
Adapted from http://www.health.gov.au/internet/immunise/publishing.nsf/Content/EE1905BC65D40BCFCA257B26007FC8CA/$File/nip-schedule-card-hib-menc-update.pdf

There may also be a greater risk of acute deterioration in the following cases:

- neonates and small infants
- children with congenital or genetic disorders
- children with chronic disease
- immunodeficiency, as in a child undergoing chemotherapy.

The key to success in managing seriously ill children is early recognition. The outcome from paediatric cardiac arrest is extremely poor, as most children who arrest do so from progressive unrecognised hypoxia or through inadequate or inappropriate resuscitation.

When assessing children, attention should focus on the 3 major systems—respiratory, cardiovascular and central nervous system (CNS)—to identify the very sick child early.

RESPIRATORY

Increased breathing effort is a sign of increasing respiratory insufficiency and is characterised by tachypnoea, the use of accessory muscles, expiratory grunting, stridor, wheezing, nasal flare, dyspnoea and cyanosis. Other important but often forgotten signs of impending respiratory embarrassment in children are irritability/lethargy/obtundation, exhaustion and apnoea.

Monitor closely:

- respiratory rate
- effort of breathing
- colour
- mental state
- oxygen saturation using a pulse oximeter.

CARDIOVASCULAR

A child's haemodynamic status is assessed by examining pulses, capillary refill time, blood pressure, mental status and urine output. It must be remembered that in children the ability to compensate through vasoconstriction is strong; changes in blood pressure are always one of the last indicators of a decompensated haemodynamic state.

The signs of shock are:

- tachycardia/bradycardia
- decreased pulse volume
- poor peripheral perfusion (colour/mottling, temperature)
- abnormal mental state (see below)
- oliguria
- hypotension.

CNS

The level of consciousness in children may be impaired for many reasons. However, invariably in the seriously ill child it is due to hypoxia. Mental state change is one of the most consistent features of shock and generally occurs when cerebral perfusion is being compromised. Neurological assessment therefore involves the following checks.

1 Level of consciousness—the AVPU scale:
   A—Alert
   V—responds only to Vocal stimuli
   P—responds only to Painful stimuli
   U—Unresponsive
   Studies comparing the AVPU scale and the Glasgow Coma Scale (GCS) demonstrate that a response only to pain equates with a GCS of 9. Therefore, children unresponsive to painful stimuli are very likely to have difficulty with their airway and ventilation.
2 Pupils. Pupillary size, reaction to light and inequality need to be assessed. Fixed, dilated pupils are a sign of severe cerebral injury.
3 Posture. Tone and posture need to be assessed. Decorticate (flexed arms, extended legs) or decerebrate (extended arms, extended legs) posture indicates severe cerebral injury.

THE PRINCIPLES OF RESUSCITATION—ABCDE

These are similar in children and in adults (see Chapter 1). When CPR is performed in children, how it is performed is determined by the child's size and age (see Chapter 1, 'Cardiopulmonary resuscitation').

A—airway

In children the goals are to recognise and relieve obstruction, to prevent aspiration and to allow adequate oxygenation. This can be done via the same manoeuvres and types of equipment that are available to adults, using the appropriate size for the child's age and weight. Intubation of a child requires knowledge of the different anatomy of the child's airway and thus the variations in technique for this intervention.

B—breathing

If breathing is laboured or poor in children, it should be supported with either a bag–valve–mask device or through intubation with mechanical ventilation. Remember that children are more susceptible to barotrauma than adults.

C—circulation

The rate-limiting step in many resuscitative efforts in children is achieving IV access. If unsuccessful after an initial attempt, an intraosseous (IO) line should be promptly attempted. An initial fluid bolus to resuscitate a shocked child is 20 mL/kg of isotonic crystalloid solution (normal saline or Hartmann's solution).

D—disability

A decreased level of consciousness may be an indication of a primary airway, breathing or circulatory problem, or a primary neurological problem. In either case, supporting the airway, breathing and circulation is the most appropriate way to stabilise a neurological problem.

Hypoglycaemia is a problem especially in the young child, and should be tested for and treated vigorously.

Drugs

When using drugs in resuscitation in children, it is important to be aware that their effect depends on:

- appropriate dosage on a weight-determined basis
- how they are delivered, e.g. diluted or undiluted
- the route of administration, e.g. IV, endotracheal, rectal
- how they are absorbed and metabolised, e.g. endotracheal adrenaline
- whether there are any unwanted effects in children, e.g. verapamil may precipitate asystole in infants.

E—environment

In children it is important to consider hypothermia, hypoglycaemia and other reversible causes early in the process of resuscitation.

Identifying the sick child

Identifying the sick child can be difficult even for experienced staff. The younger the child, the more difficult it can be, particularly when trying to exclude focal bacterial infections. The following guidelines provide a useful approach to detecting serious illness in the child < 36 months of age.

- Single signs are not as useful as considering the full complement of symptoms and signs, and may be misleading; combinations of serious symptoms are very concerning. Similarly, repeated assessment of children over time during a period of observation is more useful than a single evaluation. No child should be sent home from the ED without having had a thorough assessment, appropriate investigations and preferably a period of observation.
- Other features of concern include fever, apnoea, convulsions, a petechial rash, cyanosis and the rapid onset of symptoms. Antibiotic use, prolonged symptoms and chronic illness are important features to note. Do not ignore the signs of bile-stained vomiting or blood in the stools, alone or in the presence of abdominal pain.

Airway emergencies

CROUP

- Croup is a viral laryngotracheobronchitis characterised by a barking cough. Often several days of upper respiratory tract symptoms (coryza) precede the cough. The associated respiratory distress is worse at night and with anxiety in the child or parent. Spasmodic croup occurs without accompanying infective symptoms and is often recurrent.
- Stridor at rest is an indication of severity sufficient to warrant acute assessment and treatment, while cyanosis is a pre-arrest state. Lateral airways X-rays are not needed and are dangerous as the child is unstable.
- A calming environment with the child on the mother's lap is therapeutic.
- If there is moderate or severe airway obstruction, most commonly manifesting as stridor at rest, nebulised adrenaline (0.5 mL/kg of 1:1000, maximum 5 mL) can be used as a temporising measure. Oral dexamethasone (0.15 mg/kg) or prednisolone (1 mg/kg) reduces the risk of intubation and in moderate cases may allow the child to be discharged with review arranged. If this is not tolerated, IV/IM dexamethasone 0.6 mg/kg as a single dose or nebulised budesonide 2 mg can be given.
- Attention to hydration of the child with croup is important.
- All children should be observed for at least 4 hours to ensure there is no rebound following the dose of adrenaline. This is unlikely to occur if steroids are administered early. It is often wise to admit these children overnight. However, if a child has no stridor after a period of observation and it appears safe to do so (e.g. the home environment is supportive of home observation with the ability to enact a prompt return/summon an ambulance if the child deteriorates), then discharge home with follow-up the next day is possible.

BACTERIAL TRACHEITIS

- This is a rare infection presenting similarly to croup, with acute upper airway compromise. Usually the child appears toxic. The disease is usually rapidly progressive over hours and the child drools, is unable to phonate and assumes the 'sniffing the air' position to maximise the airway calibre. Cyanosis is a late, pre-arrest state.

- **Epiglottitis** is a severe bacterial infection of the epiglottis very rarely encountered in present times due to *Haemophilus influenzae* immunisation.
- Interventions should be avoided unless the child is pre-arrest. The initial treatment is rapid transfer to the operating suite for administration of an inhalational anaesthetic and intubation. If there is doubt about the condition, this can be diagnostic.
- If a respiratory arrest occurs before an inhalational anaesthetic is available, bag-and-mask ventilation, intubation with sedation only or needle cricothyroidotomy is needed.
- Muscle relaxants must not be used with the anaesthetic or the airway will be lost.
- Once the airway is controlled, take a swab and commence IV 3rd-generation cefalosporins.

FOREIGN-BODY INHALATION

This causes an acute onset of respiratory distress, often in a child aged between 6 months and 2 years. If the object is in the upper airway, complete or partial obstruction may be present.

- If the child is moving air or coughing, removal under inhalational anaesthetic by skilled personnel is advisable.
- If the airway is completely obstructed, rapid back-blows in an infant or the Heimlich manoeuvre in an older child should be performed. Direct visualisation and removal of the object with Magill's forceps may be possible. If this is not successful, a needle cricothyroidotomy should be performed.

WHAT ELSE COULD IT BE?

- Peritonsillar or retropharyngeal abscess
- Anaphylaxis

Respiratory emergencies

ASTHMA

Asthma in childhood is a common condition.

- Signs of respiratory distress indicating severity include tachypnoea, intercostal recession, use of accessory muscles, prolonged expiration, cyanosis and altered level of consciousness.
- Exacerbations are treated with salbutamol, initially with spacers or nebulised if moderately severe bronchospasm or worse prevents adequate inspiration. In severe cases, IV salbutamol

initially as a bolus, or an infusion if improvement is not maintained, enables stabilisation. Except in mild cases nebulised ipratropium bromide is also given.

- A short course of oral steroids for 3–5 days is given; by the IV route in severely ill patients.
- Respiratory support with either continuous positive airway pressure (CPAP) or intubation, often with assistance with expiration, is needed with apnoea or altered level of consciousness. There is a high attendant risk of barotrauma. Inhalational anaesthetics can also be used as bronchodilators.
- Long-term preventative therapy aims to reduce the incidence and severity of exacerbations, inhaled steroids such as fluticasone or ciclesonide or a fluticasone + salmetrol combination such as Seretide in more difficult cases.

PNEUMONIA

This also presents with respiratory distress. Auscultatory signs may be subtle, especially in the younger child, and an X-ray may be needed to confirm the diagnosis. Some children may present misleadingly with abdominal pain. Treatment is with antibiotics, either oral or IV.

Common organisms causing pneumonia include:

- bacterial—*Streptococcus pneumoniae, Staphylococcus aureus* (in those aged < 5 years), *Mycoplasma pneumonia* (> 3 years)
- viral—parainfluenza, influenza, respiratory syncytial virus (RSV), Epstein–Barr virus (EBV).

BRONCHIOLITIS

Viral bronchiolitis of infancy is a lower respiratory tract infection which produces small-airway obstruction with air trapping and respiratory difficulty.

- Bronchiolitis occurs particularly in children aged 2–6 months, and is caused by RSV in 90% of infants. After 1–2 days of coryza, increasing respiratory distress with tachypnoea, nasal flaring, wheezing and fever is seen and lasts from several days to > 1 week. There may be apnoea (especially in neonates or young infants) or difficulty feeding, requiring IV hydration. Chest X-ray is normal or shows hyperinflated lungs with peribronchial cuffing in approximately 50% of cases.
- Treatment involves supplemental oxygen, if required, aiming at > 94% saturation during the acute phase. During recovery, accept 90–92% if not distressed and feeding well. Use

humidification where possible. In those infants with severe respiratory distress, the use of humidified high-flow oxygen via nasal prongs to deliver positive airway pressure may make them more comfortable. For infants having or potentially likely to develop apnoea, non-invasive ventilation should be considered. They will need early high-dependency/ICU referral.
- Feed infants with mild disease normally; reserve intragastric feeds for the recovery phase. Use IV fluids if the infant is in severe respiratory distress.
- Bronchodilators and steroids are of no proven benefit, but a trial of bronchodilators may be warranted in the older infant.
- Patients who are discharged need early review by their local doctor.

Pertussis is associated with spasms of coughing (paroxysmal coughing), an inspiratory whoop in older children, which is frequently followed by a vomit. Apnoea may be the only symptom in the infant < 3 months old. Between coughing paroxysms the child is often asymptomatic. There is often a leucocytosis of 20,000–50,000 with a predominance of lymphocytes. Chest X-rays are usually normal. Treat with oxygen during spasms, IV rehydration if necessary and erythromycin if the patient is in the early phase or for prophylaxis of contacts.

Cystic fibrosis patients commonly present with respiratory decompensation related to infection. Diagnosis is almost always made from the newborn screening heel-prick blood test; undiagnosed new cases are very rare. Patients have a chronic cough and purulent sputum, and benefit from chest physiotherapy and IV antibiotics.

The unconscious child

Remember that the brain is more commonly the target of insult than the primary cause. Always consider and treat those conditions that are correctable, such as hypoxia and hypoglycaemia. Always examine the whole child in the light of a thorough history where possible.

IMMEDIATELY

- Administer oxygen via face mask at 4–6 L/minute.
- Support and maintain the airway.
  - If trauma is likely, take appropriate precautions to stabilise the cervical spine.

  - If the airway is unmaintainable, consider repositioning and jaw thrust.
  - Suction the oropharynx if this is available.
  - Insert an oral airway.
  - Intubation: this can be performed cold in the deeply unconscious child, or the rapid-sequence induction (RSI) technique may be utilised if the child is only lightly unconscious.
- Support ventilation if inadequate or impaired.
- If the circulation is compromised:
  - establish IV access (IO access may be necessary)
  - give a bolus of isotonic crystalloid: 20 mL/kg.
- Reassess the child regularly.
- Check blood glucose.

LOOK FOR

- Rashes (especially petechiae)
- Fever or hypothermia
- Evidence of head injury
- High or low blood glucose
- Blood pressure abnormalities
- State of hydration
- Evidence of raised intracranial pressure
- Abnormal neurological signs

ASK ABOUT

- Events prior to the child's presentation
- Past medical history
- Medication the child may be taking or may have been exposed to
- Specifically, accidental ingestion, diabetes, whether there has been a convulsion

MANAGEMENT

- After initial stabilisation, consider the need for airway protection.
- Check a glucose stick, and if low administer 5 mL/kg 10% dextrose solution.
- Consider poisoning and antidotes, e.g. naloxone, flumazenil.
- Consider sepsis and administer antibiotics if necessary.
- Consider dexamethasone 0.6 mg/kg before antibiotics if meningitis is likely.
- Consider adding aciclovir 10 mg/kg if encephalitis is likely.

INVESTIGATIONS TO BE CONSIDERED

- Full blood count
- Blood culture
- Formal blood glucose
- Electrolytes and urea
- Urine for glucose, ketones and drug assay
- Lumbar puncture if meningitis is considered and no evidence of raised intracranial pressure exists and patient is not obtunded
- Chest X-ray
- CT scan of the head if focal neurological signs are present

MONITOR CLOSELY

- Level of consciousness
- Respiratory rate, oxygen saturation
- Perfusion, blood pressure, heart rate
- Urine output, temperature.

Re-evaluate and reassess regularly.

The febrile child

Fever is one of the most common causes of presentation to an ED. Most fevers are due to viral infections, but care must be taken to exclude a bacterial infection.

- Diagnosis can often be difficult, particularly in the younger child. The febrile child without a clear focus presents a real challenge.
- In children who are fully immunised the risk of serious bacterial infection is low, although pneumococcal and meningococcal infection are incompletely covered and should always be considered in any child who is unwell.
- Various approaches are advised in the literature, ranging from cautious assessment and observation through to aggressive management (see Figure 33.1, below).

When dealing with children suspected of having an infectious disease, it is essential that infection-control measures are implemented to prevent cross-contamination and spread. Hand-washing is important in all situations. Isolation may be required (e.g. varicella, meningococcal disease and measles).

Note that:

1. Fever is the body's natural response to infection. It enhances the child's immunological defences against infection. However, parents/carers are often fearful of fever and will need reassurance and explanation.

2. The most important part of managing fever is to seek the underlying cause, especially in infants.
3. Children with fever are often unsettled and miserable. They may have discomfort and/or pain from the fever or from the cause of the fever. Commonly used antipyretic/analgesic drugs may relieve these symptoms.
4. Febrile convulsions are a common manifestation of fever (3% of children experience a febrile convulsion). Simple febrile convulsions are not harmful to the brain and do not necessarily indicate epilepsy (see below).

The response to antipyretics is independent of whether the illness is due to bacterial or viral infection. It should *not* be used as a diagnostic tool to try to differentiate bacterial from viral infection. Although temperatures in febrile children fluctuate and may be modified by antipyretics and the technique of measurement, children with higher temperatures are more likely to have a serious focus.

Factors to consider when assessing a febrile child:

- the age of the child
- signs of toxicity (sepsis)
- symptoms and signs of a focus of infection (respiratory, meningitis, urinary tract, ears/throat).

Neonates and young infants may not have the characteristic signs of serious infection (the temperature can be high or low), and localising features may be absent. They can deteriorate rapidly. They may be infected with organisms from the birth canal, especially group B streptococcal organisms; a history of maternal group B streptococcal colonisation and the subsequent administration of antibiotics during labour should be sought.

Young infants with fever, especially those under 3 months of age, need rapid assessment, investigation and admission to hospital. Consult a senior colleague about the extent of investigations (full blood count, cultures of blood, urine and CSF, chest X-ray) and the administration of antibiotics.

Older infants/toddlers localise infection better than neonates, but may still be pre-verbal. They are frequently exposed to infectious diseases in group childcare and get viral infections. The incidence of previously 'typical' bacterial infections (*Pneumococcus*, *Meningococcus* and *H. influenzae*) infections has been significantly lessened by immunisation.

IS THE CHILD TOXIC?

'Toxicity' is a term used to describe the clinical picture produced by the body's response to exotoxins and endotoxins (the lipopolysaccharide cell wall of Gram-negative organisms). It is often difficult to detect. The best approach to evaluating a child for toxicity is to use the ABCD approach:

A Arousal, Alertness and Activity
B Breathing difficulties
C poor Colour (pale/mottled) and poor Circulation (cold peripheries)
D Decreased fluid intake (less than half normal) and Decreased urine output (fewer than 4 wet nappies a day).

Abnormality of any of these signs places the child at higher risk of serious bacterial illness. The presence of more than 1 sign increases the risk.

It is much better to use the term 'toxic' than to describe a febrile child as being 'sick' or 'not sick'. In particular, there is the risk of a parent overhearing these terms and misinterpreting them as a dismissal of their concerns over their child who might have a viral illness, generating a negative reaction from the parent.

INVESTIGATIONS

The decision whether or not to perform investigations is not always simple, but generally depends on the child's age and the clinical presentation. A complete set of investigations, the so-called 'full septic work-up', includes a full blood count, blood culture, chest X-ray, urine microscopy and culture, and lumbar puncture.

- All children who are toxic with a potential for underlying serious bacterial infection should have a full septic work-up, as should very young children, especially those < 3 months of age.
  - Another group of children where investigations should be considered are those where there is the possibility of meningitis or where the child is on antibiotics and may have partially treated meningitis.
  - In all cases ensure appropriate observation, review and, if in doubt, seek further consultation.
  - The dilemma of when and where to treat and which antibiotic to use depends upon the individual and the local environment. It is better to err on the side of over-investigating and treating, particularly when infants are involved.

- Children with a definite focus of infection should have specific investigations of that focus unless they are very young or toxic. Very young and toxic children require empirical antibiotics and a full septic work-up, in that order. Remember, in some conditions such as meningococcaemia, delay in the administration of antibiotics may result in a poor clinical outcome.
- The most common cause of serious bacterial illness in infants is urinary tract infection and if the child is toxic, consider the possibility of underlying pyelonephritis. An ultrasound examination of the kidneys may be very useful in making the diagnosis and directing treatment.

TREATMENT

Figure 33.1 outlines one possible approach to management of the febrile child. Any child who is toxic requires urgent resuscitation (see 'Resuscitation' section, above). In particular, they are at risk of septic shock and require urgent attention to prevent circulatory collapse. This involves rapid IV or IO access, the delivery of boluses of normal saline or another isotonic crystalloid solution such as Hartmann's solution and perhaps inotropic support. In such cases, urgent consultation with paediatric specialists and intensivists should be obtained. The child should ultimately be transferred to a facility appropriate to deal with the situation.

Antibiotic choice depends on your patient population and local resistance rates. The antibiotics listed in Table 33.3 overleaf are suggested only as a starting point; we strongly recommend you discuss this with a senior colleague, paediatrician or infectious disease consultant.

WHAT ELSE COULD IT BE?

Always think of underlying metabolic, cardiac and endocrine problems. The fever may be the simple harbinger of acute deterioration in these patients (a simple viral illness causing the underlying metabolic problem to become unstable).

PROLONGED FEVER OF UNKNOWN ORIGIN

Most children in whom fever has been prolonged for 7 days or more will be found to have infectious diseases. The most common infection to consider is Epstein–Barr virus infection; however, other viruses may be found as the cause for fever. Autoimmune disorders, Kawasaki disease and malignancy should be considered. In these cases early consultation and hospital admission should be considered.

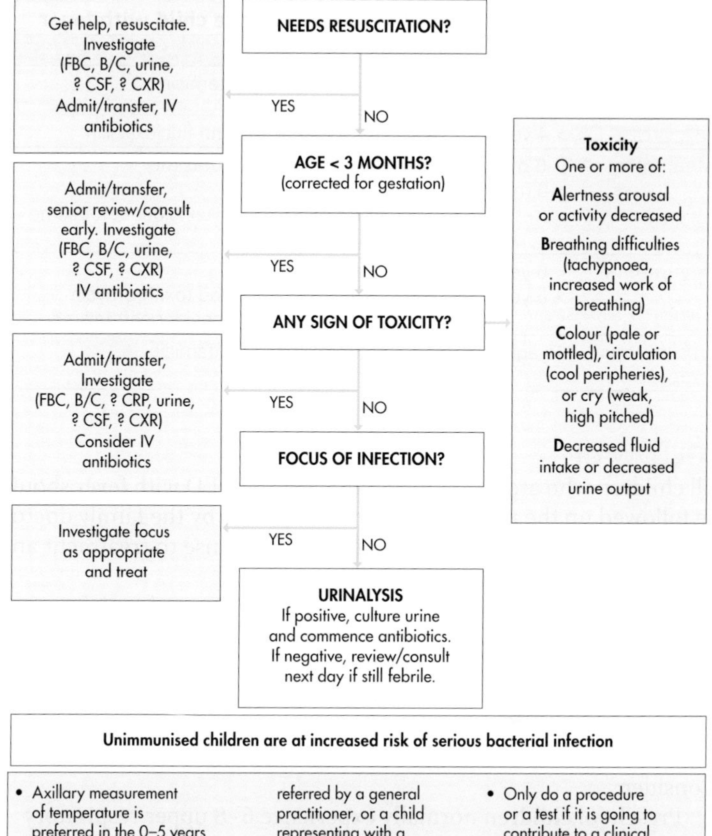

Unimmunised children are at increased risk of serious bacterial infection

- Axillary measurement of temperature is preferred in the 0–5 years age group
- Oral and rectal measurements are not recommended because of safety concerns
- Tympanic measurements may be inaccurate
- When in doubt, ask for advice. No febrile child should be discharged from an Emergency Department without senior advice, particularly a child referred by a general practitioner, or a child representing with a febrile illness
- At discharge the patient(s) should be educated on the detection and significance of toxicity, arrangements made for review and a Fever Fact sheet and discharge summary provided
- Err on the side of caution. If you are worried, admit/transfer the child
- Only do a procedure or a test if it is going to contribute to a clinical decision. Use the flowchart to work out what tests you need. If in doubt about a child's clinical condition, consult with someone more experienced such as a paediatric specialist. If a specialist is not available, call NETS (the Newborn and paediatric Emergency Transport Service) on 1300 36 2500

Figure 33.1 An approach to the febrile child < 5 years old

B/C, blood culture; CSF, cerebrospinal fluid; CXR, chest X-ray; FBC, full blood count; IV; intravenous

From NSW Health Clinical Practice Guidelines—Infants and children: acute management of fever, 2ed, p. 6. Issued October 2010.

Table 33.3 Initial choice of antibiotics in the child with fever

Condition	Age	Antibiotic
Fever with no focus	0–3 months 4 months–4 years > 4 years	Penicillin and gentamicin Benzyl penicillin Benzyl penicillin and flucloxacillin
Meningitis	0–6 months > 6 months	Ampicillin and cefotaxime Cefotaxime If *Pneumococcus*, consider cefotaxime and vancomycin
Pneumonia	< 6 years > 6 years	Benzyl penicillin Benzyl penicillin and roxithromycin In severe cases consider cefotaxime
Urinary tract infection	All ages	Ampicillin and gentamicin

FOLLOW-UP

All children who are discharged home from the ED with fever should be followed up the next day, either in the ED or by the family doctor. This is to detect progression of infection, response to treatment and results of investigations.

Parents should be encouraged to look for signs of toxicity every 4–6 hours, and to seek clinical review if the child becomes toxic or unwell. Clear communication from a doctor with empathy for the parents may enhance safety and improve the functioning of stressed families.

Common infections

Consider:

- Preschool children normally experience 6–8 upper respiratory tract infections (URTIs) per annum.
- Antibiotics neither cure viral URTIs nor prevent complications.
- Exclude common and dangerous causes:
  - otitis media
  - tonsillitis
  - bronchiolitis
  - pneumonia
  - meningitis
  - urinary tract infection.
- Decongestants and antihistamines are of dubious value.
- Take an immunisation history.
- Paediatric symptoms are often non-specific—fever, diarrhoea, off feeds, etc.

The common exanthemata (measles, rubella/German measles, varicella, scarlet fever, erythema infectiosum and roseola infantum) are not always easy to diagnose, and have significant morbidity and mortality. You should be familiar with the classical presentations. If in doubt, consult.

The use of **paracetamol** in febrile illnesses is controversial (fever has an active role in the anti-infection cascade). Vigorous control of fever will not necessarily prevent febrile convulsions. Fever control may be of assistance in a child who is in obvious discomfort in whom the fever exceeds 38.5°C (> 38.0°C axillary). Be cautious in your prescribing. Occasionally you may use doses of paracetamol of up to 15 mg/kg, but mostly 10 mg/kg 6-hourly is adequate. Remember there is a real risk of hepatotoxicity, so limit the daily dosage to 60 mg/kg (maximum 3 g/day) and do not use for more than 72 hours. If fever is persistent, the child should be reassessed.

Aspirin for the management of fever is contraindicated in childhood.

Convulsions

The most common seizures encountered in children are simple febrile convulsions. However, there are a number of other causes of seizures; in these cases there is an urgent need to attempt to identify and treat the cause.

UNCOMPLICATED FEBRILE CONVULSIONS

Uncomplicated febrile convulsions have the following characteristics:

- age 6 months to 5 years
- onset as fever rapidly rises to temperatures > 38.5°C
- generalised (not focal)
- short duration, less than 15 minutes
- single, isolated seizure in a 24-hour period
- no neurological sequelae (residual weakness or persistent decrease in level of consciousness)
- normal neurological development.

Siblings of children with febrile convulsions have an approximately 10% risk of also suffering a febrile convulsion. This risk increases to almost 50% if there is a parent with a family history. The genetics of this association are not known.

Subsequent to the recovery, children with febrile convulsions have a normal EEG and other investigations. They have an increased chance of further febrile convulsions up until approximately their fifth birthday. There is a small increase in their baseline risk of eventually suffering epilepsy; this is not due to the febrile convulsion itself. No effect on intelligence has been demonstrated.

There are a number of differentials to febrile convulsions, including:
- true afebrile convulsions, with their various individual aetiologies (see below)
- breath-holding attacks (which may be followed by a generalised seizure)
- syncope
- dystonic reactions (in particular as a reaction to various antiemetics)
- pseudoseizures (to be considered a diagnosis of exclusion).

General management

- If the seizure is continuing, triage to the resuscitation bay or similar area
- Maintain the airway
- Give oxygen
- Obtain IV access

Aborting the convulsion

- Remember, most febrile convulsions do not continue for more than 1 minute. However, most clinicians will attempt to abort a febrile seizure after a few minutes. In afebrile seizures, aborting the seizure is more urgent.
- Midazolam 0.15 mg/kg/dose, either IV or IM; repeat every 5 minutes as needed (beware of airway and breathing compromise). Alternatively, diazepam 0.2 mg/kg IV can be considered. Do not give diazepam IM.
- Buccal/intranasal midazolam (maximum buccal dose 10 mg) can be used (or rectal diazepam). Note that the IV preparation is used.
- If a prolonged seizure or status epilepticus develops (seizure lasting more than 30 minutes or multiple seizures without full recovery between events), consider:
  - > 3 months old: phenytoin 15–20 mg/kg IV over 20 minutes (cardiac monitor), then 3 mg/kg IV 6-hourly
  - < 3 months old: phenobarbitone 20 mg/kg diluted in normal saline or dextrose over 20 minutes (500 mg maximum), then 5 mg/kg/day 8-hourly.

Consider treatable causes—urgent

- Hypoglycaemia
- Herpes simplex encephalitis (focal seizure, cold-sores)
- Electrolyte disturbance (especially sodium—persistent vomiting and diarrhoea)
- Meningitis
- Trauma (accidental or non-accidental), possibly leading to intracranial haemorrhage.

Above all, listen to parents (previous management, treatable causes, etc). Recognise that they may experience significant distress, especially if this is the first seizure they have witnessed, and provide support.

Gastroenteritis

Gastroenteritis is a common childhood complaint, the commonest complication of which is dehydration. Most cases will be viral. Bloody diarrhoea often suggests a bacterial cause.

Organisms to consider include:

- viruses—rotavirus, enteroviruses, enteric adenovirus, norovirus
- bacteria—*Salmonella, Shigella, Campylobacter, Yersinia, Escherichia coli*
- protozoa—*Giardia*, amoebae.

Clinical manifestations include vomiting, diarrhoea, fever and abdominal pain. The diarrhoea with rotavirus and adenoviruses often lasts for 5–12 days, and that of bacterial diarrhoea (especially *Campylobacter*) is often bloodstained. *Giardia* infection commonly causes an epidemic and is complicated by asymptomatic carriers. Beware of attributing vomiting without diarrhoea to gastroenteritis.

ASSESSMENT

- Assessment should include (1) confirmation of the diagnosis and exclusion of differential diagnoses, and (2) determination of the degree of dehydration.
- Evidence of sepsis is important, especially in the young infant. Of children under 3 months of age with *Salmonella* infection, 5–10% are bacteraemic. *Salmonella* can also cause focal infections in children with sickle-cell anaemia.
- Abdominal X-ray commonly shows multiple fluid levels representing ileus: it is rarely helpful unless obstruction is suspected.
- Stool culture is advisable when bacterial or parasitic infections are suspected.

Signs of dehydration

Signs of dehydration can become more evident with the extent of fluid imbalance, but are altered in hypernatraemia. Percentages of fluid loss give a guide to the rate at which fluids need to be given, but frequent reassessment of the child's fluid state is vital.

- Mild dehydration:
  - 3% dehydration manifests with reduced urine output and thirst but no clinical signs.
- Moderate dehydration
  - 5% presents with sunken eyes, dry mucous membranes and reduced skin turgor.
  - 7% manifests with a more severe presentation of the above signs and irritability, lethargy and tachycardia.
- Severe dehydration
  - 10% presents with marked lethargy, irritability and even coma, plus cardiovascular compromise with tachycardia, hypotension, coldness and sweating.

These signs are difficult to appreciate at times and even experienced clinicians are only able to determine mild/moderate/severe dehydration rather than percentages. Accurate weights (performed on the same set of scales without the contribution of clothing/nappies) are accurate but rarely available.

What else could it be?

- Surgical conditions:
  - intussusception
  - appendicitis.
- Infections
  - urinary tract infection
  - sepsis, otitis media.
- Haemolytic uraemic syndrome; an uncommon condition presenting usually 5–10 days after gastroenteritis, caused by enteropathic *E. coli.* It can also occur after upper respiratory tract infection. It is manifest by microangiopathic haemolysis, low platelets, raised urea, poor urine output, hypertension and renal failure.
- Diabetic ketoacidosis.
- Metabolic disorders.
- Head injury (raised intracranial pressure).

TREATMENT OF GASTROENTERITIS

- **Rehydration** via the oral route is the best route to provide fluids for children. Try oral rehydration solution in small frequent sips at a rate of 1 mL/kg every 10 minutes. Dispensing by oral syringe is often effective where a child does not wish to drink. Oral rehydration ice preparations are available and may be more readily accepted by children.
  - Ondansetron has been demonstrated to decrease the chance of vomiting with rehydration in mild gastroenteritis. A single dose may be given as a therapeutic trial. Other antiemetics are contraindicated, especially in small children, due to the risk of a dystonic reaction.
- If the above fails, commence nasogastric tube rehydration with an oral rehydration solution. If this is not tolerated, commence IV rehydration, remembering to check the glucose and sodium levels. Volumes to replace the fluid deficit and volumes for maintenance requirements should be calculated separately, added together, then divided by 24 to get the hourly rate (see below).
- Frequent reassessment to monitor progress is important.
- **Antibiotics** (3rd-generation cefalosporins) are recommended for *Salmonella* in the young septic infant, or one with a prolonged, severe course of illness. Otherwise they do not convey any benefit, as they do not shorten the course or reduce the infectivity of the patient with *Salmonella*.
  Campylobacter infection should be treated with erythromycin only if the symptoms are prolonged.
  Giardia infection causing symptoms should be treated with metronidazole.

When not to treat at home

- Dehydration
- Diagnosis in doubt
- Family not coping
- Persistent vomiting
- No consultation available
- Deterioration
- Anticipated deterioration

Think again if

- Vomiting bile or blood
- Severe abdominal pain
- Toxic, high fever

- Abdominal signs: distension; tenderness, guarding; mass, visceromegaly
- Neonates
- Failure to thrive

Fluid therapy

Children can rapidly become dehydrated because of their small size and large, insensible fluid loss (they have a high surface area to volume ratio). The aim of fluid therapy is to continue maintenance fluid intake and replace fluid in the dehydrated child. Common causes of fluid loss are gastroenteritis, fever, blood loss and poor oral intake in respiratory distress.

MAINTENANCE FLUIDS

- Maintenance fluids can be estimated using:
  - 100 mL/kg for the first 10 kg
  - 50 mL/kg for the next 10 kg
  - 20 mL/kg for every subsequent kg.
- Maintenance fluids should be 0.45% saline + 2.5% dextrose (for neonates 0.45% saline + 5% dextrose or more).
- Potassium requirements of 2–3 mmol/kg/day should also be met, provided normal renal function is present.

Rehydration

Acute resuscitation of the child with cardiovascular compromise (i.e. shock) should include a bolus of fluid, 20 mL/kg of crystalloid such as normal saline or Hartmann's solution. Hypotonic solutions such as half normal (0.45%) and quarter normal (0.225%) saline should not be used for resuscitation.

The volume required to replace the fluid deficit can be estimated using:

$$\% \text{ dehydration} \times \text{weight (in kg)} \times 10 = \text{volume required (in mL)}$$

Once shock has been addressed, rehydration can commence in a slower, controlled fashion. More sodium is needed in rehydration replacement fluid than in maintenance therapy, so 0.45% saline + 2.5% dextrose is used. This should be administered over 24 hours and regularly reviewed to allow for further losses to be replaced.

In the case of hypernatraemia, slower rehydration over 48–72 hours is essential to avoid severe neurological complications. The only exception to this rule is if hypernatraemic seizures occur.

Remember:

- Decreased oral intake or vomiting may rapidly lead to dehydration in a child.
- Serum electrolytes, urea and creatinine should be checked if rehydrating intravenously.
- Rehydrate slowly in hypernatraemia.
- Reassess the child clinically and monitor the urine output to see if the fluid therapy is appropriate.
- If no improvement, consider repeating electrolytes and an alternative diagnosis.

Diabetic ketoacidosis and hypoglycaemia

These are not uncommon problems, but are best managed in a children's centre experienced in such specialised care; hence early referral is recommended.

Children with diabetic ketoacidosis (DKA) at diagnosis of their diabetes have often been unwell for 4–6 weeks with progressive weight loss, dehydration and altered mental state. Because of this, mistakes in diagnosis can be made early in the acute phase.

DIABETIC KETOACIDOSIS

Presentation

- Polyuria
- Polydipsia
- Weight loss
- Dehydration
- Altered mental state

Beware of the following common misdiagnoses:

- chest infection: rapid breathing due to metabolic acidosis
- urinary tract infection: polyuria (always check urine for glucose and ketones)
- gastroenteritis: dehydration
- enuresis: polyuria (always check urine for glucose and ketones).

Always take a thorough history and completely examine the child.

Management

1. If child is shocked, ensure adequate airway and ventilation while administering high-flow oxygen via a face mask. Administer 20 mL/kg of 0.9% saline rapidly and then reassess the child's haemodynamic status.
   Note: This should be reserved for children in shock; remember,

children are at risk of cerebral oedema if fluid resuscitation is too aggressive.

Then:

2 Assess the degree of dehydration.
3 Commence replacing water and sodium with 0.9% saline and aim to correct over 48 hours (not 24 hours). *Be careful not to give too much fluid too soon,* as children are prone to developing cerebral oedema.
4 Add potassium to rehydration fluids 5 mmol/kg/day once urine has been passed.
5 After rehydration has commenced, commence insulin infusion at a rate of 0.05 units/kg/h, aiming to lower blood glucose 4–5 mmol/L/h. A larger drop in the first hour is acceptable, as fluid alone would lower the blood glucose to some extent.
6 When the blood glucose falls below 12 mmol/L, change IV fluid to 0.45% saline and 5% dextrose. Maintain the blood glucose level between 5 and 10 mmol/L. If blood glucose falls below 5 mmol/L, do not decrease the insulin infusion but rather increase the amount of glucose in the infusion.
7 Strict fluid balance is essential.

Investigations

- Collect venous blood for:
  - glucose
  - sodium, potassium, chloride, urea, creatinine
  - pH, PCO_2, HCO_3^-, base deficit
  - full blood count.
- Test all urine for glucose and ketones.

Monitor closely

- Hourly to 2-hourly formal glucose, potassium, sodium
- Hourly pulse rate, respiratory rate, blood pressure, blood glucose and neurological observation
- Accurate fluid balance
- All urine for ketones until clear

Cerebral oedema/brainstem herniation

Brainstem herniation is a sudden and unpredictable complication of therapy for DKA; it occurs during the first 24 hours of treatment. Monitor all patients for evidence of raised intracranial pressure, with particular attention to those most at risk:

- severe dehydration

- severe acidosis with low potassium
- hypernatraemia
- deteriorating conscious state
- severe hyperosmolality on presentation (> 320 mOsm/L).

The onset of headache should be taken seriously.

Transfer to an ICU and arrange neurological assessment and CT head scan, provided the patient is stable enough. Management should be aimed at aggressively controlling any elevation in intracranial pressure. Urgent expert consultation should be sought.

HYPOGLYCAEMIA

Blood glucose levels of < 2.5 mmol/L. In diabetic children, hypoglycaemic symptoms often occur at blood glucose levels < 3 mmol/L. Prolonged hypoglycaemia can cause irreversible brain damage.

In children, substrate deficiency is the most common cause, either as a result of prolonged fasting or gastroenteritis or due to specific conditions such as ketotic hypoglycaemia. Young children in particular may be unable to mobilise adequate glycogen stores under acute stress conditions. Other important causes include hepatic disorders, metabolic disorders and, rarely, insulin excess (Beckwith syndrome, nesidioblastosis).

Presentation

- Anxiety, irritability, flushing
- Nausea/vomiting
- Pallor
- Sweating
- Trembling, weakness
- Tachycardia
- Confusion, drowsiness or coma

Investigations

- Blood glucose
- Sodium, potassium, urea, creatinine.

After consultation, further special tests may be necessary: alanine, cortisol, growth hormone, amino acids, free fatty acids, ammonia, etc.

Management

1. Resuscitate as necessary.
2. Check blood glucose, draw blood for investigations.
3. In some cases where a child is awake and cooperative, oral glucose drinks/sweets may be satisfactory. However, if there is

any doubt administer a glucose bolus 0.5 g/kg as 5 mL/kg 10% glucose or 2 mL/kg 25% glucose IV if patient is symptomatic and the blood glucose is < 2.5 mmol/L. After recovery, if necessary continue a 10% glucose infusion at maintenance rate.
If unable to secure IV access, glucagon 0.03 mg/kg IM may be used to a maximum of 1 mg (ineffective in hepatic disease).

4. Early referral to a specialist children's centre is recommended in difficult or refractory cases.
5. Monitor closely.

Development

Assessing normal development is a skill acquired only from constant practice and observation. Always consider seriously parents' concerns of loss of recently acquired skills or slow development of others. If you are not confident of your own skills in assessing development, do not dismiss parents' concerns but rather refer appropriately. See Table 33.4 (overleaf) for the normal developmental milestones.

Feeding

- Feeding problems are rarely acute 'emergencies'. The notable exception is the parental offering that the child is 'going off his feeds'. This can be the result of any illness, from a cold to congestive cardiac failure.
- History and examination are paramount: (1) to elucidate a cause (infection, surgical condition, etc); or (2) to assess effect (weight loss, dehydration, etc).
- It is important to be familiar with basic feeding practices and to be able to support a breastfeeding mother through a crisis when her child is unwell. Milk allergies and intolerances are not common. Resist changing milk formulas for the lack of better inspiration. Rather than give inappropriate advice, refer the infant and mother to their local doctor, paediatrician, community health centre or, in some instances, an appropriate mothercraft centre.

The inconsolable infant

The inconsolable infant will test the patience of all attendants. The condition is always worse in the quiet of night. Listen to the parents. Don't be dismissive—they are at the end of their tether, sometimes dangerously so for the child. Occasionally, a cause may be found which is of gravity.

Consider physical causes of pain and discomfort, especially treatable conditions such as:

- intussusception/malrotation volvulus
- otitis media
- dental problems (rarely 'teething')
- hair tourniquets (check toes and fingers)
- peptic ulceration (oesophagitis secondary to clinical reflux)
- missed fractures (intentional or accidental)
- stones—renal/gall bladder
- infection (paradoxically, sepsis often leads to quietening)
- ischaemic heart disease (anomalous coronary arteries—rare).

There is a group of children (infants) for whom no physical cause can be elucidated. Their parents require immense support.

Consider admission if:

- There is a physical condition to treat.
- Children are at risk from tired, frustrated carers.

Always acknowledge carers' concerns and frustrations. This often resolves 50% of problems. Plug them into 'the system' (for ongoing support) if you intend sending the child home.

Jaundice

Neonatal jaundice is an increasing concern in EDs with the advent of early-discharge obstetric programs. Although most cases are physiological, kernicterus (significant brain damage due to jaundice) can occur with high levels of unconjugated (indirect) bilirubin. There is an increasing incidence of this problem.

Be concerned by:

- Jaundice in the first 24 hours of life
- Bilirubin greater than 240 micromol/L
- Conjugated bilirubin greater than 30 micromol/L
- Jaundice present after day 10 of life
- Jaundice in an unwell infant

Consider:

- Haemolysis (Rhesus, spherocytes, cephalhaematomas, other)
- Infection:
  - intrauterine—toxoplasmosis, cytomegalovirus (CMV), rubella, other
  - sepsis, especially urinary tract infection (UTI)

Table 33.4 Normal developmental milestones

Age	Gross motor	Vision and fine motor	Social and understanding	Hearing and speech
Newborn	Prone: pelvis high, knees under abdomen, turns face to side	Can fix on a visual object and follow it briefly horizontally		Variable response to sound
1 month	Lifts head momentarily when held in ventral suspension	Follows visual object through 90°	Quietens when picked up	Soft guttural noises when content
6 weeks	Head lag not complete when pulled to sit	Hands often open	Social smiling	Quietens in response to soft sound 15 cm from ear
3 months	Prone: lifts chest off bed taking weight on forearms Only slight head lag when pulled to sit	Holds rattle placed in hand Hand regard begins	Pleasurable response to familiar, enjoyable situations (bottle, bath)	Turns head to sound at ear level
6 months	No head lag when pulled to sit Prone: lifts chest on extended arms, rolls onto back	Hand regard goes Transfers objects between hands	Shows fear of strangers Can imitate (e.g. cough)	Visually locates soft sounds at 45 cm at ear level
9 months	Crawls Stands, holding onto support Sits unsupported for 10 minutes	Pincer grip developing	Looks for toy fallen out of sight Shouts to attract attention	Deliberate vocalisation to try to communicate Localises soft sounds above and below ear at 1 metre

12 months	Walks with one hand held Can let self down from standing position	Casts objects on floor repeatedly	Claps hands Knows and turns to own name	Says 2 or 3 words with meaning
18 months	Jumps using both feet Walks backwards	Spontaneous scribble Tower of 3 or 4 cubes	Knows 2 or 3 parts of body Indicates toilet needs	6–20 recognisable words Understands many more
2 years	Runs well Kicks ball without overbalancing	Copies vertical and circular strokes Tower of 6 or 7 cubes	Parallel play with other children Mainly dry by day	Names 4 toys 2- and 3-word phrases
3 years	Rides tricycle Stands on 1 foot momentarily	Copies circle, 9 cube tower	Mainly dry by night Competent with fork and spoon	Knows full name and sex Uses plurals
4 years	Hops on 1 foot for 3–5 seconds	Copies cross Draws men with 3 parts Matches 4 primary colours	Very imaginative play Picks longer of 2 lines	Asks many questions
5 years	Skips on alternate feet	Copies square Man of 6 parts Names primary colours	Understands rules of play Washes and dries face and hands	Knows full name, address and age

- Surgical causes, some treatable (ideally early):
  - biliary atresia
  - choledochal cysts
- Genetic causes and inborn errors of metabolism:
  - hypothyroidism
  - G6PD deficiency
  - galactosaemia
  - alpha$_1$-antitrypsin deficiency
- Cystic fibrosis
- Bilirubin metabolism syndromes (Gilbert's, Crigler–Najjar, Dubin–Johnson, Lucy Driscoll)

INVESTIGATIONS

- Bilirubin, total and direct
- Haemoglobin, film, haematocrit, blood cultures, group, Coombs' test, reticulocytes
- TORCH titres (toxoplasmosis, rubella, cytomegalovirus, herpes simplex and HIV)
- Urine microscopy, culture and sensitivity, reducing substances
- Check neonatal screen for
  - thyroid function
  - galactosaemia screen
  - other inborn errors of metabolism

PHYSIOLOGICAL JAUNDICE AND 'BREAST MILK' JAUNDICE

Physiological jaundice (slow maturation of glucuronyl transferase, among other factors) and 'breast-milk' jaundice (competitive use of glucuronyl transferase) should be considered diagnoses of exclusion; they are not diagnoses of convenience. Continue to monitor the child or arrange for follow-up until either a cause is found or the jaundice disappears.

Child abuse

This is an unfortunately common problem. It should be in the differential diagnosis of all injuries, burns, poisonings and genital injuries in both sexes. There is no social or racial group immune from child abuse.

Suspect child abuse if:

- The physical findings are inconsistent with the explanation given for the injury.

- There is delay in seeking medical attention.
- The explanation for the injury varies.
- There are multiple injuries at different stages of healing.
- There is a spiral fracture (an unusual fracture in childhood, suggesting a twisting, shearing force) or metaphyseal chip fractures.
- There are two black eyes and/or haematomas on the ears.
- Retinal haemorrhages are present.
- There is fingerprint bruising (e.g. on upper arms, cheeks or trunk) caused by violent gripping.
- Bruising is in soft-tissue areas not normally injured in play.
- There are burns on the buttocks and perineum (from dunking in boiling water) or discrete burns in other areas consistent with cigarette burns.
- There is vaginal or anal bleeding or injury in the absence of an adequate explanation.

MANAGEMENT

- Take a full social history.
- Avoid having the child interviewed on multiple occasions. Questions must not be suggestive or leading. Consult a paediatrician and a social worker experienced in this area.
- Assess the child's development and behaviour.
- Carefully perform a thorough, detailed examination and record all findings and conversations accurately in the hospital record (they and you may be required in court later).
- Take appropriate forensic specimens for semen/saliva/other DNA and check for sexually transmitted diseases (use sexual assault kit).
- Obtain clinical photographs.
- Treat the injuries.
- Do skeletal survey and radionuclide scan in children under 2 years of age, looking for old fractures at different stages of healing.
- Consider CT for subdural haematoma.
- Admit the child to hospital for protection and treatment.
- Notify the statutory authority in those places that have mandatory notification laws.

Sudden infant death syndrome (SIDS)

- By definition, in SIDS there is no evident cause of death. The diagnosis thus cannot be confirmed until after the autopsy. These facts dictate management.

- Resuscitation attempts are dictated by the clinical situation. Be alert for treatable conditions.
- Parents and family, including siblings, should not be excluded from the resuscitation despite the uneasiness this may cause staff. Family counselling should involve the most experienced staff available. Note the necessity of police interviews because of the coroner's involvement.
- The family should be able to stay with the deceased infant as long as they wish, preferably in a quiet room and supported by staff.
- Photographs and hand and foot prints are often appreciated at a later date. However, taking samples such as hair is illegal in most jurisdictions.
- Follow-up for the parents is important. This may need to be organised later.
- It is often useful to involve your local SIDS association.

PREVENTION

- Position infants on their backs.
- Do not overheat.
- Provide loose-fitting clothes.
- Provide a smoke-free environment.

Surgical abdominal emergencies

Abdominal pain may be difficult to assess in a young child. Examination requires warm hands and a gentle approach to gain the child's trust. Often, asking the child to take deep breaths, move or even palpate their own abdomen will provide invaluable clues. The examination will be limited once pain has been elicited. Consider analgesia to aid examination.

INTUSSUSCEPTION

Intussusception classically presents between 3 months and 5 years of age. It frequently follows a minor viral illness, and involves intussusception of a lymphoid follicle through the bowel, causing intermittent screaming with pallor and vomiting, usually without diarrhoea. Increasing lethargy develops between exacerbations of pain. The abdomen is usually tender and a sausage-shaped mass is often palpable in the right upper quadrant. Blood in the stools and shock are traditionally considered late presentations, but may be surprisingly early. X-ray may reveal an area of paucity of gas or obstruction; however, 30% of cases have normal X-rays. Abdominal ultrasound can be diagnostic.

Treatment involves reduction under surgical supervision, preferably in a paediatric facility, by air enema under radiological visualisation. Cases that present late or may have perforation require reduction (and repair) in theatre.

Be aware that intussusception may present masquerading as a cerebrally depressed child; pursue this avenue (CT head, cerebrospinal fluid, drug screen) until all return normal, then think of other possibilities e.g. intussusception.

INGUINAL HERNIAS

Inguinal hernias are common in the first year of life and need early correction as they are liable to become incarcerated. Gentle reduction is often possible in the ED. If they become irreducible, IV fluid therapy and urgent surgery are required.

HENOCH–SCHÖNLEIN PURPURA

This is a vasculitis which commonly occurs in the bowel, causing intermittent abdominal pain in children aged 3–5 years. It is also associated with a purpuric rash developing on the buttocks, and arthropathy and haematuria signify renal involvement. Management is usually conservative.

HIRSCHSPRUNG'S DISEASE

Hirschsprung's disease is the absence of intramural ganglion cells, usually in the rectosigmoid region. It is 4 times more common in males. It presents early in life with increasing constipation and abdominal distension from the newborn period to early childhood; passage of stool within the first 24 hours is reassuring in most cases. Rectal examination often reveals explosive release of stool under pressure. Abdominal X-ray shows faecal loading.

The complications are enterocolitis and perforation. The treatment is surgical.

APPENDICITIS

Appendicitis can occur at any age. Under 2 years, the appendix is an intra-abdominal organ. Appendicitis is difficult to diagnose and the appendix is often perforated at the time of surgery. The child has abdominal tenderness and sometimes fever, vomiting and diarrhoea.

PYLORIC STENOSIS

Pyloric stenosis occurs from 1 week to 3 months of age, with males 4 times more commonly affected than females. Patients present with increasing vomiting, dehydration and hypokalaemia, with a hypochloraemic metabolic alkalosis. A pyloric mass can often be felt, particularly at the end of a test feed; ultrasound or barium meal can confirm this.

The child needs IV fluids and operative treatment after the electrolyte imbalance has been corrected.

WHAT ELSE COULD IT BE?

- Urinary tract infection
- Mesenteric adenitis
- Gastroenteritis
- Child abuse
- Constipation
- Diabetic ketoacidosis

Burns

Burns are common in the paediatric age group. Most burns in toddlers are due to scalds. In adolescents, flame burns predominate. Most are due to accidents, but they can be an intentional injury.

FIRST AID

- Remove the child's clothing over the burned areas.
- Cool the affected areas with water, ideally running tap water at room temperature for 20 minutes. Do not use creams, gels or home remedies such as butter, toothpaste, etc. Do not use ice; this will cause vasoconstriction and worsening/extension of the burn.
- Keep the rest of the child warm, especially in winter in cool regions.

RESUSCITATION

For severe burns:

- maintain a clear airway (in the case of airway burns, any hint of airway compromise indicates the urgent need for early intubation)
- support breathing with oxygen, and
- treat shock.

Remember that severe burns may be just a single part of a multiple-injury trauma, especially if explosions or falls were involved.

ASSESSING THE BURN

- The **surface area** involved may be calculated using surface area charts designed for children. Alternatively, for small areas or areas of irregular shape the child's palm (the palmar surface of the hand from the distal wrist crease to the tips of the fingers, including the thumb) may be used to represent 1% of their body surface area (BSA).

- The **depth** of the burn may be assessed according to the following system:
  - **superficial/erythema**—red, painful, not blistered, blanches readily to digital pressure and rapid capillary refill occurs once the finger is removed. These areas should not be counted in fluid calculations for burns.
  - **partial-thickness**—red, painful, blistered, still blanches and refills to digital pressure. The deeper the burn, the less blanching and the more sluggish the refill. Deep dermal burns may be quite red due to staining by escaped red blood cells (rather like a cooked lobster).
  - **full-thickness**—often black/white, may be less painful/with no pain. Deeper full-thickness burns may penetrate through to fascia, muscle or even bone.

TREATMENT

- Clean the burned areas with aqueous chlorhexidine solution.
- Elevate burned extremities.
- Ensure tetanus prophylaxis is current.
- Consider the need to transfer the patient if:
  - very young patients
  - full-thickness burns covering more than 5% of BSA
  - burns of any type deeper than superficial covering 10% or more of BSA
  - burns of special areas (hands/feet/airway/perineum/ears)
  - comorbidities such as intercurrent illness or multiple injuries
  - suspected non-accidental injury.
- Dress with a bactericidal dressing if the burn is going to be treated locally; Bactigras™ dressings or similar are appropriate. Wrap in clean plastic food-wrap (beware circumferential wraps constricting blood supply to the limbs) or saline wraps if the patient is to be transferred within 24 hours (a full burns dressing with silver-based agents is not required unless there is considerable delay).

In all cases, a specialist burns treatment unit is available to which you can direct questions. Do not hesitate to use this resource.

Orthopaedic problems

SEPTIC ARTHRITIS

Septic arthritis can occur in any joint and is characterised by pain, restricted joint movement and sometimes fever, raised white cell count and raised inflammatory markers (C-reactive protein (CRP) and erythrocyte sedimentation rate (ESR)). Suspicion requires confirmation and treatment by surgical drainage in theatre, culture of the fluid, irrigation and intravenous antibiotics.

IRRITABLE HIP

An irritable hip commonly occurs in children and is often (but not always) associated with a viral illness. The important differential to consider is septic arthritis. Serial examination often reveals limitation of internal rotation of the hip but preservation of some hip movement, absence of constitutional symptoms and normal blood pathology. Orthopaedic opinion is required in equivocal cases.

LIMP

The child with a limp needs careful assessment to establish where the problem lies. Trauma, irritable hip, Perthes' disease, slipped capital femoral epiphyses, septic arthritis or effusion in any of the joints of the limb, tumours, leukaemia, spinal problems, soft-tissue injuries and foreign bodies in the sole of the foot must all be considered. Spinal discitis may be suggested by the child refusing to walk or sit.

PULLED ELBOW

A pulled elbow occurs when the radial head is pulled out of the annular ligament sling with traction on the arm. It sometimes occurs recurrently in children aged between 1 and 4 years. Check that the story is consistent with this diagnosis, and exclude bony injury with X-ray.

To relocate the annular ligament, feel over the radial head, and firmly supinate and extend the arm. Often a click is felt and the child begins using the arm within 10 minutes. If this does not occur, check that nothing has been missed and arrange review the following day. The natural history is for these to spontaneously relocate over a few days.

WHAT ELSE COULD IT BE?

- Child abuse
- Bony tumour
- Neuromuscular conditions (Guillain–Barré syndrome)

Pain management

Pain control during procedures and with painful conditions greatly reduces the anxiety experienced by children and parents. The techniques and medications used should be commensurate with the amount of pain experienced. Therefore, quantification of the pain is important. There are pain scoring systems available for both verbal and pre-verbal children, including neonates and infants.

Anxiety reduction minimises the pain felt and should be used with all frightening or painful procedures. A confident, caring approach to the family and enlisting the parents' support for the child is vital. Clear, non-threatening and age-appropriate explanation to the child just prior to and during the procedure reduces the fear of the unknown.

Non-medical treatments such as ice for acute injuries, cooling for burns or warm packs for abdominal pain may suffice in some situations. They may also be adjuvant treatments for more-severe pain, reducing the amount of medication required.

ANALGESICS

- Paracetamol preparations in a dose of 15 mg/kg are very effective in children.
- Ibuprofen is another commonly used simple analgesic that may be appropriate, especially for muscular injuries (but has the risk of gastritis if given on an empty stomach). Doses for the oral suspension are dependent on weight and are given in Table 33.5.
- Opioid medications may be given:
  - intranasal fentanyl is an effective and rapidly active form of analgesia
  - IV opiates (in frequent small doses) or IM or orally (morphine 0.1 mg/kg, pethidine 1 mg/kg, codeine 1 mg/kg) are effective.

Table 33.5 Ibuprofen (200 mg/5 mL) oral suspension doses

Age	Weight	Dose
5–7 years	18–22 kg	4.5–5.5 mL
7–9 years	22–28 kg	5.5–7 mL
9–12 years	28–40 kg	7–10 mL

Maximum 3 doses in 24 hours

SEDATIVES

Nitrous oxide/oxygen mixture is used with great success in experienced hands. It reduces anxiety, especially when combined with verbal relaxation methods and topical cream if necessary, while consciousness is maintained. A maximum of 70% N_2O can be used if a variable-flow delivery system is available. The main-side effect is vomiting. This can be minimised by having the child fast for at least 2 hours before proceeding.

Midazolam can be given orally to a maximum of 15 mg (in juice or frozen in ice-blocks to disguise the taste), nasally at a dose of 0.5 mg/kg to a maximum of 10 mg or intravenously at 0.1–0.2 mg/kg. It is effective in about 70% of children. The main side-effect is respiratory depression, especially after the noxious stimulus is withdrawn. Recovery with careful observation and oximetry for 2 hours after the procedure is important.

Ketamine, a dissociative anaesthetic given IV or IM, is very effective. Paediatric airway expertise should be present, as should venous access. The airway is maintained but there is an increase in salivation. Its side-effects include occasional prolonged vomiting and hallucinations. This agent is not commonly used in paediatrics but may be useful in the adolescent.

ANAESTHETICS

Topical lignocaine with prilocaine creams (e.g. EMLA cream) reduce the pain felt during procedures involving needles (IV cannulas, blood taking, lumbar punctures). They are safe, but should not be used under 6 months of age because of toxicity and methaemoglobinaemia. The area should be completely occluded with a dressing once the cream is applied and left for 45 minutes to ensure maximal efficacy. The cream cannot be applied to mucosal areas or areas of broken skin. Topical mixtures such as TAC (tetracaine, adrenaline and cocaine in a gel preparation) are very effective for lacerations, but should not be used in end-organ areas.

General anaesthetics should be available, especially for procedures involving intricate work and the cooperation of a small child. These should be administered by practitioners experienced in paediatric anaesthesia.

Prescribing for the paediatric patient

When prescribing for the paediatric patient, oral therapy is preferred where possible. If parenteral antibiotics need to be given, avoid IM injections. Plan ahead by leaving a cannula in situ when taking blood. Dosages should be based on weight and the manufacturers' instructions carefully adhered to. There are many useful pocket guides available.

Special care should be taken with newborns. Maximum doses should be calculated based on a patient's weight ***not exceeding 50 kg***.

Parents should be given clear written instructions on dosage and guidance on administration. Children mostly do not enjoy taking medications and will not always cooperate. When a child refuses to take medication, gentle restraint, recruiting another adult to assist or using a syringe (without needle) to instil the medication into the buccal cleft may all help.

Procedures

WHAT SIZE TUBE?

Most items of equipment vary depending upon the age, weight and size of the patient. Table 33.6 provides a guide only to the size of commonly used items of equipment for use in emergency circumstances. In certain circumstances it may be necessary to modify the tube size (e.g. a child with croup may need a smaller tube).

OBTAINING BLOOD

It is always possible to get sufficient blood from paediatric patients for all tests—it is a matter of patience and having the right equipment and technique. Depending on the laboratory, you may be able to use smaller samples.

A superficial peripheral vein is the preferred location. If inserting an IV line, plan your investigations so that you can take blood for investigations at the same time to avoid unnecessarily hurting the

Table 33.6 A guide to equipment sizes for children

Age	ETT size (ID) to try first (mm)	Distance to insert ETT at lips (cm)	Chest tube (Fr)	Nasogastric tube (Fr)	Foley's catheter (Fr)	Laryngoscope blade
Neonate	3	10	8	6	6	1
6 months	3.5	11	8	6–8	6	1
1 year	4	12	12	8	6–8	1.5
2 years	4.5	13	12	8	6–8	2
4 years	5	15	14	10	8	2
6 years	5.5	16	20	10	8	2
8 years	6	18	20	10	8	2
10 years	6.5	19	20	12	10	2
12 years	7	20	28	12	12	3

ETT, endotracheal tube; Fr, French gauge; ID, inner diameter.

child and taking more time and effort. Use topical anaesthetics if time allows.

Tips for obtaining blood

- Appropriate reassurance, distraction techniques and restraint are the secrets to success. Therefore, having enough staff and/or the parents involved is essential.
- Consider additional analgesia such as nitrous oxide.
- Be prepared and always have an assistant.
- Hand over after 2 failures.
- Do not overconstrict, or you will prevent venous filling.
- Small veins collapse more easily—2 mL syringes are better than 5 mL.
- Unless taking blood for cultures, free flowback often gives a better volume than aspiration.
- If not siting an IV and aspiration is difficult, use a needle with the hub removed: the 'broken needle' technique. The hub promotes coagulation when the flow is slow.
- Consider scalp veins in the neonate.
- Do not use the femoral or neck veins as first options. It may be preferable to resort to arterial sampling instead.
- If leaving a cannula in situ, proper splinting is required, but avoid a tourniquet effect.

URINE SAMPLING

To adequately diagnose a urinary tract infection (UTI), a sterile sample must be collected. Midstream urines are only of value in the older child. Bag urines are inadequate. Younger children require either a suprapubic aspirate or catheterisation. Over 1 year of age, catheterisation is preferred.

Suprapubic aspiration

1. Ensure that the bladder is full by percussion/bladder scanner/ultrasound and that the child has not passed urine for 60 minutes.
2. Use EMLA cream in anticipation.
3. Be prepared with appropriate equipment and an assistant.
4. Gently restrain the child supine, with legs held at the knees.
5. Prepare the site. Cleansing may lead to urination—be prepared to catch a midstream sample.
6. Insert a 23 gauge, 32 mm needle on a 5 mL syringe 1 cm above the symphysis in the midline. Direct the needle caudally at a 20° angle to the vertical. Gently aspirate while advancing.

7 Repeat the procedure once only if unsuccessful, by withdrawing the needle just below the skin and advancing it with a slightly greater degree of angulation caudally.

Urinary catheterisation

Urinary catheterisation is an acceptable alternative to suprapubic aspiration. The procedure is essentially no different to that in adults. Use aseptic techniques, have an assistant, be prepared and, most importantly, be gentle. In young females be familiar with the anatomical landmarks. If you are unable to identify the urethra, do not proceed. Some girls have fused labia, also a contraindication to proceeding.

Urinary tract infection

Criteria for the diagnosis of a UTI are:

- 10^5 organisms (pure growth of a single organism)
- 100 white cells/high-power field
- positive leucocytes and nitrites on urine test strips (dipsticks)—should not be relied on as a screening test
- negative microscopy does not exclude UTI
- up to 20% of children with UTIs have negative dipstick analysis.

LUMBAR PUNCTURE

- No child will cooperate willingly with a lumbar puncture. Use EMLA cream in anticipation, but local infiltration is still preferable. Ensure adequate restraint with proper positioning.
- Consider nitrous oxide in children over 1 year of age.
- Position the patient in the lateral decubitus position, making sure the patient is well flexed and the back is vertical to the bed.
- Prepare the skin and drape the site.
- Identify the L3/4 interspace (at the level of the superior edge of the iliac crest).
- Insert spinal needle (with stylet) in interspinous space, directed slightly cephalad towards the umbilicus.
- Advance the needle slowly. A ‘give’ may be felt as the dura is penetrated.
- Remove stylet and, if no fluid is obtained, rotate the needle 90° so that the bevel is pointing in a cephalad direction.
- If CSF does not flow freely, replace the stylet and advance the needle until fluid is obtained.
- Pressures should be measured using a manometer.
- Collect adequate samples for testing. If blood-stained fluid is obtained, use the last tube for microscopy.

Contraindications

- Obtunded patient
- Raised intracranial pressure
- Infection at the site
- Bleeding diathesis, including thrombocytopenia

Toxicology, poisoning and envenomation

There are 3 major patterns of childhood poisoning to consider given that envenomation can occur at any age:

1. Accidental ingestion of insecurely stored household drugs and other agents (cleaning, pesticides and volatile liquids) tends to occur in inquisitive infants and children in the preschool age group.
2. Intentional self-ingestion as teenagers grapple with their changing lives. It may be frankly suicidal, experimentation gone awry or 'a call for help'.
3. Usually in the younger age group, a degree of suspicion is essential so that the child who is intentionally poisoned by a carer (or other) is not missed with possible later untoward sequelae. Notification to DOCS (Department of Community Services) in NSW or the local child welfare agency is essential.

There are excellent cross-references to recognition and management of poisonings in the Quick Reference section ('Toxicology' and 'Paediatrics'), and in Chapter 28, 'Poisoning, overdosage, drugs and alcohol' and Chapter 30, 'Envenomation'.

It is difficult to recall the detail of so many poisonings. Help is at hand at the end of the phone Australia-wide, 24 hours each day:

13 11 26

This is the National Poisons Centre, with immediate assistance available from pharmacists and scientists with toxicologists on call at all hours.

Editorial Comment

In dealing with children there is need for a combination of clinical science, listening to parents, 'soft' clues and suspicions ('rule out'), which always totally justifies a conservative and cautious approach.

Chapter 34
Geriatric care

Nick Brennan and Jeremy Fry

Geriatrics is an evolving area of emergency medicine. Emergency departments have traditionally been designed and staffed for the care of the acutely ill and injured patient rather than the needs of more complex and functionally impaired older patients. Population projections suggest that by the year 2051, persons over the age of 65 could double to more than 24% of the population which has major implications for the health system, especially the ED. Older patients come to hospital more often by ambulance, wait longer in the ED, have a much higher rate of admission to hospital, have increased mortality, undergo more investigations and cost more money to treat. They are at increased risk of further deterioration or re-admission after discharge from the ED. Older people already make up some 35% of hospital admissions.

Older people come to the ED for a wide variety of reasons. Their presentation will most commonly be due to an acute medical illness, but sometimes there will not be an obvious 'medical' emergency, simply a crisis. The many physiological changes that occur with normal ageing complicate diagnosis and management and mandate a carefully tailored approach to the older patient. Taking a careful history, which includes speaking to family, carers, friends and the local doctor, is time-consuming but crucial to accurate diagnosis.

This chapter is a guide to help you assess older patients who present to the ED with a variety of common presentations. There is also discussion on physiological changes in geriatric patients, geriatric trauma and resuscitation.

Editorial Comment

Get to like and be comfortable with older patients. It is a large and important part of our practice. A big tip is give them time—to answer, remember. Sit down—do not be rushed, get to know them; then quickly you will define issues: ? critically ill, ? acute deterioration, ? comorbidities, what are ADL issues, what are they worried about? It becomes rewarding for both of you—not 'another difficult geri patient'. Try it, it works!

Physiological changes

Geriatric medicine is not simply general medicine in old people. There are significant differences in the approach to care, diagnosis and decision making in the frail aged. The body undergoes major physiological changes as we age that render the elderly more susceptible to disease processes and cloud the presentation of illness. In addition, multiple pharmacotherapies dampen these already compromised physiological responses, which makes interpretation of clinical symptoms, signs and investigations difficult.

For example, physiological changes in cardiac function necessitate a modified approach to resuscitation and treatment of heart failure. As we age, the number of cardiac myocytes declines and there is increased deposition of cardiac collagen. This causes an increased risk of arrhythmias, bundle branch block and sick sinus syndrome. There is a diminished capacity to increase cardiac output by increasing heart rate. Antiarrhythmic therapy exacerbates these already diminished physiological responses. Ventricular compliance falls, and raises the potential for causing heart failure with aggressive fluid therapy. Diastolic failure is common and the presence of a normal systolic ejection fraction on echocardiography does not exclude a diagnosis of cardiac failure. Minor hypovolaemia can cause precipitous falls in cardiac function in older patients, but, at the same time, overly aggressive intravenous fluid replacement can precipitate cardiac failure.

Respiratory function changes as well. Decreased mucociliary clearance and T-cell function increases rates of pneumonia. Dampened cough reflex and changes in oesophageal motility increase the risk of aspiration. Reduced lung compliance, as well as impaired responses to hypercapnia and hypoxia, make ventilation difficult and increase the chance of ventilatory failure.

Neurological changes with ageing account for a significant number of presentations. Diminished reflexes, balance and sensation, and changes in cognition and vision, mean increased falls and accidents. A decline in brain mass causes stretching of the bridging vessels overlying the surface of the brain, making them more susceptible to tearing under shear forces. Thus, the elderly have a heightened risk of subdural and extradural haemorrhage, even with relatively minor injury. The concomitant use of anticoagulant therapy heightens the risk of serious bleeding complications.

Declining gastrointestinal motility, as well as senescence of sensory function and omental shrinking, make the diagnosis of serious abdominal

Table 34.1 **Some physiological changes with ageing**

System	Physiological changes	Pathological changes
Cardiovascular	↑ systolic and diastolic BP ↓ heart rate, cardiac output ↓ myocyte size/elasticity ↓ beta-adrenergic response	↓ compensation for shock Ischaemic heart disease Congestive cardiac failure Arrhythmias Bundle branch block
Respiratory	↓ compliance, diffusing capacity ↓ functional residual capacity ↓ mucociliary clearance	Chronic obstructive pulmonary disease Pneumonia Ventilation difficulties
Neurological	↑ cerebral atrophy ↓ cognition, reflexes, balance ↓ blood flow	Falls, accidents Cerebrovascular accident Traumatic brain injury (subdural haemorrhage)
Musculoskeletal	↓ muscle mass, bone density ↓ spinal column mobility	Fractures Spinal cord injury Falls
Renal	Renal atrophy ↓ glomerular filtration rate, acidification	↑ susceptibility to renotoxic drugs Infection Chronic renal failure
Gastrointestinal	↓ peristalsis ↓ Ca^{2+}/Fe^{2+} absorption	Aspiration Obstruction Anaemia Diverticulitis
Skin	Atrophy, thinning; ↓ sebaceous glands	Infection, trauma Decubitus ulcers
Immune	Immunosenescence ↓T-cell function	Infection

pathology in the elderly both more likely and more difficult. Older patients have an increased risk of bowel obstruction and infection, but they may present with vague abdominal complaints and commonly have poorly localised signs that mask serious underlying pathology.

The many physiological changes in the genitourinary tract increase the risk of lower urinary tract infection, pyelonephritis and incontinence. The decline of glomerular filtration rate (GFR) by approximately 40% by age 80 mandates special consideration when prescribing medications and administration of intravenous fluids. Older patients are particularly susceptible to fluid overload when administering normal saline as fluid replacement therapy.

Changes to the integumentary system increase the risk of infection, as well as making older patients more susceptible to even minor trauma. There is loss of sebaceous glands, thinning of the skin, loss of elasticity and reduced wound healing. Loss of thermoregulation increases heat loss and the risk of hypothermia.

The approach to the elderly patient

In addition to conventional history taking and examination, ED geriatric assessment requires detailed assessment of cognition, functional status and social context. There is added reliance on corroborative history and special emphasis on past medical history, current medications (including recent changes and compliance), social history and current functional status. Up to 1 in 4 admissions to hospital in older patients is related to medication error, overcompliance or undercompliance. It is also important to note hearing and vision impairment, nutritional status and dental hygiene. It is important that you familiarise yourself with the post-acute-care services or supported discharge programs that are available at the ED. The need to 'check the facts' with family and caregivers or any other reliable source of information cannot be overemphasised, especially when discharging patients directly home.

Common presentations

ACUTE CONFUSION

Atypical presentation of disease is common in the older patient, and the presentation of a new disease often depends on the weakest organ system, not the newly diseased organ system. This is very true in delirium, where new onset of confusion will more likely be due to infection in the urinary tract or chest rather than new pathology in the brain.

Delirium is defined as an acute, fluctuating change in cognition, accompanied by impaired consciousness and attention. Geriatric patients who present with acute confusion require a full medical assessment, especially an accurate history of events leading to the presentation, which is usually not available from the patient themselves. Baseline and contributing factors should be assessed (Figure 34.1).

It is often said that delirium is a medical emergency, a statement which emphasises the importance of first recognising delirium, as it is a condition that is often overlooked by doctors and nurses. The Confusion Assessment Method (Figure 34.2, overleaf) is a brief tool that helps to diagnose delirium. This is used in conjunction with the Mini Mental Status Examination (MMSE, Box 34.1) which should

Baseline factors		Precipitating factors	
Brain disease (dementia, stroke, head injury)	☐	Trauma/injuries	☐
Use of sedatives and anticholinergics	☐	Recent introduction of new medications	☐
Visual or hearing impairment	☐	Dehydration	☐
Malnutrition	☐	Pain	☐
Severe disability	☐	Drug withdrawal	☐

Figure 34.1 Acute confusion—why is this patient confused now?
Creasey H. Acute confusion in the elderly. Curr Therapeut 1996;Aug:21–7.

Box 34.1 Folstein Mini Mental Status Examination (MMSE)

Year	1	State	1
Season	1	City	1
Date	1	Suburb	1
Month	1	Hospital	1
Day of the week	1	Floor	1

Registration of 3 items	3
Spell WORLD backwards or serial sevens	5
Recall of three items at one minute	3
Able to name two objects (pen and watch)	2
Able to repeat 'no ifs, ands, or buts'	1
Able to follow three-stage command	3
Able to read and obey 'close your eyes'	1
Write a sentence	1
Copy intersecting pentagons or draw a clock face	1
Total	**30**

Folstein MF, Folstein SE, McHugh PR. The Mini-Mental State Examination: a practical method for grading the cognitive state of patients for the clinician. J Psychiatr Res 1975;12:189–98.

be completed in all cases to objectively document the current level of cognitive impairment.

Symptoms

- Acute deterioration, fluctuations or change in mental status: there is a continuum from hypervigilance to lethargy and/or stupor (so-called hypoactive delirium, which is more common)
- Attention deficit
- Visual hallucinations and delusions

Feature		Yes = 1, No = 0
Acute onset and fluctuating course Ask a family member or carer the following questions:	Is there evidence of acute change in mental status from the patient's baseline? Did the abnormal behaviour fluctuate during the day, that is, tend to come and go, or increase or decrease in severity?	
Inattention This feature is shown by a positive response to the following question:	Did the patient have difficulty focussing attention, for example being easily distractable, or having difficulty keeping track of what is being said?	
Disorganised thinking This feature is shown by a positive response to the following question:	Was the patient's thinking disorganised or incoherent, such as rambling or irrelevant conversation, unclear or illogical flow of ideas, or unpredictable switching from subject to subject?	
Altered level of consciousness This feature is shown by any answer other than "alert":	Alert (normal) = 0 Vigilant (hyperalert) Lethargic (drowsy, easily aroused) Stupor Coma	

The diagnosis of delirium by CAM requires the presence of features 1 and 2 with either 3 or 4.

Complete the MMSE and basic investigations.

Delirium management

ANSWER THIS QUESTION
Is the patient at risk of harm from falling, restlessness, wandering,
AND/OR is there a risk of harm to others due to agitation or aggressive behaviour?

YES	NO
Close supervision—use special nurse, family member or expedite admission to secure environment. Commence risperidone 0.5 mg, preferably given late afternoon, further doses of 0.5 mg given PRN.	Close supervision; remember that delirium fluctuates. The situation may be stable now, but will possibly deteriorate at night.

Figure 34.2 Confusion Assessment Method
From Inouye SK, van Dyck CH, Alessi CA et al. Clarifying confusion: the Confusion Assessment Method; a new method for detection of delirium. Ann Intern Med 1990; 113:941–8.

- Altered sleep–wake patterns (e.g. 'sundowning'—confusion at night-time)
- Underlying medical illness should be present by definition:
  - ± non-focal neurological deficits
  - ± localising signs of infection/pathology

Differential diagnosis

- Dementia with fluctuations
- Primary psychiatric disorder (especially agitated depression)
- Acute psychosis

Causes

There is a wide range of potential causes for delirium in the elderly, but acute infection, medication changes and metabolic derangements are the commonest causal factors. Table 34.2 lists the many potential causes of delirium, but infection accounts for up to 50% overall.

Table 34.2 Causes of delirium in elderly patients

Aetiology	Cause
Systemic	Infection (lung, urinary tract, skin, etc) Cardiovascular (acute coronary syndrome, congestive cardiac failure, shock, arrhythmia) Respiratory failure (↓ oxygen, ↑ carbon dioxide) Liver/renal decompensation Electrolyte imbalance (sodium, glucose, calcium); dehydration
Primary CNS	Cerebrovascular accident Encephalitis, meningitis Subdural haemorrhage, extradural haematoma, trauma Hypertension Malignancy Seizures
Medications (Side-effects, changes)	Anticholinergics Antihistamines Opiates Sedative-hypnotics
Withdrawal	Alcohol, sedative-hypnotics

Adapted from Wilber ST. Altered mental status in older emergency department patients. Emerg Med Clin N Am 2006;24:299–316.

Assessment and investigations

Physical examination remains a very important component of the initial assessment and can sometimes quickly reveal the underlying problem, such as acute retention of urine, faecal impaction or even acute pain from a broken bone. However, the presentation of myocardial infarction, surgical abdomen and sepsis may be subtle and easily missed in delirious elderly patients.[1] Agitated, uncooperative, confused patients are often not easy to examine.

Tests should be tailored to the presenting symptoms if they point to a likely cause for the delirium. Studies have shown that CT scanning of the brain in patients presenting with delirium without focal neurological deficits has a low diagnostic yield. Performing a CT brain scan in the emergency setting often requires the agitated patient to be sedated, and is therefore a second-line investigation, unless there is evidence of objective neurological signs or a high index of suspicion for possible recent head injury, especially in those cases presenting with a fall.

- Bedside: ECG, BSL, BP, HR, SpO_2, urine culture
- Lab: VBG, FBC, UEC, CRP, LFT, blood cultures, troponin, TFTs
- Imaging: CXR (all patients); ± CT of brain

Management

- Broad-spectrum IV antibiotics should be commenced if there is any evidence of infection (neutrophil leucocytosis, raised CRP, elevated temperature, cultures positive), but only after urine, wound and blood cultures have been collected.
- Avoid iatrogenic precipitants (such as indwelling urinary catheters, addition of multiple medications, use of restraints).
- Individual nursing is probably the most effective 'treatment'—it prevents problems such as falls and wandering, and reduces the need for sedating medications.
- Families can play a crucial role in helping to orientate patients to their current surroundings.
- If wandering patients cannot be safely contained within the ED, there is a priority to move them to a safe environment within the hospital. Physical restraint is almost never indicated, and remains overused in Australian hospitals. The vast majority of patients with delirium settle within 24–48 hours if managed appropriately.
- Careful use of low dosage of major tranquillisers such as risperidone (0.5–1 mg) or haloperidol (0.5–1 mg) is appropriate to manage paranoid and persecutory delusions or aggressive behaviour. However, the use of emergency psychiatric protocols for sedation and alcohol withdrawal need to be applied with caution in the elderly, as over-sedation increases the risks of falls, aspiration pneumonia and prolongation of the delirium. Consultation with senior ED staff, the duty geriatrician or the medical registrar should always be sought if you are considering the use of parenteral sedation for a very agitated patient.

DEMENTIA

Dementia, depression and delirium frequently co-exist, and it can be very difficult to separate them. In general, *delirium* is an acute change in cognition, attention and consciousness while *dementia* is a slower, more gradual and progressive deterioration in global brain function that typically affects memory, language, personality and behaviour. The timeline of change can often be elucidated by a careful corroborative history taken from family and caregivers, but there is often a vague history of gradual decline followed by a recent exacerbation, making the distinction between dementia and delirium difficult.

Many dementia syndromes are characterised by fluctuations that may be misinterpreted as delirium, which is why they may present as an 'emergency'. Patients with dementia are prone to falls, wandering and accidents. Worsening dementia symptoms, especially the emergence of behaviour problems such as wandering or aggression, create a crisis for the family and caregivers and lead them to seek urgent assistance. While these problems may not constitute a genuine medical emergency, they do require thoughtful assessment and care planning to ensure safe discharge from hospital back into the community. Aged-care teams are an invaluable resource for this purpose and one should be familiar with the availability of these services within the hospital.

The presence of dementia creates many barriers in providing good care in the ED, such as unreliable or unavailable history, poor compliance with treatment and many discharge dilemmas. The noisy, busy environment of the ED is particularly challenging to patients with dementia, who readily misinterpret their surroundings and feel threatened. The patient's family also feels stressed and threatened and caregivers are often at the end of their tether. Many of these presentations to the ED are a watershed event in a long struggle to provide care at home and result in admission to hospital and eventual placement in a residential care facility. It is usually neither possible nor appropriate to arrange a new admission to a residential aged care facility directly from the ED, even if it is apparent that this is needed.

DEPRESSION

The spectrum of depressive disorders is slightly different in the elderly. Major depression occurs in only 1.5% of the general population, but depression of clinical significance occurs in up to 13.5% of the older population. In addition, depressive symptoms including anxiety symptoms, phobias and somatisation are extremely common in older patients and by themselves do not constitute a diagnosis of depression of clinical significance; treatment for such symptoms should not be commenced in the ED.

There is a very strong correlation between depressive symptoms and use of health services, and the rate at which older people develop depression is highly dependent on preceding disability. Accidents causing pain or immobility and minor medical problems can threaten independence and result in the development of a reactive mood disorder with the patient giving up, feeling they have become a burden and wanting to die. Many such patients improve with treatment of their symptoms and, given time and rehabilitation, most do not need antidepressant therapy. For these patients, the main role for the ED is to address community supports, assess safety for discharge home and arrange appropriate follow-up.

In contrast, major depression is a serious condition in the older patient presenting to the ED and will usually need initial therapy to be commenced in hospital under supervision; it may even require the patient to be detained involuntarily under the Mental Health Act.

Management of depression

- It is important to perform a full mental status examination on geriatric patients, especially when you suspect depression, self-neglect, squalor syndrome or excessive alcohol intake.
- Assess cognition using the MMSE. Remember that depression and dementia can be very difficult to differentiate.
- The Geriatric Depression Scale (GDS, Box 34.2) may help you decide whether there is a likelihood of depression being present.
- Assess degree of suicidality (passive and active) and decide whether you feel that either is present. Older patients will commonly tell you that they wish they were dead, especially in the setting of acute illness, pain and disability.
- It is never appropriate to institute antidepressant therapy in the ED without first consulting the duty geriatrician or psychiatrist.
- The presence of passive suicidal ideation or depressed mood should prompt discussions with family and a referral to the ED social worker for psychological support and assessment of safety for discharge.
- If the patient is to be sent home, involvement of social supports (both family and community) is essential to reduce the risk of self-harm.

ABDOMINAL PAIN

Geriatric patients are twice as likely to require surgical intervention for abdominal complaints compared with younger patients. They are also more likely to present with vague and poorly localised abdominal

Box 34.2 The Geriatric Depression Scale

Are you basically satisfied with your life?	X	No
Have you dropped many of your interests and activities?	Yes	X
Do you feel that your life is empty?	Yes	X
Do you often get bored?	Yes	X
Are you in good spirits most of the time?	X	No
Are you afraid that something bad is going to happen to you?	Yes	X
Do you feel happy most of the time?	X	No
Do you often feel helpless?	Yes	X
Do you prefer to stay at home rather than going out and doing new things?	Yes	X
Do you feel that you have more problems with your memory than most?	Yes	X
Do you feel it is wonderful to be alive now?	X	No
Do you feel pretty worthless the way you are now?	Yes	X
Do you feel full of energy?	X	No
Do you feel that your situation is pretty hopeless?	Yes	X
Do you think that most people are better off than you are?	Yes	X
Total score (one point per question answered)		**15**

Yesavage J, Brink T, Rose T et al. Development and validation of a geriatric depression screening scale: a preliminary report. J Psychiatr Res 1983;17:37–49.

symptoms and signs, which in part explains why geriatric patients have higher mortality from abdominal pathology.[1] Therefore, you should have a low threshold for the use of diagnostic imaging (CT, abdominal X-ray and ultrasound) in older patients presenting with abdominal pain. Table 34.3 lists some of the classic presentations of serious abdominal emergencies that should always be considered.

Table 34.3 Serious abdominal syndromes in the elderly

Symptom	Pathology
Abdominal pain + syncope/hypotension	AAA, perforation
Vague abdominal pain + AF, CCF	Ischaemic bowel
Abdominal pain, distension, BNO	Obstruction, volvulus
Abdominal pain + neurological symptoms	Dissection, AAA

AAA, abdominal aortic aneurysm; AF, atrial fibrillation; BNO, bowels not open; CCF, congestive cardiac failure.

Symptoms and signs

- High incidence of asymptomatic intra-abdominal disease
- Abdominal pain—is often absent, vague and/or poorly localised
- ± Delirium

- ± Syncope
- Bloating
- Vomiting
- Change in bowel habit; rectal bleeding
- Rectal examination for faecal impaction, fresh blood, melaena or rectal mass
- Classic signs of localised tenderness and guarding, peritonism and rebound tenderness may be present or absent
- Absent or tinkling bowel sounds

Differential diagnosis

There is a wide differential diagnosis for the elderly patient with abdominal pain, which includes similar pathology to younger age groups as well as important causes that become more common with ageing. Alterations in bowel habit and rectal bleeding can be the first signs of colonic malignancy, which is more common in older patients. Chronic constipation is a very common condition in older patients and may coexist with acute pathology, rather than being the primary cause of the pain itself. However, severe constipation with or without faecal impaction is still a common cause of acute abdominal pain in older patients presenting to the ED.

- Abdominal aortic aneurysm (AAA), dissection, mesenteric ischaemia
- Biliary tract disease
- Appendicitis, diverticulitis
- Peptic ulcer disease
- Gastroenteritis
- Large- or small-bowel obstruction
- Renal tract disease (stone, urinary tract infection)
- Malignancy
- Pneumonia
- Acute coronary syndrome
- Constipation
  Tip: Remember that constipation is a diagnosis of exclusion and serious causes for a patient's presentation should be actively sought.

Note: Abdominal pain with syncope is AAA until proven otherwise!

Investigations

- Bedside: ECG, BSL, BP, HR, urinalysis, faecal occult blood; ED ultrasound is useful to screen for AAA.

- Lab: VBG (lactate); FBC, UEC, LFT, CRP, amylase, lipase, coagulation screen
  Tip: A normal serum lactate does not exclude bowel ischaemia.
- Imaging: AXR (erect and supine), CXR; CT of abdomen–pelvis
  Tip: A CT KUB is a useful and rapid screening tool in suspected AAA, perforation or renal colic in the stable patient.

Geriatric trauma

FALLS

Falling is the leading cause of accidental death in those older than 85 years and is the most common cause for trauma in older patients presenting to ED (60.7%), followed by motor vehicle crashes (21.5%).[2] The incidence of falls increases with age and one-third of all people older than 65 years will fall every year, with half of these falling repeatedly. 5% of falls lead to a fracture and 10% of fallers sustain other serious injuries. Falls also cause pain, fear, suffering and restriction of activities of daily living (ADLs), which can significantly affect future quality of life. After a fall and fracture, 1 in 4 older people will never regain their previous mobility.

Elderly fallers are different from their healthy, age-matched counterparts. Although some have medical conditions that cause the fall, most have no single diagnosis but rather a combination of risk factors for falls (Box 34.3). The more risk factors present, the greater the likelihood of further falls. Interventions targeted at these risk factors have been shown to reduce the rate of further falls.

Editorial Comment

Many elderly patients are on aspirin, let alone anticoagulation. They bleed easily, especially venous bleeding—subdural haematoma may occur after minimal head trauma (due to brain atrophy and bridging veins). This is often not clinically evident within < 4 hours, or in early CT! Have a low threshold to admit and observe.

Causes

A cause for the patient's fall should be actively sought. Obtaining a careful history of the circumstances of the fall and any preceding symptoms or possible environmental factors is key to accurate diagnosis.

- Common 'medical' causes of falls include delirium, syncope, acute medical conditions and recent medication changes.

Box 34.3 Some factors contributing to falls in the elderly

Chronic medical conditions	Acute medical conditions	Environmental factors
• Osteoarthritis, osteoporosis • Ischaemic heart disease, cerebrovascular accident, hypertension • Anaemia • Diabetes • Gait/balance disturbances; Parkinson's disease (not common) • Dementia • Visual impairment • Polypharmacy	• Delirium, infection • Cerebrovascular accident, acute coronary syndrome, transient ischaemic attack • Syncope • Arrhythmias • Hypoglycaemia • Electrolyte imbalances • New medications	• Rugs • Poor lighting • Stairs • Wet floor, bathtubs • Walking aids **Other** • Older age • Female • Alcohol, drug abuse • Elder abuse

Adapted from Aschkenasy MT, Rothenhaus TC. Trauma and falls in the elderly. Emerg Med Clin N Am 2006; 24:413–32.

- Simple 'mechanical falls' can be indicative of poor mobility and chronic medical conditions that put the patient at heightened risk of future falls and trauma.
- Presentation with facial fractures and head injuries is very suggestive of syncope or arrhythmia, and a period of cardiac monitoring may help confirm the diagnosis (refer to the section on syncope, below).

Investigations

As a general rule, radiographs should be ordered of any apparent injuries. The most common fracture sustained is the wrist, followed by neck of femur (NOF). Patients sustaining NOF fractures or other injuries requiring an operative intervention should have CXR and baseline bloods performed, as well as group and hold.

Delirious patients or those with non-mechanical falls should have targeted investigations performed. Cardiac monitoring is an appropriate investigation if syncope is suspected.

If a patient has remained on the ground for some time before help arrived, special attention should be paid to the duration of time spent on the ground: the so-called 'long lie'. Such patients can develop pressure ulcers, dehydration, hypothermia and muscle breakdown leading to rhabdomyolysis in a relatively short period of time, all of which must be investigated and managed accordingly. Respiratory or urine infection is a common sequelae in these patients.

- Bedside: ECG, BSL, postural BP, urine
- Lab: FBC, UEC, LFTs, CRP, troponin; coagulation/INR if patient is warfarinised or for theatre; CK for 'long lie', blood cultures
- Imaging: site of injury ± CXR; CT of brain

Management

Appropriate management depends largely on whether or not significant injuries have been sustained and whether the patient requires admission for acute or chronic medical conditions. Many elderly patients with relatively minor injuries may require hospital admission due to difficulties in mobilisation owing to slings, casts, pain and loss of confidence.

For those who can be discharged:

- Complete a simplified falls risk assessment (Figure 34.3, overleaf) of all older patients who present after having a fall.
- Exclude postural hypotension.
- Check vision.
- Perform a neurological assessment.
- Perform a gait assessment, including the time to 'Up & Go' test (Box 34.4) and review adequacy of footwear. Consult with the physiotherapist in the ED regarding the gait assessment and provision of a mobility aid where appropriate.
- Review all medications (in particular hypnosedative agents) and reduce medications where possible. However, medications that are often implicated in falls, such as beta-blockers or antidepressants, should not be ceased abruptly by the ED resident without appropriate consultation.
- A follow-up occupational therapy home visit should be organised, as 50% of falls are due to extrinsic (environmental) factors.

Box 34.4 The time to 'Up & Go' test

The time to 'Up & Go' test is a useful bedside test that correlates well with more-sophisticated falls risk assessment. The patient should be able to arise from a chair, walk 6 metres and return to the seated position within 15 seconds. Failure to do so within this time limit constitutes an abnormal test and indicates a high risk of further falls.

Podsialdo D, Richardson S. The time to 'Up & Go': a test of basic functional mobility for frail elderly persons. J Am Geriatr Soc 1991;39:142–8.

Baseline factors (tick box if present)		Suggested action by RMO
Postural hypotension	☐	Measure erect & supine BP
Hypno-sedative agent	☐	Discuss with consultant
Use of ≥ 4 medications	☐	Medication review; discuss with consultant
Environmental hazards	☐	Consider OT assessment
Any impairment of gait	☐	Mobilise the patient
Any impairment of balance or transfers	☐	Observe transfers and test standing balance
Impairment of leg or arm muscle strength or ROM	☐	Neurological examination

ANSWER THIS QUESTION
Is the patient at risk of harm from falling over again now?

YES

- Close supervision especially if confused and falling
- Physiotherapy assessment for provision of walking aid and indication of mobility status
- Daily supervised mobilisation if possible
- Do not send home without further consultation

NO

Consider future risks; referral to community team for OT assessment; referral to outpatients for falls risk assessment and exercise program

About half of patients who fall will do so repeatedly. Your task is to prevent another fall; falls risk assessment coupled with appropriate interventions can reduce the risk of further falls and injury.

Figure 34.3 Falls risk assessment
From Tinetti ME, Speechley M, Ginter SF. Risk factors for falls among elderly persons living in the community. N Engl J Med 1988;319:1701–7.

HEAD INJURY AND CERVICAL SPINE INJURY

The potential for significant intracranial injury warrants special attention in the elderly patient who has fallen or sustained other trauma. The elderly are at increased risk for subdural, extradural and traumatic subarachnoid haemorrhage. The presence of anti-platelet medication or warfarin compounds the potential for significant morbidity and mortality. Reductions in brain mass can mean delays in symptoms for hours to days, and head injury is the highest cause of mortality related to falls in the elderly.[3] Given this background, there should be a high index of suspicion for intracranial injury in any patient over the age of 70 who has sustained a head injury, even for those who have fallen and not obviously struck their head. As a rule, CT of the brain is indicated in any patient over 70 who has sustained a head injury and is on a blood-thinning agent. CT scans on patients who are taking warfarin should be done as a matter of some urgency, as prompt reversal of anticoagulation can be life-saving.

Similarly, owing to fusion of vertebrae, reduced spinal capacity for flexion, and other osteoarthritic and osteoporotic changes in the cervical spine of the older patient, a high index of suspicion should be held for an asymptomatic vertebral fracture or even a spinal injury without fracture in any trauma patient. A CT scan of the cervical spine is the initial investigation of choice. Older patients are at elevated risk of C1 and C2 fractures, as well as the 'central cord syndrome' which is caused by hyperextension of the cervical spine in a person with pre-existing cervical spondylosis. For screening purposes, the NEXUS criteria have been validated in elderly patients (see 'Online resources').

Note: Due to the high incidence of C1–2 fractures, it is reasonable to perform CT of the cervical spine of all geriatric trauma patients undergoing CT of the brain.

MOTOR VEHICLE CRASHES

Owing to slowed gait, visual/auditory impairment, impaired reflexes, and in some cases impaired cognition and judgment, older pedestrians are at increased risk of being struck by motor vehicles. There is significantly increased mortality in these individuals—most commonly from head injuries or major vascular damage. Elderly patients sustain twice as many lower-limb injuries as younger victims, and injuries to all areas of the body (except for intra-abdominal) increase with age. Patterns of injury in older persons in other motor vehicle crashes are relatively similar to those seen in younger persons, apart from an increased risk of sternal fracture.

Management of the trauma patient is covered in detail elsewhere in this book; however, there are several specific things to consider when managing the geriatric trauma patient:

- physiological changes mean less capability to compensate for blood loss/injury
- ↑ risk of cardiac/cerebral ischaemia from hypotension
- ↑ risk of aspiration when lying supine
- ↑ risk of fluid overload from rapid volume infusion
- ↓ basal metabolic rate (BMR) elevates risk of hypothermia
- pre-morbid medical conditions may affect compensatory responses

- ↑ use of medications (especially antiarrhythmics and antihypertensives which can mask tachycardia and worsen the effect of hypovolaemia)
- different patterns of injury and greater injuries sustained from minor trauma.

RIB FRACTURES

Rib fractures are commonly sustained after falling and require a considered approach to pain management and an awareness of possible complications. Rib fractures are frequently missed on plain radiographs, and specific views need to be requested if rib fracture is suspected. They are often more easily visible on a chest CT scan.

The older patient is not only more susceptible to fracturing ribs from simple falls, but is also more likely to develop aspiration pneumonia or atelectasis owing to reduced lung compliance and other physiological changes in the lung and chest wall.

Achieving adequate pain control can be difficult given the heightened susceptibility to sedation and respiratory depression from opiate analgesics in older patients. Non-steroidal anti-inflammatory drugs (NSAIDs) should not be used in frail, elderly patients because of the risk of precipitating heart failure, renal failure and upper gastrointestinal bleeding.

Patients on warfarin are at increased risk of developing a haemothorax following a rib fracture.

Investigations

- Bedside: SpO_2, ECG
- Lab: VBG (hypercapnia, hypoxia)
- Imaging: CXR ± CT of chest

Management

- Supplemental oxygen
- Analgesia—avoid IV opiates unless necessary; oxycodone is well tolerated in elderly patients
- Low threshold for admission for analgesia and respiratory monitoring

Syncope

Syncope is one of the most common presentations to the ED. The incidence of syncope rises with increasing age. 3% of all geriatric visits to the ED and up to 6% of hospital admissions are syncope related.[4] Although syncope is most commonly benign, the incidence of life-threatening causes rises with age.[5]

Pre-syncopal symptoms of dizziness and light-headedness, etc should be sought in taking the history, but the investigation of pre-syncope should follow the same approach as for syncope, and the two shall be considered together here. Pre-syncope may be difficult to differentiate from vertigo, although the rotational symptoms seen in true vertigo are atypical in pre-syncope/syncope. The cause of syncope remains undiagnosed in up to 50% of cases, though it has been argued that this can be narrowed to 20% with thorough and detailed history and examination.[6]

The goals of syncope investigations are to identify potential life-threatening causes and to stratify the risk of further episodes. Older patients have more comorbidity and risk factors than younger patients and are more likely to have underlying life-threatening pathology as a cause for their syncope. Older patients are also less likely to present with typical symptoms, even in the presence of significant pathology. However, the converse also holds true, in that relatively minor illness can present as syncope in frail older patients with impaired physiological reserves.

CAUSES

The causes of syncope (Box 34.5, overleaf) are usually defined as:

- neurocardiogenic (vasovagal, or 'faint')—most common (35–40%)
- orthostatic—orthostatic hypotension is present in 40% of elderly patients, is a common side effect of many medications and is often asymptomatic
- cardiogenic—arrhythmia is the most frequent life-threatening cause of syncope
- neurological—TIA does not commonly present as syncope
- other.

HISTORY

Almost 50% of syncope/pre-syncope can be diagnosed on history and examination alone. In some patients this can be somewhat difficult owing to co-existing dementia or acute confusion. Corroborative history from witnesses and family is imperative. The existence of prodromal symptoms (warmth, nausea, light-headedness) is more frequently associated with benign causes, whereas a lack of prodrome or sudden loss of consciousness resulting in injury are more common with arrhythmias. However, there are many exceptions to these rules.

Box 34.5 Common causes of syncope

(Vasovagal) Neurocardiogenic	Orthostatic
• Pain • Fear • Cough • Micturition • Defecation • Carotid sinus hypersensitivity • Postprandial	• Dehydration • Blood loss • Sepsis • Medications
Cardiogenic	**Neurological**
• Arrhythmia — ventricular fibrillation, ventricular tachycardia — sick sinus syndrome — bradycardia — atrioventricular dissociation — heart block • Structural — cardiomyopathy • Obstructive — hypertrophic obstructive cardiomyopathy — pulmonary embolism — tamponade • Valvular — aortic stenosis — mitral stenosis • Ischaemia • Other: dissection	• Subarachnoid haemorrhage • Migraine • Transient ischaemic attack • Subclavian steal • Seizures **Other** • Psychiatric

Key points in history

- Prodromal symptoms
- Triggers (emotion, fear, pain, cough, micturition)
- Position (lying, standing)
- Activities (e.g. related to exertion)
- Environment (hot room, weather)
- Associated symptoms (chest pain, palpitations, headache, shortness of breath, abdominal pain, infective symptoms, blood loss)
- Previous history
- Past medical history, e.g. arrhythmias, heart failure, cardiomyopathy
- Medications (especially antihypertensives and antidepressants, recent changes or additions)
- Social situation (including walking aids, use of alcohol, level of independence, support at home)

RISK STRATIFICATION

Older patients generally fall into the high-risk categories in most risk stratification protocols, which highlights the importance of clinical judgment and taking an accurate history. Several scoring criteria exist for the evaluation of syncope, though there is some question about their validity in the Australian setting.[7] The CHESS criteria (or San Francisco syncope rule) were shown to reduce admissions when applied in American EDs, but actually increase the admission rate when applied in Australian EDs. The conflicting results are perhaps due to different patterns of admission in the US, based on many other factors. In Australia, no scoring system has currently been shown to be any better than clinical judgment.

PHYSICAL EXAMINATION

Particularly in the elderly patient, examination should focus on cardiovascular and neurological status, abdominal examination and careful assessment for any injuries sustained from the syncope.

- Murmurs can indicate structural or valvular heart disease (HOCM, aortic stenosis). Extra heart sounds (S_3, S_4) can suggest heart failure.
- Peritonism, peri-umbilical or flank bruising or distension may suggest intra-abdominal pathology/haemorrhage as a source of syncope.
- The presence of neurological deficits may rule out syncope in favour of stroke, TIA or other intra-cranial cause.
- Traumatic injuries sustained from a syncope do not necessarily differentiate between benign and life-threatening causes, but do favour the latter. Remember that intra-cranial haemorrhage can occur in minor head injuries in the elderly—especially in those patients taking antiplatelet or anticoagulant therapy. Fractured neck of femur and upper limb and facial fractures are common sequelae of syncope in the geriatric population.

INVESTIGATIONS

In general, investigations should be tailored to the presenting history. Troponin is a low-yield test and should not be routinely performed, as a positive result will be difficult to interpret. Unfortunately, routine blood tests find the cause in only 2–3% of syncope presentations. Cardiac syncope due to myocardial infarction in the absence of prodromal symptoms or ECG changes is exceedingly rare, although silent myocardial infarction is not an uncommon finding in frail elderly patients who develop serious illness from any cause.

- Bedside: BSL, ECG, BP (including postural), urinalysis
- Blood: UEC, FBC (haemoglobin/haematocrit Hb/Hct)

- Imaging: CXR, echocardiogram (only if a new or significant cardiac murmur is present)
- Cardiac monitoring by telemetry or ambulatory Holter monitoring if arrhythmia is suspected or ECG is suggestive of conduction defects

ADMISSION/DISCHARGE

Discharge of elderly patients with benign causes of syncope should be done with careful consideration of pre-morbid status, social situation and appropriate follow-up. Geriatric patients prone to orthostatic hypotension or vasovagal syncope will be at heightened risk of significant falls and injuries. There should be a low threshold for admission of the geriatric patient with pre-syncope or syncope if safety at home cannot be assured. Patients who are still driving should be advised to discontinue until reviewed by their GP or until specialist follow-up investigations have been arranged. Those patients whose syncope is symptomatic of a more serious underlying medical condition (such as malignancy causing anaemia) will usually need admission to hospital for further investigation and management.

The 'not-coping' patient

You will be encouraged to send both young and old patients directly home from the ED and help avoid their admission to hospital. This is not a bad thing, as admission to hospital is associated with physical, cognitive and functional decline in the elderly. However, older patients are often seen as 'bed blocking' or not really sick enough to warrant hospital admission. This is especially the case when there is a shortage of inpatient beds (which is most of the time) and when the performance of EDs is measured in terms of hours spent in the department. This combination of bed shortage, performance targets and the subacute, atypical presentation of older patients can lead to hasty and poor discharge decisions.

You should be very wary of the frail elderly patient whose triage assessment lists social factors or 'not coping' as the main presenting problem. Such patients commonly have a combination of identifiable medical conditions that are collectively responsible for their current inability to manage their ADLs, and appropriate medical treatments often improve these patients to the point where they can continue to cope at home. This is often actually the aim of a geriatric admission to hospital. What may initially present as a simple case of 'not coping' will often result in a period of hospitalisation, treatment and rehabilitation, with the patient eventually returning home. Obviously, this is not a role for the ED as these things take time. Nonetheless, you should become familiar with a brief assessment of ADLs (Figure 34.4) which should become part of your routine medical assessment, because being dependent in basic ADLs is a powerful predictor of poor health outcomes from acute illness.

Involvement of the ED social worker is important in the early stages, especially if you are planning to send the patient directly home. Many EDs now have specific aged-care teams available to help coordinate services on discharge. Your patient may temporarily need services to cope once they go home, but do not assume that appropriate services can be arranged immediately (especially after-hours and on weekends). Your primary responsibility is to your patient. If you feel that discharge is unsafe, you should discuss the case with a senior consultant or duty geriatrician in order to admit the patient, even if there is no room in the inn!

Personal activity of daily living (tick box if patient needs help in ADL)		Instrumental activity of daily living (tick box if patient needs help in ADL)	
Bladder or bowel function	☐	Shopping	☐
Feeding	☐	Meal preparation	☐
Dressing	☐	Housekeeping	☐
Transfers	☐	Taking medications	☐
Bathing	☐	Transport	☐
Mobility	☐	Finances	☐

ANSWER THIS QUESTION
Have you ticked any of the boxes?

YES

- Referral to social worker
- Do not send home without further consultation
- Confirm the history with family, carer or GP
- Test for cognitive impairment

NO

Can you be sure?
Is there evidence of cognitive impairment?
Have you confirmed the history with the family, carer or GP?

Being dependent in activities of daily living is strongly predictive of deterioration after being sent home from the emergency department. Patients themselves will often overestimate their level of independence. Always check the history with family or friends. Do not send the patient home with new medications unless you are sure that they will be taken correctly.

Figure 34.4 Dependency in activities of daily living (ADLs)

Resuscitation[8]

Resuscitation in older patients presents both ethical and practical challenges in the ED setting. You may be presented with a frail elderly patient from a nursing home 'in extremis' with little or no background history immediately available, where advanced life support including resuscitation is urgently required. What do you do?

The general principles of resuscitation apply to elderly patients; however, there are several important caveats. As outlined in Table 34.4, important physiological changes alter the expected response to normal resuscitation protocols and special care must be exercised when approaching geriatric resuscitation.

Table 34.4 Changes affecting resuscitation in the elderly

Change	Problem
Poor dentition; bridges, dentures, edentulous	Difficulty in intubation, bag–mask ventilation; poor seal
Cervical spine immobility	Poor view for intubation; spinal injury from forced neck extension
↓ Lung compliance, diffusing capacity	Ventilation difficulties; risk of barotrauma
↓ Oxygen tension, hypercapnic response	Occult ventilatory failure
Reduced cardiac/renal function	20–40% reduction in induction agents required
Reduced cardiac reserve	↓ Response to hypovolaemia, sepsis, trauma
Osteoporosis	Rib/vertebral fractures with CPR

MANAGEMENT

Special care should be taken in the management of geriatric resuscitation, as follows.

Airway:

- Dentures can remain in situ until intubation to aid in obtaining a good mask seal
- Take care with mouth opening and with loose teeth
- Ensure use of appropriate laryngoscope (e.g. Miller blade)
- Ensure use of adjunctive airways

Breathing:

- Measured use of supplemental oxygen
- Avoidance of high airway pressures
- Be aware of low respiratory rates
- Elevation of the patient to at least 30° to minimise aspiration

Circulation:

- Use multiple small 250 mL fluid boluses with constant reassessment to avoid overload
- Reduce induction agents by 20–40%
- Avoidance of hypothermia important.

Some studies have shown that the age of patients receiving CPR in hospital was not a significant determinant of survival. Independent of age, the presence of asystole or electromechanical dissociation (EMD) and multiple comorbidities were associated with decreased survival. This remains true for older patients. Thus, it seems reasonable to provide advanced life support and CPR to older patients who are highly functional and have relatively few comorbidities. The main problem is actually determining the patient's pre-morbid level of functioning and quality of life in the emergency setting, where there is often no history immediately available.

ETHICS OF RESUSCITATION/NFR ORDERS[8]

Any approach to emergency treatments and resuscitation in any patient must consider several, sometimes competing, issues:

- the wishes of the patient
- the wishes of the family
- pre-existing advance care directives (ACDs) (if available)
- likelihood of success
- possible futility of any resuscitation attempt.

All of this must be conducted within the rubric of *primum non nocere.*

Older people, their families and GPs are increasingly being encouraged to prepare ACDs to indicate their preferences for invasive medical therapies before the event. However, where there has been no ACD made or there has been a reluctance to discuss issues of resuscitation etc with a patient before he/she comes to hospital, it increasingly falls to the ED doctor to broach the subject. This task is generally best done by a senior ED clinician, but junior doctors should not shy away from being actively involved in end-of-life discussions. Inclusion of the family is a must and contact with the local GP or other treating doctors can yield valuable insight into pre-existing medical conditions and quality of life. Often the patient is too unwell or unable to participate in these discussions, so that surrogate decision making by doctors, families and caregivers is required.

All discussions of this nature need careful documentation in the patient's notes. Increasingly, Australian hospitals are creating 'NFR orders' whereby documentation is made of any limitations to further treatment. These documents often include a section for the doctor to determine not-for-resuscitation (NFR) status based on the futility of such interventions, but they should also include clear instruction as to which treatments are still appropriate, even if this includes palliative measures only.

Futile attempts at resuscitation should be avoidable with good communication and planning, but in the emergency setting where there is limited information to hand, you often have little choice other than to resuscitate and ask questions later. It is important never to make assumptions about another individual's quality of life until you have either sought the patient's views directly yourself or interviewed family, caregivers or other health professionals who have known the patient for some time.

References

1. Bryan ED. Abdominal pain in elderly persons, http://emedicine.medscape.com/article/776663-overview
2. Kahn JH, Magauran B. Trends in geriatric emergency medicine, Emerg Med Clin N Am 2006;24:243–60.
3. Marx JA, ed. Rosen's Emergency medicine: concepts and clinical practice, 7th ed. Philadelphia: Mosby, 2010.
4. Hood R. Syncope in the elderly. Clin Geriatr Med 2007;23:351–61.
5. Kessler C, Tristano JM, De Lorenzo R. The emergency department approach to syncope: evidence-based guidelines and prediction rules. Emerg Med Clin N Am 2010;28:487–500.
6. Ouyang H, Quinn J. Diagnosis and evaluation of syncope in the emergency department. Emerg Med Clin N Am 2010;28:471–85.
7. Cosgriff TM, Kelly AM, Kerr D. External validation of the San Francisco Syncope Rule in the Australian context. Can J Emerg Med 2007;9(3):157–61.
8. Naran AT, Sikka R. Resuscitation of the elderly. Emerg Med Clin N Am 2006;24:261–72.

Online resources

Cervical spine X-rays in trauma, including NEXUS criteria
www.nhmrc.gov.au/nics/nics-programs/emergency-care-community-practice/emergency-care-evidence-practice-series-cervica

Chapter 35
Gynaecological emergencies

Nikki Woods

General principles

- History includes last normal menstrual period (LMP), past pregnancy history, sexual activity, contraception, pregnancy signs and symptoms, preventative health strategies (Pap smear, breast examination) as well as characteristics of presenting symptoms (commonly pain, abnormal vaginal bleeding ± pregnancy, vaginal discharge, fever).
- Investigations often will involve quantitative serum beta-human chorionic gonadotrophin (beta-hCG; see Table 35.1, overleaf) and pelvic ultrasound.
- Management includes excluding pregnancy for every female of reproductive age, and early attention to vital signs, anticipating that certain conditions are associated with immediately life-threatening presentations.
- Sensitivity and attention to patient comfort mandates conducting gynaecological history and pelvic examinations in a private area (when the patient's condition is stable), using a chaperone if male, using a warmed speculum and offering analgesia early.

Common presentations

PAIN

Ruptured ectopic pregnancy

Incidence of ectopic pregnancy is increasing worldwide, mainly due to the increased incidence of pelvic inflammatory disease (PID) caused by *Chlamydia trachomatis* and assisted reproductive techniques. Ectopic pregnancy occurs at a rate of about 11 in 1000 diagnosed pregnancies.

Risk factors include past history of tubal damage or tubal surgery, previous ectopic pregnancy, PID, assisted reproductive techniques, increased age, smoking, progesterone-only contraception, intrauterine contraceptive device (IUD).

History includes abdominal pain (97%), missed period (80%), vaginal bleeding (79%), which is rarely heavy, and syncope. Patients

Table 35.1 Interpretation of quantitative serum beta-hCG results

Reference intervals		
	Serum beta-hCG (U/L)	
Females	< 2.0	Pre-menopausal
	< 10	Post-menopausal
Males	< 2.0	
Pregnancy test		
	Serum beta-hCG (U/L)	**Interpretation**
	< 2	Negative (if taken after first missed period)
	2–25	Borderline result (suggest repeat in 48 hours)
	> 25	Consistent with pregnancy
Pregnancy staging		
Weeks since LMP	**Approximate hCG range (U/L)**	**Comment**
3–4	0–130	Week prior to first missed period
4–5	75–2600	Week after first missed period
5–6	850–20,800	
6–7	4000–200,000	
7–12	11,500–289,000	
12–16	18,300–137,000	
16–29	1400–53,000	Second trimester
29–41	940–60,000	Third trimester

LMP, last normal menstrual period

commonly present between the 5th and 8th week following the LMP. Presenting signs of ruptured ectopic pregnancy include abdominal tenderness, adnexal tenderness and, less frequently, shoulder tip pain, syncope and hypovolaemic shock.

Investigations

Diagnosis is made by positive beta-hCG (see Table 35.1) and an ultrasound negative for intrauterine pregnancy. (Heterotopic pregnancy—an ectopic pregnancy together with an intrauterine pregnancy—occurs in approximately 1 in 3800 pregnancies, and up to 1 in 100 in those who have undergone assisted reproduction.)

Other investigations include a full blood count (FBC) and cross-match in any haemodynamically unstable patient. Blood group and Rhesus factor should be determined on all patients.

Management

Haemodynamically unstable patients: oxygen, large-bore cannula, IV fluids, cross-match blood, urgent obstetrics and gynaecological (O&G) consult for operative management.

Haemodynamically stable patients: insert IVC, perform group-and-hold (G&H), O&G consult. Management may be expectant, medical or surgical, depending on initial serum titre of beta-hCG and trend in titres, and local practice.

Acute salpingitis (PID)

(See also the section 'Pelvic inflammatory disease' in Chapter 41, 'Infectious diseases'.)

- Encompasses endometritis, salpingitis, tubo-ovarian abscess and/or pelvic peritonitis.
- Risk factors include history of previous episode, multiple sexual partners, instrumentation, adolescence and an IUCD.
- Often sexually acquired. Infection is usually due to *Chlamydia trachomatis* or *Neisseria gonorrhoea*. Infection may be caused by mixed pathogens including anaerobes, facultative bacteria and *Mycoplasma* species.
- May result from mechanical interruption of the normal cervical barrier, e.g. post-termination, postpartum, postoperative infection, or in association with IUDs.
- Presenting symptoms include lower abdominal pain, purulent or mucopurulent vaginal discharge, low-grade fever, generalised malaise, dyspareunia and abnormal vaginal bleeding. There is no correlation between extent of disease and symptom severity.
- On examination there may be abdominal tenderness and adnexal and cervical motion tenderness (95% sensitivity).

Investigations

Diagnosis is made by a combination of clinical findings and some or all of the following: positive microbiology from endocervical swabs or positive urine PCR (for *N. gonococcus* and *Chlamydia*), leucocytosis, ultrasound documenting inflammatory adnexal mass or retained products.

Management of acute salpingitis

1 **Severe infection or systemically unwell** or requires removal of retained products or IUD: admit for IV antibiotics
   — sexually acquired—doxycycline 100 mg PO 12-hourly, metronidazole 500 mg IV 12-hourly plus ceftriaxone 1 g IV 8-hourly while awaiting culture results.
   — non-sexually acquired—ampicillin 2 g IV 6-hourly, metronidazole 500 mg IV 12-hourly plus gentamicin 4–6 mg/kg IV once daily.

2 **Milder infections** may be discharged on oral therapy
   — sexually acquired—azithromycin 1 g PO stat dose, doxycycline 100 mg 12-hourly PO for 14 days plus metronidazole 400 mg PO 12-hourly for 14 days.
   — non-sexually acquired—amoxycillin + clavulanate 875 mg + 125 mg PO 12-hourly, plus doxycycline 100 mg PO 12-hourly, both for 14 days.

3 Must treat sexual partner(s).

4 *Chlamydia* and *Gonorrhoea* are notifiable diseases.

5 If associated with IUD or retained products, removal is necessary.

Long-term sequelae may include tubo-ovarian abscess, chronic pelvic pain, dyspareunia, infertility and increased risk of ectopic pregnancy.

Adnexal cyst or mass complications

Ruptured ovarian cyst

- Ovarian cysts are asymptomatic until complications occur.
- Physiological cysts such as corpus luteum cysts (in pregnant or non-pregnant women) and follicular cysts rupture at different points in the menstrual cycle, giving a clue to aetiology:
  — Rupture of a follicular cyst with the extrusion of an ovum occurs midcycle, and gives rise to the unilateral pain of mittelschmerz. Discomfort may last 2–3 days, and may be associated with mild general malaise and/or vaginal spotting.
  — Corpus luteal cyst rupture in the non-pregnant woman occurs just prior to menses and is usually associated with some intraperitoneal bleeding, which may be significant. Ectopic pregnancy must be excluded.
  — In pregnancy, the corpus luteum may persist until 10 weeks, so that spontaneous rupture typically occurs during the first trimester.
- Presenting symptoms and signs are unilateral pain and adnexal tenderness; fever and leucocytosis are uncommon

(approximately 20%). Diffuse peritoneal irritation occurs with spillage of fluid into peritoneal cavity.

Investigations:

- Ectopic pregnancy must be excluded: serum beta-hCG and pelvic ultrasound.

Management:

- Resuscitation with IV fluids and oxygen if haemodynamically unstable
- Exclude pregnancy
- Analgesia
- Laparoscopy may be indicated

Torsion of ovarian or tubal mass

- This is usually associated with a diseased ovary or fallopian tube. Torsion occurs when these structures twist on their supportive appendages, causing compromise to their vascular supply.
- Clinical features include the sudden onset of sharp, unilateral pain which is intermittent and which becomes increasingly severe. There may have been previous similar episodes. There may be associated nausea, vomiting, low-grade fever and leucocytosis and, infrequently, amenorrhoea or abnormal vaginal bleeding.
- Examination findings vary from unilateral lower abdominal tenderness to peritonitis.

Investigations:

- Ultrasound reveals reduced perfusion of the torted mass.

Management:

- Analgesia, resuscitation as appropriate and laparoscopy or laparotomy.
- Complications include ovarian necrosis and shock.

Other gynaecological causes of lower abdominal or pelvic pain

Endometriosis: initially the pain is cyclic and associated with menses. Later it can become continuous as adhesions develop. Diagnosis is made at laparoscopy.

Uterine perforation: typically after intrauterine instrumentation, may present acutely due to intraperitoneal irritation secondary to intraperitoneal blood or as delayed diffuse pain with diffuse peritonitis.

Severe dysmenorrhoea: manage with antiprostaglandins, e.g. NSAIDs, and paracetamol.

Denial of pregnancy and unanticipated labour: estimated at 1 in 2000–5000 births, the diagnosis is made when the woman presents in labour, putting both mother and fetus at risk.

Vulvovaginitis: common causes are infection, irritation, allergy, systemic disease. Treatment depends on the likely cause.

BLEEDING

In early pregnancy

Ectopic pregnancy

See 'Ruptured ectopic pregnancy' section above.

Spontaneous abortion or miscarriage

- Approximately 25% of all pregnancies are associated with bleeding in the first trimester. 50% of these will be due to a failed pregnancy.
- Presenting symptoms include intermittent vaginal spotting progressing to heavy bleeding with passage of clots and gestational tissue; midline, cramping abdominal discomfort occurring after bleeding has commenced. On examination there may be midline, suprapubic tenderness on deep palpation, uterine enlargement consistent with pregnancy or the abdominal examination may be unremarkable.
- Shock or bradycardia can occur due to products sitting in the cervical os. These will require urgent gentle removal after direct visualisation on speculum examination. Vaginal speculum examination is necessary to assess the cervical os, i.e. open or closed?
- Several stages of spontaneous miscarriage are recognised:
  - threatened miscarriage—cervical os closed; no products passed
  - incomplete miscarriage—cervical os open; bleeding ± products passed
  - complete miscarriage—cervical os open or closed; products of conception expelled
  - inevitable miscarriage—cervical os open; no products passed
  - missed miscarriage—cervical os closed; no products passed.

Investigations:

- Confirmation of pregnancy with serum beta-hCG level
- Assessment of state of cervical os
- Ultrasound examination to confirm diagnosis and exclude ectopic pregnancy (if not already known to have intrauterine pregnancy)

- Assessment of Rhesus (Rh) status

Management:

- Assessment of vital signs, and monitoring of blood loss
- May occasionally require IV fluids and, rarely, ergometrine or oxytocin
- Analgesia
- May require D&C after consultation with O&G
- Administration of Rh (anti-D) immunoglobulin if Rh-negative.
- Miscarriages are frequently associated with grieving, and referral for counselling should be offered to the patient.

In later pregnancy (antepartum haemorrhage, > 20 weeks' gestation)

Placental abruption and placenta praevia

Placental abruption. Separation of the placenta from the uterine wall is usually associated with characteristically dark vaginal bleeding, uterine pain and tenderness. Complications include fetal distress or death, disseminated intravascular coagulation (DIC), maternal haemorrhage.

Placenta praevia. Implantation of the placenta over, or near, the cervical os. Bleeding in this situation is usually associated with painless fresh vaginal bleeding, which may become severe with cervical probing. The uterus is typically non-tender. There may be a history of several small 'warning' bleeds.

Assessment:

- Vaginal or speculum examination is contraindicated until the placenta position is identified
- FBC, coagulation screen, Rh factor and cross-match
- Urgent ultrasound to assess placental position, fetal gestation, presentation and liquor volume. However, 50% of placental abruptions are not seen on ultrasound The diagnosis is often clinical.

Management of antepartum haemorrhage:

- Maternal and fetal monitoring
- Resuscitation with IV fluids ± blood, oxygen
- Urgent obstetric consultation; massive antepartum haemorrhage requires urgent delivery, usually by caesarean section
- Analgesia if required
- Anti-D if Rh-negative (dose dependent on gestation).

Bleeding in the non-pregnant woman

- History should include questions to elucidate the cause and severity of the bleeding. There may be history of PID, vaginal trauma, abnormal Pap smear, previous cervical surgery, recent instrumentation or childbirth.
- The timing of bleeding is important (postcoital, intermenstrual), as are associated symptoms e.g. pelvic pain, fever, dyspareunia, dysmenorrhoea.
- Symptoms and signs of systemic disease should be sought, e.g. bleeding diathesis, symptoms of hypothyroidism.
- Assessment of blood loss may be difficult, but menorrhagia is indicated by anaemia, use of 2 pads concurrently or tampon plus pad, pads/tampons changed every 1–2 hours when flow is heaviest, episodic flooding with staining of clothes or sheets, frequent clots, duration > 7 days.
- Differential diagnosis is shown in Box 35.1.

Box 35.1 Differential diagnosis of abnormal bleeding in the non-pregnant patient

- Ovulatory bleeding
- Anovulatory bleeding or dysfunctional uterine bleeding (DUB)
- Uterine and ovarian pathology:
  - — fibroids
  - — pelvic inflammatory disease
  - — endometriosis
  - — polycystic ovary syndrome
  - — endometrial polyps
  - — endometrial carcinoma
- Genital trauma or foreign body
- Iatrogenic cause:
  - — IUD
  - — Drugs, e.g. anticoagulants, chemotherapy

Investigations

- Exclude pregnancy
- Exclude pelvic infection
- FBC and coagulation studies
- Consider TFTs
- Consider pelvic ultrasound

Management

- Resuscitation if necessary
- Supportive treatment

- Specific treatment depending on identified cause ± O&G consultation or follow-up

Editorial Comment

Vaginal bleeding is a common ED presentation. In the non-pregnant female get a gynaecological opinion—even by phone works, especially as hormonal regimens or other agents such as tranexamic acid are not routinely prescribed in the ED.

Other complications of later pregnancy (> 20 weeks' gestation)

PREECLAMPSIA AND ECLAMPSIA

- **Preeclampsia** is a multisystem disorder, unique to pregnancy, which is usually associated with hypertension and significant proteinuria. It rarely presents before 20 weeks' gestation and is more common in nulliparous women.
- Hypertension in pregnancy is a systolic BP ≥ 140 mmHg and/or diastolic BP ≥ 90 mmHg.
- Features of severe preeclampsia are BP > 160/110 mmHg, proteinuria > 300 mg/day, hyperuricaemia, serum creatinine > 0.09 mmol/L.
- Other features include liver pain, elevated transaminases or bilirubin, persistent headaches, visual disturbances, hyperreflexia or clonus, thrombocytopenia.
- **Eclampsia** is the onset of seizures in pregnancy or the postnatal period, usually preceded by preeclampsia.
- Preeclampsia and eclampsia may occur up to 4 weeks postpartum.

Investigations

- FBC, blood film (haemolysis), coagulation studies, EUC, LFTs, uric acid, group-and-hold
- Urinalysis for proteinuria ± 24-hour urine collection
- CT of the brain may be indicated only to confirm a differential diagnosis or complication

Management

Severe preeclampsia and eclampsia are medical and obstetric emergencies.

1. Seizure prophylaxis or treatment:
   - Magnesium sulfate loading dose = 4 g IV over 15 minutes
   - Followed by an infusion of magnesium sulfate 1 g/h IV.

— Monitor serum magnesium levels 6-hourly and assess for clonus and deep tendon reflexes 1- to 2-hourly.

2 Blood pressure control:
   — Intravenous labetalol is the antihypertensive of choice. If unavailable, intravenous hydralazine can be used.
   — The aim is for a diastolic BP of 90–100 mmHg.
3 Urgent obstetric consultation.
4 Fetal monitoring.
5 General resuscitative measures—maintenance of airway, oxygen therapy, IV access, nurse patient on left side, IDC and fluid balance monitoring.
6 Delivery is indicated in severe preeclampsia or in a fetus > 37 weeks' gestation.

Emergency delivery

Preparation

- Call for help—O&G, paediatrics
- Obtain focused medical and obstetric history
- Perform an assessment:
  — number of fetuses
  — palpate the presenting part
  — fetal heart rate
  — cervical dilation
  — determine whether delivery is imminent
  — maternal BP, temperature

Equipment

- Chlorhexidine wash for perineum
- Gauze sponges
- Sterile gloves and gown
- Sterile clamp to clamp umbilical cord
- Umbilical cord plastic clamp
- Sterile scissors to cut cord
- Clean towels and blanket to dry and wrap neonate
- Container for placenta
- Nappy for neonate
- Neonatal resuscitation equipment
- Oxytocin 10 units

Procedure

1 Wash your hands and the patient's perineum. Put on gloves and gown.

2 Place one hand on the baby's head and apply gentle pressure to maintain it in a flexed position. Use the other hand to ease the perineum over the baby's face.
3 Feel for the umbilical cord around the baby's neck. If present, gently slip it over the baby's head.
4 With the next push guide the head downwards to deliver the anterior shoulder, then guide the head slightly upwards to deliver the posterior shoulder. The rest of the baby's body should follow immediately.
5 Wipe or suction the mouth, then the nose.
6 Place the baby on the mother's abdomen or chest, double-clamp the umbilical cord and cut in between, approximately 1–2 cm from the baby's abdomen.
7 Dry the baby and wrap in a blanket. Keep warm.
8 Resuscitate if necessary, as per neonatal resuscitation algorithm (Australian Resuscitation Council guidelines; see Figure 1.4).
9 Assign Apgar scores at 1 and 5 minutes post delivery (Table 35.2).
10 Check for undiagnosed twin.
11 Administer 10 U intramuscular oxytocin.
12 Look for signs of placental separation—lengthening of the cord, gush of blood from the vagina, change in shape of uterus fundus from discoid to globular with elevation of fundal height. Apply traction on the cord, backwards and downwards with one hand, while the other is placed suprapubically to support the uterus.
13 Inspect the placenta to ensure it is complete.

Table 35.2 Apgar score for assessment of neonates

Sign	Score 0	Score 1	Score 2	'APGAR' acronym
Colour	Blue, pale all over	Body pink, extremities blue	Body and extremities pink	Appearance
Heart rate	Absent	Slow (< 100 bpm)	> 100 bpm	Pulse
Reflex irritability	No response	Crying, some motion	Vigorous cry/ pulls away	Grimace
Muscle tone	Flaccid	Some flexion of extremities	Active motion, good flexion	Activity
Breathing	Absent	Slow, irregular, hypoventilation	Strong, cries lustily	Respiration

14 Rub over the uterus to facilitate contraction and expulsion of clots.
15 Inspect the perineum for lacerations. Apply pressure until these can be repaired.

TRAUMA IN LATE PREGNANCY

The risk to the pregnancy in 'minor' trauma is significant, with preterm labour occurring in 8%, abruption in 1% and fetal death in 1% of occurrences. In severe trauma, the fetal death rate rises to 20% or greater.

It is important to remember that there are 2 patients; however, the survival of the fetus is dependent on optimal management of the mother. Maintaining maternal oxygenation and tissue perfusion is the primary goal.

Assessment and management

- Maternal primary survey and resuscitation (ABCs with cervical spine precautions).
- Left lateral tilt if > 20 weeks' gestation (while maintaining cervical spine stability) to displace uterus and prevent vena caval compression.
- Perform secondary survey, including assessment of the uterus ± vaginal exam. If mother unstable, resuscitate and treat cause.
- Monitor mother and fetus (cardiotocography (CTG) ideally).
- Continue CTG monitoring for at least 4–6 hours. Consider ultrasound.
- Check Rhesus status.

All patients with minor trauma should be admitted to hospital for at least 24 hours.

CARDIOPULMONARY RESUSCITATION IN LATE PREGNANCY

In cardiac arrest, all the principles of basic life support (BLS) and advanced life support (ALS) apply; see Chapter 1. Specific considerations include:

- Call for help immediately—obstetrician, neonatologist, anaesthetist.
- Tilt the pelvis to the left (shoulders flat to enable cardiac compressions and a wedge under woman's right hip).
- Secure the airway early.
- Perform chest compressions slightly above the centre of the sternum.

- Consider preparation for emergency Caesarean section within 4 minutes of cardiac arrest if gestation is estimated to be > 24 weeks.

Prescribing in pregnancy

- All drugs should be avoided if possible during the first trimester.
- Drugs should be prescribed in pregnancy only if the expected benefit to the mother is thought to be greater than the risk to the fetus.
- Drugs that have been extensively used in pregnancy and appear to be usually safe (category A) should be prescribed in preference to new or untried drugs; and the smallest effective dose should be used.
- For information regarding specific drugs, MIMS should be consulted.

Anti-D prophylaxis

Rh_o(D) immunoglobulin (anti-D) is administered for prophylaxis against haemolytic disease of the newborn. Current indications and doses include potentially sensitising events, e.g. miscarriage, ectopic pregnancy during the first trimester (250 IU Rh_o(D) immunoglobulin); potentially sensitising events during the 2nd and 3rd trimesters (625 IU Rh_o(D) immunoglobulin, plus additional doses as indicated from the assessment of the extent of feto-maternal haemorrhage).

Sexual assault

Sexual assault is a common, and under-reported, violent crime. Women presenting to the ED following a sexual assault are preferably referred to a sexual assault service, where expertise in obtaining forensic samples, documenting the physical examination, offering pregnancy and STD prophylaxis and providing psychological support exists. Occasionally, victims require management of other injuries prior to assessment by the sexual assault service.

Post-coital contraception: morning-after pill

- Give levonorgestrel 0.75 mg orally at presentation and repeat dose at 12 hours.
- If administered within 72 hours of unprotected intercourse, pregnancy rate is approximately 1.1%.
- Antiemetics should always be given, and a spare dose of hormone tablets, should vomiting occur.

Advice given with emergency contraception should include risk of failure, risk of sexually transmitted infections and appropriate follow-up and counselling regarding contraceptive use.

Online resources

Australian Resuscitation Council (ARC) guidelines
    www.resus.org.au
eTG Therapeutic Guidelines
    www.ciap.health.nsw.gov.au
MIMS Online
    www.ciap.health.nsw.gov.au
Royal Women's Hospital, Melbourne, Victoria
    www.thewomens.org.au

Acknowledgement

The work of the previous author of this chapter, Dr Sally McCarthy, is acknowledged with thanks.

Chapter 36
Ophthalmic emergencies

Michael R Delaney and Iromi Samarasinghe

Principles of examination

1 All cases of suspected eye injuries need a good history and examination of:
— visual acuity—visual loss sudden/gradual; central/peripheral; monocular/binocular
— pupillary reactions
— the fundus
— ocular movement
— fields to confrontation
— lids and ocular adnexae.

2 Do not put pressure on the eye to examine it (especially if there is a possible penetrating injury).

3 Use a short-acting mydriatic, e.g. tropicamide 1% (duration of action 60 minutes), and only if essential.

4 Cyclopplegics are not used when examining the eye due to their long duration of action. Only use a short-acting cycloplegic, if necessary for comfort, e.g. cyclopentolate 1% (effective for 4–8 hours) or homatropine 2% (effective for 8–12 hours).

5 CT scan or X-ray the orbits in all cases of a suspected intraocular foreign body, especially if the patient was using a hammer on metal, e.g. a chisel.
Note: Request X-ray with eyes in up and down gazes.

See 'Common Pitfalls' overleaf.

Use of the slit lamp

These remarks apply to the Haag Streit slit lamp, but the principles apply to all slit lamps.

- The patient and the examining doctor must both be seated comfortably. In particular, the patient should not be straining to keep the chin on the chin rest, and the patient's forehead must rest comfortably against the forehead strap.
- The eye should be at the level of the black mark on the side of the two columns that hold the chin rest and forehead strap; this

Common Pitfalls

- Never use steroid drops in the ED in initial treatment. Refer for further assessment.
- Do not use atropine drops to dilate the pupil.
- Do not use mydriatics in cases where the ocular state and optic nerve function may need to be monitored.
- Eye swabs need to be plated out directly.
- Avoid contaminated diagnostic medications. Use only sterile drop solutions.
- Always pad an eye after instilling local anaesthetic.
- Never give local anaesthetic drops to the patient to take away and use.
- Do not apply ointment in cases of suspected penetrating injury.
- Do not persist in trying to remove a corneal foreign body if it is not easily removed—refer for ophthalmology review.
- Always provide adequate systemic analgesia in cases of corneal injury.
- When in doubt seek an ophthalmic consultation.

is achieved by adjusting the height of the chin rest. The slit lamp should then be adjusted so that it is in its mid position, allowing a full range of vertical and horizontal movement. This position is adjusted by rotating the joystick which controls the height of the slit lamp (by rotating the handle alone) as well as the movement of the slit lamp in all directions, thereby controlling its focus.

- After the patient is positioned correctly, the eye can be examined. Turn power on at base of slit lamp table; adjust eye pieces to zero if no refractory error adjustments are required for the examiner; set magnification by adjusting swing lever between eye pieces.
- On the bottom of the rotating light-source column of the slit lamp is a knob that controls the width of the slit beam; the knob on the left side can be adjusted with the examiner's left hand. Further up near the top of the light-source column, immediately under the globe-housing, is a control to adjust the intensity of the light; use the neutral-density filter (mid-position) to reduce discomfort for the patient from the brightness of the light. This same control also allows the insertion of a cobalt blue filter into the light, producing the characteristic blue light used to detect corneal ulcers with fluorescein dye. Below this control is another control knob that adjusts the height of the slit beam.
- Focus the slit beam on the eye before looking through the viewfinder. Move the joystick with one hand while looking

through the viewfinder till the cornea comes into focus. Keep the other hand free for handling the eye.

- The slit lamp can be used in many ways.
  - The easiest is simply to use it as a high-powered illumination source with magnification using the broad beam; this is particularly useful to detect corneal ulceration after instilling fluorescein dye and using the cobalt blue filter.
  - To detect and assess iritis, a narrow slit beam can be shone through the anterior chamber; this will highlight any flare or cells.
  - A slit beam can be shone directly through the pupil to retro-illuminate the iris using the red reflex; this is also a useful way of assessing the clarity of the media.
- Intraocular pressures are measured using the application tonometer, which is either attached to the slit lamp on a swinging arm or is detached from the slit lamp and is placed on the platform immediately in front of the eye pieces.

Trauma

FOREIGN BODY (FB)

Conjunctiva

Carefully examine posterior lid surfaces and fornices by everting the upper lid. Remove FB with moist swabstick or fine forceps.

Cornea

- Remove FB with a sterile swab stick or sterile 25-gauge needle. Do not attempt to remove any rust ring. Apply antibiotic ointment and pad firmly.
- Topical antibiotic drops are often preferred to ointment by patients following the initial management.
- Patients with a residual rust ring and foreign body remnants must be referred to an ophthalmologist according to your hospital's practice.

Intraocular

- Always suspect FB if there has been an eye injury after using a metal hammer on metal, or where there have been high-velocity particles.
- There are often minimal signs. CT scan or X-ray of the orbit is mandatory.
- Treat as a penetrating injury (see below) and organise urgent ophthalmic consultation.

CORNEAL ABRASIONS

- Examine the eye under cobalt blue light after instilling local anaesthetic drops (amethocaine 0.5% [also known as tetracaine]) and fluorescein.
- Check for subtarsal FB.
- Treat with chloromphenicol 1% antibiotic ointment and firm pad for 24 hours and provide adequate analgesia.

LID LACERATIONS

- All lid lacerations must be carefully assessed to exclude penetrating eye injury.
- Lacerations nasal to the punctum on the upper or the lower eyelids should be referred to an ophthalmologist to exclude damage to the nasolacrimal drainage system.
- Inspect punctum and look for lacerations to the canaliculus, which require prompt repair.
- Lacerations through the lid margin need meticulous repair to prevent lid notching. Refer to ophthalmology service according to your hospital's practice.

BURNS

Chemical: acid or alkali

1. Immediate irrigation with copious amounts of water or saline solution for at least 30 minutes until the pH neutralises to 7.5. Use universal indicator paper (if available) to check corneal pH in the forniceal space after every litre of fluid irrigation.
2. If pain limits eye opening, instil local anaesthetic drops (amethocaine [tetracaine] 0.5%).
3. Alkali burns from lime, mortar and plaster are the most damaging of all chemical injuries. All particles of lime must be removed using a cotton bud or fine forceps. Evert lids to inspect fornices.
4. Acid burns commonly result from exposure to car battery fluid, toilet cleaners and pool cleaners.
5. All chemical burns should be referred to ophthalmology on the same day. Systemic analgesia is often required.

Thermal burns

Remove any obvious loose FBs after instilling anaesthetic drops. Start antibiotic drops and pad if possible.

Flash burns

- Symptoms appear hours after exposure to sunlamps or welding arcs without eye protection. These are intensely painful with

blepharospasm, tearing and redness. Pain can start up to 6–12 hours after injury and last for 24 hours.
- Examination is only possible after topical anaesthesia. Slit lamp examination with fluorescein will show widespread epithelial defects bilaterally.

Management

1. Apply chloramphenicol 1% ointment and pad. Cycloplegics may be needed to minimise severe eye pain (homatropine 2% BD for 3 days). Systemic analgesia and sedation are usually needed.
2. Ophthalmic review in 24 hours.

BLUNT OCULAR TRAUMA

Severe injuries can be easily missed. The history is not always a good guide to the severity of the injuries.

Subconjunctival haemorrhage

- The appearance is alarming. No treatment is needed except reassurance.
- Examine the eye to exclude any other injuries.

Hyphaema

Blood in anterior chamber following blunt trauma involving punch or cricket/squash ball to eye. Consider lymphoma, leukaemia and child abuse if bleed is 'spontaneous'.

Management

1. Admit to hospital for bed rest, head elevation to 30–45° and limit eye movement with pad. Bed rest at home if circumstances are appropriate. Arrange for urgent ophthalmic consultation within 24 hours.
2. Rule out orbital fracture and ruptured globe with CT of orbits and facial bones.
3. Provide adequate analgesia, avoiding aspirin.
4. After ophthalmic consultation control intraocular pressure (IOP) with:
   - prostaglandin analogues, e.g. latanoprost 1 drop daily *AND/OR*
   - beta-blockers, e.g. timolol 0.5% 1 drop BD *OR*
   - acetazolamide 250–1000 mg/day *OR*
   - mannitol 20% in 500 mL IV in severe cases.

5 Complications include:
— a more severe secondary haemorrhage in 30% of cases, 2–5 days after the initial bleed (especially in children)
— secondary glaucoma due to outflow obstruction
— raised IOP
— missed blowout fractures of orbit.

Traumatic mydriasis and iridodialysis

No treatment is available. Often associated with hyphaema. Remember as a cause of abnormal pupillary reactions in cases with head and eye injuries.

Lens and retinal injuries

These need referral within 24 hours. See the section 'Retinal detachment' under 'Sudden painless monocular visual loss', below.

Ruptured globe

Occurs following blunt trauma with sufficient force, resulting in rupture at thinnest point of scleral wall, usually near corneal limbus.

- Examination may be significantly limited by oedema. Assess visual acuity and extraocular movements. Ophthalmoscopy may often reveal loss of red reflex due to vitreal haemorrhage.
- Urgent CT scan of orbits to exclude blowout fracture and referral to ophthalmologist, if otherwise stable from trauma point of view.
- Ensure eye is lightly padded and patient has adequate analgesia.

Traumatic vitreous haemorrhage and choroidal haemorrhage

Advise bed rest at home. Arrange ophthalmology referral within 24 hours to exclude retinal detachment. See the section 'Vitreous haemorrhage' under 'Sudden painless monocular visual loss' below.

ORBITAL FRACTURES AND HAEMORRHAGE

Blowout fractures

Mechanism of injury involves punch or squash/cricket ball to orbit. Often associated with fractures of malar complex and of middle 3rd of face.

- Pain on vertical eye movement and local tenderness along orbital margin. Suspect if there is restriction of extraocular movement, enophthalmos or the patient complains of double vision (restricted up and down gaze).

- Assess infraorbital nerve involvement by testing sensation on unilateral cheek and upper incisors. The eye must be examined during initial assessment.
- Investigations include CT scan of brain and orbital reconstructions (coronal views most useful).

Management

1. Admit if other injuries require treatment. Otherwise needs referral within 24 hours for evaluation of diplopia and enophthalmos.
2. Start oral antibiotics (cefalexin 500 mg QID).
3. Instruct patient not to blow nose and to avoid Valsalva manoeuvres in 1st week. Nasal decongestants for 7–10 days.
4. Surgical repair is usually done after 7–14 days.

Orbital haemorrhage

- Often associated with orbital fractures.
- Can be sight-threatening. Needs urgent consultation if severe or the patient has reduced vision, non-reacting pupils or ophthalmoplegia (diplopia on up and down gaze) and proptosis.
- May need urgent orbital decompression.

Optic canal fractures

- Often cause total visual loss due to compression of the optic nerve. Diagnosed on CT scans of brain and orbits.
- Needs urgent referral to ophthalmic surgeon.

PENETRATING INJURIES

- Suspect from history, especially hammering on metal.
- Examine very gently. Do not put pressure on the eye. Check visual acuity; red reflex; slit lamp examination for anterior chamber and corneal disruptions should only be done if trauma is not obvious.

Management

1. Keep nil by mouth. Provide adequate parenteral narcotics with antiemetics. Check tetanus immunisation and update as appropriate. Start systemic antibiotics (ceftriaxone 1 g daily) and local antibiotic drops (do not use ointment). Gently shield (do not pad) the eye.
2. Obtain X-ray or CT scan of the orbit if there is any possibility of intraocular FB.
3. Admit to hospital for bed rest or refer for urgent ophthalmology review according to your hospital's practice.

The painful red eye

ACUTE BLEPHARITIS

Localised eyelid inflammation. Can present as chalazion or stye.

- Treat with topical antibiotics and warm compresses. Routine referral to ophthalmologist.

CORNEAL FOREIGN BODY OR ABRASION

(Discussed above.)

ACUTE CONJUNCTIVITIS

Red inflamed eye, less congested towards the limbus. May be allergic, viral or bacterial. Often gritty with copious mucopurulent discharge in bacterial infections. Copious serous discharge in viral infections. Highly contagious.

Management

1. Observe strict hand hygiene.
2. Swab for culture and polymerase chain reaction (PCR).
3. Start broad-spectrum antibiotic drops every 1–2 hours, e.g. chloramphenicol 0.5% drops or ciprofloxacin drops in contact-lens wearers.
4. If viral conjunctivitis suspected, treat with antihistamine drops or another suitable OTC preparation to reduce chemosis and itching.
5. Patient should avoid wearing contact lenses for duration of treatment.
6. Does not need ophthalmic review unless photophobia is associated with decreased visual acuity, or protracted inflammation longer than 3 weeks, or swabs reveal *Chlamydia*.

ACUTE KERATITIS (HERPES SIMPLEX)

- Painful eye often with blurred vision, diffuse conjunctival injection and watery discharge.
- Look for dendrite using fluorescein stain and cobalt blue light of ophthalmoscope or slit lamp. Branching dendritic pattern of herpes simplex ulceration of cornea will appear green.

Management

- Herpes simplex ulceration is treated with aciclovir 3% ointment 5 times a day for 14 days plus antibiotic drops 4 times a day. Do not patch due to risk of *Pseudomonas* infection. Refer for ophthalmology review on following day.

- In non-herpetic keratitis, start antibiotic drops 4–6 times a day.
- Refer for urgent ophthalmology review if history of contact-lens use.

HERPES ZOSTER OPHTHALMICUS

- Shingles in trigeminal nerve distribution involving ophthalmic branch.
- Vesicular rash noted on forehead or upper eyelid. Hutchinson's sign is a vesicle on the tip of the nose.
- On corneal examination, 'pseudodendritic' ulcer may be seen.

Management

1. Treat with famciclovir 250 mg TDS or aciclovir 800 mg every 4 waking hours for 7 days.
2. Ophthalmology referral if visual acuity affected or eye is red.

ACUTE IRITIS (UVEITIS)

- Dull pain, photophobia and red eye; ciliary injection (more injected near the limbus).
- Sluggish small pupil and blurred vision.
- Hypopyon (collection of white cells in anterior chamber) may be seen in severe uveitis.
- Slit lamp examination essential: anterior chamber appears cloudy from cells and flare.
- Intraocular pressure is normal.

Management

1. Dilate pupil with short-acting cycloplegic drops, e.g. cyclopentolate 1% 3 times a day and local steroid drops 4–6 times a day after consultation with ophthalmologist.
2. Analgesia and dark glasses may be required.

ACUTE NARROW-ANGLE (ANGLE-CLOSURE) GLAUCOMA

- Severe pain in unilateral red eye. Poor vision associated with headache, nausea and vomiting.
- Semi-dilated non-reacting pupil. Cornea appears hazy.
- Intraocular pressure is markedly raised. Eye is tender and tense to palpation.
- Headache, nausea and vomiting may be systemic features.
- The main differential diagnosis is acute iritis, which can cause secondary glaucoma.

Management

1 Urgent referral to ophthalmologist, as acute glaucoma is a sight-threatening condition.
2 Start miotic drops—pilocarpine 2% every 5 minutes for 1 hour; then hourly. In addition timolol 0.5% twice daily plus prednisolone 0.5% 4 times a day topical to affected eye.
3 Acetazolamide 500 mg IV, then 250 mg every 8 hours (orally if tolerated).
4 Narcotic analgesia for pain management, e.g. morphine 5–10 mg IM injection.
5 Admit under care of ophthalmologist.

PERIORBITAL CELLULITIS

Periocular superficial cellulitis involving pre-septal tissue. Eye not involved. Requires systemic antibiotics and observation. Usually due to *Staphylococcus aureus, Streptococcus pneumoniae* or *Haemophilus influenzae* (if unimmunised) in children with otitis media.

- Examination of the eye may be difficult due to marked swelling. In children, especially, may require examination under general anaesthetic to exclude eye involvement. CT of the orbits is an essential part of investigations.
- Consider admitting for intravenous flucloxacillin 12.5 mg/kg QID or cephazolin 12.5 mg/kg QID. Can usually be managed with oral antibiotics and good follow-up.

ORBITAL CELLULITIS

Potentially life-threatening eye infection.

- Oedema and swelling of eyelids and conjunctiva. Often with proptosis, restriction of eye movement, dull pain and fever. There may be altered pupillary response; reduced visual acuity is a late sign. Usually secondary to trauma or orbital extension of paranasal sinusitis.
- Commonly due to *Staphylococcus aureus, Haemophilus influenzae* or *Streptococcus pneumoniae.*

Management

1 Swab any wounds, start high-dose IV antibiotics: dicloxacillin 2 g QID plus ceftriaxone 2 g daily in adults.
2 CT scan of orbits and paranasal sinuses to exclude cavernous sinus thrombosis.
3 Admit to hospital and observe the vision and the eye. Urgent ophthalmology referral.

Sudden painless monocular visual loss

AMAUROSIS FUGAX

Sudden painless visual loss, usually partial and transient, due to embolic occlusion of retinal artery in transient ischaemic attack. Visual loss lasts minutes and returns to normal by the time of presentation to the ED.

- Fundoscopic examination essentially normal. Often not associated with history of dysphasia or hemiparesis.
- Requires timely referral to neurologist for appropriate investigations, including CT cerebral angiogram, echo, carotid duplex scans, cerebral perfusion scans and interventions in stroke management. Stroke pathway work-up is indicated if presenting within 4.5 hours of onset of symptoms.

CENTRAL RETINAL ARTERY OCCLUSION

- Sudden painless total or partial loss of vision, more often in the elderly. Visual acuity < 6/60.
- Fundoscopic findings: pale disc, retinal oedema, cherry red spot on the macula and narrowed arteries.
- This is an ophthalmological emergency—likely embolic cause.
- Consider differential diagnoses, especially giant cell arteritis (see below).

Initial treatment

If seen within 2 hours of onset of symptoms:

1. Lower IOP with digital massage and acetazolamide 500 mg IV.
2. Attempt to dilate blood vessels by breathing carbogen (95% O_2 and 5% CO_2) via mask, or re-breathing from a paper bag.
3. Continue treatment for at least 30 minutes.
4. Do urgent ESR and CRP to exclude giant cell arteritis.
5. Obtain urgent ophthalmology consultation for treatment options. Admit to hospital.

GIANT CELL ARTERITIS (TEMPORAL ARTERITIS)

- An ophthalmological emergency with similar presentation to central retinal artery occlusion (see above).
- Giant cell arteritis (GCA) is an ischaemic optic neuropathy characterised by blurred vision and temporal headache, generally in the elderly.
- GCA results in progressive blindness in both eyes if treatment is not instituted early.

Initial treatment of GCA

1 Attempt to reduce intraocular pressure and vasodilate:
  - Lower IOP with digital massage and acetazolamide 500 mg IV.
  - Attempt to dilate blood vessels by breathing carbogen (95% O_2 and 5% CO_2) via mask, or re-breathing from a paper bag.
  - Continue treatment for at least 30 minutes.

2 Do urgent ESR and CRP to assist diagnosis.

3 Obtain urgent ophthalmology consultation for treatment options and rheumatology consultation for diagnostic temporal artery biopsy.

4 Admit to hospital.

5 Commence high-dose steroids: methylprednisone 1000 mg/day IV infusion over 1 hour or prednisone 1–2 mg/kg/day (maximum 150 mg) PO. High-dose steroids should commence on clinical suspicion prior to biopsy results being available. GCA is associated with a high incidence of blindness and the aim of steroids is to stop progression of visual impairment in the affected eye and prevent blindness in the other eye.

RETINAL VEIN OCCLUSION

Sudden and painless loss of vision that is usually incomplete and variable. Commonly seen in the elderly, diabetics and hypertensives.

- Fundoscopy shows dilated retinal veins with multiple haemorrhages throughout the retina; optic disc often swollen. Referred to as 'blood and thunder' fundus if severe.
- Urgent ophthalmology consultation.
- No treatment.

OPTIC NEURITIS

Loss of vision over hours to days, usually painless but pain may occur with eye movement.

- Common presenting feature of multiple sclerosis. Examine for other focal neurological defects.
- Variable visual loss, more frequently central field loss.
- Afferent pupillary defect and marked loss of red saturation, i.e. reduced visual acuity affecting colour and contrast vision.
- Urgent ophthalmology referral for investigation, including MRI.
- No initial or urgent treatment, but may respond to intravenous corticosteroids or immune modulators after appropriate consultation. There is no indication for oral steroids.

RETINAL DETACHMENT

- Painless visual loss with partial field loss, after a recent history of visual flashes and floaters. More common in myopic and aphakic (lens-extracted) patients; often occurs after blunt trauma.
- Grey, elevated veil-like retina seen. Red reflex is lost.

Management

1. If macula still not detached, admit to hospital for bed rest and urgent ophthalmic assessment.
2. If macula detached (visual acuity is reduced), refer for assessment within 24 hours.

VITREOUS HAEMORRHAGE

- Often preceded by large black floaters. Vision may vary up to complete visual loss.
- Advise bed rest at home. Needs referral within 24 hours to exclude retinal detachment.

Postoperative problems

VITREORETINAL SURGERY

Intraocular gases used in retinal surgery to tamponade and flatten the retina can create symptoms of a row of bubbles in the visual field, which the patient may mistake for a recurrent retinal detachment.

- Fundoscopy to exclude retinal detachment and visualise air bubbles on retina.
- Get patient to sit up and then lie on their side. The patient will note that the direction of the bubbles has changed, as the row of gas bubbles will always remain parallel to the floor.
- Reassure patient as the air bubbles will resorb in about 5 days postoperatively; other intraocular gases may take from 2 to 8 weeks to resorb.
- Flying is an absolute contraindication until gas bubbles are completely resorbed, as intraocular gas expansion can cause central retinal artery occlusion.
- Nitrous oxide anaesthetic is contraindicated as it can cause expansion of the gas bubbles with similar complications from rising IOP.
- Silicon oil, used instead of intraocular gases, can cause acute open-angle glaucoma; but cornea remains clear, unlike in glaucoma. Silicon oil may be seen in the anterior chamber or the vitreous cavity, on slit lamp examination. Treatment

is as for open-angle glaucoma, but the pupil is dilated with cyclopentolate or homatropine to allow oil to move back into the vitreous cavity.

REFRACTIVE SURGERY

Dislocation of the corneal flap following laser eye surgery (Lasik) is a surgical emergency.

- Blurred vision and a foreign-body sensation following laser surgery.
- Do not attempt to manipulate or reposition flap.
- Instil local anaesthetic (tetracaine) to relieve pain and lid spasm. Cover eye with clear shield. Do not pad or apply any pressure to eye.
- Refer for urgent ophthalmological consultation.

CATARACT SURGERY

Cataract surgery is one of the most common operations performed; patients present with symptoms of floaters and flashes and reduced vision.

- Check visual acuity.
- The pupil should be dilated prior to fundoscopy to look for retinal detachment or vitreous haemorrhage.
- Urgent ophthalmological consultation if significant findings.

Ophthalmic conditions needing referral

Acute dacryocystitis. Treat with warm compresses and massage of tear sac. Start antibiotics.

Squints in children. Need to be seen by an ophthalmologist without delay. Perform cover test to diagnose.

Chronic glaucoma. Patient needs full assessment and institution of therapy. Refer without delay.

Meibomian gland cyst/abscess. Treat with hot compresses plus local antibiotic drops (oral antibiotics if severe). Refer.

Common ophthalmic medications

Antibiotics. Availability and use varies from country to country. A routine course of treatment would be 1 or 2 drops, 4–5 times a day for 4 days. Intensive treatment needs drops every 1 or 2 hours during waking hours with ointment at night. Antibiotics suitable for initial treatment: sulfacetamide 10%; chloramphenicol 0.5%; gentamicin 0.3%; tobramycin 0.3%, ciprofloxacin 3 mg/mL.

Antiviral agents. Aciclovir 30 mg/g (3%) ophthalmic ointment.

Local anaesthetics. Tetracaine hydrochloride 0.5% (available as Minims; also known as amethocaine); proxymetacaine hydrochloride 0.5%.

Mydriatics. Fundal observation is best carried out using 1 drop of tropicamide 0.5% (Mydriacyl) and waiting about 15 minutes. Reverse with pilocarpine 2% drops.

Cycloplegics. Use short-acting preparations, e.g. cyclopentolate 1% or homatropine 2%, 1–3 times a day. Do not use atropine.

Miotics. Pilocarpine 2% is the most commonly used strength.

Glaucoma preparations. Latanoprost; bimatoprost; brimonidine tartrate; apraclonidine HCl; pilocarpine HCl 1%, 2%, 4%; acetazolamide 250 mg PO.

Non-steroidal anti-inflammatory drugs (NSAIDs). Diclofenac; ketoralac.

Steroids. Fluorometholone 0.1%; prednisolone 0.5%, 1%; dexamethasone 0.1%.

Frequency of use. Remember to tell the patient to wait 5 minutes between different drops.

Chapter 37
Ear, nose and throat (ENT) emergencies

Shalini Arunanthy

The care of these patients requires an organised approach and some basic equipment (see Box 37.1).

Box 37.1 ENT equipment

- Head light
- Nasal speculum
- Ear speculum
- Jobson Horne curette
- Packing forceps
- Alligator forceps
- Magill's forceps
- Suction catheters—including fine metal sucker
- Co-phenylcaine spray (lignocaine 5% + phenylephidrine 0.5%)
- Tampons (Merocel)—ear, nasal
- Rapid Rhino devices—anterior and posterior

Ear emergencies

OTITIS EXTERNA

Clinical features

- Ear pain
- History of water exposure or trauma—commonly cotton tips
- Oedema of canal, with debris

Organisms

- *Pseudomonas*
- *Staphylococcus*
- Rarely fungal

Management

1 Analgesia.
2 Remove debris gently—suction catheter or cotton-wool swab.
3 Insert Merocel tampon (ear).

4 Instil antibiotic/steroid drops (Otodex, Sofradex).
5 ENT consult for admission and IV antibiotics if has spread outside ear canal. Otherwise outpatient ENT follow-up.

OTITIS MEDIA

Clinical features

- Common in children
- Ear ache ± fever
- Pulling at pinna
- Injection of tympanic membrane with bulging of membrane
- Effusion behind membrane
- Purulent discharge if tympanic membrane ruptured (leads to relief of pain)

Organisms

- Viral
- *Streptococcus pneumoniae*
- *Haemophilus influenzae*
- *Moraxella catarrhalis*

Management

1 Analgesia.
2 Antibiotics if < 6 months old or if systemic features (fever, vomiting).
3 Otherwise wait for 48 hours.
4 Review and start antibiotics if not improving.
5 Antibiotic of choice is amoxycillin.[1]

Note: Antibiotics are no longer routinely recommended for all patients with acute otitis media.[2]

Complications

- Ruptured tympanic membrane usually heals spontaneously without complications within 2–3 weeks. Advise to keep dry and avoid instilling any drops.
- Recurrent infections/otitis media with effusion—refer to ENT as outpatient.
- Mastoiditis—see 'Mastoiditis' section below.
- Intracranial complications such as epidural abscess, meningitis are rare.

MASTOIDITIS

Mastoiditis is a rare but significant complication of otitis media.

Clinical features of mastoiditis

- Symptoms of otitis media
- Pain over mastoid region
- Fever
- Erythematous, bulging ear drum
- Tenderness ± swelling over mastoid
- Elevated white cell count (WCC), C-reactive protein (CRP)
- CT scan shows changes of mastoiditis (mainly fluid in mastoid air cells)

Organisms

Similar to acute otitis media.

Management

1. IV antibiotics—usually ceftriaxone plus flucloxacillin.
2. Analgesia.
3. ENT referral for admission ± surgery.

PERICHONDRITIS

Becoming more common due to infected ear piercings involving cartilage (high piercings).

Clinical features

- Painful auricle
- Erythema and swelling of auricle
- Fever

Organisms

- *Pseudomonas aeruginosa*
- *Staphylococcus aureus*
- *Streptococcus pyogenes*

Management

1. Analgesia.
2. Remove ear piercing—use auricular block (see Fig 37.1 below), if embedded
3. Antibiotics—flucloxacillin and gentamicin.
4. ENT referral for admission ± drainage.
5. Explain to patient the possibility of necrosis of cartilage with associated deformity.

RUPTURED TYMPANIC MEMBRANE

Caused by otitis media, blows to the ear or direct trauma, usually due to objects used to clean ear canal.

Clinical features

- Hearing loss—conductive
- If associated with infection, acute pain; relieved once membrane has ruptured
- Discharge from ear also if associated with infection
- Visible tear of membrane on otoscopy

Management

Most perforations do not require specific treatment and will heal spontaneously, especially if a central perforation.

1. Keep ear dry—the most important instruction for the patient.
2. Oral antibiotics if associated with infection.
3. Hearing test.
4. Refer to ENT outpatient for follow-up.
5. Refer to ENT immediately if associated tinnitus or vertigo, as this signifies inner ear injury.

AURICULAR HAEMATOMA

Clinical features

Patient presents with a swollen, painful pinna following blunt trauma.

Management

ENT referral for drainage and pressure dressing to prevent further bleeding.

Complication

If not treated adequately, the cartilage undergoes necrosis and a 'cauliflower ear' will result.

AURICULAR LACERATIONS

Simple lacerations may be repaired in the ED. Complex wounds should be referred to the ENT or plastic surgeon for repair.

Refer the following wounds:

- loss of skin
- multiple lacerations
- exposed cartilage
- involvement of external auditory canal
- avulsion or near-avulsion of ear.

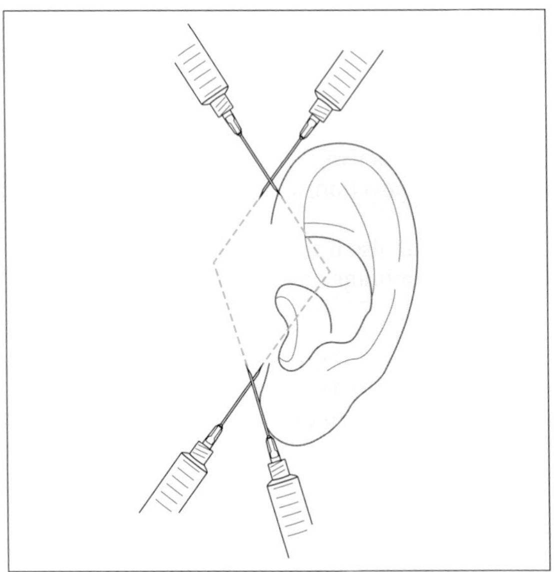

Figure 37.1 Anaesthetic block of the ear

Management of simple lacerations

1 Irrigate with saline (place gauze in canal to reduce amount of saline going into external ear).
2 Anaesthetise with a block rather than local infiltration into the pinna (see Figure 37.1).
   - Insert needle just above the attachment of the ear to the head. Direct the needle first anteriorly towards the tragus and inject local anaesthetic, then withdraw to point of insertion and inject posteriorly behind ear.
   - Do the same at inferior attachment of ear.
   - DO NOT inject into pinna.
3 Repair cartilage with 5/0 absorbable suture.
4 Repair skin with 5/0 or 6/0 non-absorbable suture.
5 Pressure dressing.
6 Remove sutures in 5 days.

TEMPORAL BONE FRACTURES

Temporal bone fractures are reported to be included in 15–20% of all skull fractures. This injury has a low priority in the multi-trauma patient, but should not be forgotten.

Clinical features

- CSF or blood in ear canal
- Battle sign—post auricular haematoma
- Facial nerve palsy
- Vertigo
- Deafness
- CT scan with fine cuts through the temporal bone is required for evaluation

Management

1. Most important is to look for the injury in the secondary survey.
2. ENT referral.
3. Most are managed conservatively.

FOREIGN BODIES—EAR

- Common in children. Usually beads, bits of toys, seeds, paper.
- In adults may be insects or cotton off the tip of a cotton bud.

Clinical features

- Pain
- Discharge if left unattended and gets infected
- Visible foreign body on otoscopy

Management

1. Most important is a cooperative patient. A child may require sedation, e.g. with nitrous oxide. Explain procedure to parents and get them to calm the child.
2. If insect, drown in lignocaine and then remove with alligator forceps.
3. If non-organic foreign body and tympanic membrane intact, trial of irrigation.
4. Try suction with small catheter if irrigation fails or as first choice.
5. If unsuccessful, use an angled hook or curette to get behind the object and then move the object out along the canal (see Figure 37.2).
6. If unable to remove object, refer to ENT.

Note: DO NOT try to grab a hard round object with forceps, as this is likely to push it further into the auditory canal.

VERTIGO

Vertigo is the sensation of spinning of self or surroundings. Causes may be central or peripheral. Peripheral causes are labyrinthitis,

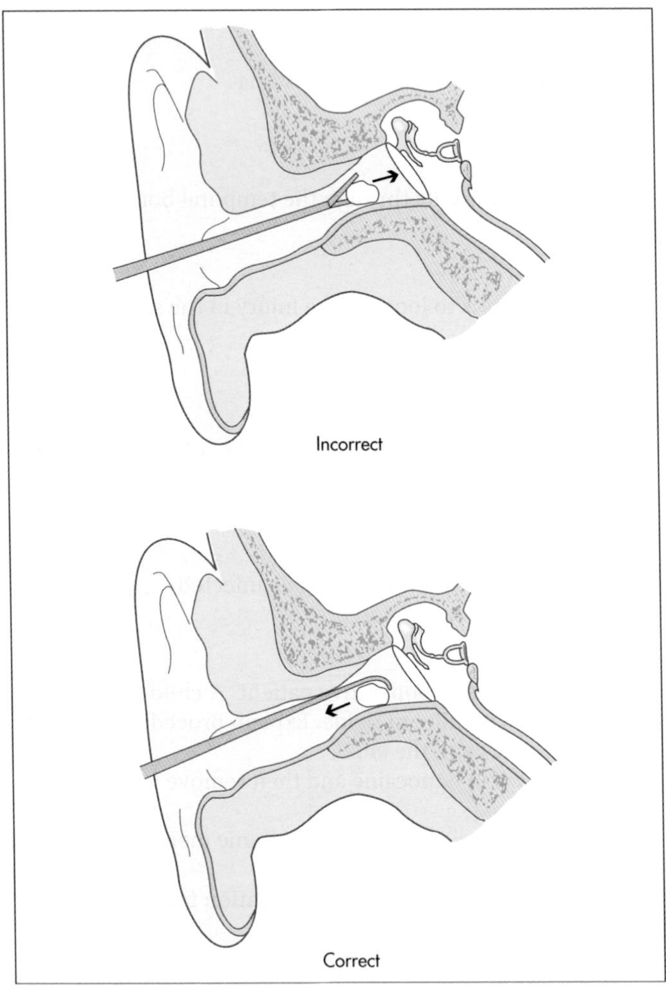

Figure 37.2 Incorrect and correct ways to remove a foreign body from the ear

vestibular neuronitis, Ménière's disease and benign paroxysmal positional vertigo (BPPV). This section will deal only with the peripheral causes of vertigo.

Clinical features

- Onset of vertigo is sudden and severe.
- May be paroxysmal and brought on by change in position of head in BPPV.
- Associated with nausea and vomiting.
- Tinnitus and deafness, especially in Ménière's disease.
- Exclude central causes with a complete neurological examination.
- Examine the ears for infection/inflammation.

Management

1. Symptomatic: with diazepam and/or prochlorperazine.
2. IV fluids if vomiting/dehydrated.
3. Diagnose BPPV with Dix–Hallpike manoeuvre and use trial of Epley manoeuvre for treatment[3]—see below.
4. If not settling and due to a peripheral cause, refer to ENT or neurology service for admission until symptoms settle.

Dix–Hallpike manoeuvre

To diagnose BPPV, use Dix–Hallpike manoeuvre.

Indications

Peripheral vertigo.

Contraindications

- Neck injury
- Cervical spondylosis
- Vertebrobasilar insufficiency, transient ischaemic attack, cerebrovascular accident
- Carotid bruits

Method

1. Warn patient that this may provoke/worsen vertigo.
2. Sit patient up in bed so that should they be lying their head is off the end of the bed.
3. Turn patient's head 45° to one side.
4. Ask patient to keep the eyes open.
5. Lie patient flat rapidly with head over end of bed by 20°.
6. Look for nystagmus—rotatory nystagmus indicates a positive test on that side.
7. Sit the patient back up.
8. Repeat with head turned to other side.

Epley manoeuvre

Indications

BPPV with positive Dix–Hallpike test.

Contraindications:

As for Dix–Hallpike, above.

Method

1. Warn patient that this may worsen or provoke symptoms temporarily or may be ineffective.
2. Sit patient as for the Dix–Hallpike manoeuvre.
3. Turn the patient's head to the side that was positive on the Dix–Hallpike test.
4. Gently lower patient to lying position with head hanging over the end of the bed by around 20°.
5. Leave patient in this position for a few minutes (3–5 minutes).
6. Turn patient's head to face the midline.
7. Turn patient's head 45° to opposite side.
8. Turn patient onto shoulder so that head faces a further 45° to that side.
9. Sit patient up and return head to midline.

Nose emergencies

ACUTE SINUSITIS

Most cases are viral—approximately 90% of patients with upper respiratory tract infection (URTI) have involvement of the paranasal sinuses. However, only 0.5–2% of these proceed to have bacterial infection.[4]

Clinical features

- Symptoms of viral URTI not resolved after 10 days
- Purulent nasal discharge
- Facial or maxillary dental pain
- Fever
- Post nasal drip
- Tenderness over sinuses
- CT of sinuses confirms sinusitis

Organisms

- *Streptococcus pneumoniae*
- *Haemophilus influenzae*
- *Moraxella catarrhalis*

Management

1. Analgesia.
2. Antibiotics—combination amoxycillin + clavulanate is the drug of choice, but is likely to have more side-effects, especially diarrhoea. A recent Cochrane review found minimal effect in patients with uncomplicated acute sinusitis of more than 7 days' duration.[5]
3. Intranasal corticosteroids—there is limited evidence to support use as monotherapy or adjunct with antibiotics.[6]
4. Intranasal saline douches/spray—there is evidence that this is helpful in chronic sinusitis,[7] also recommended in acute sinusitis.
5. Oral steroids are sometimes used and may be effective.[8]

Complications

- Periorbital and orbital cellulitis
- Meningitis
- Brain abscess

EPISTAXIS

One of the commonest ENT emergencies. Approximately 90% are anterior bleeds from Little's area of the septum. Posterior bleeds are harder to visualise, more difficult to treat and occur in older patients with co-existing cardiovascular disease.

Clinical features

- Bleeding from nostril
- Blood in the oropharynx
- Airway usually intact
- May be haemodynamically compromised

Management

1. Protect yourself with gloves, gown and goggles.
2. Assess and manage ABCs initially.
3. Insert large-bore IV cannula and take blood for FBC, coagulation studies and group-and-hold.

Anterior bleeds

1. Ask patient to compress anterior nares between thumb and forefinger, applying constant pressure for 10–15 minutes.
2. Sit the patient up, leaning forwards, and ask the patient to hold a kidney dish below the mouth and spit into this.

3 Now inspect the nose to identify bleeding point.
4 Apply cotton-wool pledgets soaked in co-phenylcaine to visible bleeding spot or vessel.
5 If bleeding controlled and bleeding point identified, use a silver nitrate stick to cauterise the area. Be careful not to apply to large area and do not apply on both sides of the septum as this could lead to necrosis of the cartilage.
6 Observe patient for a few hours and, if no further bleeding, patient may be discharged with outpatient ENT follow-up.
7 If bleeding is too heavy, spray with co-phenylcaine and then use a nasal (Merocel) tampon (see Box 37.2) or a Rapid Rhino device (inflatable balloon covered with hydrocolloid fabric, see Box 37.3).
8 If above not available, pack with gauze (see Figure 37.3).
9 Depending on hospital policy, patient may require admission if packing left in situ.
10 Prophylactic antibiotics if packing left in situ.

Posterior bleeds

Bleeding site is usually not visible.

1 Options are:
   - Merocel nasal tampon (see Box 37.2)—may not be effective in posterior bleeds
   - Rapid Rhino posterior device (see Box 37.3)
   - Epistat nasal balloon (see Box 37.4)—not used very often now
   - Foley catheter and Vaseline gauze pack (see Figure 37.4).
2 May need to pack both sides to stop bleeding.
3 All patients need admission under the care of the ENT team.
4 Prophylactic antibiotics.

Box 37.2 To insert Merocel nasal tampon

1. For anterior bleeds use shorter tampon; use the longer ones for posterior bleeds
2. Use co-phenylcaine spray
3. Lubricate tip with water-soluble gel (KY gel)
4. Advance as far as possible along floor of nasal cavity
5. When soaked with blood, will expand to fill nasal cavity
6. Tape attached thread to side of face
7. To remove soak with saline, remove tape and slide gently out

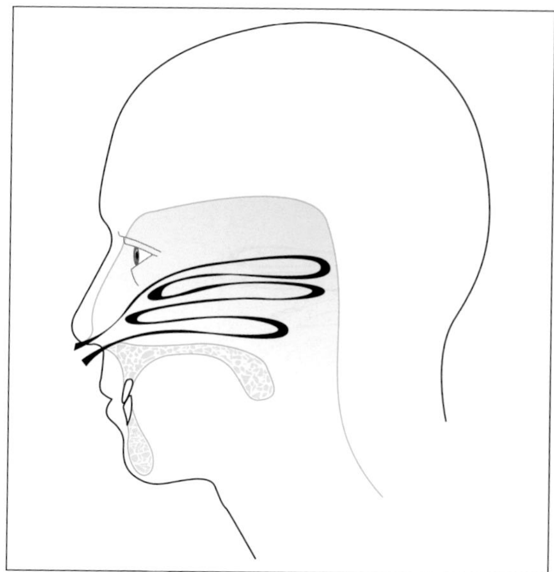

Figure 37.3 Correct placement of Vaseline gauze packing, with antibiotics commenced (possible bacteraemia in presence of nasal packing)

Box 37.3 To insert Rapid Rhino device

1. Soak in sterile water for 30 seconds
2. Get patient to blow nose to expel clots/blood
3. Use co-phenylcaine spray
4. Use 20 mL syringe to inflate with air until pilot cuff firm. Device will expand to fit nasal cavity
5. Tape pilot cuff to side of face

Box 37.4 To insert Epistat nasal balloon

1. Use co-phenylcaine spray
2. Lubricate device and insert to full length
3. Inflate posterior balloon with approximately 5 mL of air
4. Pull forward gently till fits against posterior choana
5. Fill anterior balloon till tamponade achieved
6. Tape to side of face

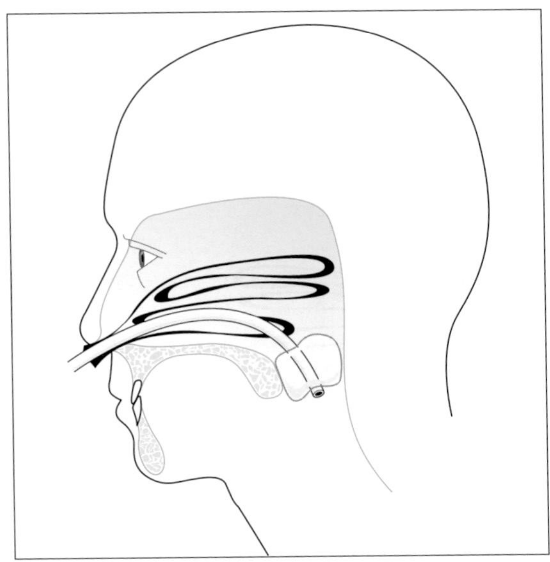

Figure 37.4 Foley's catheter used as postnasal balloon packing, with gauze anterior pack

FOREIGN BODIES—NOSE

Usually seen in children. Beads, parts of toys, paper, seeds, pebbles are some of the objects inserted by children. Usually present soon after as child tells parent or parent/sibling witnesses the child putting something in the nose. If presentation delayed, may present with offensive unilateral nasal discharge.

Note: Button batteries should be removed as soon as possible. If left for any length of time, they lead to a corrosive injury.

Management

1. Ask the parent to blow hard into the child's mouth (or use bag–mask to give positive pressure over mouth only) while occluding the normal nostril—the FB may be expelled by the positive pressure. Worth trying before the other methods, especially for things like beads.
2. Spray co-phenylcaine into nostril.
3. Sedate child if not cooperative.
4. Get a good view using headlight (if available).
5. If hard, round object, use angled hook to get behind object and pull out.

6 If soft, irregular and can be grasped by forceps, use these.
7 Other methods described include using a Foley or Fogarty catheter to get behind the object, then blowing balloon up and pulling object out; or using a suction catheter to apply suction on object and bring it out.
8 Once removed, re-inspect nostril to make sure object is removed completely and no other objects are present.

FRACTURED NASAL BONES

One of the commonest bones fractured in the body.

Note: Diagnosis of nasal fractures is a clinical one, and X-rays are rarely if ever indicated.

Clinical features

- History of direct trauma to nose
- Patient may have noticed an immediate deformity if fracture with displacement
- Swelling of nose
- Epistaxis
- May have a palpable step in the bone
- X-rays are difficult to interpret

Management

1. Treat any life-threatening injuries first.
2. Exclude other facial bone injuries.
3. Manage epistaxis if present with pressure or packing.
4. Inspect for septal haematoma—cherry-red swelling arising from septum. If present, the patient should be immediately referred to the ENT service for drainage. If left untreated, may lead to necrosis of cartilage with resultant saddle nose deformity.
5. The fracture is left for a few days until the swelling has gone down.
6. If deformity is present at that time, should be referred to ENT or plastic surgeon for reduction.

Throat emergencies

PHARYNGITIS/TONSILLITIS

- More common in children.
- It is difficult to differentiate clinically between bacterial and viral infections. However, it is important to try to differentiate between group B haemolytic streptococcal infection and other causes of sore throat.

Aetiology of pharyngitis/tonsilitis

- Viral including Epstein–Barr virus (EBV)
- Group B beta-haemolytic *Streptococcus* (GBHS)
- Other bacteria including other *Streptococcus, Chlamydiae, Gonococcus*

Clinical features

- Sore throat
- Fever
- Odynophagia
- Generalised symptoms of headache, malaise—thought to be more likely bacterial but often viral, especially EBV
- Associated runny nose, cough—more likely with viral infection
- Inflamed pharynx, enlarged tonsils with or without exudate/pus upon examination
- Cervical lymphadenopathy
- Hepatosplenomegaly usually indicates EBV
- Raised WCC, CRP
- Lymphocytosis with atypical lymphocytes—viral, especially EBV
- Abnormal liver function tests (LFTs)—EBV
- Throat swab for GBHS
- Monospot, EBV serology.

Of the above, a combination of fever with temperatures > 38°C, tender cervical lymphadenopathy, tonsillar exudate and no cough is suggestive of GBHS sore throat.

Management

1. Analgesia.
2. IV fluids, as patients are often dehydrated.
3. Steroids are often used to reduce symptoms, but there is not much evidence to support this. Dexamethasone 4–8 mg as a one-off dose is used.[9]
4. Penicillin for GBHS if there is a high index of clinical suspicion or is confirmed on throat swab PCR or culture.
5. If uncomplicated, patient may be discharged after symptomatic treatment.

Complications

- Airway compromise—unusual if not complicated. Requires admission to high-dependency unit under the care of the ENT team. Nasendoscopy performed by ENT to assess degree of swelling/obstruction. Rarely requires airway intervention.
- Peritonsillar abscess—see below.

PERITONSILLAR ABSCESS (QUINSY)

Starts as a pharyngitis or tonsillitis and progresses to form abscess. Common in young adults. Usually polymicrobial with a mixture of aerobic and anaerobic organisms.

Clinical features

- Starts like a sore throat, but gets progressively worse.
- Difficulty swallowing, opening mouth and talking.
- Fever and systemic symptoms more marked.
- Examination reveals a unilateral swelling displacing the tonsil inferomedially.
- Uvula is displaced to the contralateral side.
- Enlarged cervical lymph nodes.

Management

1 Analgesia.
2 IV fluids.
3 Antibiotics—combination of penicillin and metronidazole.[1]
4 Clindamycin may be used instead of metronidazole.[1]
5 Anaesthetise with co-phenylcaine spray.
6 Needle aspiration (see Box 37.5) is generally curative, and incision and drainage is rarely indicated.
7 ENT referral for 24-hour admission or for follow-up if discharged from ED.
8 Use of steroids is controversial.[10]

Box 37.5 Needle aspiration of quinsy

1. Have patient sitting up with kidney dish under chin
2. Use a large-bore needle on a 10 mL syringe and insert at area of maximal pointing while applying continuous negative pressure. You will feel a 'give' when you enter the abscess cavity
3. Aspirate pus and send for culture

Epiglottitis

Inflammation of the supraglottic region, including epiglottis, should be called supraglottitis.

Epiglottitis used to be a disease of childhood. After immunisation against *H. influenzae* B was started, it is now usually seen in adults.

Clinical features

- Sore throat—pain is lower than in tonsillitis
- Muffled voice

- Difficulty swallowing
- Fever
- Acute onset in children, may have prodromal URTI symptoms in adults
- Examination reveals a toxic-looking patient
- Drooling of saliva in children
- Cervical lymphadenopathy may be present
- Stridor is a late sign
- Lateral soft-tissue X-ray of neck may show classic 'thumb print'

Organisms

- *H. influenzae*, type B
- *Streptococcus pneumonia*e
- *Streptococcus pyogenes*
- *Staphylococcus aureus* and Gram-negatives are less common

Management of epiglottitis

1. If respiratory distress with stridor, consult anaesthetics and ENT and organise urgent transfer to operating theatre for gaseous induction and intubation.
2. If intubation fails, cricothyroidotomy or tracheostomy will need to be performed.
3. In adults who are not in respiratory distress, refer for ENT consultation for nasendoscopy.
4. Airway intervention is rarely required in adults.
5. IVC inserted and bloods taken for FBC, electrolytes, urea and creatinine (EUC), blood cultures.
6. Ceftriaxone is the antibiotic of choice.
7. Steroids may be used to reduce swelling.
8. Admit to high-dependency unit or ICU for close observation and airway intervention if required.
9. If patient has a respiratory arrest, commence bag–valve–mask ventilation and then intubation should be attempted. If this fails, proceed to a cricothyroidotomy.

FOREIGN BODIES—OROPHARYNGEAL

Usually an adult who has eaten chicken or fish and has a bone stuck in the pharynx.

Note: Button battery if swallowed is an emergency, and the ENT service should be called immediately.

Clinical features and examination

- History as above
- Feeling of foreign body (FB) stuck in throat
- Examine neck for surgical emphysema
- Inspect pharynx with headlight to visualise object if able
- X-ray lateral soft tissue of neck, looking for FB and retropharyngeal air

Management

1. If FB visible with headlight and tongue depressor, anaesthetise with lignocaine spray and remove with Magill's forceps.
2. If not visualised but visible on X-ray, refer to ENT for endoscopic removal.
3. If not visualised on inspection and not visible on X-ray, an FB may still be present or the patient may feel a scratch on the mucosa as an FB. These patients will also require endoscopy if the feeling of FB is persistent.

Complications

If left unattended, may perforate and lead to retropharyngeal infection and mediastinitis.

FOREIGN BODIES—OESOPHAGEAL

Depending on the hospital policy, these may be dealt with by ENT or gastroenterology. Upper oesophageal objects are commonly dealt with by the ENT service. In adults usually a food bolus and in children a coin are the commonest objects. Beware of button batteries in children, as this is an emergency to prevent perforation of the oesophagus.

Clinical features

- Sensation of FB
- Inability to swallow—varying degrees depending on degree of obstruction
- Drooling in complete obstruction
- Chest X-ray ± lateral soft tissue of neck, depending on level of obstruction.

Note: Coin in oesophagus appears in coronal plane (front on) on X-ray. Coin in airway appears in sagittal plane (side on) due to incomplete tracheal rings posteriorly.

Management

1. Trial of glucagon 1–2 mg IV ± carbonated beverage if foreign body is food bolus or coin. Do not attempt if sharp object or button battery.
2. If above method unsuccessful or sharp object/button battery, requires urgent ENT referral for endoscopic removal.
3. Keep patient nil by mouth (NBM).
4. Pre-anaesthetic work-up if indicated.

Complications

Oesophageal perforation and mediastinitis.

FOREIGN BODIES—AIRWAY

Common in children and the very elderly. Usually aspirated and lodged in right main or lower lobe bronchus. Complete airway obstruction is a life-threatening emergency and should be treated with back blows.

Clinical features

- History of choking, coughing, gagging
- If aspirated, child may be minimally symptomatic initially and only have a cough or wheeze, especially unilateral wheeze
- Stridor
- Respiratory distress if causing upper airway obstruction
- Chest X-ray may reveal FB if radio-opaque or unilateral hypertranslucency, atelectasis or consolidation

Management

1. Supportive therapy till endoscopic removal—oxygen, IV access and monitoring.
2. Urgent ENT referral for endoscopy.
3. If patient has complete obstruction and respiratory arrest, intubate and push tube as far as possible, thus pushing object into one bronchus. Then withdraw the tube to normal position to ventilate until endoscopic removal is organised.

POST-TONSILLECTOMY BLEED

Secondary haemorrhage may occur after 24 hours, but commonly between 5 and 10 days. Can be fatal from airway obstruction or haemorrhagic shock.

Management

1. Keep patient seated upright with kidney dish to spit into.
2. Monitor haemodynamics and oxygen saturation.

3 Keep NBM.
4 Obtain large-bore IV access and send blood for FBC, UEC, coagulation studies and group-and-hold.
5 Resuscitate as required including airway protection if necessary. Be prepared to perform surgical airway if unable to intubate.
6 Notify ENT team immediately.
7 Commence IV penicillin and metronidazole.
8 Hydrogen peroxide gargles are prescribed, but there is no evidence to support their use.

References

1. Antibiotic guidelines eTG complete [Internet]. Melbourne: Therapeutic Guidelines Limited; 2010.
2. Sanders S, Glasziou P, Del Mar C, Rovers M. Antibiotics for acute otitis media in children. Cochrane Database Syst Rev 2010, Issue 1. Art. No.: CD000219. DOI: 10.1002/14651858.CD000219.pub2
3. http://emedicine.medscape.com/article/791414-clinical#a0217
4. Gwaltney JM. Acute community-acquired sinusitis. Clin Infect Dis 1996;23(6):1209–23.
5. Ahovuo-Saloranta A, Borisenko OV, Kovanen N et al. Antibiotics for acute maxillary sinusitis. Cochrane Database Syst Rev 2008, Issue 2. Art. No. CD000243. DOI: 10.1002/14651858.CD000243.pub2.
6. Zalmanovici Trestioreanu A, Yaphe J. Steroids for acute sinusitis. Cochrane Database Syst Rev 2009, DOI: 10.1002/14651858.CD005149.pub3.
7. Harvey R, Hannan SA, Badia L et al. Nasal saline irrigations for the symptoms of chronic rhinosinusitis. Cochrane Database Syst Rev 2007, Issue 3. Art. No.: CD006394. DOI: 10.1002/14651858.CD006394.pub2.
8. Venekamp RP et al, Systemic corticosteroids for acute sinusitis. Cochrane Database Syst Rev 2011, DOI: 10.1002/14651858.CD008115.pub2.
9. Bulloch B, Kabani A, Tenenbein M. Oral dexamethasone for the treatment of pain in children with acute pharyngitis: a randomized, double-blind, placebo-controlled trial. Ann Emerg Med 2003;41(5):601–8.
10. Ozbek C, Aygenc E, Tuna EU et al. Use of steroids in the treatment of peritonsillar abscess. J Laryngol Otol 2004;118(6):439–42.

Chapter 38

Management of dental emergencies

Peter Foltyn

There are many kinds of dental emergencies, some of which can be extremely subjective. Whereas a small carious lesion or infected extraction socket may cause excruciating pain for one person, a fractured jaw may be asymptomatic and only discovered as an incidental finding after routine X-rays. Emergency departments in teaching hospitals will nearly always have an accredited on-call dentist, or in rural settings may refer all dental emergencies to a local dental emergency service or individual dentist. As dental emergencies are rarely life-threatening, commonsense measures such as antibiotics, sedatives and analgesics where appropriate should get the patient through the night or weekend until an appointment can be arranged for the next working day.

It would be an inappropriate utilisation of resources to ask an on-call dentist to personally attend all cases of dental or oral pain. Many dental problems are the result of dental neglect, which would have initially presented many days or weeks earlier.

If the patient is to be admitted or there is doubt about management, contact the on-call dentist. Always have any relevant medical history at hand and try to establish a history for the dental problem. The dental history should include duration and nature of any pain or swelling and any measures taken to counter the problem by the patient's own doctor, dentist or by themselves.

Toothache

In the majority of instances toothache can be narrowed down to a specific tooth, which may be tender to the touch and is often a direct result of tooth decay. However, pain can be referred to adjacent teeth, the opposing jaw, facial areas or the neck but does not generally extend across the midline except when the origin is the anterior teeth. As ED imaging may be limited to taking orthopantomogram (OPG) X-rays or standard views of facial bones, the source of the toothache may not be immediately evident.

Clinical examination by ED staff may prove unrewarding without some training in oral examination. A strong light source, dental mirror and probe and an air source are required (wall-outlet medical air or oxygen or cylinder gases and tubing would normally be available in all EDs).

DENTAL CARIES

Dental caries may be minor or extensive and may undermine an existing dental restoration or artificial crown.

Response/Advice

Provide adequate analgesia until the next working day.

EROSION OR ABRASION AT THE TOOTH/GUM JUNCTION

Such areas may produce extreme hypersensitivity.

Response/Advice

Provide adequate analgesia until the next working day and suggest an anti-hypersensitivity toothpaste such as Sensodyne or Colgate Gel-Kam.

DENTAL PULP INVOLVEMENT

Dental pulp (nerve) involvement is often an extension of decay in the body or branches of the dental pulp. Invasion by microorganisms into the dental pulp often leads to an initial acute pulpitis which may settle and return as a chronic, more diffuse pain many weeks or even months or years later. The microorganisms which invaded the dental pulp may now extend beyond the tooth apex and be responsible for dental abscess formation. (See also section 'Facial swellings', below.)

Response/Advice

Provide adequate analgesia until the next working day; however, antibiotics may also be required if there is established lymphadenopathy, pyrexia or visible dental abscess formation on X-ray. Advise the patient to attend a dentist as a matter of urgency.

FRACTURED OR SPLIT TEETH

Fractured or split teeth may be a result of trauma or a heavily filled tooth giving way. In some instances intact teeth may fracture as a result of an anatomical irregularity in their formation or as a result of an occlusal or bite discrepancy.

Response/Advice

Provide adequate analgesia until the next working day. Advise the patient to attend a dentist as soon as possible. See also 'Traumatic injuries to teeth', below.

Infected gums

GINGIVITIS/PERIODONTITIS

- Poor oral health may lead initially to marginal gingivitis, progressing over many years to moderate or severe periodontitis and associated problems with the bone surrounding the teeth.
- Advanced periodontal disease may lead to tooth mobility, bad breath, oral bleeding, periodontal abscess formation, extrusion, drifting or exfoliation of teeth and generalised mouth pain.
- Periodontal disease may be an early clinical clue for systemic diseases such as HIV infection and diabetes, or may follow treatment in the case of graft-versus-host disease (GVHD) in bone marrow transplantation and radiation therapy of the head and neck.

Response/Advice

Provide adequate analgesia until the next working day; however, antibiotics may also be required. A chlorhexidine mouth rinse, preferably one which is alcohol-free and not associated with discolouration (e.g. Curasept), will reduce microorganism numbers. Advise the patient to attend a dentist as soon as possible.

ACUTE NECROTISING ULCERATIVE GINGIVITIS (ANUG)

ANUG is a severe gingival infection often characterised by severe pain, pyrexia, bad breath, with punched-out and ulcerated interdental papillae. It can be found in otherwise healthy mouths and is often associated with stress. ANUG is often found around examination time or in times of partnership breakdown.

Response /Advice

Provide adequate analgesia until the next working day and prescribe metronidazole (Flagyl) or tinidazole (Fasigyn). A chlorhexidine mouth rinse, preferably one which is alcohol-free and not associated with discolouration (e.g. Curasept), will reduce microorganism numbers. Advise the patient to attend a dentist as soon as possible.

Impacted teeth

The usual age for eruption of wisdom teeth or 3rd molars is 17–22 years; however, eruption can occur as early as age 15.

In the past, when oral health was poor and fluoridation of water supplies had not commenced, it was common for young adults to have had a number of teeth removed due to tooth decay before the end of their teenage years. Today, most young adults born and raised in communities with fluoridated water are rarely missing any teeth and also have had a minimal number of teeth restored. A consequence of having good teeth is that for many there is little room for their orderly eruption. This has now led to a significant increase in impaction of not only wisdom teeth but occasionally other teeth as well, especially when there is a discrepancy between tooth and mouth size.

Impacted teeth can cause pain for numerous reasons. In most instances the cause of pain is a result of local infection which often leads to regional lymphadenopathy. Carious breakdown with acute pulpitis and pressure on an adjacent tooth can also cause severe pain.

RESPONSE/ADVICE

Provide adequate analgesia until the next working day; however, antibiotics may also be required if there is established lymphadenopathy or pyrexia. Advise the patient to attend a dentist or a specialist oral surgeon as soon as possible.

Mouth sores and ulceration

- Oral ulceration and mouth sores may be the result of a myriad of precipitating factors including stress, acidic foods and even specific foods. Sodium lauryl sulfate (SLS), a detergent commonly found in toothpastes, has also been implicated.
- Random aphthous and traumatic ulceration is not uncommon; however, ulceration as an oral manifestation of a systemic disease can also occur.
- Severe mouth sores also occur in GVHD following bone marrow transplantation and canker sores during head and neck irradiation.
- Nutritional deficiencies in the aged and unwell may also lead to oral ulceration.
- Denture wearers who have lost 5–10 kg or more since the dentures were initially fabricated may have experienced shrinkage of alveolar ridges and other changes within their mouths, altering the once good fit of their dentures. As shrinkage of oral tissues is not uniform, the denture may impinge or dig in at various locations.

RESPONSE/ADVICE

- Good oral hygiene and reducing stress is a starting point for limiting the recurrence of oral ulceration.
- Rinsing or topical application of lignocaine oral gel (e.g. Xylocaine Viscous) with a cotton bud to a specific ulcer may help.
- Chlorhexidine mouth rinse and topical steroids, such as Kenalog in Orabase, should be prescribed until the patient can get to their dentist.
- Thalidomide has been shown to reduce pain in large intractable ulcers found in immunocompromised patients, as has nicotine-containing gum (Nicorette) in non-smokers suffering random aphthous ulceration.

Neoplasia

The average age of a person with an oral cancer in Australia is 64 years; however, young people are regularly being diagnosed with oral-based malignancies. An area of induration, leucoplakia or erythroplasia, which has progressed in size or has been managed topically or systemically without resolution, requires urgent attention.

Long-term immunosuppression is closely linked to a higher risk for a neoplasm. Any lumps and bumps in and around the mouth for a person who has been HIV-positive for 10 or more years should be carefully assessed. Unusual and aggressive lymphomas are appearing in this cohort. Similarly, any person who has received solid-organ transplantation should have any unusual swellings quickly assessed.

RESPONSE/ADVICE

As the consequences of delay in providing a definitive diagnosis of an oral cancer may compromise the patient in many ways, biopsy of the suspect lesion should be carried out as soon as possible. Punch biopsy or excisional biopsy can be carried out by a surgical or plastics registrar or on-call dentist.

Facial swellings

The most common cause of facial swellings is dental abscess formation.

- A dental abscess is an infection around the root of a tooth or in the gum which causes an accumulation of pus. At this stage there is often associated pain but not necessarily swelling.
- If the infection is left unchecked, the accumulated pus attempts to drain and will track via the path of least resistance and

accumulate further as a intra- or extra-oral swelling which may not necessarily be overlying the abscessed tooth.
- Local lymphadenopathy is common with marked facial swellings caused by dental abscess formation.

RESPONSE/ADVICE

- Provide adequate analgesia until the next working day, together with antibiotics if the swelling is slight and there is no concern for airway obstruction or progression to cellulitis.
- Have the patient rinse their mouth with warm salty water every hour or as needed to ease the pain. If the patient is able, they can cover the handle of a teaspoon with cotton-wool, immerse this in hot salty water and press it on the swelling. This may help to establish drainage.
- Using ice packs or a bag of frozen peas, 20 minutes on and 10 minutes off, over the affected area may also help to relieve the pain.
- The patient should be advised to return to the ED if
  - there is increased swelling in their face, jaw, cheek, eye
  - swelling spreads to their neck or chest
  - there are any symptoms of airway obstruction
  - the pain becomes worse
  - they develop pyrexia.
- Should the swelling be significant or have spread to the eye, neck or chest, or there is concern for potential airway obstruction (Ludwig's angina) the patient should be admitted and commenced immediately on IV antibiotics.
  - Give benzylpenicillin 1.2 g 6-hourly. In the more severe or unresponsive cases, add metronidazole 500 mg 12-hourly.
  - For patients hypersensitive to penicillin, give clindamycin 300 mg 8-hourly or lincomycin 600 mg 8-hourly.
  - IV fluids should also be considered.
  - Contact the on-call dentist; however, if the swelling is significant and CT or X-rays are available, fine-cut views in the area of the swelling will help determine whether there is an accumulation of pus and whether incision and drainage is required.

Heart disease and dental care

The following recommendations from the St Vincent's Hospital Dental Department are based on guidelines and antibiotic regimens which have been endorsed by all Australian state and Commonwealth health departments, the Cardiac Society of Australia and New Zealand and the Australian Dental Association.

Several heart conditions require the patient and dentist to take special precautions. These recommendations are especially important for:

- people with artificial heart valves (aortic, mitral)
- people with a previous history of heart valve infection
- people born with or who acquire heart problems such as
  - most at-birth heart malformations
  - damaged heart valves
  - thickened heart muscle
- cardiac transplantation recipients with cardiac valvular disease.

Someone with a heart problem has 3 responsibilities:

1. They need to establish and maintain a clean and healthy mouth. That means practising good oral hygiene and visiting their dentist regularly.
2. They need to make sure that their dentist and their doctor know that they have a heart problem.
3. They must carefully follow both their doctor's and their dentist's instructions when prescribed any medications and in particular antibiotics.

Antibiotic guidelines for dental procedures in high-risk patients[1]

- Amoxycillin 2 g (children: 50 mg/kg, up to 2 g) orally as a single dose 1 hour before the procedure. (*Note:* the Australian Guidelines are now 2 g, not 3 g.)
- For patients hypersensitive to penicillin, on long-term penicillin therapy or having taken penicillin or a related beta-lactam antibiotic more than once in the previous month, use clindamycin 600 mg (children: 10 mg/kg, up to 600 mg), not erythromycin or tetracyclines, orally as a single dose 1 hour before the procedure commences.

Post-extraction instructions

Often teeth need to be removed due to excessive dental decay or formation of a dental abscess. Immediately following a tooth extraction, the patient should be advised to keep biting on the rolled gauze which has been placed in their mouth for at least 20–30 minutes. If they are still bleeding, provide extra gauze.

RESPONSE/ADVICE

General

1 Do not smoke or rinse the mouth vigorously.
2 Do not spit or continually wipe away blood.
3 Do not drink through a straw for 24 hours.
4 Do not suck on the extraction site.

These activities may disturb the healing blood clot.

Immediately after a tooth is extracted, the patient may experience discomfort and notice some swelling. This is normal. The initial healing period typically takes from 1 to 2 weeks, and some swelling and residual bleeding should be expected in the 24 hours following an extraction.

It is important not to dislodge the blood clot that forms on the wound. Occasionally this clot can break down, leaving what is known as a dry socket (see below). This can cause temporary pain and discomfort that will subside as the socket heals through a secondary healing process.

To limit swelling

1 Place ice packs or a bag of frozen peas on the area of the face overlying the extraction site, 20 minutes on and 10 minutes off for 2–3 hours.
2 Should there still be bleeding after 2–3 hours, place a dry tea bag on the extraction site and bite down on it firmly but without rupturing the bag.
3 Reduce strenuous activity for 24 hours.
4 Drink plenty of fluids and maintain as normal a diet as possible, which may be limited to soft foods for the first few days.
5 Avoid alcoholic beverages and hot liquids.
6 Brush and floss as normal, being extra careful around the extraction area.
7 On day after extraction, gently rinse the mouth with warm salt water (half a teaspoon in one glass of water).
8 Medication may be prescribed to help control pain and infection.

Dry socket

Alveolar osteitis or dry socket is often a severe pain following a recent extraction. It is the result of disintegration of the blood clot formed in the socket after the extraction and may not be relieved by over-the-counter analgesics. The pain may radiate to the ear and is often accompanied by fetor oris or bad breath. When the usual process of healing is disturbed the blood clot may be dislodged, leaving bone within the socket exposed to saliva, food and other mouth debris rather than surrounded by an organising blood clot. If a dry socket occurs it usually does so immediately following the extraction, although breakdown of the blood clot occasionally occurs after several days of uneventful healing.

RESPONSE/ADVICE

Provide adequate analgesia, which may include the addition of a non-steroidal anti-inflammatory drug (NSAID), until the next working day; however, antibiotics may also be required if there is established lymphadenopathy or pyrexia. Advise the patient to attend a dentist as soon as possible to have the dry socket irrigated and dressed.

Oral bleeding

Generally, warfarin or antiplatelet medications need not be ceased prior to dental extractions or deep cleaning; however, appropriate local measures should be adopted in addition to checking with the patient's cardiologist in the case of an underlying cardiovascular disease, or haematologist if the concern is due to a blood dyscrasia. Most patients can be managed in a general dental practice setting and do not need to be admitted to hospital. St Vincent's Hospital has adopted as the basis for new prescribing and formulary guidelines dental recommendations from the United Kingdom.[2,3]

Patients being treated with oral anticoagulant medication who have an International Normalisation Ratio (INR) below 4.0 may have dental extractions without interruption to their treatment. Local measures, which include suturing and packing the extraction site with absorbable gelatine sponge, are generally sufficient to prevent post-extraction bleeding.

Excessive post-extraction or oral bleeding for other reasons may still occur. The most common cause of post-extraction bleeding for the patient with no known systemic problems is failure to follow instructions from the dentist.

RESPONSE/ADVICE

If bleeding persists in spite of repeating local measures as described in the section above, or if a bleeding disorder or dyscrasia is suspected, follow the St Vincent's Hospital Dental Department Protocol for local anti-fibrinolytic treatment as follows.

1 Obtain tranexamic acid IV solution.
2 Wet but don't saturate a sterile gauze square in undiluted

tranexamic acid. Fold or roll the gauze so that it can be placed on the extraction site.

3 Ensure that the gauze is exerting pressure on the site.
4 Repeat after half an hour or as required.
5 If being discharged, give patient the remaining tranexamic acid and additional bite pads to repeat at home if required.
6 Have the patient use an alcohol/phenol-free mouth wash twice daily, commencing after 24 hours.

Traumatic injuries to teeth

In 2010 the Danish Dental Association, supported by the International Association for Dental Traumatology, established a website for evidence-based management of dental trauma (www.dentaltraumaguide.org). This excellent interactive guide utilises drop-down boxes with the description, aetiology, diagnosis, treatment, prognosis and references for every conceivable dental trauma.[4]

FRACTURE

Traumatic injuries to teeth can be divided into 5 categories:

Grade 1—involved minor chipping of the incisal edge limited to enamel

Grade 2—involves fracture through to dentine without pulpal or nerve exposure

Grade 3—fracture with pulpal or nerve exposure

Grade 4—root fracture

Grade 5—complex.

Response/Advice

- If the traumatic injury is the result of a minor accident, provide analgesia if required until the next working day.
- If, however, the injury is the result of a motor vehicle crash, assault or other significant incident, an OPG X-ray should be taken, if available. Often, displaced and asymptomatic fractures of the body of the mandible, ramus, condylar head or coronoid process may be detected with an OPG.
- With grade 3–5 fractures where there are no other bodily injuries present other than minor local lacerations, provide analgesia until the next working day.
- Should the patient be admitted or require observation in the ED for any length of time, contact the on-call dentist.

LUXATION

A tooth is considered luxated when it has been moved, often occupying a position other than its original one. Luxated teeth can be divided into five categories:

Grade 1—tooth loosened but still in its original position (subluxation)
Grade 2—loosened and out of position
Grade 3—significantly out of position
Grade 4—pushed into upper or lower jaw
Grade 5—complex (out of its original position with a grade 2–5 tooth fracture).

Response/Advice

Except for a grade 1 luxation, always contact the on-call dentist as soon as possible. If there are no other bodily injuries precluding dental management, repositioning and splinting of the loosened teeth will generally be required.

AVULSION

Evidence suggests that avulsed or knocked-out teeth which have been re-implanted within 30–45 minutes have a reasonable chance of long-term retention. However, after 2 hours out of the mouth the prospects are diminished significantly. Correct handling, transportation and storage of the knocked-out tooth is critical.

Response/Advice

- Ideally, the patient should be encouraged to push the tooth back into the socket, even if it is out of alignment and loose. If this is too painful or not possible, holding the tooth in the floor of the mouth will keep the root bathed in the patient's own saliva.
- Should other injuries or the patient's mental state preclude the above, immediate storage in UHT milk is preferred to whole milk or water.
- Only handle avulsed teeth by the enamel and do not rinse in any disinfectant solution.
- Always contact the on-call dentist as soon as possible, as implantation, repositioning and splinting of an avulsed tooth will be required.
- Should the dentist be unavailable immediately, small rectangular strips of ConvaTec Stomahesive® wafer can be used to provisionally hold the tooth. This will provide additional working time for the dentist and could save the patient many thousands of dollars.
  - Hold the tooth only by the crown.

- Try not to touch the root.
- Remove visible debris by gently washing with saline.
- Replace back in the dental socket as soon as possible.
- Use a single rectangular piece of ConvaTec Stomahesive®. Wetting the wafer first can help it adhere.
- It may take 10–15 minutes for the wafer to feel secure.
- When securely in place, the wafer can last several hours.

The case shown in Figure 38.1 was jointly managed by both the Emergency Department and the Dental Department at St Vincent's Hospital.

A

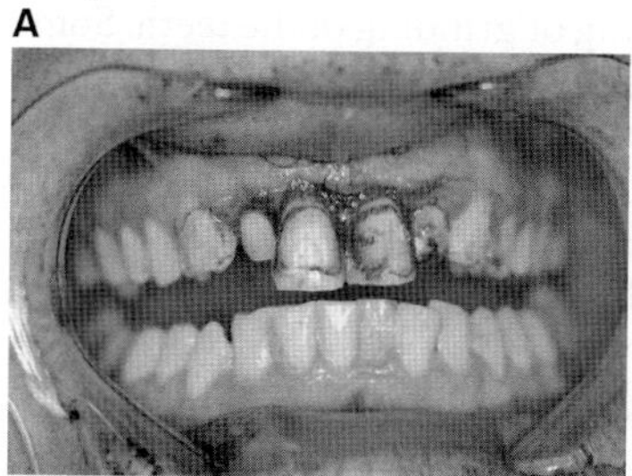

B

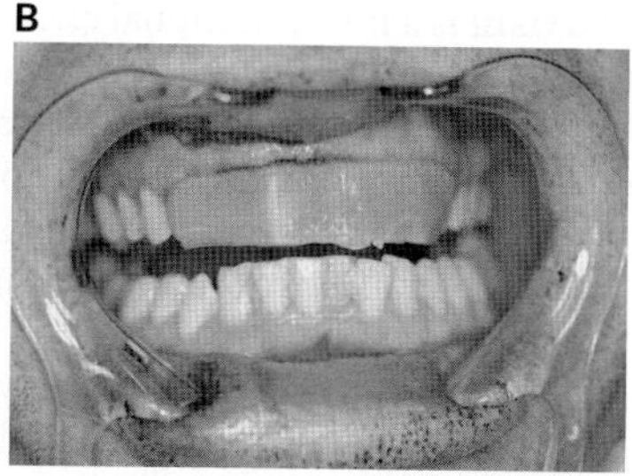

Figure 38.1A and B Upper central incisor teeth were avulsed following an assault. They were placed back in their sockets and secured using ConvaTec Stomahesive® wafer

C

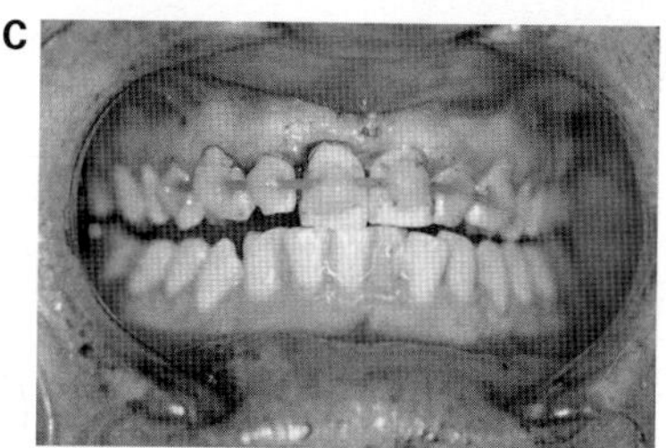

Figure 38.1C The upper central incisor teeth were splinted using flexible nylon and flowable composite resin

Trismus and temperomandibular joint (TMJ) dysfunction

Many people have pain or discomfort in and around the TMJ at some time during their lives.

- The symptoms may include pain, tenderness, spasm, clicking or crepitus, as well as direct or referred pain in the muscles of the face, neck, shoulder and ears.

- TMJ dysfunction may lead to loss of jaw function, with pain ranging from a mild discomfort in the morning to a chronic debilitating pain rendering the patient unable to open their mouth by the afternoon.
- Conservative treatment (NSAIDs plus alternating hot and cold packs or compresses and rest) may prove effective following acute trauma to the jaw following a motor vehicle crash, fall or assault.
- Direct trauma to the TMJ area or either jaw may also cause chronic or latent damage which may eventually contribute to a TMJ problem, often years later.

Bruxism is a non-functional clenching or grinding of the teeth. Some people will brux during waking hours; however, bruxing is generally carried out subconsciously while asleep.

- Although bruxing while asleep is extremely common and can lead to enamel wear, pathological bruxing can lead to significant TMJ damage over time, especially when the dentition is less than optimal in the first place.
- Dentists can fabricate a variety of splints which the patient will generally wear at night and will help in either alleviating the symptoms of TMJ dysfunction or in the retraining of the facial musculature.

Dental nomenclature

The international numbering system for teeth (FDI notation) should be used in any written or verbal communication.

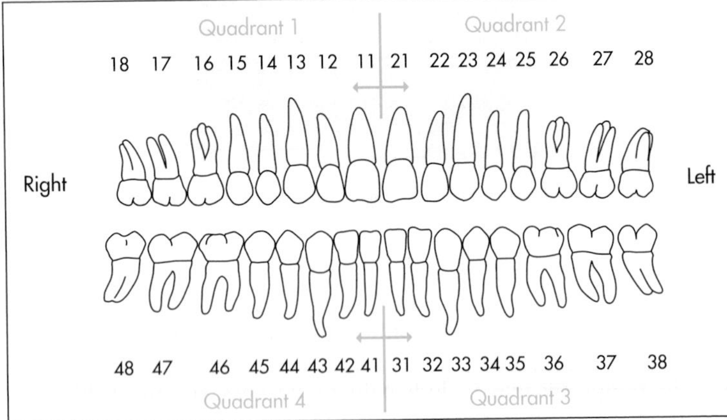

Figure 38.2 Adult dental nomenclature

The mouth can be divided into four quadrants. In the adult dentition (Figure 38.2) the maxillary right is quadrant 1, the maxillary left quadrant 2, the mandibular left quadrant 3 and the mandibular right quadrant 4. The individual teeth are numbered from the central incisor outwards to the 3rd molar. This provides an easy-to-use (and communicate) two-digit code to indicate the tooth or region of concern.

Deciduous or baby teeth follow a similar pattern. Starting from the maxillary right, the quadrants are numbered 5, 6, 7 and 8 (in place of 1, 2, 3 and 4 in the adult); individual teeth are numbered outwards from the central incisors in the same manner. The complete deciduous dentition has only 5 teeth in each quadrant as opposed to 8 teeth in each quadrant in the adult dentition.

Additional resources

Copies of information sheets referred to are available from:

Dr Peter Foltyn
Consultant Dentist, Dental Department
St Vincent's Hospital
pfoltyn@stvincents.com.au

References

1. Therapeutic Guidelines—Oral and Dental (2007 Version 1). Available from:
   Therapeutic Guidelines Limited
   Level 2, 55 Flemington Road
   North Melbourne, Victoria 3051
   (03) 9329 1566
   (03) 9326 5632
   e-mail sales@tg.com.au
   Website www.tg.com.au
2. Randall C, ed, for UK Medicines Information and NHS, 2004. Surgical management of the primary care patient on warfarin. Online. Available at www.ukmi.nhs.uk/med_info/documents/Dental_Patient_on_Warfarin.pdf 18 Apr 2013.
3. Randall C, ed, for UK Medicines Information and NHS, 2004. Surgical management of the primary care dental patient on antiplatelet medication. Online. Available at www.ukmi.nhs.uk/med_info/documents/Dental_Patient_on_Antiplatelet_Medication.pdf 18 Apr 2013.
4. The Dental Trauma Guide. Online. Available at www.dentaltraumaguide.org.

Chapter 39
Psychiatric presentations

Paul Preisz and Beaver Hudson

Mental health presentations to emergency departments are common and encompass a wide variety of issues either as principal reasons for attendance or as important comorbidities. Problems with mental health, drugs and alcohol, social disability and medical illness frequently co-exist, complicating assessment, management and disposition. The more common primary mental health presentations include:

- thoughts of or attempts at deliberate self-harm
- aggressive, threatening or bizarre behaviour
- depressed and withdrawn behaviour
- anxiety
- psychosis
- exacerbations of chronic mental illness
- combinations of the above.

Editorial Comment

As mental health is now being mainstreamed through EDs, it has become easier but no less important to ensure that the patient does not have an organic illness/cause contributing to their behaviour, i.e. a delirium. Also, the patient must be assessed for any risk that their therapy may present. Medical clearance is a clumsy term; the modern approach is for mental health and emergency doctors to simultaneously and collaboratively assess the patient.

Triage

Triage should be performed as with all ED patients along standardised lines (see Table 39.1). A team approach for the reception of involuntary patients should involve mental health, medical, nursing, security and other staff, working with established and practised protocols. Police, when initially present, should stay until safety and control

Table 39.1 Mental health triage guidelines—triage codes 1–5

Description	Typical presentation	General principles of management
1—Treatment acuity: immediate		
Definite danger to life (self or others)	**OBSERVED** Violent behaviour Possession of weapon Self-destructive behaviour in ED	**SUPERVISION** Continuous visual surveillance* **ACTION** Provide safe environment for patient and others Ensure adequate personnel to provide restraint/detention **Consider** 1 to 1 observation Alert mental health team Consult mental health specialist
2—Treatment acuity: emergency within 10 minutes		
Probable risk of danger to self or others Severe behavioural disturbance	**OBSERVED** Extreme agitation/restlessness Physically/verbally aggressive Confused/unable to cooperate Requires restraint **REPORTED** Attempt at self-harm/threat of self-harm Threat of harm to others	**SUPERVISION** Continuous visual surveillance* **ACTION** Provide safe environment for patient and others Ensure adequate personnel to provide restraint/detention **Consider** 1 to 1 observation Alert mental health team Consult mental health specialist

Continues overleaf

Table 39.1 Mental health triage guidelines—triage codes 1–5 continued

Description	Typical presentation	General principles of management
3—Treatment acuity: urgent within 30 minutes		
Possible danger to self or others Moderate behaviour disturbance Severe distress	OBSERVED Agitation/restlessness Intrusive behaviour Bizarre/disorganised behaviour Confusion Withdrawn and uncommunicative Ambivalence about treatment REPORTED Suicidal ideation Presence of psychotic symptoms: —hallucinations —delusions —paranoid ideas —thought disorder —bizarre/agitated behaviour Presence of affective disturbance: —severe symptoms of depression/ anxiety —elevated or irritable mood	SUPERVISION Close observation* ACTION **Consider** Consult mental health specialist Re-triage if evidence of increasing behavioural disturbance: —restlessness —intrusiveness —agitation —aggressiveness —increasing distress

Description	Typical presentation	General principles of management
4—Treatment acuity: semi-urgent within 60 minutes		
Moderate distress	**OBSERVED** No agitation/restlessness Irritability without aggression Cooperative Gives coherent history **REPORTED** Symptoms of anxiety or depression without suicidal ideation	**SUPERVISION** Intermittent observation* **ACTION** **Consider** Re-triage if evidence of increasing behavioural disturbance: —restlessness —intrusiveness —agitation —aggressiveness —increasing distress
5—Treatment acuity: non-urgent within 120 minutes		
No danger to self or others No acute distress No behavioural disturbance	**OBSERVED** Cooperative Communicative Compliant with instructions **REPORTED** Known patient with chronic psychotic symptoms Known patient with chronic unexplained somatic complaints Request for medication Minor adverse effect of medication Financial/social/accommodation/ relationship problems	**SUPERVISION** General observation* **ACTION** **Consider** Referral to mental health specialist/social worker Mobilise or establish support network—community team/LMO/family

have been established. A rapid sedation protocol should be used as required (see Figure 39.1, overleaf).

Safety must be taken into consideration. Physical environments must be assessed for potential hazards to either patients or clinicians. Assessment rooms specifically set up for this kind of examination are essential. Security and other staff should be trained in aggression minimisation and de-escalation techniques, and protocols should include routine security checks for possible weapons or dangerous objects at the time of triage.

Interviewing the potentially violent patient needs to be undertaken in a manner that minimises the chances of escalation while maintaining your safety and that of the patient. This is best done in an environment which has at least 2 exits and which can be observed by other staff (this may need to be done discreetly, out of respect for the patient's privacy). The presence of potential dangers should be considered and appropriate steps taken:

- Furniture should be too heavy to throw and anything that could be used as a weapon (e.g. IV poles) should be removed
- Consider removing neckties/necklaces, stethoscopes, pens, etc from your person.
- Tell others where you will be and who you are with.
- Carry a 'personal duress alarm' and make sure you know how to activate it.

The **initial contact** is aimed at defusing the situation, but this will often depend on elucidating and treating the underlying cause. Therefore, history taking, assessment of mental state and looking for other diagnostic clues should proceed simultaneously. Your approach should be empathic and non-confrontational; avoid making the patient feel verbally threatened (e.g. by using ultimatums) or physically threatened (e.g. by standing over a seated patient or blocking their exit).

Control of aggression

There are a number of different ways of controlling aggression, ranging from verbal de-escalation to pharmacological and/or physical restraint. Often a number of strategies will need to be employed. The underlying cause, especially if it is organic in nature, needs to be identified and treated.

- **Verbal de-escalation** and distraction is almost invariably the initial means of approaching the aggressive patient. This needs to be done in a non-judgmental and non-confrontational manner; allow the patient to state their concerns while stating

your desire to sort things out in the manner most appropriate for everyone.
  - Although there is often a role for the setting of limits of acceptable behaviour, issuing ultimatums will frequently result in escalation of the situation.
  - Avoid getting drawn into long-term grievances or issues beyond your control.
  - Simple courtesies, such as offering something to eat or drink (this should be avoided if sedation is likely to be required) or somewhere to sit, may assist you in establishing a rapport with the patient.
  - If appropriate, try to get the patient to accept help such as psychiatric assessment or to voluntarily take oral sedative/antipsychotic medication.
- Should this approach fail a '**show of force**' may be necessary, such as the obvious presence of security/police officers to back up the clinician, with the aim being to convince the patient that further escalation is unwise and in the hope that they will then agree to take medication.
  - One person (usually the clinician involved) should lead the staff and interact with the patient.
  - A fallback plan should always be in place at this stage: if the violence/aggression appears to be due to a medical or psychiatric condition and physical/pharmacological restraint is legally justifiable, it should be the next step; if not, the patient/subject should be escorted from the department by security or police.
- **Physical restraint** should only be performed in an emergency situation in the initial treatment of a delirious or psychiatrically unwell patient. In these cases, it must be done in a manner aimed at minimising the chance of injury to patient or staff, and should always be followed by pharmacological sedation.
  - There must be sufficient staff with well-defined roles. Usually 7 staff are required; one to immobilise each limb, one for the head and neck, one to administer medication and a runner/scribe.
  - One person should be in charge; they will nominate when immobilisation will take place and will be responsible for talking to the patient.
  - Throughout, extreme care must be taken to avoid injury to staff (e.g. punching, biting, spitting by patient) or to

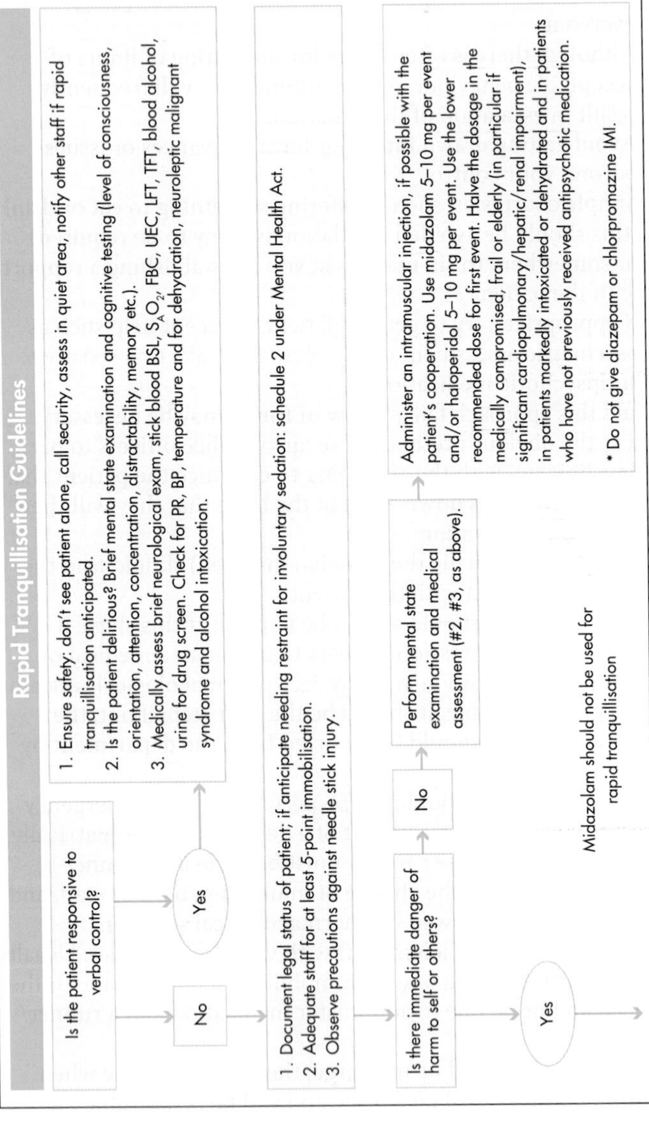
Rapid Tranquillisation Guidelines
Is the patient responsive to verbal control?
Yes
1. Ensure safety: don't see patient alone, call security, assess in quiet area, notify other staff if rapid tranquillisation anticipated.
2. Is the patient delirious? Brief mental state examination and cognitive testing (level of consciousness, orientation, attention, concentration, distractability, memory etc.).
3. Medically assess brief neurological exam, stick blood BSL, S_AO_2, FBC, UEC, LFT, TFT, blood alcohol, urine for drug screen. Check for PR, BP, temperature and for dehydration, neuroleptic malignant syndrome and alcohol intoxication.
No
1. Document legal status of patient; if anticipate needing restraint for involuntary sedation: schedule 2 under Mental Health Act.
2. Adequate staff for at least 5-point immobilisation.
3. Observe precautions against needle stick injury.
Is there immediate danger of harm to self or others?
No
Perform mental state examination and medical assessment (#2, #3, as above).
Yes
Administer an intramuscular injection, if possible with the patient's cooperation. Use midazolam 5–10 mg per event and/or haloperidol 5–10 mg per event. Use the lower recommended dose for first event. Halve the dosage in the medically compromised, frail or elderly (in particular if significant cardiopulmonary/hepatic/renal impairment), in patients markedly intoxicated or dehydrated and in patients who have not previously received antipsychotic medication.
* Do not give diazepam or chlorpromazine IMI.
Midazolam should not be used for rapid tranquillisation

1. Rapid tranquillisation is best performed on a mattress on the floor in an open area cleared of other patients/equipment etc.
2. Gain intravenous access via a large superficial antecubital/forearm vein.
3. Give bolus dose of diazepam 5–10 mg, followed by 5–10 mg of haloperidol. This may be repeated after a 2-minute interval. The dose should be titrated slowly against S_AO_2, respiratory rate, level of consciousness and BP. Diazepam should be given at a rate not exceeding 5 mg/min.
4. If additional sedation is required, add further diazepam, if there are no signs of respiratory depression or hypotension. Maximum 60 mg diazepam per event.
5. If additional sedation is required, add further haloperidol (5–10 mg). Maximum 20 mg haloperidol per event.
6. Watch for acute dystonia from haloperidol. Treat with benztropine 1–2 mg IVI but not prophylactically.
7. Difficult patients:
   Markedly intoxicated: significant risk of respiratory depression with benzodiazepines. Titrate slowly and, if necessary, use maximum doses of haloperidol (20 mg per event). Avoid fumazenil if oversedated as reversal of benzodiazepines can precipitate seizures or unmask the effect of other agents already ingested. Benzodiazepine tolerant: do not proceed past response plateau or 60 mg diazepam without consultation with psychiatrist. Use maximum doses of haloperidol (20 mg per event).
8. The patient should be asleep but rousable at the end of rapid tranquillisation.

Subsequent monitoring:

1. Observe PR, BP, level of consciousness, airway, S_AO_2 and for dystonic reactions at least every 10 min for 60 min after sedation.
2. Nurse in the coma position.
3. Give parenteral benztropine 2 mg for dystonic reactions.
4. If even mildly dehydrated, ensure adequate IVI rehydration while sedated.
5. Document immediately both the use of restraint and the nature of sedation in the case notes and on the medication chart.
6. Ensure clear documentation of observations and nursing level of care/supervision required.

Figure 39.1 St Vincent's Hospital Emergency Department rapid tranquillisation guidelines

BP, blood pressure; BSL, blood sugar level; FBC, full blood count; IMI, intramuscular injection; IVI, intravenous injection; LFT, liver function test; PR, pulse rate; S_AO_2, alveolar partial pressure of oxygen; TFT, thyroid function test; UEC, urea, electrolytes and creatinine.

the patient (e.g. asphyxia, broken limbs during restraint). Universal precautions, such as gloves and face masks, should be used and great care should be taken with sharps.

As many of these patients may be frequent re-presenters, an 'alerts system' may be worthwhile to warn of potential violence risk as well as other important information, such as adverse reactions to drugs or concurrent chronic physical illness. For patients who present very often, an agreed multidisciplinary management plan may be prepared and kept in the medical record or in a linked database. It is important that such plans are regularly reviewed and do not prejudice or limit care.

History and assessment

The most important aspects of psychiatric assessment are a comprehensive history and the mental state assessment.

- Gathering reliable information can be very difficult and may be important for medical and legal reasons, as involuntary admission and treatment may be required. Documentation from ambulance, police and others must be completed.
- If a friend, relative, case-worker or health professional has accompanied the patient, this will help the assessment process; however, the patient should be asked if they would prefer privacy initially. Some people in psychosocial distress will feel more willing to share personal information when given this option.
- The psychiatric history should include:
  - identification of the patient
  - the presenting issues
  - questioning about other psychiatric symptoms
  - past mental health history, particularly with regard to treatment and admission, personal and family life history, drugs and alcohol, forensic history, information about hobbies and habits and some assessment of personality features.
- A medical history and physical examination should be performed. Basic blood tests are indicated in most new patients. As is the case with many presentations in emergency medicine, assessment may need to proceed concurrently with treatment; indeed, thorough history taking, mental state and physical examination may need to be deferred until the acute situation is under control. More-involved investigations, including cerebral CT scanning and drug or septic screening, may sometimes be required.

- There are many medical conditions that can give the appearance of mental illness or may be concurrently present. Particular care is required in the presence of:
  - pyrexia
  - impaired, clouded or depressed levels of consciousness
  - recent and abrupt onset of confusion, disorientation and impaired memory
  - visual and tactile hallucinations
  - periods of complete inactivity during which time there is a loss of awareness of surroundings
  - known diabetes or other major illness
  - history of seizure, recent head injury or drug ingestion.

There are many causes of aggressive behaviour, which vary from psychosis and antisocial/borderline personality traits to organic causes such as head injury, delirium, drugs, sepsis and post-ictal states. Use of a Mini Mental State Examination (MMSE; see Box 34.1 in Chapter 34, 'Geriatric care') will help to identify cognitive deficits or a possible delirium. It can be especially useful if a change over time can be identified and this can also help you decide whether the patient is too sedated, sleepy or disorientated to provide a valid history.

Initial approach

In the ED the following points will help you to rapidly assess psychosocial distress for potential mental health problems, establish the degree of urgency for psychiatric referral and identify any need for safety and/or security measures to be instituted.

Establish the nature of the problem and whether immediate action is needed to prevent the patient from self-discharging or failing to wait for a thorough psychiatric assessment. Consider:

- suicidal ideation
- anxiety/panic
- depression
- thoughts disordered
- bizarre behaviour
- hallucinating
- aggression
- 'stress'
- alcohol or other drug withdrawal
- delusional
- agitation.

Establish why this problem requires attention *now*:

- self-referral
- general practitioner referral
- police referral
- concern from others
- deliberate self-harm
- uncommunicative patient
- personal crisis
- involuntary—mental health legislation.

Context is important: why here and why now? Preliminary information gathering can significantly expedite the assessment process. In some instances there may be an existing 'management plan'. Early enquiries and review of previous presentations or an existing mental health record can reveal valuable information regarding the involvement of other healthcare providers or provide an established working diagnosis.

Corroborative history from others is especially valuable; however, you will need to seek the patient's consent if not under a Mental Health Act. People/places to approach are:

- family, friends or significant others
- general practitioner
- community health centre
- voluntary or non-government agencies
- case managers, psychiatrists, counsellors and psychologists
- in the waiting room (enquire about children, and where they are now).

WHAT DOES THE PATIENT WANT?

Most patients who present in distress will have an idea of what they feel they need or want. Determine what this might be at the outset. Once again, this will further assist you in getting to the core of the problem and a possible solution quickly. Does the patient want:

- medication?
- accommodation?
- someone to talk to?
- psychiatric treatment as an inpatient or an outpatient?
- detoxification from alcohol or other drugs?
- they have no idea ...?

ESTABLISH THE DEGREE OF URGENCY

This will depend on:

- the immediate needs the patient has at that moment

- whether the patient requires specialist psychiatric consultation now
- whether the information you have is accurate and sufficient to refer to psychiatry
- whether the patient could be discharged safely
- how the patient will be followed up
- support and back-up available to the patient.

THE MENTAL HEALTH INTERVIEW

It is important to maintain a professional but empathic attitude to develop a rapport with the patient. Questions should be conversational, yet direct. Asking about suicidal thoughts or plans will often elicit a sense of relief from the person who has been thinking about such acts.

Risk of self-harm

Some of the questions that will determine risk of harm to self are:

- Have you been thinking life is not worth living?
- Have you thought about harming yourself?
- Are you thinking of killing yourself?
- Have you thought about how you would do it?
- Have you already done anything to harm yourself?
- Have you tried to harm yourself before?
- How many times have you tried before?
- When was the most recent time?

Other relevant questions are:

- How often are you getting these thoughts?
- Do you have the means of taking your life and are they accessible?
- When would you intend to take your life?
- Is there anything that would stop you from taking your own life?
- Do you know anyone who has died by suicide?
- Do you have access to a firearm or other weapon?
  Note: If you suspect the patient to be in possession of any weapon(s), the interview should be terminated and security called immediately!

Suicide attempt

Where a suicide attempt has already been made:

- Does the patient still have access to the method used?
- Did the patient use alcohol or other drugs prior to the attempt?

Degree of risk to patient

Some factors to be aware of when determining the increased degree of risk are:

- definite plan
- hopelessness
- severe depression
- psychotic symptoms (command hallucinations)
- recent discharge from a psychiatric facility
- use of alcohol and/or other drugs (especially if there is recent escalation in use)
- recent suicide attempt
- single men who are young or elderly or homeless
- medical illness
- history of sexual/physical abuse
- recent suicide of friend or family member
- temporary effects of alcohol and/or other drugs.

Editorial Comment

There are several risk assessment tools. A commonly used one is the SAD Persons Scale (Table 39.2).

Table 39.2 The SAD PERSONS scale

Factor		Points
S	Sex (male)	1
A	Age (< 19 or > 45 years)	1
D	Depression	1
P	Previous suicide attempt	1
E	Ethanol abuse	1
R	Rational thinking loss	1
S	Social supports lacking	1
O	Organised plan	1
N	No spouse	1
S	Sickness (chronic debilitating disease)	1

Score less than 2: discharge with outpatient psychiatric evaluation
Score of 3 to 6: consider for hospitalisation or at least very close follow-up
Score of 7 or greater: hospitalisation

From Patterson WM, Dohn HH, Bird J, et al. Evaluation of suicidal patients: the SAD PERSONS scale. Psychosomatics 1983 Apr;24(4):343–5, 348–9

Degree of risk to others

Questions to determine the degree of risk to others:

- Have you been thinking of hurting anyone else?
- Have you ever acted on these thoughts?
- Have you been involved in any fights recently?
- Were you using alcohol or other drugs at that time?
- Were you ever assaulted as a child or an adult?
- Have the police ever charged you with assault?

Predictors of violence

Predictors of violence may include:

- history of violence
- history of impulsivity
- alcohol and other drug use
- violent father
- criminal charges for violence
- antisocial behaviour.

Psychotic symptoms

Some questions to elicit psychotic symptoms:

- Do you feel safe at the moment? (May elicit paranoid ideas.)
- Do you hear a voice(s) that others do not hear? (Auditory hallucinations)
- Does this voice(s) tell you what you must do? (Command hallucinations)
- Has your relationship to religion changed recently? (Religious delusions)
- What are your energy levels like? (Psychomotor excitation/ retardation)
- Do you feel you or your thoughts are being controlled? (Ideas of passivity)
- Do you receive communications from the TV, radio etc? (Ideas of reference)

Should the patient respond with garbled or illogical answers, it is likely they are experiencing thought disorder. It is important to try to keep the patient on the subject if possible and give time for them to respond to questions. This may also uncover possible thought-blocking—another form of thought disorder.

KEY POINTS

- Consider physical safety!

- Is there a physical explanation or medical component for the behaviour?
- Preliminary information gathering and corroborative history is essential.
- Will the patient be safe if left alone?
- Most patients will have an idea of what they feel they need or want.
- Conduct a mental state examination (see below).
- Questions should be conversational, yet direct.
- The patient who has been having suicidal thoughts or plans will often have a sense of relief when asked directly.
- If you suspect the patient to be in possession of any weapon(s), the interview should be terminated and security involved immediately!

Further assessment and management

Having formulated provisional diagnoses, medical and psychiatric management should be commenced concurrently when required. For patients with significant comorbidities, inpatient care in a medical setting with mental health consultation is often safer.

- Treating medical issues (e.g. sepsis, pain) may well lead to improvement in mental health symptoms.
- Management of intoxication or withdrawal states, such as with methamphetamine or alcohol (see Figure 39.2 overleaf), is important.
- Basic needs such as food and personal hygiene need to be addressed.
- Psychiatric medication should be instituted (or re-instituted) with care and ideally with specialist consultation. A basic understanding of antipsychotics, antidepressants, sedatives and neuroleptics as well as their interactions is required (see Table 39.3, below).

Ideally, use defined criteria to assign a care level to each patient to ensure appropriate supervision and observation (see Box 39.1 below). Documentation should clearly explain the reasons that sedation and/or restraint were required, and the doses, routes of administration and timing of any medications used. At the earliest possible time, fill out the legal forms (schedules) if indicated.

THE MENTAL STATE EXAMINATION

The mental status examination is a set of observations made throughout the psychiatric interview. These observations can then be articulated to describe the person's mental state.

1 Appearance and behaviour
  — Dress, hygiene and motor activity
2 Speech
  — Rate, quantity and volume
3 Mood and affect
  — Depressed, euphoric, euthymic, suspicious
  — Blunted, restricted, flat
4 Form of thought
  — Rate of production
  — Continuity
  — Disturbances
5 Thought content
  — Delusions
  — Preoccupations (suicide/homicide)
6 Perception
  — Hallucinations
  — Perceptual disturbances (depersonalisation)
7 Sensorium and cognition
  — Glasgow Coma Scale, MMSE (see Chapter 34, Box 34.1)
8 Insight
  — Demonstrated level of awareness of the problem

Common drugs used in psychiatry

See Table 39.3.

MONITORING

If rapid sedation is used, the sedated patient should be moved to an appropriate medical assessment and monitoring area. Physical examination and adequate tests to identify and manage organic illness should be instigated. Nursing care, including cardiovascular and neurological observation, should be regularly performed. The sedated patient should be closely observed, given supplemental oxygen and have pulse oximetry ± non-invasive blood pressure (NIBP), temperature and ECG monitoring in place.

DISPOSITION

Physical restraints should be removed once chemical control is achieved. Medical documentation must be clear and detailed and should include history and physical findings, test results and dosage and timing of all medications given. Legal forms should be completed and arrangements for further management and disposition clearly stated.

Promoting a safe environment Early detection and intervention	Maintaining a safe environment Risk management and planning for safety	Restoring a safe environment Psychiatric emergency crisis intervention
Level 1 Definition: amphetamine identified as likely cause Behaviours: anxiety/agitation Mildly aroused, pacing, still willing to talk reasonably or may be moderately aroused	Level 2 Definition: escalation of aggressive behaviour with reduced capacity to control emotions and behaviour Behaviours: verbal aggression Not dangerous or violent. Moderately aroused, agitated, becoming more vocal, unreasonable and hostile or may be highly aroused	Level 3 Definition: aggressive behaviour poses an imminent threat to the safety of all Behaviours: violence or danger is imminent or physically aggressive. Highly aroused, distressed and agitated. Patient refuses all medication
ACTION: Aggressive behaviour monitored and controlled	**ACTION:** Clinical intervention required	**ACTION:** Crisis intervention required
• Pre-empt and intervene early. • Exercise crisis communication skills. • Address concerns and fears. • See level 1 regimen	• Coordinate intervention. • Monitor the effectiveness of continued engagement. • Continue to address concerns and fears. • See level 2 regimen	• Senior clinician coordinates an emergency response. • Ensure the safety of others in your care. • Mechanical restraint in extreme violence or combativeness • See level 3 regimen

Promoting a safe environment Early detection and intervention	Maintaining a safe environment Risk management and planning for safety	Restoring a safe environment Psychiatric emergency crisis intervention
PER ORAL LEVEL 1 Diazepam 5–10 mg *OR* Combine diazepam 5–10 mg with olanzapine 5–10 mg Review in 30 minutes and repeat × 1 if required if there is minimal clinical response. Further review by senior doctor if necessary. NOTE – DAILY MAXIMUM DOSES Daily maximum dose not to be > 60 mg diazepam Daily maximum dose not to be > 30 mg olanzapine	**PER ORAL LEVEL 1** Olanzapine 10–15 mg oral wafers with *lorazepam 1–2 mg (max 8 mg/d) or diazepam 10–20 mg Review in 30 minutes and repeat ×1 if required for suitable clinical response. Further review. LESS PREFERRED OPTION Diazepam 10–20 mg with haloperidol 5–10 mg PO Typical or atypical options may be combined with benzodiazepines and must be in keeping with the daily max dose (see Level 1) Max 40 mg/d haloperidol	**PARENTERAL INTERVENTION LEVEL 3** **Diazepam IVI 10 mg, repeated after 5 minute reviews to achieve a clinical response. Max 60 mg or until sedated with **haloperidol IVI 5–10 mg to a maximum of 20 mg per rapid tranquillisation event If IVI route is compromised in fit adult give midazolam IMI 10 mg Repeat in 10 min if necessary (max 40 mg/d). LESS PREFERRED OPTION ** IMI droperidol 5–10 mg (max 20 mg/d) NB: ** IV/IM benzodiazepines or droperidol/haloperidol used ONLY when adequate ECG/O_2 monitoring is available. ED CONSULTANT notified if clinical response inadequate after max mg/d ALL medications.

Figure 39.2 St Vincent's Hospital guidelines for the treatment of methamphetamine intoxication

Developed by Jamie Houlahan (CNC), Gary Nicholls (Clin Pharm) and Beaver Hudson (CNC) in association with Emergency, D&A, Psychiatry & Clinical Pharmacology, St Vincent's Hospital Sydney Ltd. Adapted from 'Development of clinical guidelines for the pharmacological management of behavioural disturbance and aggression in people with psychosis' by D Castles, Australian Psychiatry 2005;13(3):247–52

Table 39.3 Common drugs used in psychiatry*

Drug	Indications	Dose	Cautions
Antipsychotics			
Olanzapine	Schizophrenia and related psychoses Acute mania	5–10 mg PO	*Parkinson's disease*—risk of aggravation and potential for drug interactions
Haloperidol	Acute and chronic psychoses Acute mania Tourette's syndrome and other choreas Adjunct in treatment of alcoholic hallucinosis	5–10 mg PO	Respiratory failure—sedating antipsychotics may cause respiratory depression or worsen that associated with alcohol, benzodiazepines or barbiturates Epilepsy—antipsychotics may alter EEG or lower seizure threshold
Anxiolytics/sedatives			
Diazepam	Short-term management of anxiety, agitation Acute alcohol withdrawal Acute behavioural disturbance	5–10 mg PO 10–20 mg PO 10–20 mg PO	Respiratory depression Severe hepatic impairment, particularly when hepatic encephalopathy is present Myasthenia gravis
Lorazepam	Anxiety Short-tem treatment of insomnia associated with anxiety	1–2 mg PO	
Midazolam	Acute behaviour disturbance—adjunctive treatment with haloperidol IM injection	5–10 mg IM stat	

Drug	Indications	Dose	Cautions
Antidepressants			
Sertraline	Major depression Obsessive–compulsive disorder (>6 years) Panic disorder Social phobia Major depression	50–100 mg PO daily	Treatment with, or within 14 days of stopping, a MAOI Treatment with, or within 2 days of stopping, moclobemide Epilepsy, reduced seizure threshold—SSRIs may lower seizure threshold; use low doses and titrate slowly Bipolar disorder—all antidepressants may provoke a manic episode when used in people with bipolar disorder; some patients without a history of bipolar disorder may develop an antidepressant-induced manic episode; this does not necessarily imply a diagnosis of bipolar affective disorder People at high risk of bleeding (age > 80 years or previous upper GI bleeding) or taking drugs known to increase risk of GI bleeding (regular aspirin or NSAIDs)—likelihood of serious bleeding may be increased
Fluoxetine	Obsessive–compulsive disorder Premenstrual dysphoric disorder Bulimia nervosa Panic disorder Post-traumatic stress disorder	20 mg PO daily	
Citalopram	Major depression	20 mg PO daily	

*Disclaimer: The information contained in this table is provided as a guide only and is not to be used without appropriate clinical reference.

Box 39.1 Care levels for mental health patients

Care level 1: visual range within 1 metre

- Criteria for the allocation of care level 1:
  - High risk of self-harm suicidal intent
  - Self-harming behaviour (self-mutilation, confusional state, delirium)
  - High risk of absconding with danger to self
- Nursing responsibilities:
  - The allocation of care level 1 must be documented at least once per shift in the patient's progress notes
- Documentation is to include:
  - Requirement for care level 1
  - Rationale/symptoms for care level 1
  - Observations regarding emotional state and behaviour and any medical concerns
  - Interventions planned and/or implemented
  - Individual specifics (restrictions/alerts, visitors, telephone calls, meals)
  - Evaluation of effectiveness of care level

Care level 2: visual range outside 1 metre

- Criteria for the allocation of care level 2:
  - May require the assistance of security and assessment for rapid tranquillisation
  - High assaultative risk potential towards others
  - Severe behavioural disturbance
  - High risk of absconding with assaultative potential towards others
- Nursing responsibilities:
  - The allocation of care level 2 must be documented at least once per shift in the patient's progress notes
- Documentation is to include:
  - Requirement for care level 2
  - Rationale/symptoms for care level 2
  - Observations regarding emotional state and behaviour and any medical concerns
  - Interventions planned and/or implemented
  - Individual specifics (restrictions/alerts, visitors, telephone calls, meals)
  - Evaluation of effectiveness of care level
- The shift coordinator must ensure the person assigned to observe the patient on care level 1/2 is fully aware of his/her responsibilities:
  - That the person understands care level 1/2 is a clinical management strategy that is not open to individual clinical judgment
  - That the patient is never to be left unobserved for even brief periods

- — Issues of privacy and dignity are important but are secondary to safety and security issues
- — The 'line of vision' and 'within easy reach' rules are to be maintained at all times for those patients on care level 2 including toileting and showering

Care level 3: close observation

- Criteria for the allocation of care level 3:
  - — Potential risk towards others
  - — Potential risk to self
  - — Potential risk of absconding
  - — Confused and wandering
  - — Evolving mental state
- The decision to place a patient on nursing care level 3 is made by the senior medical officer or psychiatry registrar in consultation with the shift coordinator. Nursing staff may initiate 'close observation' while waiting to discuss the issue with the senior medical officer. Patients are placed on a 15-minute interval observation chart, which is to be completed by the allocated nurse.

Decisions regarding admission to medical or mental health units can be difficult, and early input of senior clinicians should be sought. Medical conditions and social issues may be the predominant issues or may make the decision for inpatient or outpatient care more difficult. Good follow-up is essential for ongoing care; patients may have difficulty arranging and keeping appointments themselves—it may be necessary for you to notify other healthcare providers right away by phone/fax/email.

When available, admission to a short-stay combined medical and mental health facility (psychiatric emergency care centre) may be an option. These units ideally have joint admission processes under the care of a psychiatrist and an emergency or other doctor. Ideally they should have clearly defined inclusion and exclusion criteria and streamed clinical pathways. Community mental health, GPs, psychiatrists, social workers and drug and alcohol professionals will usually be involved.

Diagnoses in psychiatry

Classification systems in psychiatry are evolving and being updated. The Diagnostic and Statistical Manual of Mental Disorders (DSM) and the International Classification of Diseases (ICD) are both widely used. Adult psychiatric disorders are also sometimes divided into Organic, Schizophrenias, Bipolar, Depression, Anxiety and Personality groupings.

Anxiety

Anxiety is a subjective experience and one which can be manifested in a number of clinical conditions.

- It may be accompanied by autonomic symptoms such as palpitations, chest pain, shortness of breath and diaphoresis.
- The patient may report a sense of unpleasant unease or impending doom which may induce them to seek emergency care.
- Symptoms can occur suddenly (as in a panic attack); or develop gradually, increasing over a period of time.
- There are significant common characteristics between serious medical conditions and anxiety, e.g. respiratory disorders such as airway limitation disease, cardiovascular disorders such as arrhythmia, neurological conditions such as transient ischaemic attack and side-effects from substances such as caffeine or medications such as SSRIs.
- Anxiety can have physical causes, e.g. alcohol withdrawal; or other psychiatric causes, e.g. schizophrenia or depression.
- When approaching the patient with anxiety it is important to present a reassuring and confident manner while demonstrating real concern. Anxiety can give rise to rash impulsive behaviour, therefore safety must be considered.
- Longitudinal history taking will establish first onset of symptoms, triggers, family history and coexistent medical conditions.
- Treatment may involve reassurance, medication or other therapy and may sometimes require hospital admission.

Editorial Comment

Australia has one of the world's highest rates of youth suicide. Mental health problems during all segments of the patient's life are increasing. Know and practise your standard approach to these common ED patients.

Online resources

American Psychiatric Association news
psychnews.psychiatryonline.org
Beyond Blue—National Organisation for Depression and Anxiety Treatment and Management
www.beyondblue.org.au
Black Dog Institute
www.blackdoginstitute.org.au
Mental Health for Emergency Departments—NSW Health
www.health.nsw.gov.au/resources/mhdao/pdf/mhemergency.pdf
National Youth Mental Health Association
www.headspace.org.au
Sane Australia
www.sane.org

Chapter 40
Dermatological presentations to emergency

John R Sullivan, Veronica A Preda
and Margot J Whitfield

Dermatology presentations to the emergency department are common, accounting for 15–20% of visits,[1] with the majority of presentations due to an infective aetiology or the result of drug reactions. Overall, there are 4 basic categories of dermatological presentation to the ED (see Table 40.1).

Assessing patients with dermatological emergency presentations

DERMATOLOGICAL HISTORY

Note: Take advantage of being able to readily and concurrently evaluate and examine the skin early in the consultation process to assist in the provision of an expedient and clinically focused and relevant medical assessment.

- Where: site(s) of initial lesion, then subsequent lesions.
- Associated dermatological symptoms: e.g. irritable, pruritic, burning or tender skin.
- Temporal disease course/exposures:
  - onset/duration—acute, exacerbation of a chronic or an intermittent condition
  - recent medication and medical history (weeks–months)
  - travel (rural/farm or overseas)
  - change in symptoms over time.
- Prior similar episodes/reactions to medications.
- Any other family members/colleagues/school friends affected.
- Personal and family history of skin disease.
- Cutaneous changes warning of a potentially severe cutaneous reaction/disease and/or systemic reaction/disease, such as a previously itchy skin eruption that becomes tender and/or blisters.
- Other dermatological symptoms and manifestations suggesting/warning of associated mucosal involvement preceding,

Table 40.1 **Isolated dermatological disorders**

Reason for presentation	Common or important clinical examples
New onset or flare	Eczema (atopic dermatitis) Papular urticaria—mainly a paediatric emergency presentation usually representing an exaggerated local hypersensitivity to an insect bite which can be clinically dramatic and/or severe, such as a blistering skin reaction
Subacute or chronic with complication	Impetiginised scabies, eczema
Dermatological presentations with systemic associations	
Fifth disease	Pregnant woman—increased risk of hydrops fetalis or aplastic crisis if underlying haematological disorder
Systemic disorders resulting in acute presentations with prominent cutaneous manifestations	
SLE/PAN/cholesterol emboli	Vasculitis, trash foot, broken livedoid eruption
Systemic disorders with associated cutaneous changes or disorders	
Inflammatory bowel disease and/or inflammatory arthritis	Pyoderma gangrenosum
Systemic disorders with unrelated/incidental cutaneous findings	
Common presentations	Seborrhoeic dermatitis (> 50% are elderly but also more common in particular clinical settings, e.g. advanced HIV/AIDS or neurological disorders, especially Parkinson's disease)

HIV/AIDS, human immunodeficiency virus/acquired immune deficiency syndrome; PAN, polyarteritis nodosa; SLE, systemic lupus erythematosus

coinciding or following onset of skin changes (e.g. sore throat/pharyngitis, gritty eyes/periorbital puffiness or head and neck swelling/enlarged cervical glands).

- Presence or absence of associated symptoms suggesting skin involvement by a systemic disease/associated internal organ involvement/toxicity (e.g. high fever/night sweats, anorexia, arthritis).
- Occupational history (e.g. a possibly infective presentation and work history exploring animal exposures) and/or work/close contact with an elderly family member living in a nursing home (e.g. if scabies considered in a patient with an acute/subacute ± itchy skin reaction).

- Home environment/activities: blistering, extremely itchy, streaky inflammatory eruption mainly and most severely involving upper limbs and other exposed skin areas starting hours after gardening.
- Treatments tried and any associated temporal changes in disease symptoms.

EXAMINATION

- Dermatological: distribution, morphology, pattern.
- Where relevant, also examine mucosal surfaces e.g. for oropharyngeal inflammation/erosion/ulceration.
- General examination (tailor and target to presentation as illustrated by the following examples):
  - arterial examination including abdominal examination specifically checking for an acutely dissecting abdominal aortic aneurysm as the source of cholesterol emboli in a person presenting with lower back pain and a tender, dusky, ischaemic reticulate lower leg eruption
  - examination for presence or absence of tender lymphadenopathy of draining lymph nodes with cutaneous infections and/or an infective complication of skin disease.

Important emergencies are listed in Box 40.1, and terminology is defined in Table 40.2.

Box 40.1 Dermatological emergencies: what not to miss!

- Angio-oedema/anaphylaxis
- Adult varicella zoster
- Meningococcal
- Staphylococcal scalded skin syndrome
- Necrotising fasciitis
- Exfoliative erythroderma
- Stevens–Johnson syndrome (SJS)
- Toxic epidermal necrolysis (TEN)
- Haemangiomas (children)

DIAGNOSIS

See Table 40.3. Infective complications in immunocompetent patients are outlined in Table 40.4.

Table 40.2 **Terminology for skin lesions**

Lesion	Description
Bulla(e)	Large fluid-filled lesion > 0.5 cm in diameter
Cyst	Closed cavity/sac with epithelial lining containing solids or fluids
Discoid	Disc-shaped (nummular)
Erythema	Redness of the skin from vascular congestion or increased flow such as in inflammation
Macule	Flat alteration in colour and/or texture of the skin, e.g. colour change due to skin inflammation including erythema and/or hyper/hypopigmentation (change in melanin, haemosiderin); if larger than several centimetres, referred to as a patch
Nodule	Solid mass > 0.5 cm in diameter, palpable
Papule	Solid elevation of the skin < 0.5 cm in diameter
Petechiae	Pinpoint, flat, round, purplish red spots caused by intradermal or submucosal haemorrhage
Plaque	Solid, elevated lesion; may be formed by coalescence of papules
Purpura	Bleeding into the dermis; may be macular or papular
Pustule	Circumscribed collection of pus, commonly staphylococcal, but may be sterile in inflammatory and autoimmune dermatoses, e.g. pustular psoriasis
Telangiectasia(e)	Tiny visible blood vessels in the upper dermis ± inflammation
Verrucous	Rough, warty
Vesicle	Visible accumulation of fluid within or beneath the epidermis, < 0.5 cm
Wheal	Transient area of dermal oedema, pale, compressible, papular or plaque-like
Surface characteristics	
Scale, crust, horn, excoriation, maceration, lichenification	

Morphological classification of dermatological presentations

1 URTICARIA (HIVES) ± ANGIO-OEDEMA ± ANAPHYLAXIS

- Cutaneous versus systemic reaction.
- Common condition: 15–25% of people have an episode of urticaria ± angio-oedema at some stage in their life. Usually it is acute.[2]

Table 40.3 Diagnosis of dermatological disease

Diagnosis	
Accurate characterisation of skin eruption	E.g. exanthematic eruption, skin rash due to or mimicking a viral infection
Isolated skin presentation versus any worrisome systemic involvement; concerning symptoms or associated findings	E.g. high fever (temperature > 40°C) or 'sick' patient presentation
Differential diagnosis	
Infection: viral, bacterial, fungal Drug eruption: isolated (simple) exanthematic hypersensitivity reaction (and/or the manifestation of a systemic hypersensitivity reaction) Connective tissue disease, graft-versus-host disease (due to an acute disease flare and/or active inadequately controlled disease)	
Drug and other exposures	
Medications history	When medications, including over-the-counter and alternative or natural therapies, were started and/or stopped; any previous reactions to similar or crossreacting medications, vaccinations or injections
Other exposure	IVDU, environmental exposure, history of infective symptoms, travel
Diagnostic testing	
Diagnosis	Most diagnoses are suspected in emergency but confirmed at a later date. e.g. drug reactions are largely a diagnosis of exclusion
Differential diagnosis	May require baseline (acute) viral and autoimmune serology ALWAYS perform a bacterial culture for M/C/S if itchy/weeping/crusted/purulent, ± viral culture if painful
Associated diseases/ toxicities/complications	E.g. hepatitis, nephritis as part of a drug hypersensitivity syndrome and/or connective tissue disease flare. Drug hypersensitivity reactions are more common in those living with HIV/AIDS, lymphoma ± CTD
Determine probabilities	
Paediatric	Infectious aetiology more likely
Adult	Consider comorbidities and always consider drug causes, especially in the elderly
Dermatologist consult	
Urgent	E.g. suspected SJS/TEN
Organise follow-up/discuss	

CTD, connective tissue disease; IVDU, intravenous drug use; M/C/S, microculture and sensitivity; SJS, Stevens-Johnson syndrome; TEN, toxic epidermal necrolysis

Table 40.4 Infective complications of dermatoses in immunocompetent patients

Bacterial	*Staphylococcus aureus* (approximately 90%); always consider risk factors for methicillin-resistant *S. aureus* (MRSA) *Streptococcus pyogenes*; always consider nephritogenic strain, especially in Indigenous populations Mixed
Viral	Herpes simplex virus 1, 2
Fungal	*Trichophyton rubrum* and *T. tonsurans* (especially in rural and remote Indigenous populations)

History

Onset of hives, swelling and itch in relation to stimulus. Acute presentations are typically seen in acute infections and hypersensitivity reactions to foods, medications or insect bites. See Table 40.5, overleaf for classification of causes.

Clinical features

- Urticaria: intensely itchy, swollen, red rounded lesions with pale raised centres, often with bizarre shapes and typically moving around every few hours. (Mild forms may present with just itch and/or dermographism.)
- Angio-oedema: generalised swelling of the soft tissues. Commonly most dramatic, noticeable and symptomatic in the loose-tissue areas, e.g. periorbital, perioral, pressure areas (waistline, soles of feet) and genitalia. Typically the angio-oedema is non-pruritic but burning[1,2] and/or tender when involving pressure areas.
- Upper airway involvement: check for impending upper airway obstruction (due to angio-oedema involving soft tissue of perimucosal areas).
- Anaphylaxis: shock—hypotension, tachycardia, bronchospasm, i.e. cardiorespiratory compromise. Perform auscultation for added sounds/silent chest, peak flow if appropriate.

Differential diagnosis: erythema multiforme (EM)

- Clinical features of EM:
  - acute, self-limiting, mucocutaneous reaction
  - classic 'iris' or target lesion: round or oval area of redness, dusky purplish centre ± blisters ± mucosal involvement. The lesions may vary. Appear on extensor surfaces of the arms and legs, including the palms and soles.

Table 40.5 Classification of causes of erythema multiforme, urticaria, angio-oedema and anaphylaxis

Acute (minutes to hours)	Subacute (days)	Chronic	Rare syndromes
(Major concern is anaphylaxis) IgE-dependent path Hypersensitivity syndromes —Drug allergy: penicillins, sulfonamides, diuretics, muscle relaxants, allopurinol, NSAIDs (rarely IgE) —Food allergy: milk, egg, peanuts, tree nuts, seafood —Insect allergy	IgG-dependent path —Serum sickness	Autoimmune (35–40% of chronic urticaria)	Cold-induced disorders
Idiopathic acute	**Idiopathic subacute**	**Idiopathic chronic**	**Urticaria pigmentosa and systemic mastocytosis**
(Rare cause of acute, e.g. exercise-induced anaphylaxis) IgE-independent path (clinically looks the same), 'pseudoallergic reactions' —Drugs: opioids, vancomycin, NSAIDs, beta-blockers —Foods other than those above —Viral infections, e.g. in children as part of inflammatory processes produced by viral illness; enteroviruses are the commonest cause of childhood urticaria; other examples —Other causes: HBV, EBV, HIV —Bacterial associations: streptococcal-related urticaria	IgE independent path —Serum-sickness-like reaction (usually urticarial, occasionally exanthematic) —Radiocontrast dyes—with the current agents usually onset is delayed 48–72 hours and not usually anaphylactic (i.e. consider alternative triggers in the context of recent IV contrast)	(35–40% of chronic urticaria) Physical (20%) —Dermatographism —Cholinergic: after exercise or exposure to heat, i.e. with a rise in basal body temperature —Exercise-induced anaphylaxis —Delayed pressure —Solar vs cold —Vibratory —Aquagenic	Hereditary angio-oedema (atopic dermatitis, AD)

Idiopathic acute	Idiopathic subacute	Idiopathic chronic	Urticaria pigmentosa and systemic mastocytosis
Toxic reaction		Systemic disease—presumed immune-complex-induced: —Thyroid disease —Urticarial vasculitis —Malignancy-associated (e.g. B cell lymphoproliferative) —Collagen vascular disease	ACE inhibitors are contraindicated in patients with C1INH deficiency
Contact urticaria: —Latex —Animal saliva —Processing foods/biologicals		Ingestants, e.g. food intolerance (10–20% of chronic urticaria patients intolerant to amines and salicylates): food, drugs, dietary supplements Infections: e.g. multicellular parasites in endemic areas Hormonal changes	
Immune complex: —Serum sickness —Transfusion-related	Immune complex (re-exposure): —Serum sickness —Transfusion-related —Postviral		

ACE, angiotensin-converting enzyme; AD, Addison's disease; C1INH, C1-inhibitor; EBV, Epstein–Barr virus; HBV, hepatitis B virus; HIV, human immunodeficiency virus; Ig, immunoglobulin; NSAIDs, non-steroidal anti-inflammatory drugs.

Amar SM, Dreskin SC. Urticaria. Prim Care Clin Office Pract 2008;35:141–57.

- Triggers: herpes simplex virus is the most common trigger.
- Causes: see Table 40.5.
- Clinical spectrum: mild EM to minor to severe which can be Stevens–Johnson syndrome (SJS) or toxic epidermal necrolysis (TEN).
- Management of EM: symptomatic treatment ± aciclovir ± nutritional supplementation if there is significant mucosal involvement.

Management

Refer to the flow chart, which includes anaphylaxis management, in Figure 40.1. Table 40.6 lists medications used in angio-oedema, anaphylaxis and acute/'subacute' urticaria, and Table 40.7 outlines treatment of chronic urticaria.

2 'SPOTTY, BLANCHING' EXANTHEMATIC ERUPTIONS

Infection-associated skin eruption or other disease with skin changes mimicking those of an infective exanthem.

Exanthematic eruption

Generalised cutaneous eruption usually associated with a primary systemic infection, often accompanied by oral mucosal lesions (an exanthem).

Clinical features

- Lesion morphology: flat, erythematous macules or papular, less frequently vesicles, pustules, petechiae and itch.
- Systemic features: consider the seriousness of the presentation (not the aetiology) to differentiate isolated 'skin changes only' versus symptomatic.
  - 'Skin changes only'—no fever, no systemic symptoms, no systemic findings, normal lab tests.
  - Symptomatic—unwell with fever ± hypotension, internal organ involvement; ± lymphadenopathy ± hepatosplenomegaly.
- Associated exanthem: severe mucosal changes are predictors of serious systemic disease, e.g. oropharyngeal ulceration, especially haemorrhagic changes and/or eye or genitourinary.
- Characteristic mucosal changes include:
  - drug eruptions
  - inflammatory disease
  - Koplick spots, red strawberry tongue, mouth changes in Kawasaki's disease, etc.

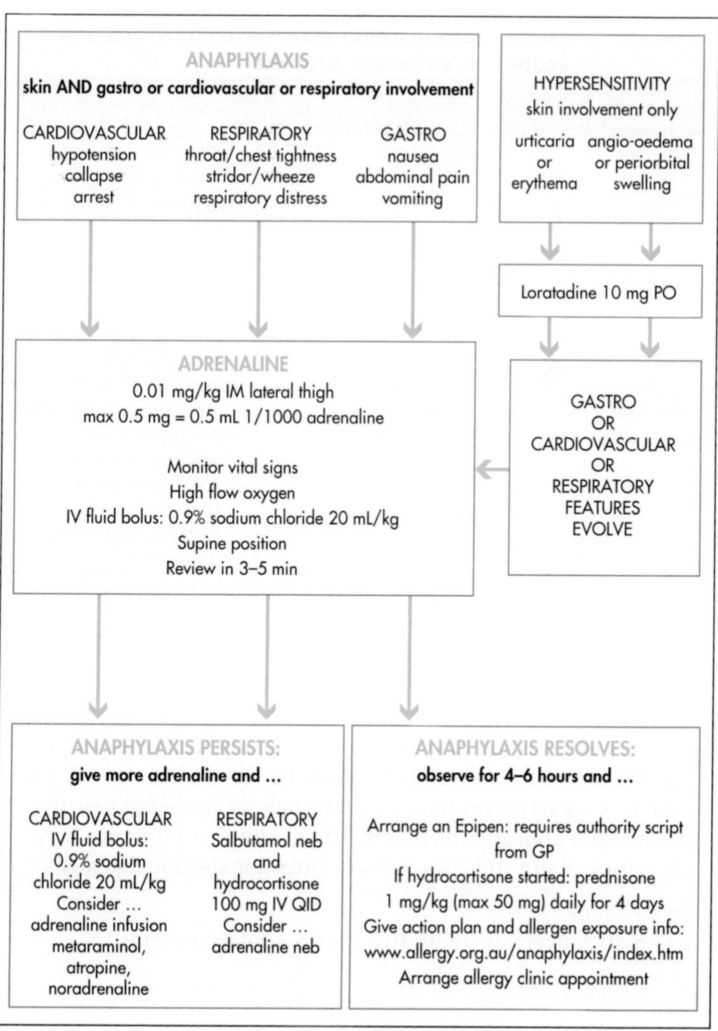

Figure 40.1 Allergic reactions: 3-step management
Adapted from Amar SM, Dreskin SC. Urticaria. Prim Care Clin Office Pract 2008;35:141–57

Note: For exanthematic 'spotty, blanching' eruptions, ALWAYS consider the seriousness of the presentation: skin changes ± mucosal features ± systemic features, i.e. eruption plus systemically well versus eruption plus systemically unwell patient.

Table 40.6 Medications in angio-oedema, anaphylaxis and acute and 'subacute' urticaria

Medication	Recommended adult dose	Comment
Adrenaline	0.5–1.0 mL of 1:1000 IM	Used if evidence of anaphylaxis
H_1 antihistamines		Mainstay of therapy
Dexchlorpheniramine (Polaramine)	2 mg q6h	Sedating in 50% of patients
Diphenhydramine	4 mg q4–6h, max 24 mg/day	
H_1 antihistamines, 2nd generation		Reasonable to continue antihistamines for approximately 72 hours after acute presentation
Loratadine	10 mg daily	Although caution required, medications are safe in general long-term and can be used in higher doses for urticaria
Fexofenadine	180 mg daily	
Cetirizine HCl	10 mg daily	
Steroids		Acute severe episodes, avoid chronic use, especially in patients with chronic urticaria
Hydrocortisone	100 mg IV	
Prednisone	20–40 mg/day, max 80 mg/day	

Investigations

- If there is suspicion of systemic involvement: full blood count (FBC), urea, electrolytes and creatinine (UEC), liver function test (LFT), C-reactive protein (CRP), urinalysis, urine microscopy
- Cultures if appropriate: blood, urine, ± lumbar puncture (LP)
- Serology: acute and convalescent titres for specific diagnosis

Differential diagnosis

See Box 40.2, overleaf. Table 40.8 covers viral exanthems.

Kawasaki's disease

- Mucocutaneous lymph node syndrome.
- Cutaneous features of an exanthematic eruption, with prominent peeling hands and feet. Often the differential is that of an infective illness, but usually fever for > 5 days unresponsive to antipyretics suggests Kawasaki's.
- Large- and medium-vessel vasculitis in children < 10 years (usually < 5 years), predilection for Japanese children.
- Cardiac sequelae.

Table 40.7 Treatment of chronic urticaria (often a distressed patient with chronic symptoms presenting with a flare)

Treatment/medication	Recommended adult dose	Comment
Simple measures	Keep cool, loose clothing	
H_1 antihistamines		Mainstay of therapy Sedating in 50% of patients
Dexchlorpheniramine (Polaramine)	2 mg q6h	
Diphenhydramine	4 mg q4–6 h, max 24 mg/day	
H_2 antihistamines		Useful in chronic urticaria in addition to H_1 antihistamines
Ranitidine	150 mg BD	
Cimetidine	400 mg BD	
Famotidine	20 mg BD	
Omeprazole	20–40 mg daily	
Cyproheptadine	4 mg TDS	Sedating antihistamine plays an important role in chronic urticaria, e.g. with nocturnal exacerbations or insomnia due to urticaria, and appetite stimulant
Doxepin	10–50 mg/day	H_1- and H_2-blocking properties, sedating, appetite stimulant, higher doses have anxiolytic and antidepressive effects
Steroids		Acute severe episodes, avoid chronic use, especially in patients with chronic urticaria
Hydrocortisone	100 mg IV	
Prednisone	20–40 mg/day, max 80 mg/day	
Other immunosuppressives	For immunologist referral	

Clinical features

- History is typically > 5 days (usually has been unresponsive to antibiotics in the community) and 4 out of 5 elements of the mnemonic CRASH:
  - **C** Conjunctivitis, Cervical lymphadenopathy (> 1.5 cm)
  - **R** Rash (mostly truncal polymorphic morbilliform)
  - **A** Aneurysms of the coronary arteries
  - **S** Strawberry tongue, crusting of the lips, fissuring of the mouth and oropharyngeal erythema
  - **H** Hands and feet have induration, erythema of the palms and soles, desquamation of the digits.

Box 40.2 Differential diagnosis, exanthematic eruption	
Paediatric exanthematic eruption • Infection-related—most commonly in children and usually well: — viral (see Table 40.8 for management) — bacterial — parasitic — fungal • Drugs—common nuisance drug eruptions (see section later in chapter) **Things not to miss** • Meningitis—meningococcal can present atypically • Serious drug eruption • Reye's syndrome • Kawasaki's disease	**Adult exanthematic eruption** • Drugs[2]—just about all medications but particularly: — antibiotics — antivirals — anti-inflammatories — anticonvulsants — antipsychotics[3] • Inflammatory—includes connective tissue disease; otherwise as part of a flare or warning of disease activity in the context of systemic illness • Infection-related: — viral—including adult varicella zoster, seroconversion illness in HIV[4] — rickettsial infections, e.g. *Rickettsia australis*[5]—'recurrent mild chicken pox in an adult' — bacterial e.g. *Streptococcus pyogenes* causing toxic shock syndrome — parasitic — fungal **Things not to miss** • Serious drug eruption • Autoimmune causes—rheumatoid arthritis, systemic lupus erythematosus • Malignancy e.g. lymphoma • Adult varicella zoster

Diagnosis of Kawasaki's disease

- Confused with scarlet fever, but scarlet fever does not have fissured lips and does have a positive streptococcal throat test.
- It is important to ask parents about eye changes occurring prior to other symptoms in the 7 days before, as these may be transient.
- Complications: cardiac, 10–40% untreated cases have coronary vasculitis (dilation/aneurysm) within the first weeks of the illness.

Table 40.8 Features and management of common viral exanthems in paediatric patients

Disease/virus	Signs/symptoms	Management
Enterovirus	Commonly respiratory or gastroenterology presentations ± exanthem or urticaria	Presentation-dependent
Varicella—chicken pox/ Varicella zoster virus (VZV) Reactivation → herpes zoster (HZ)	Incubation 10–21 days Mid-prodrome—pruritic vesicles that break and crust, starts centrally or facially and spreads to the extremities New lesions appear 3–5 days, typically take 3 days to crust Contagious for 24 h prior to rash onset and until lesions crust	Immunocompromised children with VZV are given VZ immunoglobulin (VZIG) within 96 h of exposure Aciclovir for immunocompromised children with disseminated VZ or HZ
Measles (rubeola)/ paramyxovirus	Prodrome fever, malaise, coryza, conjunctivitis, cough; then erythematous maculopapular rash on face, trunk, legs, buccal mucosal lesions, Koplick spots Incubation 8–12 days	Symptomatic management, contact considerations, vaccinations
Rubella (German measles)/ RNA togavirus	No prodrome during incubation 14–21 days	Symptomatic, consider contacts including pregnant contacts
Roseola infantum/ HHV6	Infants 6–8 months—high fever, relatively well; multiple pale pink macules/papules as fever breaks	Supportive
Erythema infectiosum (fifth disease)/ parvovirus B19 'slapped cheeks'	Sore throat, cough, headache, nausea, fever with rash, slapped-cheek appearance followed by lace-like erythema on the extremities and buttocks	Supportive but consider concurrent haematological disease or exposure of pregnant contacts
Scarlet fever/toxins from *Streptococcus pyogenes*	Commonly confused with Kawasaki's disease Child 4–8 years—high fever, sore throat, headache, vomiting Exanthem 1–2 days post—small papules with diffuse erythema (continues overleaf)	If suspected treat with penicillin, (clindamycin or erythromycin if allergic)

Continues

Table 40.8 Features and management of common viral exanthems in paediatric patients (continued)

Disease/virus	Signs/symptoms	Management
Scarlet fever/toxins continued	Skin may feel rough, like sandpaper Linea petechiae = Pastia's lines in the axillae and groin. Desquamation 7–10 days post, hand and feet worse Strawberry tongue; lips normal; tonsils/pharynx usual site of infection ± surgical wounds Investigations include anti-DNase B, anti-streptolysin O titre	Management is to avoid complications, e.g. rheumatic heart disease
Mumps	Morbilliform rash with lymphadenopathy, an issue in young males with potential infertility	Despite vaccination consider occurrence
Mycoplasma pneumoniae	Skin changes may be macular papular or present as purpura Mainly in school children, cough, coryza Skin eruptions in approximately 10% of children with mycoplasma Swab throat—polymerase chain reaction	Antimicrobial therapy for *Mycoplasma*, e.g. rifampicin
Hand, foot and mouth disease (HFMD)/ enterovirus, coxsackievirus	Generally mild clinical course Distinct clinical presentation of oral and distal extremity lesions Highly contagious, faecal–oral spread Usually in children < 10 years, can affect adults Hands, feet and buttocks involved; 2–10 mm erythematous macules, with central grey oval vesicle Skin lesions asymptomatic, resolve in 3–7 days Mucosal oral ulcers are painful Associated fever, malaise, diarrhoea, systemic involvement can progress to myocarditis, pneumonia, meningoencephalitis	Symptomatic management *Note:* Can be serious, especially in the immunosuppressed population

Investigations

- FBC, UEC, LFT, CRP, ESR.
- Evaluate patient 1 week post-discharge and repeat 3–6 weeks after fever; if no coronary abnormality is seen, then nothing further is required.

Management

- Aspirin and immediate IVIG to prevent coronary vasculitis.

Note: High-dose corticosteroids are contraindicated.

Simple exanthematic drug eruptions (common nuisance)

- The common classic 'maculopapular' drug rash = morbilliform, rubelliform, scarlatiniform
- Red spotty changes, flat ± raised ± itch
- Onset mostly within the first 5–14 days of therapy
- Patient is otherwise systemically well, and is asymptomatic to very pruritic
- Resolution occurs with a change in colour from bright red to a brownish red, sometimes followed by scaling or desquamation.

Clinical features

Clinical features are outlined in Box 40.3.

Box 40.3 Clinical features of simple exanthematic drug eruptions

- Facial involvement minimal
- No periorbital/facial oedema
- No lymphadenopathy
- No lip, mouth or eye involvement
- Rash spotty, non-confluent
- Peaks in days, then settles (10–14 days)

Onset:

- Typically 5–14 days after starting the drug
- Can begin up to several days after the drug causing it has been stopped (within hours with rechallenge)

Associated drugs:

Essentially all; especially antibiotics, antivirals, anti-inflammatories, anticonvulsants.

Course/resolution:

- Worsens for several days after drug cause is stopped.
- Then progressively resolves over 7–14 days.

- Treatment—antihistamine (cetirizine), cortisone cream (e.g. 0.5% betamethasone valerate).

Note: An infection-like skin eruption may be the tip of an iceberg—it may warn of serious life-threatening skin reactions, e.g. SJS, TEN or internal toxicities.

Management of 'non-serious or simple' exanthematic eruptions:

- History
- Examination
- Investigations to confirm diagnosis, exclude important and serious differential diagnosis
- Management of cause

Symptomatic management:

- Moisturiser
- Moderate-potency topical steroid cream, e.g. betamethasone valerate cream 0.02% TDS
- Antihistamine (non-sedating during daytime, e.g. loratadine 10 mg; ± sedating at night, e.g. promethazine 10–25 mg)

Serious drug eruptions

Clinical features are given in Box 40.4, with examples in Box 40.5.

Box 40.4 Clinical features of serious drug eruptions

- Associated with systemic symptoms and/or high fever; precede/coincide/follow eruption onset
- Eruption:
  - — confluent
  - — associated periorbital puffiness and/or facial swelling
  - — tender or painful eruption
  - — mucous membrane symptoms or signs, e.g. crusting and erosion of lips, gritty eyes

Box 40.5 Examples of serious drug eruptions

- Drug hypersensitivity eruptions
- Serum sickness—versus serum-sickness-like eruptions
- Blistering disorders; Stevens–Johnson syndrome (SJS), toxic epidermal necrolysis (TEN)
- Acute generalised exanthematic pustulosis (AGEP)
- Drug-induced lupus (may be considerably delayed) ± polyarteritis nodosa (PAN)

Box 40.6 Drug hypersensitivity syndrome (DRESS): commonly implicated drugs

- Aromatic anticonvulsants (phenytoin, phenobarbitone, carbamazepine), lamotrigine
- Sulfonamide antibiotics, dapsone, trimethoprim, minocycline, metronidazole
- Azathioprine
- Allopurinol
- Alternative therapies including Chinese herbal remedies
- Abacavir, nevirapine

Drug hypersensitivity syndrome (DRESS)

- Commonly implicated drugs are listed in Box 40.6.
- Presents with triad of:
  1. high fever
  2. skin eruption
  3. internal organ involvement.
- Prodrome: fever, malaise, sore throat (i.e. mimics upper respiratory tract infection).
- Skin eruption is most commonly exanthematic but can evolve to erythroderma or SJS/TEN (when an originally itchy rash turns tender/painful and blisters); see relevant sections under 'Blistering/shedding of skin'.
- Internal toxicities include:
  — lymphadenopathy
  — hepatitis
  — nephritis
  — pneumonitis (e.g. minocycline); with SJS/TEN, significant desquamation of the mucosal lining; can occur acutely with associated pulmonary obstruction
  — pancreatitis (e.g. azathioprine)
  — meningitis (especially NSAIDs, trimethoprim), encephalitis
  — haematological (early—atypical lymphocytosis, neutrophilia; later—eosinophilia, cytopenias (red, white, platelets))
  — deaths—colitis, carditis, arrhythmias (most commonly reported with the anticonvulsants), massive hepatic necrosis
  — arthralgias that are not arthritis.
- Onset: typically 1–8 weeks, occasionally months (especially anticonvulsants and allopurinol); recurrence in hours to days on rechallenge.

Serum-sickness-like reaction (SSLR)

- SSLR has multiple causes, including drug-induced by cefaclor, amoxycillin, minocycline, etc.
- Differential diagnosis: autoimmune connective tissue disease, infections such as hepatitis B or C and infective endocarditis, and lymphoma due to cryoglobulins and/or circulating immune complexes.

See Table 40.9.

Table 40.9 Comparison of serum sickness versus serum-sickness-like reaction (SSLR)

	Serum sickness	SSLR
Skin: eruption	Urticarial and vasculitic	Exanthematic and urticarial
Fever	✓	✓
Arthritis	✓	– (arthralgia only)
Renal involvement	✓ (nephritis)	–
Serositis/carditis	✓	–
Associated drugs	Streptokinase, antivenoms, digoxin immune Fab	Cefaclor, buspirone, infliximab, rituximab, griseofulvin
Histopathology	Systemic vasculitis	Inflammatory or unknown
Management	Admission and specialist care Symptomatic relief ± immunosuppressive therapy	Symptomatic Paracetamol Topical steroids

Management of suspected potentially serious drug eruptions

1. Stop all suspected or potentially causal medications or drugs.
2. Admission.
3. Supportive management.
4. Specialist care.

Note the overlapping potential internal toxicities of SJS/TEN, DRESS and AGEP:

- respiratory compromise
- carditis (± arrhythmias)
- hepatitis
- renal involvement.

3 GENERALLY RED, INFLAMED AND SCALY: ERYTHRODERMA[6]

Causes of erythroderma are given in Box 40.7.

Box 40.7 Causes of erythroderma

- Exfoliative erythroderma syndrome
- Psoriasis flare
- Eczematous dermatitis—atopic dermatitis flare, contact dermatitis
- Drug hypersensitivity reaction—antiepileptics, penicillins, sulfonamides, NSAIDs
- Acute graft-versus-host disease (AGVHD)
- TEN, SJS, erythema multiforme (EM)
- Lymphomas, e.g. cutaneous T cell lymphoma

Exfoliative erythroderma

Clinical features

Generalised red, inflamed and scaly skin eruption ± lymphadenopathy. Pruritus is usually the initial symptom, and malaise and fever may subsequently develop owing to excessive vasodilation. Fluid and protein loss through the skin can lead to life-threatening hypotension, electrolyte imbalance, congestive heart failure and enteropathy. Potentially fatal.

Causes

Many cases are idiopathic, but can be associated with a diverse range of underlying dermatoses, including:

- eczema
- psoriasis
- drug reaction, e.g. allopurinol, calcium-channel blockers, anticonvulsants and lithium
- cutaneous T-cell lymphoma or leukaemia
- pityriasis rubra pilaris
- paraneoplastic syndrome
- dermatomyositis.

Management

1. The cause should be determined and, if a drug reaction is suspected, the offending medication stopped.
2. Management includes supportive therapy, hospital admission, proper hydration, nutrition, electrolyte and cardiac monitoring and temperature support by nursing in a warm room.
3. Skin biopsies can be obtained to help establish the diagnosis.

4. Skin care involves the use of emollients and compresses as well as topical corticosteroid therapy and antihistamines for pruritus. Antibiotic therapy should be administered if signs of infection develop.

Atopic dermatitis (AD) flare[7]

Atopic dermatitis (eczema) is a common inflammatory skin condition especially of childhood.

- Relapsing course, severe pruritus.
- Frequently complicated by secondary skin infections, often bacterial colonisation with *Staphylococcus aureus*.

Clinical features

- Dry, erythematous, pruritic skin lesions. Chronic skin change of lichenification, thickened, hyperpigmented epidermis.
- Mostly involving flexural areas.
- History of atopy, asthma, hayfever and family history of atopy.
- AD flare and erythroderma: relapsing and remitting episodes with severe itching and failure of routine topical therapies ± superinfection.

Consider admission in patients with:

- generalised erythema and exfoliation—erythroderma
- severe, generalised itching who have failed outpatient topical therapies
- severe skin infections.

Differential diagnosis

Contact dermatitis allergic or irritant, photodermatitis and contact urticaria.

Management

1. Use soap-free products.
2. Avoid skin irritants; use cotton clothing as much as possible.
3. Apply wet dressings/wraps of topical corticosteroid or topical calcineurin inhibitor to affected areas and hypoallergenic moisturiser, e.g. Sorbolene, to the asymptomatic areas. Ointment-based medications are better used in the flare setting.
4. Antihistamines; non-sedating for during the day, e.g. cetirizine, and sedating, e.g. promethazine, at night.
5. Topical calcineurin inhibitors, e.g. pimecrolimus cream, are particularly useful non-steroid topical immunosuppressants for AD in the thinner areas, e.g. face, groin, axillae.

Infections

Staphylococcus aureus is the most common cause of bacterial infections in children with AD. Severity ranges from minor local skin infections to cellulitis, abscesses, bacteraemia and sepsis. Secondary skin infections may present as erythema with oozing, honey-coloured crusts. Topical mupirocin can be considered for local infected lesions. The main presentation of secondary infection is simply worsening with increased exudation of the eczema.

- **Clinical features:** secondary *S. aureus* infection is usually a worsening, increased exudation of the eczema. Fever, malaise, disseminated eruptions of dome-shaped vesicles that may or may not be superimposed on areas of eczematous change. Head and neck are frequently affected. Lesions may spread rapidly to involve extensive areas of the skin. Systemically unwell in some cases, ± lymphadenopathy.
- **Management:** oral antibiotics, wet dressings and topical steroids.
- **Eczema herpeticum:** widespread herpes simplex virus infection accompanying atopic eczema can occur in children and adults affected by atopic dermatitis. In severe cases, treat with IV aciclovir; refer for ophthalmology review if there is suspected eye involvement.

Follow up with dermatologist and/or immunologist as many of these children have food allergy, allergic rhinitis and asthma.

Sunburn ('photo-distributed'/'exposed')

Clinical features

Skin exposed to too much UVB smarts, and becomes red a couple of hours later. Severe sunburn is painful, may blister in 24 hours and settles in 2–3 days.

Cause

UVB rays penetrate the epidermis and superficial dermis, stimulating the production and release of prostaglandin (PG), histamine, interleukin and tumour necrosis factor (TNF)-alpha. This stimulates the production of inducible nitric oxide synthetase enzyme → high concentrations of nitric oxide → dermal vasodilation and erythema.

Differential diagnosis

Phototoxic reactions caused by drugs (Box 40.8) are similar to an exaggerated sunburn.

Box 40.8 Drugs commonly causing photosensitivity

- Amiodarone
- Oral contraceptive pill (OCP)
- Phenothiazines
- Psoralens
- Sulfonamides
- Tetracyclines
- Thiazides

Treatment

- Symptomatic: baths; cooling; oily lotions, oil-in-water lotions/creams for comfort; potent topical steroids briefly and used early; oral aspirin; sprays, gels or creams containing lignocaine relieve pain, occasionally sensitise.
- If the skin reacts badly to light through glass, then think drugs or porphyria and sunscreens usually ineffective.

Photodermatitis

- Similar appearance to sunburn.
- May appear after contact with plants—phytophotodermatitis; plants containing psoralens e.g. lemons, limes, celery, parsley, parsnips, figs.
- Sunscreens as a group may alternatively cause photoallergic contact dermatitis; contained in foundation, moisturisers, cosmetics.
- Rash is similar to sunburn with pain, vesiculation, erythema.

Acute allergic contact dermatitis

- Causes of more-severe allergic contact dermatitis presenting to the ED are often plants (e.g. rhus tree, grevillea Robyn Gordon).
- Exposed areas appear streaky, can disseminate; initially there is acute blistering. When more severe, skin is eczematised with dissemination.
- Worsens for days.
- In more severe reactions, check for associated glomerulonephritis.

Management

Potent topical corticosteroids, systemic steroids (e.g. prednisolone, usual adult dose 20–40 mg/day up to 80 mg/day then reduced as per schedule), calcineurin inhibitors (e.g. oral cyclosporin 3–4 mg/kg/day weaned and stopped over 2–4 weeks).

Other causes of photosensitivity

Drug-induced lupus erythematosus.

4 BLISTERING/SHEDDING OF SKIN

Presentations of blistering/shedding of skin are outlined in Table 40.10.

Varicella zoster/herpes zoster

Note: Always suspect herpes in any neonate with a vesiculobullous or eroded weeping eruption.

Clinical features

- Prodrome: with a unilateral ache, soreness or neuritic shooting pain which may be non-specific.

Table 40.10 Presentations of blistering/shedding of skin

Presentation	Neonate	Child	Adult
Acute illness; systemically unwell (often a history of prodromal illness of days)	Neonatal herpes Epidermolysis bullosa (EB)	Stevens–Johnson syndrome/ toxic epidermal necrolysis (SJS/ TEN)	SJS/TEN Acute generalised exanthematous pustulosis (AGEP)
Acute-on-chronic or subacute history; systemically unwell	EB (many variants in severity, type and systemic associations)		Staphylococcal scalded skin syndrome (SSSS) Bullous lupus*
Isolated skin change; systemically stable	Impetigo SSSS EB	Bullous insect bites Bullous contact reaction (especially plant) Impetigo SSSS** AGEP	Bullous contact reaction (especially plant) Bullous pemphigoid Pemphigus vulgaris
Esoteric (to be made following admission under dermatology)		Chronic bullous disease of childhood BP—very rare	Linear immunoglobulin A disease

*Active systemic lupus erythematosus (SLE) with widespread epidermal shedding rather than bullous pemphigoid–lupus overlap etc.

**SSSS may occur in neonates and children not necessarily systemically unwell or behaving septically, as there may be a minor focus of *Staphylococcus* infection and illness is mediated by exotoxins excreted renally (immature renal function) versus adults where SSSS presents with overwhelming sepsis and/or renal impairment.

- Skin changes: early on little or nothing to see, then erythematous or cellulitic presentation or the classic vesiculobullous eruption in a dermatomal distribution.

Pearls and Pitfalls

- If shingles/zoster is suspected treat early, especially in a patient at risk. This includes the immunocompromised, very young, sick or elderly.
- Other important features include dermatomal distribution—head and neck including periorbital and tip of nose (nasociliary branch)—or a severe and prolonged prodrome which heralds a postherpetic neuralgia.
- Beware any signs of disseminated disease, i.e. lesions beyond 3 dermatomes and lesions outside the confines of a dermatome.

Investigations

Diagnosis is clinical; however, confirmation is by polymerase chain reaction (PCR). The highest yield is from a fresh vesicle by breaking it aseptically with a 19-gauge needle and scraping from the base with a viral culture swab.

Management

- Valaciclovir or famciclovir both have excellent oral availability. Have a low threshold for admission if there is concern about oral intake or absorption. Systemic aciclovir works best if given early in the course of the disease.
- Look for an underlying cause if there is dissemination outside the main affected dermatomes.

Staphylococcal scalded skin syndrome (SSSS)

Aetiology

- *Staphylococcus*-toxin-mediated disease
- Adult risk factors: deficits in cell-mediated immunity e.g. HIV, malignancy, malnutrition, renal failure (exfoliative toxins are renally excreted)

Clinical features and focus of infection are given in Table 40.11.

Investigations

- Biopsy of the lesions is the gold standard for differentiation.
- Avoid biopsy in children, but in the ED a frozen section of the shed skin can differentiate SSSS from SJS/TEN.

Table 40.11 Clinical features and focus of SSSS

Child	Adult
Clinical features: 'Miserable' but not obtunded, skin tender to the touch, i.e. child withdraws to touch Cutaneous involvement often begins in the flexural creases, i.e. neck, axillae, inguinal area, knees Most common in children aged < 5 years	Clinical features: Only seen in a patient who is immunocompromised with significant renal failure and/or overwhelming sepsis
Focus of infection often difficult to find	Focus of infection usually obvious, in contradistinction to children

Management

Admit both children (important to exclude all the life-threatening differentials) and adults and arrange specialist consultation.

In adults:

- supportive therapy to treat electrolyte imbalance, hypotension and potential multiorgan failure; inciting factor cessation
- cultures—peripheral, central and swabs
- antimicrobial therapy with dicloxacillin or flucloxacillin 2 g IV q6h, rare reports of MRSA.

Serious cutaneous adverse reaction (SCAR)

SCAR includes Stevens–Johnson syndrome (SJS) and toxic epidermal necrolysis (TEN). *Note: If SJS or TEN is suspected, urgent specialist review is required.*

- TEN is rare but most severe, and leads to extensive painful full-thickness epidermal skin death with blistering and sheet-like shedding of > 30% of the epidermis.
- SJS, which is more common, leads to < 10% full-thickness epidermal death and shedding, and a 5% mortality. SJS–TEN overlap cases shed 10–30% of the epidermis. The more severe the skin changes, the more likely it is to be drug-induced and the higher the mortality.

The differential between SJS and TEN is difficult to distinguish until the ultimate extent of skin disease is known, usually 7–10 days from onset.

SCAR is potentially life-threatening due to multisystem involvement and skin-barrier breakdown.

- Epithelial loss predisposes to bacterial and fungal infections, septicaemia and severe fluid loss with electrolyte disturbance. Mortality ranges from 5% in SJS to 30% in TEN.
- Mucous membranes are usually involved, with erythema and erosions of buccal, genital and ocular mucosa.
- Severe ophthalmic involvement may lead to permanent scarring and blindness.

Early clinical features of SCAR are given in Box 40.9.

It is commonly drug-induced (see Box 40.10); rarely reported post-vaccination (e.g. MMR), post exposure to industrial chemicals, post-mycobacterial infections, post Chinese herbal remedies; very rarely idiopathic.

The pathogenesis is thought to involve an impaired capacity to detoxify intermediate drug metabolites and genetic susceptibility. Drug administration typically precedes the rash by 1–3 weeks.

Box 40.9 Early clinical features of SCAR

Mucous membrane involvement, especially if:

- Multiple areas involved
- Erosive, ulcerative or haemorrhagic
- Early changes including crusting of the lips

Skin changes that include:

- Confluent extensive skin involvement
- Prominent central facial or head and neck involvement, especially if periorbital puffiness or facial swelling
- Dusky purpuric macules ± tenderness

Box 40.10 Causes of SCAR

- Infectious: e.g. *Mycoplasma pneumoniae*, herpes simplex
- Common medications responsible for SJS and TEN:[8]
  — sulfonamides
  — anticonvulsants (e.g. phenytoin, carbamazepine, phenobarbitone)
  — allopurinol
  — NSAIDs

Investigations

FBC, including differential with eosinophilia, UEC, LFT, CRP, immunofluorescence, skin swabs, blood cultures, urinalysis, chest X-ray.

Management

Note: **Stop** potentially causal drugs as soon as the diagnosis is suspected. This saves lives and is especially so for longer-acting medications, e.g. traditional aromatic anticonvulsants (phenytoin, carbamazepine, phenobarbitone along with lamotrigine).

1 SJS and TEN:
- — Admission to a burns unit if necessary.
- — Identify and withdraw all possible causative and/or interacting medications (e.g. stop both lamotrigine and sodium valproate when lamotrigine is suspected as causal).
- — Supportive measures which include: intravenous fluid administration, maintenance of electrolyte and temperature homeostasis, enteral feeding, analgesia and ophthalmological assessment in case of ocular involvement.
- — In addition apply emollients, anticipate and treat infection.
- — Have a low threshold to involve clinical pharmacologist and dermatologist early.

2 Skin care consists of
- — proper wound dressings (e.g. hydrocolloid dressings or saline-soaked gauze)
- — oral hygiene (i.e. chlorhexidine rinses)
- — oral antihistamine and topical corticosteroid therapy for pruritus
- — antimicrobial therapy in cases of superinfection due to skin-barrier breakdown. Some centres use high doses of IV immunoglobulin and plasmaphoresis.[9]

3 Frequent culture of skin, urine, blood and intravenous catheter site, as the major causes of sepsis are *Staphylococcus aureus* and *Pseudomonas aeruginosa*. Avoid systemic corticosteroids.

Pemphigus vulgaris

- Clinical features: most have a chronic or subacute presentation. Rare forms present acutely through the ED with painful blistering of the mucous membranes.
- Differential diagnosis: other blistering disorders (see Table 40.12).
- Management:
  - — Acute presentation of any blistering eruption requires admission.
  - — Corticosteroids topical and systemic ± other immunosuppressants.
  - — Referral to a dermatologist.

Table 40.12 Differential diagnosis of blistering disorders

Bullous disease	Fever	Mucositis	Morphology	Onset	Other	Immuno-fluoresence
Staphylococcal scalded skin syndrome (SSSS)	✓	Absent	Erythema, skin tenderness, periorificial crusting	Acute	Children < 5 years, adults on dialysis; patients on immunosuppressants	Negative
Acute generalised exanthematous pustulosis (AGEP)	✓	Rare	Superficial sterile pustules, resembles pustular psoriasis	Acute	Self-limiting on stopping drug, usually due to antimicrobials	Negative
Acute graft-versus-host disease (AGVHD)	✓	✓	Morbilliform rash, bullae, erosions	Acute	Closely resembles TEN Prominent gastrointestinal and mucosal involvement	Negative
Bullous lupus	✓	✓	Erythema, tenderness, blistering and shedding of skin	Acute	May have background of SLE ± acute presentation	Positive
Paraneoplastic pemphigus	✓	✓	Often mixed morphology overlapping lupus, SJS/TEN and pemphigus	Acute or subacute	Underlying haematological malignancy known or unknown	Positive (special tests to confirm)

From Hertzberg M, Schifter M, Sullivan J et al. Paraneoplastic pemphigus in two patients with B-cell non-Hodgkin's lymphoma: significant responses to cyclophosphamide and prednisolone. Am J Hematol 2000;63(2):105–6.

Bullous pemphigoid

- Clinical features: blistering skin disease of the elderly with large tense bullae arising on normal or erythematous skin. Early inflammatory disease presents with urticaria-like lesions. Oral mucosal lesions. Characterised by intense itch.
- Causes: immunobullous disorder of the skin.
- Management: in itself not usually a cause for admission, but usually occurs in the elderly with a complication, e.g. ± cellulitis. In isolation it is not an emergency, but rather treat the secondary infection.
  - Specific management is recommended to be individualised and specialist dermatology input is required.
  - Stop the antecedent cause if possible, e.g. drug ± corticosteroids.

Grade 4 acute graft versus host disease (AGVHD)

- Clinical features: usually an inpatient. Usually recent bone marrow transplant or recent procedure from overseas. Similar clinical, pathological and immunological features as TEN. See the section 'Serious cutaneous adverse reaction (SCAR)'; refer to Table 40.12.
- Differential: refer to Table 40.12.
- Management is supportive and requires specialist collaboration.

5 VASCULITIS/PURPURIC VERSUS ISCHAEMIC/NECROTIC SKIN ± DEEPER TISSUES

Differential diagnosis is shown in Table 40.13.

Meningococcaemia

- Meningococcal.
- Have a very low threshold to treat even if only considered a diagnostic possibility.
- Always promptly treat a patient with an infective illness, rapid deterioration or re-presentation in a patient with an infective illness.
- Skin changes are classically petechial/purpuric (i.e. do not completely blanch on pressure) but initial very early lesions may fully blanch.

Clinical features

- All ages, but especially small children and young adults.
- Approximately 60% of patients present with a characteristic

Table 40.13 Vasculitis/purpuric versus ischaemic/necrotic skin ± deeper tissues

Differential diagnosis	Clinical scenario
Meningococcaemia	Always consider, and if considered always treat
Disseminated intravascular coagulation (DIC)	Sick, septic patient reflecting underlying illness
Vasculitis (venular or usual leucocytoclastic vasculitis)—unknown infection, connective tissue disease, malignancy, drug, multifactorial, including Henoch–Schönlein purpura	Often multifactorial aetiology; recent illness, sepsis, drug-induced The three Ps of small-vessel vasculitis: painful palpable purpura
Vasculitis (larger vessel e.g. arterial, e.g. polyarteritis nodosa)	Usually systemic disorder; consider infection and drugs
Embolic; septic, cholesterol etc	Background comorbidities, e.g. ischaemic heart disease, intravenous drug use, trauma
Heparin and warfarin necrosis	Anticoagulant therapy
Haemorrhagic and bullous cellulitis	Consider deep fungal infections not only in the immunocompromised population but also in the general population
Haemorrhagic or necrotic infections of deeper 'soft' tissue, including necrotising fasciitis	General immune and immunosuppressed
Metabolic and intravascular disorders including: calciphylaxis (ischaemic tissue necrosis, ITN)/catastrophic anticardiolipin syndrome (reticulate 'dusky' or cyanotic ± painful purpuric changes early on)	*Note:* Catastrophic anticardiolipin syndrome may have prominent central nervous system symptoms and signs

petechial rash on the trunk and lower limbs, but lesions can also occur on the head, palms, soles and mucous membranes.
- — Irregular lesions, smudged appearance. Can progress to ecchymoses, bullous haemorrhage.
- — Petechial skin rash is more typical of acute meningococcaemia, can resemble viral exanthema.

- The classic presentation of meningococcaemia is the abrupt onset of maculopapular or petechial rash and flu-like symptoms—fever, chills, malaise and disorientation. Over several hours, the disease may rapidly progress to purpura,

disseminated intravascular coagulation (DIC), shock and death. Potentially fatal outcome.
- Spread through respiratory secretions; living in close quarters with infected persons puts people at increased risk.
- Predisposing factors: preceding upper respiratory tract infection or infection with *Mycoplasma*.

Cause

Neisseria meningitidis, Gram-negative diplococcus.

Differential diagnosis

Includes purpuric enterovirus exanthem.

Management

1 Any febrile patient with a petechial rash should be suspected of having meningococcaemia and treated promptly after blood cultures are obtained.
2 Besides supportive management, therapy with a 3rd-generation cephalosporin (e.g. ceftriaxone) or intravenous penicillin G (benzylpenicillin) therapy are the treatments of choice.
3 Chloramphenicol may be used for patients allergic to penicillin.

Necrotising fasciitis

- Cutaneous findings may not correlate with the extent of the necrosis as it is a spreading infection of the deep fascia, causing necrosis of the subcutaneous tissues.
- Treatment is based on clinical suspicion with broad antimicrobial cover.

Clinical features

- Rapidly developing infection with erythema, oedema and extreme pain, which may be disproportionate, ± fever.
- Lesions are typically on the extremities. Often there is a 1–2 day history of disease onset with blue discolouration associated with bullous eruption.
- The organisms can be introduced through minor cuts, burns, blunt trauma or surgical procedures.
- Type I necrotising fasciitis is caused by mixed anaerobes, Gram-negative aerobic bacilli, and enterococci are implicated in type I; type II is group A streptococci.

Risk factors include:
  - diabetes mellitus
  - peripheral vascular disease
  - immunosuppression.

Diagnosis

- Clinical predominantly—without prompt treatment, the infection may develop into frank cutaneous gangrene.
- Shock and organ failure may occur—with poor prognosis.
- When skin necrosis is not obvious, diagnosis of necrotising fasciitis must be suspected if there are signs of severe sepsis or some of the following local symptoms and signs:[10]
  - severe pain
  - indurated oedema
  - skin hyperaesthesia
  - crepitation
  - muscle weakness
  - foul-smelling exudates.
- Confirmatory imaging may be useful to assist in defining the extent of disease. This includes CT scan to confirm gas in the subcutaneous tissues.

Management

If necrotising fasciitis is suspected, early treatment while working up for surgical debridement is essential. Broad antimicrobial including antistreptococcal cover is required.

Common lower leg emergency presentations—ulcers/wounds

These are summarised in Table 40.14.

CELLULITIS

Clinical features

- Area of skin and subcutaneous tissue which is red, hot, swollen, tender ± blister formation ± skin necrosis. Frequently on the legs but other sites possible.
- Patient may feel systemically unwell, fevers, rigors ± confusion in the elderly.
- Deeper level of infection than erysipelas (see below). Organisms gain entry via minor abrasions, fissures between the toes; leg ulcers are the portal of entry in many cases (see Box 40.11 for causes of ulcers).
- Predisposing factor: oedema of the legs, e.g. cardiac, venous or lymphatic origin.
- In immunocompetent individuals, usually caused by *Streptococcus pyogenes*. *Haemophilus influenzae* may be associated in the context of facial cellulitis and otitis media in children.

Table 40.14 Common lower leg emergency presentations

Presentation	Differential	Comment
Unilateral erythematous legs	Cellulitis; bacterial, fungal, superinfection, e.g. scabies Always consider primary or secondary deep venous thrombosis (DVT)	Bacterial—staphylococcal and streptococcal infections are most common Others; in immunosuppressed or atypical presentations (e.g. bullous and haemorrhagic), consider deep fungal or atypical mycobacterium (e.g. *Cryptococcus neoformans* var *gattii*, *Mycobacterium haemophilum*)
Bilateral erythematous legs (Acute venous eczema flare presentations in the elderly are not always classical, e.g. patient may not complain of itch)	Always consider venous 'stasis' eczema (most likely underlying condition) There can be secondary staphylococcal infection but it is important to treat the eczema Always consider DVT: ? duplex ± prophylaxis and/or treatment Always consider contact allergy to product ingredients, e.g. in topical dressings, product (OTC and prescribed)	Potent topical steroid ointment (daily—TDS) sparingly, fragrance-free bland moisturiser generously over the top ± wet wraps and elevation and/or compression bandaging if compression stocking not possible (e.g. Setapress) if no significant arterial disease In isolation is not a reason for admission; however, prompt LMO follow-up ± community nursing ± dermatologist required
Other rare causes	Prothrombotic, thrombotic or occlusive vascular presentations, e.g. phlegmasia alba and cerulea dolens	Major arterial or venous events which require urgent vascular surgical review and appropriate investigation for cause with therapy

Box 40.11 Causes of ulcers

- Venous
- Arterial
- Traumatic
- Neuropathic
- Malignancy
- Infectious: viral, bacterial, fungal
- Systemic disease-related, e.g. pyoderma gangrenosum, systemic lupus erythematosus, rheumatoid arthritis
- Drug-induced
- Dermatitis artefacta
- Multifactorial

Management

1. In presumed streptococcal cellulitis, penicillin is treatment of choice, benzylpenicillin IV.
2. Elevation of the affected area and analgesia.
3. Some patients have recurrent episodes of cellulitis, each episode damaging the lymphatics and leading to further oedema. Treat with prophylactic penicillin or erythromycin.

Box 40.12 gives indications for admission.

Box 40.12 Consider admission in the context of ulcer presentation for patients with the following

- Systemic illness, e.g. significant fever and constitutional symptoms
- Pain including pain disproportionate to clinical presentation; arterial, neutrophilic including Sweet's syndrome through to pyoderma gangrenosum, serious infective cause (staphylococcal to deep fungal to mycobacterial)
- Immunocompromised population (may be multifactorial ulcer; vasculitis, infection ± deep venous thrombosis in an oncology patient)
- Rapidly progressing ulcer or involving the distal extremities, especially atypical locations for a chronic arterial, venous or neuropathic ulcer; consider complicating deep-tissue infection, tendonitis, fasciitis, compartment syndrome, osteomyelitis

Consider admission and appropriate emergency investigations: full blood count, differential, swab—microculture and sensitivity, imaging—plain X-rays and ultrasound

PYODERMA GANGRENOSUM

In any patient presenting with a painful, rapidly progressive inflammatory ulcer, always consider pyoderma gangrenosum. This warrants an urgent dermatological consult as the diagnosis is one of exclusion, but it is an inflammatory rather than an infective condition requiring relatively heavy immunosuppression. Thus, ruling out infection either clinically by a dermatologist and/or concurrently covering major infective possibilities while awaiting dermatology input is essential.

Other common skin infections

These are summarised in Table 40.15, overleaf.

Bites[11]

- Animal bites are common.
- Mortality from bites is low.
- Morbidity is common, with both dog and cat bites potentially becoming infected with *Pasteurella multocida*. Consider rabies with bites from bats.

COMPLICATIONS FROM BITES

Dog bite: may be complicated by infections—*Staphylococcus, Streptococcus, Eikenella, Pasteurella, Proteus, Klebsiella, Haemophilus, Enterobacter, Bacteroides* and *Capnocytophaga*.

Cat bite: may be complicated by infections—*Pasteurella, Actinomyces, Propionibacterium, Bacteroides, Fusobacterium, Clostridium, Wolinella, Peptostreptococcus* and *Streptococcus* species.

Human bite: high risk of infection. Cover the mix of anaerobes and aerobic organisms.

HISTORY

Patient's tetanus status.

CLINICAL FEATURES

On examination: breach of the skin, and foreign bodies. If the bite is deep, examine neurovascular supply, muscle and tendon integrity and injury to any bones.

INVESTIGATIONS

- Cultures if appropriate and, if infection with *P. multocida* is suspected, send for Gram stain.
- Plain X-rays to exclude fractures or osteomyelitis if presentation is delayed.

Table 40.15 Common skin infections elsewhere

Disease	Signs/symptoms	Management
Erysipelas	Superficial streptococcal cellulitis with a well demarcated edge. On face is common *Haemophilus influenzae* is important cause of facial cellulitis in children, often associated with ipsilateral otitis media Immunocompromised patients have a variety of potential bacteria Often strikes in the same place twice	Recurrent bouts need long-term prophylactic penicillin; consider referral to infectious diseases service
Impetigo: superficial skin infection of the epidermis *Staphylococcus aureus* or *Streptococcus pyogenes*	Honey-crusted lesions or vesicles, usually in children around nose and mouth, may be bullous or non-bullous	Cefalexin, mupirocin Always ensure microculture and sensitivity, patient follow-up by LMO (if *S. pyogenes*, requires 10 days of therapy)
Abscess: localised collection of pus, e.g. hidradenitis suppurativa, venous access; iatrogenic, intravenous drug use	Often febrile and neutrophilia, however elderly/diabetic/ immunocompromised may not mount a white cell response or fever; low threshold to treat, especially for lower-leg infection	With foot infections always consider portal of entry e.g. interdigital tinea, ± peripheral neuropathy
Furuncle: pus collection in 1 hair follicle, often *S. aureus* Carbuncle: pus collection involving many hair follicles	Wash bedsheets and clothing in hot water, etc For recurrent episodes of staphylococcal infections with furunculosis, referral to infectious diseases or dermatology is recommended to address predisposing factors	Incision and drainage or 1st-generation cephalosporin and/or consider at risk for MRSA Consider risk of NORSA—non-multiresistant oxacillin-resistant *S. aureus* Community strain of MRSA—most appropriate antibiotic, clindamycin

Disease	Signs/symptoms	Management
Cellulitis: spreading subcutaneous infection usually *Staphylococcus* or *Streptococcus*	Cardinal signs of inflammation: red, hot, swollen, tender, loss of function	Depending on severity and risk, beta-lactam, e.g. dicloxacillin or flucloxacillin or 1st-generation cephalosporin
Lymphangitis	Traditionally streptococcal, but always cover	Penicillin
Necrotising fasciitis: infection along the fascial planes *S. pyogenes* (group A) or *Clostridium perfringens*	Pain, fever, ↑ white cell count, systemically unwell	Immediate extensive surgical debridement, add penicillin and clindamycin to prevent spread High mortality without rapid, extensive debridement

MANAGEMENT

1. Good wound care is essential; irrigate and if possible leave open for healing.
2. Surgical consult if the injuries are extensive or involve the hand.
3. Treatment is instituted based on the history of dog or cat bite with amoxycillin and clavulanate for 7–10 days; close follow-up is required.
4. If rabies is suspected, consider rabies immune globulin or rabies virus vaccine.
5. Snake bites may require treatment with antivenom if serious.

Itching/pruritus[7]

This is a common topic; not really an emergency issue unless in the context of more-complicated disease already addressed above. Common causes are listed in Box 40.13 and screening investigations in Box 40.14.

- Pruritus varies in duration, localisation and severity.
- **Treatment:** treat the cause. If no apparent underlying reason can be found, then use soap sparingly, topical steroid, topical emollients, non-sedating antihistamine during the day, sedating antihistamine at night.

Note: Scabies is an important diagnosis not to miss, especially in the context of a patient admitted with another illness (especially infective) and/or patients requiring surgery where staphylococcal infection may complicate.

Box 40.13 Common causes of itching

- Urticaria
- Chronic skin disorders: eczema, psoriasis, lichen sclerosis
- Contact dermatitis
- Infestations: scabies, lice, fleas
- Drug ingestion: especially opiates (action on mast cells), oestrogens and phenothiazines (cholestasis)
- Haematological disorders: iron deficiency, polycythaemia rubra vera
- Cholestatic liver disease: extrahepatic obstruction, hepatitis, drug-induced cholestasis, primary biliary cirrhosis
- Chronic renal failure
- Thyroid disease: thyrotoxicosis, myxoedema
- Malignancy: lymphomas, leukaemias, carcinomas
- Pregnancy
- 'Senile' pruritus (unknown cause)
- Psychological

Box 40.14 Screening for generalised pruritus

- Full history and examination—to rule out secondary causes
- FBC, LFT, UEC, ESR, iron studies, TFTs
- Urine protein
- Chest X-ray

SCABIES

When to suspect scabies:

- Recent onset of an itchy rash (weeks to months)
- Other friends, partners or family members are also itchy
- Itchy pustules on the hands or feet of young children and infants
- Development of an itchy rash after contact with someone diagnosed with scabies

Clinical features

- Itching, typically worse at night.
- There are 2 types of skin lesions in scabies: the burrow and the scabies rash.
  - Burrows are principally on the hands and feet, sides of the fingers and toes, toe-web spaces, wrists and insteps. Burrows on the trunk are more common in the elderly. Male genitalia with burrows and inflammatory papules are pathopneumonic.
  - Rash of scabies is an eruption of tiny inflammatory papules mainly around the axillae and umbilicus. It is the allergic reaction to the mites.

Diagnosis

Scabies should be suspected in anyone with an unexplained itch of recent onset (weeks to months). It is common in children and young adults, also the elderly, and is acquired by close physical contact with another individual.

Definitive diagnosis is by demonstrating mites microscopically via skin scraping. You cannot see the mite without magnification. The mite leaves squiggly burrows in the skin, which are usually less than a centimetre long. These are most commonly found on the hands (particularly between the fingers), wrists and feet. Scrapings from a number of burrows will reveal the mite, eggs or faeces when examined under magnification. Itchy lumps or nodules can occur on the penis and are characteristic of scabies.

Management

All close contacts of a person who has scabies should be treated, to prevent re-infestation and recurrence of the itchy rash.

- All members of an affected household should be treated, not just those that are itchy, plus anyone else who has been in close physical contact with members of an infested household. In extended families this will include grandparents, uncles, aunts and other relatives who have had significant physical contact with affected people.
- Infestations in nursing homes, other institutions and large close-knit communities can be a major logistical challenge to eradicate.
- All members of the same house should be treated at the same time.
- If the patient is pregnant, or there is a chance of pregnancy, this should be discussed before use of any cream or tablet to treat scabies. Similarly, discuss treatment of babies, young infants and the old and frail, as special precautions may be required.
- Permethrin is the treatment of choice in Australia because of its effectiveness and proven safety. Apply permethrin 5% cream and leave for 8 hours; wash off with soap and water.
- Other treatments such as ivermectin (a tablet taken by mouth) may be considered in severe and complicated cases (this can interact with a number of medications which may cause potentially serious adverse effects, especially in older individuals and those with multiple medical conditions such as heart disease, AIDS, breast cancer and stroke).

Instructions to hand out to patients are given in Box 40.15.

Box 40.15 Scabies treatment instructions for patients

1. Before going to bed, apply 5% permethrin (Quellada or Lyclear) to the whole body from the neck down (infants and adults over the age of 55 years should also treat the head and neck). It takes around 30 mL or grams to cover the average adult. Permethrin is available over the counter at chemists. Make sure the cream is applied to all body parts, paying particular attention to the elbows, breasts, groin/genitals, hands and feet (including under the nails). If one burrow is spared then the infestation will persist.
2. The cream should be left on for at least 8 hours before washing. If you wash your hands during this 8-hour period, reapply cream to the hands.
3. Permethrin cream can sting and irritate. This is normal but, if this is severe, wash off the cream and contact your dermatologist to discuss other options.
4. All bed linen and clothes should then be changed and washed (wash with hot water to kill the mite and its eggs). Dry cleaning, ironing or hot clothes drying are also effective. Any clothing or bedding that cannot be washed should be put aside for 7 days before using (e.g. placed in a plastic bag). The mite and eggs will die during this time.
5. The treatment of all household members (steps 1–4) can be repeated at 7–10 days to maximise chance of eradication of the infestation. This should be discussed with your doctor.

From Sullivan J, Commens C. Patient information pages. Australasian College of Dermatologists website. www.dermcoll.asn.au/public/a-z_of_skin-scabies.asp#06

Common medications in the ED

See Box 40.16 and Table 40.16.

Box 40.16 Appropriate use of topical corticosteroids for ED presentations

- Potent topical corticosteroid use is appropriate for control of flares, e.g. atopic dermatitis (even in the context of superinfection with *Streptococcus/Staphylococcus*). Organise follow-up with LMO 5–7 days later for appropriate long-term weaning and maintenance regimen.
- BUT avoid corticosteroid use in the setting of viral skin infections such as herpes simplex and herpes zoster
- Use with caution in immunosuppressed patients, e.g. diabetes mellitus (DM).
- In groin/foot infection, cover both bacterial and fungal causes. Bacterial therapy is oral therapy; yeast/tinea is a cream containing an azole antifungal such as clotrimazole, miconazole or bifonazole

Table 40.16 **Topical steroids**

Potency*	Name	Areas of use
Low	1% hydrocortisone TDS (cream combined with moisturiser usually most appropriate)	Face, axillae, genital areas
Moderate	Betamethasone valerate 0.02%	Ointment for dry, chronic and subacute eczematous presentations Cream for where itch is the main issue rather than dry, scaly eczematous skin
High, group II/IV	Mometasone furoate (Elocon, Novasone) ointment vs cream Methylprednisolone aceponate (Advantan) lotion, cream, ointment and fatty ointment Triamcinolone (Kenalog)	Appropriate for most emergency presentations of acute/severe eczema or contact dermatitis Use cream, moisturiser and wet compressors for weeping dermatitis and ointment plus emollient for drier eczematous presentations (daily up to TDS)

* Carrier vehicles: lotion—low potency, cream—mid-potency, ointment—high potency.

Wound and ulcer care in the ED

Ulcers on lower legs are slower to heal than other body sites and in particular benefit from efforts to address underlying factors to optimise conditions for healing. See Table 40.17 for the causes of leg ulcers. In some patients they are multifactorial in their causation.

EVALUATION OF ULCERS

Assess the cause (Table 40.17) and any contributing factors ± complications:

- Cause (e.g. injury)—a typical example is loss of control of shopping trolley leading to local skin injury on the lower leg which results in an ulcerating wound.
- Contributory factors:
  — local—neuropathy (e.g. diabetic)
  — systemic—conditions that have a deleterious effect on maintaining normal healthy skin including healing, e.g. diabetes oncology patients, chemotherapy (including antimetabolites and epidermal growth factor receptor inhibitor, EGFRI), immunosuppression including iatrogenic; increasing age, debility/poor nutritional state.

Table 40.17 Ulcers—causes and clinical findings

Causes	Clinical: location and surrounding skin findings	Pain*	Comment
Common causes			
Venous ulcer	Most commonly medial lower leg/ankle Skin warm ± associated skin changes due to venous insufficiency (lipodermatosclerosis [firm and variably inflammation]), venous eczema, haemosiderin and scarring	±	Slough: usually contains yellow slough Base: usually fairly superficial Exudate: usually moderate to highly exudative
Arterial	Most commonly pretibial, feet and/or toes Cool, pale surrounding skin, reduced sweating and hair growth, dystrophic toe nails	++	± Necrotic eschar (possible slough) Edge: usually punched-out appearance Base: usually deep (e.g. down to tendons) Exudate: usually dry/minimally exudative
Neuropathic	Most commonly feet and toes (pressure/ friction areas) Surrounding skin dry ± hyperkeratotic		Edge: undermined Base: can be deep Exudate: minimal
Uncommon but important causes			
Vasculitis		±	
Pyoderma gangrenosum	Most commonly lower leg, usually painful, solitary or multiple inflammatory papular/pustular lesions that break down and ulcerate (of unknown pathogenesis) Course varies from lesions that quickly stabilise through to rapidly enlarging tissue-destructive ulcers	+++	Edge: usually raised, purple and undermined

Causes	Clinical: location and surrounding skin findings	Pain*	Comment
Infections	Non-tuberculosis mycobacteria Deep fungal infections	+++	Not necessarily immunosuppressed Refer for incisional skin biopsy + special stains + atypical mycobacteria and deep fungal cultures
Uncommon causes			
Ischaemic tissue necrosis	Dusky ischaemic tender indurated soft tissue progressing to necrotic and potentially extremely deep progressing extensive breakdown	++	Early in the clinical presentation, pain is severe and disproportionate, often subtle early clinical features
Malignancy		–	Ulcer either representing malignancy from onset and/or malignant change

* Venous ulcers are typically minimally symptomatic; infection is the main reason for venous ulcers becoming painful, or alternatively they have become partly arterial in nature. Significant pain disproportionate to lesions should suggest multifactorial aetiologies including infection.

- Complications:
  - infection
  - malignant transformation.

INVESTIGATIONS (EMERGENCY)

- Swabs—for microscopy, culture and sensitivity
- Biopsy—(on ward) consider if vasculitis, neoplasia and/or atypical infection are suspected

MANAGEMENT OF LEG ULCERS/WOUNDS

This should involve:

1. correcting or addressing underlying causes such as venous hypertension (leg elevation when resting, compression stockings/bandaging, etc) (see Table 40.18)
2. the treatment of complications or complicating factors such as clinical infection
3. wound care
4. appropriate follow-up.

Table 40.18 Treatment of leg ulcers/wounds

Treat	Example	Comment
Correct or address underlying cause	Venous hypertension	Compression is mainstay of treatment
Infection vs colonised ulcers	Treat if clinically infection, e.g. surrounding skin inflammation and/or fever	In pressure ulcers, treat infection vigorously Avoid treating colonising bacteria *Streptococcus pyogenes* should be treated

Aims of wound management

- Debride the wound of necrotic slough and debris.
- Reduce bacterial burden.
- Promote granulation tissue and subsequent re-epithelialisation.
- Pain relief.

Editorial Comment

Some patients presenting with a skin problem that is due to a drug reaction are becoming critically ill. One of the most important questions to ask is: 'Have you changed any medication in the last few weeks—started, stopped, tried—including over-the-counter, herbal, natural therapies, diets, etc?' In other words, don't just ask: 'What medications are you on?'

References

1. Freiman A, Borsuk D, Sasseville D. Dermatologic emergencies. CMAJ 2005;173(11):1317–19.
2. Shear NH, Knowles SR, Sullivan JR et al. Cutaneous reactions to drugs. In: Austen K, ed. Dermatology in general medicine (Fitzpatrick). 6th edn. New York: McGraw-Hill; 2003.
3. Calabrese JR, Sullivan JR, Bowden CL et al. Rash in multicenter trials of lamotrigine in mood disorders: clinical relevance and management. J Clin Psychiatry 2002;63(11):1012–19.
4. Sullivan JR. HIV and skin disease. Australasian College of Dermatologists website. www.dermcoll.asn.au/public/a-z_of_skin-hiv_and_the_skin.asp#01.
5. Dyer JR, Einsiedel L, Ferguson PE et al. A new focus of Rickettsia honei spotted fever in South Australia. Med J Aust 2005;182(5):231–4.
6. Graham-Brown R, Burns T. Lecture notes. Dermatology. 9th edn. Oxford: Blackwell Publishing; 2007.
7. Ong PY, Bogunewicz M. Atopic dermatitis and contact dermatitis in the emergency department. Clin Ped Emerg Med 2007;8:81–6.
8. Heymann W. Toxic epidermal necrolysis. J Am Acad Dermatol 2006;55(5):867–9.
9. Browne BJ, Edwards B, Rogers R. Dermatologic emergencies. Prim Care Clin Office Pract 2006;33:685–95.
10. Buddin D, Beddingfield F. Recognising emergent dermatologic conditions. Emerg Med 2004;3:26.
11. Schlessinger J. Animal bites. eMedicine from WebMD. Updated May 2012. Online. Available at http://emedicine.medscape.com/article/768875-overview 20 Apr 2013.

ONLINE RESOURCES

Allaboutacne website
    www.allaboutacne.info
DermNetNZ website
    www.dermnet.org.nz
Virtualskinconsult website
    www.comiteskin.com

Acknowledgements

Special thanks for assistance with this chapter go to Dr Maureen Rogers MB BS FACD, Dermatologist Consultant Emeritus, Westmead Children's Hospital.

Chapter 41
Infectious diseases

Melinda J Berry and Emma Spencer

Antibiotic prescribing

Emergency department doctors commence life-saving antibiotic therapies in large volumes during the course of their work. Good antibiotic stewardship is therefore as essential in the ED as it is on the wards.

- A history of allergic reaction (don't miss the presence of a medic alert bracelet), the use of antibiotics *prior to presentation* and the collection of appropriate and timely cultures prior to the administration of therapy are all standard-of-care considerations.
- The rise of multi-resistant organisms over the last 40 years is well known. Research has shown that up to half of all antibiotic regimens prescribed in Australian hospitals are considered inappropriate. The use of inappropriate antibiotics at inappropriate doses leads to the spread of resistant organisms in hospitals and the community. Patients with infections due to resistant bacteria experience delayed recovery, treatment failure and in some cases death.
- The use of up-to-date therapeutic guidelines and consultation with the infectious diseases and microbiology services in your hospital is essential.
- Antibiotics are not harmless; e.g. anaphylaxis and drug interaction between antibiotics and other commonly prescribed drugs can cause death.

Antibiotic recommendations in this book are largely based on eTG Therapeutic Guidelines (can be accessed via www.ciap.health.nsw.gov.au). See opposite for some 'Pearls and Pitfalls'.

CNS infections

BACTERIAL MENINGITIS

Most adult patients with bacterial meningitis present with 2 of the following:

- fever
- headache

Pearls and Pitfalls

- An accurate history and examination is essential.
- Ask about allergies to previous antibiotic regimens.
- Ask specifically about symptoms of anaphylaxis.
- Look for a medic alert bracelet.
- Drug history:
  - — co-administration of warfarin needs to be monitored closely
  - — effectiveness of the oral contraceptive pill (OCP) can be compromised by intercurrent antibiotic use, and alternative methods of contraception should be discussed with the patient for use during that cycle.
- Prescribe the simplest appropriate regimen *at the optimum dose.*
  - — Explain to the patient what the antibiotics are for, their frequency and their duration.
  - — Explain possible side-effect profiles e.g. indigestion, diarrhoea, changes in the colour of urine, etc.
- Infection with *Clostridium difficile* is a serious consequence of antibiotic usage, and all patients prescribed antibiotics should be told to cease antibiotics if they develop diarrhoea. If the diarrhoea persists, they need to seek medical review and provide a stool to exclude this as the cause.

- neck stiffness
- altered mental state.

Elderly people, especially those with chronic diseases such as diabetes and those who have had antibiotics prior to their presentation, may have a more insidious onset of lethargy with few other signs.

Immediate action

If an assessment of bacterial meningitis has been made, the following empirical antibiotics should be administered within 30 minutes of this initial assessment and should NEVER be delayed for CT or lumbar puncture. Steroids should be administered immediately prior to the antibiotics or with them.

- Ceftriaxone 4 g IV daily (or 2 g IV 12-hourly)
  plus
- Benzylpenicillin 2.4 g 4-hourly *IF* patient is at risk of *Listeria monocytogenes* (Box 41.1)
  plus
- Dexamethasone IV 10 mg (child 0.15 mg/kg, up to 10 mg)

Also:

- Add vancomycin if there is otitis media or sinusitis or Gram stain shows Gram-positive diplococci (pneumococci) or Gram-positive cocci resembling staphylococci.

Box 41.1 Patients at risk of *Listeria monocytogenes*

- Immunocompromised
- > 50 years old
- Alcohol abuse
- Pregnant
- Debilitated

Cultures

As empirical antibiotics are being drawn up and administered, it is opportune to take samples for culture:

- 2 sets of blood cultures
- swabs or aspirates of skin lesions
- urine cultures
- NAAT (nucleic acid amplification testing) on blood urine and skin aspirates/swabs should also be requested.

Computed tomography

Indications for CT scanning prior to lumbar puncture include:

- history of CNS disease
- focal neurological signs
- papilloedema
- seizure
- abnormal/deteriorating level of consciousness
- immunocompromise.

Antibiotics should already have been administered before patient proceeds to scanning.

Lumbar puncture (LP)

Early LP is essential in the diagnosis of bacterial meningitis and can be critical in determining the type, dose and duration of antibiotic.

Contraindications to LP *may* include anticoagulant therapy, bleeding problems and infection overlying the LP site. Advice should be sought *if a decision not to perform LP* is going to be made.

Note:

- Measure opening pressure.
- Take off at least 3 bottles of CSF.
- Write the clinical history clearly on the laboratory form, including HIV status, other underlying illnesses and antibiotics already given to the patient.
- Ring the lab to advise that CSF is being sent to them.

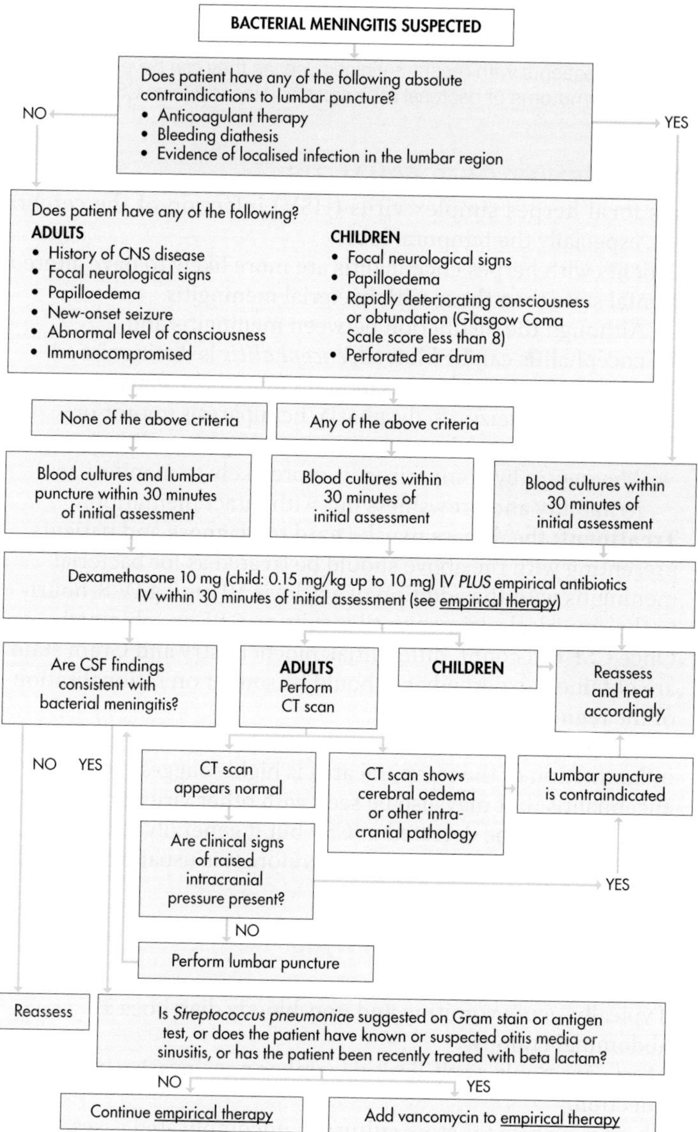

Figure 41.1 Algorithm for management of suspected bacterial meningitis in adults and children
eTG complete [Internet]. Melbourne: Therapeutic Guidelines Limited; 2012 Jul.

Pearls and Pitfalls

- Beware patients with recent antibiotic use, as they can have more-subtle symptoms of bacterial meningitis and inconclusive CSF findings.

HERPES MENINGOENCEPHALITIS

This is focal herpes simplex virus (HSV) infection of the cerebral cortex, especially the temporal lobe.

- Patients with herpes encephalitis are more likely to have altered mental state than those with bacterial meningitis.
  - Although the distinction between meningitis and encephalitis can be blurred, *encephalitis* is distinguished by specific abnormalities of brain function: e.g. focal or generalised seizures, dysphasia, hemiparesis, motor or sensory deficits, altered behaviour and personality change.
  - *Meningitis*, by comparison, is more likely to manifest as irritability and drowsiness but with intact mentation.
- **Treatment:** the disease may be hard to diagnose and patients presenting with the above should be treated as for bacterial meningitis with the addition of aciclovir 10 mg/kg IV 8-hourly to the empirical regimen until results on CSF are obtained.
- Once CSF cell count, differential, biochemistry and Gram stain are obtained, expert advice should be sought on rationalisation of the regimen.
- CT, or preferably MRI, can assist with the diagnosis acutely as inflammation of the temporal area is highly suggestive of HSV encephalitis (but may also be seen with other viruses).
- Viral DNA can be detected in CSF but it generally takes some time for the test to return, and therefore it is usually not helpful in the initial management.

Gastrointestinal infections

GASTROENTERITIS

- Typically, acute vomiting and non-bloody diarrhoea ± abdominal cramps.
- Most commonly a self-limiting viral or non-invasive bacterial infection.
- There is no role for stool culture in uncomplicated cases.
- Fever and peritoneal signs may indicate invasive disease.
- Patients with HIV infection require particular consideration (see Chapter 42, 'The immunosuppressed patient').

- Bloody diarrhoea needs to be referred to your gastroenterology service.

Management

- Hydration (oral or IV) is the cornerstone of management.
- Adults present to the ED because they feel they are unable to tolerate liquid orally, and feel significantly better after IV fluids ± an antiemetic ± an antispasmodic.
- Anti-diarrhoeal agents can relieve stomach cramping and inconvenience, e.g. loperamide 4 mg initially then 2 mg with each episode of diarrhoea, up to 16 mg/day. These agents should not be used in children, patients with inflammatory bowel disease or cases of invasive infection suggested by severe or bloody diarrhoea.

Pearls and Pitfalls

- Antibiotics often cause diarrhoea, particularly broad-spectrum antibiotics such as amoxycillin + clavulanate. Consider *Clostridium difficile* infection and send stool for culture and *C. difficile* toxin detection.
- If *C. difficile* infection is proven or highly suspected, administer oral metronidazole 400 mg 8-hourly for 7–10 days.
- Infection-control precautions will need to be initiated in the ED.
- *C. difficile* infection can be fatal and relapse is common despite adherence to the regimen.
- These patients should be referred to the gastroenterology or infectious diseases service.

Viral hepatitis

HEPATITIS A VIRUS (HAV)

- This acute self-limiting liver infection is transmitted by the faecal–oral route. It is endemic in developing countries and immunisation is recommended for travellers.
- The incubation period is 2–7 weeks. Clinical features include flu-like symptoms, fever, fatigue, nausea, then jaundice and dark urine. It is clinically indistinguishable from other causes of acute hepatitis.
- The diagnosis is serological.
- **Management** is supportive. Fulminant hepatitis is a rare complication of acute HAV infection but acute infection does not lead to chronic hepatitis.
- Immunoglobulin is used to control outbreaks in developed countries.

HEPATITIS B VIRUS (HBV)

- This blood-borne virus is transmitted by parenteral or mucosal exposure to blood or body fluids, including sexually transmitted fluids.
- The incubation period is 1–4 months.
- Acute infection:
  - Can be subclinical or non-specific hepatitis with flu-like symptoms, fatigue, nausea, right upper abdominal quadrant discomfort and jaundice.
  - Liver transaminases can be elevated over 1000 IU/L.
  - Markedly elevated prothrombin time can indicate development of fulminant liver failure.
- Serology detects HBV surface antigen and IgM antibodies to core antigen. Hepatitis B DNA and hepatitis B e antigen are markers of viral replication.
- Less than 1% of patients will develop fulminant liver failure.
- The presence of HBV surface antigen beyond 6 months indicates persistent infection. Hepatitis B e antigen indicates viral replication. These patients can develop chronic hepatitis with the risk of progressing to cirrhosis and hepatocellular carcinoma.
- 95% of immune-competent patients will clear the virus over 3–4 months, as indicated by normalisation of liver enzymes and loss of hepatitis B surface antigen. The latter is replaced by hepatitis B surface antibodies. IgM core antibodies become IgG antibodies. Hepatitis B e antigen disappears and may be replaced by e antibody. Immunity as a result of past infection is indicated by these surface and core antibodies.

Immunisation results in development of surface antibody and has been part of the universal childhood vaccination program in Australia since 1996. Adults in high-risk groups, such as healthcare workers, are also offered vaccination.

Hepatitis B immunoglobulin is also available and is used for passive immunity in non-immunised individuals following significant exposure to HBV-infected blood or body secretions. Vaccination is also commenced at this time. Be guided by your infectious diseases service, local post-exposure prophylaxis guidelines and *The Australian Immunisation Handbook* (10th edition, 2013).

HEPATITIS C VIRUS (HCV)

This blood-borne virus is transmitted predominantly by percutaneous exposure to infected blood. It is prevalent in the injecting drug user population. Sexual contact and mother-to-infant transmission is much less common than with hepatitis B infection.

- Acute infection is usually subclinical.
- Approximately 75% of those with acute HCV infection develop chronic hepatitis with the risk of cirrhosis and hepatocellular carcinoma.
- Treatment with interferon and ribavirin is successful in select patients; new medications are also becoming available.
- No vaccination is available.

HEPATITIS D VIRUS

This is found only in patients infected with hepatitis B. In developed countries, it is mostly found in the injecting drug user population. It increases the risk of fulminant hepatitis and the sequelae of chronic hepatitis.

HEPATITIS E VIRUS

Hepatitis E is an enterically transmitted self-limiting acute hepatitis similar to hepatitis A; fulminant disease is, however, more common than with hepatitis A, particularly in pregnant women. The disease is rare in developed countries.

Genitourinary infections

URINARY TRACT INFECTION (UTI)

Asymptomatic bacteriuria need not be treated, except in pregnant women. Asymptomatic bacteriuria is quite common in elderly patients.

Uncomplicated lower UTI

- Non-pregnant women
- No structural urinary tract abnormality
- No comorbidity such as diabetes
- 90% of cases are caused by *Escherichia coli*

Symptoms

- Burning on micturition
- Frequency
- Suprapubic discomfort
- Macroscopic haematuria

Investigations

Urinalysis is part of the physical examination in suspected UTI. Urine culture is not routinely necessary.

Management

- Trimethoprim 300 mg daily for 3 days.
- Over-hydration dilutes the bacteria, but also dilutes antibacterial mechanisms.
- Urinary alkalinisation can give significant symptomatic relief.

Pregnant women

- Treat all suspected UTIs in pregnancy. Infection in this group is associated with complications and a high risk of progression to pyelonephritis.
- Send urine for culture pre-therapy and 48-hours post-therapy.
- Treatment is cefalexin 500 mg 12-hourly for 5 days (TGA Pregnancy Category A).

Always consult the Therapeutic Goods and Administration category of risk posed by a particular antibiotic before prescribing it in pregnancy.

Men

Men with cystitis usually have an underlying urinary tract abnormality requiring investigation:

- Incomplete bladder emptying
- Sexually transmitted infections (STIs)
- Chronic prostatitis.

Empirical treatment is with trimethoprim 300 mg daily for 14 days.

ACUTE PYELONEPHRITIS

Symptoms of upper UTI include:

- fever, often with rigors/chills
- flank pain—bilateral or unilateral
- vomiting and dehydration are common.

Investigations

- Send urine and 2 sets of blood cultures to the laboratory.
- Routine imaging is *not* necessary in uncomplicated pyelonephritis, but renal ultrasound should be performed in:
  - all men
  - pregnant women
  - diabetic patients
  - severe flank pain unresponsive to therapy

— persistent fever
— impaired renal function.

Management

Mild infection can be treated with oral antibiotics, but often people present to the ED because these have failed or they are unable to keep the medication down.

Empirical therapy for **severe infection** is:

- gentamicin 4–6 mg/kg IV daily (in severe sepsis give 7 mg/kg IV for the first dose + ampicillin 2 g IV 6-hourly)
  OR
  ceftriaxone 1 g IV daily.
- IV fluid rehydration is essential in these cases, both for comfort of the patient and to maintain adequate circulation and protect the kidneys.
- Analgesia and antiemetics should also be administered.

Patients often feel better after a few hours and can then go home on cefalexin 500 mg 6 hourly for 10 days.

Pearls and Pitfalls

- Urosepsis can be a cause of severe sepsis and septic shock, especially in diabetics and elderly patients, so pay attention to appropriate fluid resuscitation and actively monitor blood pressure and end-organ perfusion.
- The rise of multi-resistant *E. coli* has complicated the treatment of UTIs. This makes the collection of adequate blood and urine cultures essential to guide appropriate antibiotic use.

URINARY-CATHETER-RELATED INFECTION

- Asymptomatic bacteriuria and pyuria is common with long-term catheterisation.
- Should only be treated if symptomatic.
- Catheter change or removal is essential if treatment for a catheter-associated UTI is considered necessary.

ACUTE PROSTATITIS

- Tender perineum and prostate.
- High fever, chills, back pain, perineal pain, dysuria, retention.
- Send urine for culture.
- Do not forget the possibility of an STI—take a sexual history, consider testing for gonorrhoea and chlamydia and referral to a sexual health clinic.

Management

- Trimethoprim 300 mg daily for 14 days
- Stool softeners

Sexually transmitted infection (STI)

- The presence of one STI implies potential exposure to every other STI and to pregnancy. All patients need referral to a sexual health clinic where follow-up, contact tracing, counselling and education can occur.
- Commencing treatment in the ED may have important public health benefits.
- Presenting complaints include:
  - genital lesions
  - vaginitis/vaginal/urethral discharge or dysuria
  - pelvic pain in women.

GENITAL LESIONS

Painful, vesicular lesions

- Likely to be herpes simplex infection.
- Swab base of ulcer and send for direct immunofluorescence/ PCR and culture.
- **Management:**
  - aciclovir 400 mg 8-hourly for 5 days
    OR
    valaciclovir 500 mg 12-hourly for 5 days.
  - Frequent recurrences can be treated with suppressive therapy.
  - Remember to provide pain relief such as topical lignocaine and oral analgesia, and beware of acute urinary retention in patients presenting with a first episode of genital herpes.

Solitary painless lesion

- Syphilitic chancre
- Serological diagnosis (rapid plasma reagin (RPR)/venereal disease reference laboratory test (VDRL), confirmed with *Treponema pallidum* haemagglutination assay (TPHA))
- Notifiable infection; requires referral to sexual health service
- **Treatment:**
  - benzathine penicillin 1.8 g or 2.4 million units (Bicillin LA) (painful injection)
    OR
    azithromycin 2 g PO

Wart-like lesions

- Human papilloma virus (HPV)
- Diagnosis is clinical
- Refer to sexual health clinic, gynaecologist or urologist for management

Itchy lesions

- Don't forget scabies and lice!
- **Management:**
  - Topical treatments available over-the-counter are usually sufficient. Patient's clothing and bedding should be laundered.
  - Transmission generally requires prolonged skin-to-skin contact.

VULVOVAGINITIS

- Inflamed, irritated vagina/labia with discharge
- If discharge is from cervix, manage as for cervicitis
- If there is pelvic tenderness, manage as for pelvic inflammatory disease (PID; see below)
- Send swab for culture

Trichomonas

- Not normal flora—sexually transmitted
- Purulent malodorous discharge
- Linked with pregnancy complications
- **Treatment** is metronidazole 2 g PO single dose

Candida

- Generally not sexually transmitted
- Associated with antibiotic use, high oestrogen levels (e.g. OCP) and poorly controlled diabetes
- Clinically characterised by:
  - thick white discharge
  - pruritus
  - superficial ulceration/excoriation
- **Treatment** is with topical anti-candidal creams (for 7 days in pregnancy) or fluconazole 150 mg PO single dose (not in pregnancy)

Bacterial vaginosis

- Polymicrobial overgrowth with anaerobes
- Generally not sexually transmitted

- Treat if symptomatic
- **Treatment:**
  - Metronidazole 400 mg 8-hourly for 7 days

CERVICITIS

- Non-irritating vaginal discharge, seen to come from cervical os on speculum examination
- Sexually transmitted infection—*Chlamydia trachomatis* and/or *Neisseria gonorrhoeae*
- **Investigations:**
  - Endocervical swab for PCR for gonorrhoea/chlamydia and culture.
  - PCR for both chlamydia and gonorrhoea can also be performed.
- **Management:**
  - Ceftriaxone 250 mg IM + azithromycin 1 g PO stat.
  - If there is fever or pelvic pain, manage as for PID (see below).
  - Refer to sexual health service for counselling, contact tracing and follow-up.

MALE URETHRITIS

- Urethral discharge or asymptomatic
- May be detected as pyuria
- Send swab and/or urine for chlamydia/gonorrhoea PCR
- Coincident chlamydia infection in patients with gonorrhoeal urethritis leads to recommendation for treatment of both simultaneously:
  - Ceftriaxone 250 mg IM + azithromycin 1 g PO stat.
- Refer to sexual health service for counselling, contact tracing and follow-up.

EPIDIDYMO-ORCHITIS

- Secondary to UTI or STI.
- If sexually transmitted, manage as for urethritis and refer to sexual health service.
- Otherwise, manage as per UTI in men.

PELVIC PAIN IN WOMEN

- Always exclude pregnancy by testing urine or blood, regardless of the history given.
- PID is common and often undiagnosed.
- **Beware a diagnosis of appendicitis or 'grumbling**

appendicitis' in a young woman. Urine should be sent for microculture and sensitivity and a *Gonorrhoea* and *Chlamydia* NAAT should also be requested.

Pelvic inflammatory disease (PID)

- 13% of women are infertile after a single episode
- Risk of ectopic pregnancy increases 7-fold after 1 episode
- Can also lead to pelvic adhesions and chronic pelvic pain

Clinical features of PID

- Low-grade fever
- Pelvic tenderness
- Cervical discharge
- Palpable mass suggests tubo-ovarian abscess.

Most commonly PID is from a sexually acquired infection, but it can develop after termination of pregnancy or be associated with an intra-uterine device (IUD) or other instrumentation of the uterus.

All PID is polymicrobial with endogenous flora.

Treatment

- Azithromycin 1 g PO on day 1 and day 8
  OR
- Ceftriaxone 1 g IV daily
  OR
- Metronidazole 500 mg IV 8-hourly.

All women with PID should be referred to a gynaecologist for follow-up.

Pearls and Pitfalls

- Ensure women realise that a speculum examination in this setting does not include a Pap smear. This will need to be done by their GP once any infection has subsided.

Needle-stick injuries and body fluids exposures

- Wash affected area/wound with water or saline.
- Irrigate affected mucous membranes/eyes (remove contacts) with water or saline.

RISK ASSESSMENT

- Determines need for testing and treatment
- Method of exposure, e.g. anal or vaginal insertive or receptive

intercourse, occupational needle-stick injury, sharing of injecting equipment
- Donor infection status or risk
- Immune status of recipient—e.g. HBV immunisation, tetanus immunisation.

BASELINE TESTING OF RECIPIENT

- Depends on risk assessment
- May include HIV antibody test, HBV and HCV serology, STI screen, pregnancy test
- Full blood count (FBC), liver function tests (LFTs), electrolytes for patients commencing post-exposure prophylaxis (PEP) for HIV
- Testing always requires appropriate counselling and follow-up

PROPHYLACTIC MEDICATION AND IMMUNISATIONS

Consider
- HIV, HBV, HCV (see Box 41.2)
- Tetanus immunisation
- Prophylactic STI treatment
- Pregnancy

COUNSELLING AND FOLLOW-UP

- Occupational health service
- Sexual health service

POST-SEXUAL ASSAULT PROPHYLAXIS

Refer patient to specialist sexual assault service.

Consider emergency contraception as well as STI treatment and post-exposure management as above.

COMMUNITY NEEDLE-STICK INJURIES

The risk of HIV transmission in this situation is so low that it is not measurable. Tetanus prophylaxis is indicated.

Respiratory tract infection

See Chapter 37, 'Ear, nose and throat (ENT) emergencies' for upper respiratory tract infection.

LOWER RESPIRATORY TRACT INFECTION (LRTI)

(See Chapter 9, 'Respiratory emergencies'.)
- Outpatient management of community-acquired pneumonia:
  - amoxycillin 1 g PO 8-hourly for 5–7 days
  - *If atypical organism is suspected:* roxithromycin 300 mg daily for 5 days.

Box 41.2 Prophylaxis for hepatitis B, hepatitis C and HIV

Hepatitis B

- Commence vaccination schedule if not immunised.
- If immune response post vaccination is unknown, test HBV surface antibody level.
- Consider giving HBV immunoglobulin to non-immune individuals within 72 hours if the source is, or strongly suspected to be, infected with HBV.
- Discuss with your infectious diseases service.

Hepatitis C

- Test with PCR at 1 month, antibody testing at 6 months.
- Refer to hepatologist or infectious diseases service for possible early therapy if PCR becomes positive and/or the patient develops acute HCV disease.

HIV

Situations where PEP may be appropriate:

- Occupational exposure for healthcare workers
- Sexual assault
- Unprotected sex/broken condom
- Contaminated injecting equipment.
- If PEP is indicated, it should commence as soon as possible. In general, PEP is not recommended after 72 hours.

Follow protocols within your healthcare facility.

(See also 'Post-exposure prophylaxis in HIV' in Chapter 42, 'The immunosuppressed patient'.)

- Patients with moderate to severe pneumonia require inpatient management:
  - ceftriaxone 1 g IV daily
  - *If atypical organism suspected or severe, add:* azithromycin 500 mg IV daily.

Some 'Pearls and Pitfalls' are given overleaf.

Tuberculosis (TB)

- In developed countries, TB is found in migrant populations from high-prevalence countries and the itinerant population. It is also found in the Australian Indigenous population.
- Prolonged exposure to infected respiratory droplets is usually required for transmission to occur, e.g. household contacts. Patients with acid-fast bacilli seen on sputum smear are significantly more infectious than those without.
- Cellular immunity develops 3–8 weeks following exposure, causing a positive tuberculin test, and immune response causes limitation of further infection.

Pearls and Pitfalls (LRTI)

- Patients with chronic lung disease may have known colonisation with *Pseudomonas*, which may be contributing to their current infection. Obtain sputum cultures that have been taken in the community by the GP when initial treatment has been started. This can assist in directing the antibiotic regimen after a presentation to the ED.
- Any significant pleural effusion should be considered for drainage to prevent empyema and allow for cytology and culture.
- *Burkholderia pseudomallei* is a bacteria found in the tropical north of Australia and part of South-East Asia. It particularly affects immunocompromised people such as those with non-insulin-dependent diabetes mellitus, alcohol abuse or people with severe cardiorespiratory conditions. It can affect any organ, but respiratory and genitourinary infection is common.

  It is a Gram-negative rod distinguished by its resistance to gentamicin. It is not found in southern Australian states but an accurate history of comorbidities, place of residence or travel in tropical Australia may prompt the emergency doctor to discuss this as a possible pathogen with an infectious diseases or microbiology consultant. Standard antibiotic protocols for pneumonia and urinary tract infection will not cover *B. pseudomallei* infection.

- TB can remain dormant for many years, 'latent TB infection' (LTBI), and may reactivate with immunodeficiency, immunosuppression and immunocompromise (including senescence of old age). In general, after exposure to TB infection, there is considered to be about a 5% lifetime risk of developing the disease. The first half of this risk (2.5%) is for progression to TB disease within 2 years of exposure. The other 2.5% risk is conferred lifelong, with an increasing risk in old age.
- Progressive primary infection can occur in the very young and immuno-compromised/deficient/suppressed.
- Uncontrolled haematogenous spread causes disseminated disease with widespread lung involvement (miliary TB).

CLINICAL FEATURES

- Anorexia, weight loss, fatigue
- Fever, night sweats
- Cough with purulent sputum ± haemoptysis
- Pleural effusion/consolidation

- Normochromic, normocytic anaemia
- Raised inflammatory markers.

Note: Migration from a high-prevalence country and symptoms of cough lasting > 3 weeks with systemic features is highly suggestive of TB infection. Extrapulmonary TB may also occur, and should be carefully considered in patients with a chronic illness from a high-TB-prevalence country.

Investigations

- Sputum acid-fast staining and culture.
- Specialist teams can perform PCR on relevant secretions.
- Chest X-ray:
  (chest X-ray changes can be extensive despite the patient remaining comparatively well)
  — pneumonia with hilar adenopathy suggests primary disease
  — apical changes
  — cavitating lesions
  — effusion.

Note: In the immuno-compromised/deficient/suppressed patient, the typical patterns of chest X-ray change are not sensitive. In end-stage HIV infection, 10% of people with pulmonary TB have a normal chest X-ray.

Management

TB is a notifiable disease that needs specialist management.

- Concurrent HIV infection needs to be considered.
- Public health staff perform contact tracing and prophylactic treatment of household contacts.
- Respiratory isolation/infection control should be initiated if TB is in the differential diagnosis to simplify public health measures once the diagnosis is confirmed.
- People with underlying TB can present to the ED with an intercurrent community-acquired LRTI and will need to be managed for this in addition to appropriate work-up for TB infection.
- The decision to isolate should first be addressed in the ED, and advice can be sought regarding whether this is necessary.

Severe sepsis

(See also 'Septic shock' in Chapter 12, 'Shock'.)

- Sepsis is infection with a systemic inflammatory response.

- Severe sepsis is sepsis with acute organ dysfunction.
- Septic shock (high mortality, ~30%) is defined as:
  - sepsis with hypotension refractory to an initial fluid bolus

  OR
  - evidence of tissue hypoperfusion (lactate > 4 mmol/L).

Early aggressive resuscitation in the ED has been shown to improve outcome.

MANAGEMENT

- Prompt fluid resuscitation
  - 20–30 mL/kg fluid bolus on diagnosis.
- Take at least 2 sets of blood cultures simultaneously from different sites:
  - at least 2 sets percutaneously
  - at least 1 set from a vascular access device (if present > 48 hours)
  - culture other sites as clinically indicated.
- Broad-spectrum antibiotics within 1 hour.
  - e.g. ceftriaxone 2 g IV plus vancomycin 1 g IV if MRSA suspected
- Insert central line and arterial line early.

Goals in the ED within 6 hours:

- Continue fluid resuscitation (crystalloid or colloid) to a central venous pressure (CVP) of 8–12 mmHg.
- Mean arterial BP > 65 mmHg using a vasopressor, such as a noradrenaline infusion once patient adequately fluid-resuscitated.
- Central venous oxygen saturation > 70% if sample from central venous catheter (CVC), or > 65% if mixed venous sample.
- Transfuse blood to haematocrit (HCT) ≥ 30% and/or dobutamine infusion (start at 2.5 microg/kg/min).
- Consult early with your infectious diseases service.
- Source control of infection, e.g.:
  - drainage of abscess, debridement of tissue
  - removal of foreign bodies, e.g. vascular access devices, etc.

Meningococcal infection

- Invasive meningococcal disease is life-threatening. The course can be fulminant, with patients deteriorating within hours of the onset of symptoms.

- *Neisseria meningitidis* is a Gram-negative diplococcus with many serotypes. Serotypes B and C cause disease in Australia.
  — Serotype C is now on the Australian childhood immunisation schedule.
  — There is no vaccination available for serotype B.
- Transmission is via asymptomatic nasal carriage (~ 10% of the population). The age groups 0–4 years and 15–25 years are most commonly affected by invasive disease, with a seasonal peak in winter–spring.
- Invasive infection can manifest as meningitis or more commonly as septicaemia (also referred to as meningococcaemia). Meningococcal meningitis has a high mortality rate of around 7%, but the mortality rate is even higher for meningococcal septicaemia at around 19%.

CLINICAL FINDINGS

The classic clinical findings of meningococcaemia are fever and a petechial or purpuric rash. Clinical features can be non-specific early in the course of disease, requiring a high index of suspicion and thorough clinical examination to make the diagnosis.

Early findings can also include:

- maculopapular rash that develops in the first 24 hours of illness
- myalgia which can be very painful
- cold extremities and pallor with fever.

Late signs (12–16 hours) are:

- meningism
- impaired consciousness
- shock.
- **Management:**
  — Pre-hospital antibiotics in meningococcal sepsis can be life-saving:
    - benzylpenicillin 30 mg/kg up to 1.2 g IM or IV
      OR
    - ceftriaxone 50 mg/kg up to 2 g IM or IV.

  — Draw blood cultures beforehand, but don't delay antibiotic therapy:
    - ceftriaxone 2 g IV 12-hourly

INVESTIGATIONS

- Blood culture and meningococcal PCR
- Skin scrapings of purpuric lesions for Gram stain and culture

- CSF for culture and meningococcal PCR
- FBC, coagulation and biochemistry

MANAGEMENT

- Antibiotic therapy as above.
- Further management as per severe sepsis.
- The local public health unit needs to be notified ASAP (< 12 hours) for all cases where invasive meningococcal disease is being considered. Discuss with your infectious diseases service.
- Droplet transmission precautions should be instituted for 24 hours after commencement of antibiotics.

CHEMOPROPHYLAXIS FOR MENINGOCOCCAL CONTACTS

This is the role of the public health department.

Healthcare workers

The only healthcare workers that require prophylaxis are those who:

- intubated the patient without wearing a mask
- performed mouth-to-mouth resuscitation.

Close contacts

- The main purpose is to eliminate the carrier state.
- Includes household members and intimate contacts.
- Outside the immediate family, public health authorities coordinate contact tracing and prophylaxis.

Treatment

- Ciprofloxacin 500 mg PO single dose (for adults and children > 12 years of age)
  OR
- Rifampicin 10 mg/kg (5 mg/kg in neonates) up to 600 mg PO 12-hourly for 48 hours (preferred option in children)
  OR
- Ceftriaxone 250 mg IM single dose (best option in pregnancy)

MRSA and NORSA

- Multi-resistant *Staphylococcus aureus* (MRSA) is resistant to beta-lactam antibiotics and one or more others. Initially it was only present in the healthcare setting but now it has independently evolved in the community, hence the use of the term community-acquired MRSA (CA-MRSA) versus hospital-acquired MRSA (HA-MRSA). It is all MRSA.

- Some MRSA strains are sensitive to antibiotics such as clindamycin, doxycycline or trimethoprim + sulfamethoxazole, and are therefore sometimes referred to as non-multi-resistant oxacillin-resistant *S. aureus* (NORSA). These strains manifest clinically as subcutaneous abscesses and necrotising pneumonia.
- MRSA is now so prevalent in Australia that any staphylococcal infection needs to be thought of as potentially MRSA. Appropriate specimen collection is very important.
- Skin abscesses are managed by effective incision and drainage and rarely require antibiotics even when there is some surrounding erythema.
  — If antibiotics are indicated, mild infection can be treated with a beta-lactam such as dicloxacillin while awaiting sensitivity results.
  — Severe infection, manifest as organ dysfunction, hypoperfusion or hypotension, needs treatment before sensitivities become available: vancomycin 1 g IV 12-hourly (adapted according to estimated glomerular filtration rate, eGFR).

Skin infections

(Also see Chapter 40, 'Dermatological presentations to emergency'.)

INFECTIOUS CELLULITIS

- Commonly seen in the lower limb in adults. Bilateral cellulitis is rare.
- Tinea pedis between toes is a common entry site.
- Wound-associated cellulitis is usually due to *S. aureus*, whereas 'spontaneous' cellulitis is usually group A streptococcal infection.
- Examination reveals erythema with or without lymphangitis. There may be enlarged and tender draining lymph nodes.

Management

- Management involves rest with immobilisation and elevation. Drawing a line around the border of the erythema provides some objective measure of progression or remission.
- For **mild disease:**
  — dicloxacillin 500 mg PO 6-hourly
  — alternatively, consider daily IV antibiotics in the home: cefazolin 2 g IV daily, probenecid 1 g PO daily.

- **Indications for admission** to hospital include:
  - moderate to severe infection or rapidly spreading infection
  - systemically unwell patient
  - significant comorbidities such as diabetes (see below), immunosuppression, impaired lymphatic drainage of the affected area.
  - **Treatment:** dicloxacillin 2 g IV 6-hourly. This covers methicillin-sensitive *S. aureus* and group A *Streptococcus* without needing benzylpenicillin.

Diabetic patients with infectious cellulitis

Cellulitis in diabetic patients is serious and can often become limb-threatening. Infection can progress rapidly. Have a low threshold for admitting these patients to hospital.

Infection is often polymicrobial and includes anaerobes, so a broader antimicrobial cover is needed:

- amoxycillin + clavulanate 875 mg + 125 mg PO 12-hourly
  OR
- cefazolin 1 g IV 8 hourly + metronidazole 500 mg IV 12-hourly.

In severe infection:

- ticarcillin + clavulanate 3 g + 0.1 g IV 6-hourly.

ABSCESS

- Usually due to *S. aureus*.
- Incision and drainage is the main management principle.
- If there are systemic symptoms, antibiotic therapy as for cellulitis can be used.
- Consider NORSA (as mentioned previously) in at-risk populations or unresolving infection.
- Follow-up of culture results is important to treat NORSA.
- **Treatment:**
  - clindamycin 10 mg/kg up to 600 mg PO 8-hourly
    OR
  - doxycycline 100 mg PO 12-hourly
    OR
  - trimethoprim + sulfamethoxazole 320 mg + 1600 mg PO 12-hourly.
- If **IV therapy** is required: vancomycin 1 g IV 12-hourly (adapted according to eGFR).

SCALDED SKIN SYNDROME

- This is a medical emergency; mortality in adults can be up to 60%.
- Exfoliative toxin produced by *Staphylococcus* or *Streptococcus.*
- Fever with widespread erythema, bullae and exfoliation.

Management

- Resuscitation—as for severe sepsis and septic shock
- Skin management—as for burns
- Vancomycin 1 g IV 12-hourly (adapted according to eGFR)

RAPIDLY PROGRESSING INFECTIONS (GANGRENOUS CELLULITIS)

Necrosis of the soft tissues can spread rapidly and be limb- and life-threatening.

Can be **polymicrobial** e.g.:

- Fournier's gangrene, necrotising fasciitis of scrotum that can progress to perineum, penis and abdominal wall.

Can be a **single microbe** e.g.:

- *Clostridium myonecrosis* (gas gangrene)
- *Streptococcus pyogenes*
- *Staphylococcus aureus.*

Clinical features

- Marked systemic toxicity out of proportion to local findings
- Erythema, swelling, indiscrete margins
- Very tender initially
- Crepitus cellulitis
- Anaesthesia of overlying skin
- Rapid spread (can spread widely in deep fascial planes with relative sparing of overlying skin)
- Systemic toxicity ± septic shock

Management

- Needs urgent debridement of necrotic tissue and early antibiotics:
  - meropenem 1 g IV 8-hourly
    plus
  - clindamycin 600 mg IV 8-hourly.
- Consult surgeons and infectious diseases services early in your management.

Wound infections

(Also see Chapter 40, 'Dermatological presentations to emergency'.)

- These are usually related to skin organisms and can be managed as for cellulitis (see above).
- Remove any foreign material such as sutures and clean/debride as appropriate.
- Some special circumstances are included under the following sections.

HUMAN AND OTHER ANIMAL BITE WOUND INFECTIONS

- Prophylactic antibiotics are recommended for:
  - wounds with delayed presentation
  - puncture wounds
  - wounds involving hands, feet or face
  - involvement of underlying structure.
- Amoxycillin + clavulanate 875 mg +125 mg PO 12-hourly for 5 days.
- If there is established infection, consider admission and parenteral antibiotic therapy: ceftriaxone 1 g IV daily + metronidazole 500 mg IV 12-hourly.

PENETRATING WOUNDS THROUGH FOOTWEAR

- *Pseudomonas* infection is common.
- Treat with ciprofloxacin 500 mg PO 12-hourly for 5 days.

Water-related infections

These are complicated infections and advice should be sought from your infectious diseases service.

- Salt-water exposure with cellulitis/bullous lesions or necrotic ulcers—consider *Vibrio* species infection.
  - Administer doxycycline 200 mg stat, then 100 mg 12-hourly for 5 days.
- Fresh-water infection can be *Aeromonas* infection.
  - Administer ciprofloxacin 500 mg PO 12-hourly for 5 days.
- Coral cut infections are often caused by *Streptococcus pyogenes*.
  - These are sensitive to penicillin and so can be managed as for uncomplicated cellulitis.
- Infection related to fish tank water can be *Mycobacterium marinum*, which can cause papular lesions.
  - Requires referral for biopsy and infectious diseases expertise.

Herpes zoster (shingles)

Shingles is a reactivation of varicella (chickenpox) manifesting as a vesicular rash in a dermatomal distribution. A prodrome may precede the appearance of vesicles, e.g. pain, itch or other abnormal sensation at the site.

If more than one dermatome is involved or disease is disseminated, consider underlying immunosuppression/compromise/deficiency.

MANAGEMENT

- Antiviral therapy can reduce symptoms if commenced within 72 hours of rash onset:
  - valaciclovir 1 g 8 hourly for 7 days
    OR
  - aciclovir 800 mg 5 times a day for 7 days.
- Zoster of the first division of the trigeminal nerve requires special consideration as the cornea can be involved—consult an ophthalmologist.
- Patients with shingles need pain relief to be prescribed for them.

Tetanus prophylaxis

The route of tetanus infection is commonly via contaminated puncture or laceration wounds that contain an anaerobic environment as

Table 41.1 Tetanus prophylaxis

Fully vaccinated (> 3 doses) in past	Time since vaccination or booster	Wound type	Give tetanus vaccination (ADT, DTP, tetanus toxoid)	Give tetanus immuno-globulin (< 24 h, 250 IU IM; > 24 h, 500 IU IM)
Yes	< 5 years	All wounds	No	No
	5–10 years	Minor clean wounds	No	No
		All other wounds	Yes	No
	> 10 years	All wounds	Yes	No
No	–	Minor clean wounds	Yes	No
		All other wounds	Yes	Yes

ADT, adult diphtheria and tetanus; DTP, diphtheria, tetanus and pertussis.

a result of devitalised tissue. Tetanus is a preventable disease through immunisation and wound care.

The overseas traveller

TRAVELLER'S DIARRHOEA

- Commonly caused by enterotoxigenic *Escherichia coli.*
- Usually a self-limiting illness with supportive oral rehydration.
- Antibiotics are associated with reduction of the duration and severity of the diarrhoea, and so can be used if the symptoms are not tolerable:
  - norfloxacin 800 mg PO single dose.
  - if there is fever or blood in the diarrhoea norfloxacin 400 mg PO 12-hourly for 5 days.
- Bloody diarrhoea should be referred to your gastroenterology service.

FEVER IN THE OVERSEAS TRAVELLER

Five important diagnoses to consider:

1 Malaria
2 Dengue
3 Typhoid
4 Viral hepatitis (discussed above)
5 HIV (see Chapter 42, 'The immunosuppressed patient').

Malaria

- Fever in the overseas traveller is malaria until proven otherwise.
- Five *Plasmodium* species cause human malaria—*falciparum, vivax, ovale, malariae* and *knowlesi.*
- *Falciparum* causes almost all deaths directly related to malaria and is responsible for several million deaths throughout the world each year.

Presenting symptoms

- Clinical features are protean.
- Spiking fevers with temperatures up to 40°C.
- Headache, diarrhoea, abdominal pain.
- Can be non-specific 'flu-like' symptoms.

Severe malaria is characterised by:

- altered level of consciousness and/or seizures (cerebral malaria)
- shock
- respiratory distress
- jaundice, anaemia, hypoglycaemia.

Investigations

- Thick blood film for identification of malarial parasites.
- Thin blood film to determine malaria species.
  Note: Detectable parasitaemia can lag behind symptoms; should repeat 12-hourly until malaria is diagnosed or excluded (usually 3 negative blood films).
- Other findings include: anaemia, thrombocytopenia, ↑ lactate dehydrogenase (LDH), ↑ bilirubin.
- Rapid-detection kits are available; most only detect *P. falciparum*.

Treatment

- Requires up-to-date knowledge of geographical patterns of drug resistance.
- Always seek specialist advice.
- *Falciparum* malaria can progress to life-threatening complications within hours, even after initiation of treatment. Discuss hospital admission with your infectious diseases service or medical doctor/team on call.

Severe malaria:

- artesunate 2.4 mg/kg IV (first choice if available) as 4 doses over 3 days
  OR
- quinine 20 mg/kg IV over 4 hours (note possible hypoglycaemia with quinine)

Uncomplicated *Falciparum* malaria and other malaria species from chloroquine-resistant areas:

- artemether + lumefantrine, 20 mg + 120 mg tablets (first choice if available); 4 tablets at 0, 8, 24, 36, 48 and 60 hours
  OR
- mefloquine 750 mg PO then 500 mg PO 6–8 hours later (as long as the drug is not used as prophylaxis).

Note: The combination artemether + lumefantrine is TGA-approved for adults but not children in Australia. Artesunate is not registered for use in Australia, but is available under the special access scheme and is kept in selected hospital pharmacies.

Pearls and Pitfalls

- Malaria has been eradicated from Australia; however, the vector exists in the tropical north making it possible for the disease to be introduced again in that region.
- Refugees can become unwell from malaria many weeks after arrival in Australia.

Dengue fever ('break bone fever')

Dengue is a common disease in the Asia–Pacific region. Travellers, NGO aid workers and defence personnel are often affected. Dengue is endemic in Far North Queensland.

- It is a mosquito-transmitted flavivirus with a short incubation period of 4–7 days.
- Patients usually present with various combinations of fever, myalgia, arthralgia and rash. The rash is fine and sometimes not noticed by the patient. It may involve the palms and soles.
- Thrombocytopenia is almost always present, as are elevated hepatic transaminases.
- Dengue haemorrhagic fever and dengue shock syndrome are due to a sudden increase in vascular permeability and occur in infants and secondary exposures.
- Management is supportive.

See also 'Chikungunya', below.

Chikungunya

Chikungunya is a re-emerging arbovirus seen through Asia into southern Indonesia and Timor-Leste.

- Its clinical spectrum is similar to dengue. Thrombocytopenia is less severe and progression through to haemorrhagic shock syndromes does not seem to occur.
- Dengue and chikungunya cannot be distinguished clinically and epidemics may overlap. If you are testing for dengue in a returning traveller, then it is reasonable to request chikungunya testing as well.
- Management is supportive.

Typhoid fever

- Transmitted through food or water faecally contaminated with *Salmonella typhi* or *paratyphi* subtypes.
- Vaccination efficacy is somewhere between 50% and 80%, depending on innoculum, so does not exclude the diagnosis.
- Symptoms:
  - Classically, there is fever and abdominal tenderness initially with constipation.
  - Patient may also have confusion, rose spots (faint salmon-coloured maculopapular rash on the trunk) and hepatosplenomegaly.
  - Relative bradycardia is not very sensitive or specific.
  - Untreated infection can lead to intestinal perforation.

- Diagnose by culturing blood and stool.
- **Treatment** is ciprofloxacin 500 mg PO for 5–7 days or ceftriaxone 2 g IV daily.
- There is quinolone resistance in some countries (e.g. in India and Vietnam), so discussion with the infectious diseases service is recommended.

Acknowledgements

The authors wish to acknowledge the content used from the previous edition of *Emergency Medicine* which was provided by Dr Mark A Boyd.

Online resources

Australian Immunisation Handbook, 10th edn
www.health.gov.au/internet/immunise/publishing.nsf/Content/Handbook10-home

CIAP
www.ciap.health.nsw.gov.au

National guidelines for post-exposure prophylaxis after non-occupational exposure to HIV. Approved March 2007 (undergoing revision in 2013). Commonwealth of Australia.
www.ashm.org.au/uploads/2007nationalNPEPguidelines2.pdf (2007 guidelines)
www.ashm.org.au/default2.asp?active_page_id=251 (draft guidelines 2013)

Therapeutic Guidelines Australia
www.tg.org.au

Chapter 42

The immunosuppressed patient

Judy Alford and Anthony Kelleher

Overview

Patients with immunosuppression present with emergencies related to their increased susceptibility to infection and to their underlying condition.

- The most frequently encountered causes of immunocompromise vary according to the location and specialisation of the institution, with cancer, AIDS and solid-organ transplant being the commonest conditions.
- Other causes of immunocompromise are immunosuppressive and/or cytotoxic therapy for non-malignant disease, post splenectomy, congenital immune defects and marrow failure due to drugs or infection.

The signs and symptoms of infection are often diminished and patients may present with subtle and non-specific findings and deteriorate rapidly. Fever may be the sole presenting symptom, but even that may be masked by the presence of drugs such as corticosteroids. Therefore, infection must be considered in the differential diagnosis of the immunocompromised patient presenting with non-specific symptoms.

IMMUNE SYSTEM FAILURE

The immune system consists of *innate* and *adaptive* components.

- Innate immunity stems from intact epithelial barriers, phagocytic cells (neutrophils and macrophages), natural killer cells and the complement system. Innate immunity does not require prior exposure to the infective agent for rapid activation.
- Adaptive immunity is conferred by lymphocytes and their products.
  — T-cells act against intracellular microbes and provide cell-mediated immunity.
  — Humoral immunity is conferred by B-cells and the antibodies they produce, which are active against extracellular microbes.

Failure of a component of the immune system leads to vulnerability to different infective agents.

- T-cell defects occur in acquired immune deficiency syndrome (AIDS), immunosuppressive therapy and congenital severe combined immune deficiency (SCID) and leave patients susceptible to:
  - bacterial sepsis
  - infections with intracellular bacteria (tuberculosis (TB), *Listeria*)
  - viral infections (cytomegalovirus (CMV), Epstein–Barr virus (EBV), varicella)
  - fungal infections (*Candida, Cryptococcus, Pneumocystis*), and
  - protozoal infections (*Toxoplasma*).
- B-cell defects occur in haematological malignancies, myeloma, AIDS and congenital disorders such as common variable immune deficiency.
  - Patients are predisposed to infection by encapsulated bacteria (*Streptococcus pneumoniae, Haemophilus influenzae, Neisseria*), staphylococci, *Giardia* and enterovirus.
- Granulocyte defects including neutropenia result from chemotherapy, marrow aplasia or infiltration, drug reactions, myelodysplasia and rarely from congenital defects. Patients are vulnerable to infection by:
  - Gram-negative bacilli including *Pseudomonas*
  - Gram-positive cocci such as staphylococci and viridans streptococci, and
  - fungi such as *Candida* and *Aspergillus*.
- Complement defects lead to susceptibility to infection with *Neisseria* and pyogenic bacteria, as well as predisposing to autoimmunity.
- Asplenia predisposes to severe infections due to encapsulated bacteria including *S. pneumoniae, H. influenzae* and *N. meningitidis*.

In addition to infections, fever in the immunocompromised patient may be due to malignancy, drugs and allograft rejection.

MANAGEMENT

Improvements in the management of the conditions associated with immunodeficiency have led to improved long-term survival and better quality of life for these patients. Nonetheless, there remains the potential for severe infections with rapid deterioration and death.

- Early aggressive care is essential, which includes early, rapid investigation, early institution of broad-spectrum antibiotics, application of treatment protocols for sepsis and the use of ventilatory support where indicated.
- Non-infective causes such as rejection must be considered, especially in transplant patients.
- Early ICU referral and a team approach involving treating haematologists, oncologists, HIV specialists or transplant doctors is essential in the deteriorating patient.
- The patient's wishes should be ascertained early, particularly in those with severe advanced disease or chronic progressive conditions that have been unresponsive to intervention.

Cancer patients

Cancer patients are at risk of severe infection due to immunosuppression induced by their disease and its treatment. Most at risk are patients undergoing therapy for haematological malignancies or stem-cell transplant, who have severe and prolonged neutropenia. The risk of infection rises as the neutrophil count falls.

FEBRILE NEUTROPENIA

Clinical features

Febrile neutropenia is defined as fever with temperatures above 38.0°C in a patient with a neutrophil count $< 0.5 \times 10^9$/L or $< 1.0 \times 10^9$/L with a predicted decline to $< 0.5 \times 10^9$/L.

- Associated signs of infection may be present, such as tachypnoea, tachycardia, altered mental state, dehydration and acidosis.
- Localising signs may be absent; however, a thorough examination of the lungs, oropharynx, skin, catheters, perineum and perianal area, sinuses and urinary tract is essential and may reveal the site of infection.

Non-specific symptoms in the absence of fever may still indicate infection, especially if the patient is on high-dose corticosteroids.

Investigations

- Investigations should include:
  - urea, electrolytes and creatinine (UEC)
  - full blood count (FBC)
  - liver function tests (LFTs)
  - chest X-ray

  - urinalysis
  - swabs from any skin lesions.
- Two sets of blood cultures should be obtained, one from any indwelling catheter that may be present. Swabs should be sent from any lesions or catheter insertion sites. There should be a low threshold for the collection of specimens for culture.
- Cerebrospinal fluid (CSF) is not routinely cultured, but should be if CNS infection is suspected. However, in the rapidly deteriorating patient, or in those with a coagulopathy, lumbar puncture may need to be delayed or forgone. Antibiotic administration should not be delayed by the need for lumbar puncture.
- Stool should be sent for culture if diarrhoea is present. The patient with abdominal signs will require imaging by ultrasound or computed tomography (CT); however, this should not delay surgical consultation, as signs of peritonitis are minimal in the neutropenic patient.
- CT scans of the sinuses should be obtained if there is facial pain or swelling, as severe, invasive fungal sinusitis occurs in these patients.

Management

Broad-spectrum antibiotics

Broad-spectrum antibiotics should be started immediately after cultures have been obtained. Delay in initiating appropriate antibiotic therapy is associated with increased mortality. Coverage for Gram-negatives, including *Pseudomonas aeruginosa,* is essential.

Recommended regimens vary between institutions. The following antibiotics are suitable:

- ceftazidime 2 g IV 8-hourly
  OR
- piperacillin 4 g + tazobactam 0.5 g IV 8-hourly
  OR
- ticarcillin 3 g + clavulanate 0.1 g IV 6-hourly
  plus gentamicin 4–6 mg/kg IV daily
  OR
- cefepime 2 g IV 12-hourly.

Vancomycin

Gram-positive bacteraemia due to *Staphylococcus epidermidis, S. aureus,* viridans streptococci and enterococci is very common. The routine use of vancomycin is not recommended, although it should be given if the patient is in shock, is known to have methicillin-resistant *S. aureus* (MRSA) or has a clinically infected catheter.

- The recommended dose is 30 mg/kg up to 1.5 g IV 12-hourly, with adjustment according to renal function and serum levels.
- Vancomycin is often added if fever persists beyond 48 hours.

Antifungals

Antifungals are not routinely used in the initial treatment of febrile neutropenia, unless there is evidence of fungal infection such as sinusitis. They may be introduced when fever persists beyond 96 hours, especially in patients with pulmonary infiltrates.

A subgroup of low-risk neutropenic patients may be managed at home with oral therapy. This should only be done in consultation with the treating haematologist or oncologist.

Colony-stimulating growth factors

Recombinant colony-stimulating growth factors may be used in high-risk patients with sepsis or organ failure, after consultation with a haematologist or the patient's treating doctor.

Non-invasive ventilation (NIV)

NIV used early in the course of hypoxaemic respiratory failure may reduce the need for intubation and improve survival.

FEVER IN THE NON-NEUTROPENIC CANCER PATIENT

Cancer patients with a normal granulocyte count remain susceptible to infections when their adaptive immune response is impaired by treatment with steroids or chemotherapy, or by haematological malignancy.

- T-cell defects increase the risk of infection with intracellular pathogens like *Listeria*, *Salmonella*, mycobacteria and fungi.
- Patients with impaired humoral immunity are at risk of infection by encapsulated bacteria, often manifesting as pneumonia.

Non-infectious complications of cancer and its treatment

SPINAL CORD COMPRESSION

This is most common in the thoracic spine (70% of cases), although it may involve any level. It is most frequently due to metastatic breast, lung or prostate cancer, or lymphoma. An epidural abscess or discitis should be considered in patients who have had lumbar puncture or intrathecal therapy, or who are at risk of bacteraemia.

Pain usually occurs before the development of neurological symptoms. Once symptoms such as weakness, sensory loss and sphincter dysfunction begin, treatment must occur within hours to give the patient a chance of recovery.

Investigations

- Plain films of the spine show tumour in 70–90% of cases.
- Urgent MRI will localise the lesion.

Management

1. Obtaining MRI images should not delay treatment with corticosteroids in the patient with neurological signs. An initial dose of dexamethasone 20 mg IV is followed by 4 mg IV 6-hourly.
2. Radiotherapy to the affected area is the treatment of choice, with surgery used in selected cases with spinal instability.

HYPERCALCAEMIA

- Increased osteolysis releases calcium and phosphate into the circulation. This can be caused by primary (myeloma or leukaemia) or metastatic (commonly breast or lung) bone lesions, or by the action of paraneoplastic-hormone-like substances.
- The severity of symptoms depends on the rate of increase of calcium, with more-acute hypercalcaemia causing worse symptoms for a given level of serum calcium.
- CNS symptoms range from lethargy and weakness to coma. Polyuria and renal impairment occur, along with gastrointestinal disturbance (nausea, vomiting, constipation and abdominal pain).
- The diagnosis is made by measuring the serum ionised calcium. The ionised calcium can be calculated from the total serum calcium (Ca):

$$\text{corrected Ca (in mmol/L)} = \text{serum Ca} + [0.02 \times (40 - \text{serum albumin (in g/L)})]$$

- Hypokalaemia is common. The patient may be significantly dehydrated and have renal impairment.

Management

1. Hydration with oral fluids or normal saline is the initial step in treatment, and may be sufficient in mild cases.

2 Once dehydration has been corrected, diuretics may be used to promote calciuria.
3 Bisphosphonates (pamidronate 90 mg infusion over 4–24 hours or zolendronate 1–4 mg over not less than 15 minutes) can be used to reduce the calcium level further.

SUPERIOR VENA CAVA (SVC) OBSTRUCTION

The SVC may be obstructed by compression, infiltration or thrombosis, and this is usually a complication of malignancy (particularly lung, breast or testicular cancer or lymphoma). Occasionally it occurs as a complication of a central venous catheter (CVC), or from a benign lesion such as a goitre, constrictive pericarditis or aortic aneurysm.

- Symptoms and signs are more prominent when the patient is supine, including periorbital and facial oedema (also trunk, arms), shortness of breath (SOB), cough, chest pain and dysphagia.
- On examination there may be neck vein distension, facial plethora and cyanosis, along with tachypnoea.

Investigations

- An important differential diagnosis is pericardial tamponade. A bedside ultrasound scan can rule out an effusion.
- Chest X-ray usually reveals a mass in the mediastinum, which may be accompanied by pulmonary lesions or a pleural effusion.

Management

1 Treatment is directed at the tumour and involves radiotherapy or chemotherapy.
2 Elevating the head of the bed can alleviate some symptoms. Corticosteroids may be useful if the tumour is sensitive.
3 SVC stenting is a further treatment option.

TUMOUR LYSIS SYNDROME

This occurs within days of commencing treatment for sensitive tumours, although it may occur spontaneously. Rapid cell death releases products of cell breakdown into the circulation, leading to hyperuricaemia, hyperkalaemia, hyperphosphataemia and hypocalcaemia. Renal failure and metabolic acidosis may develop. It most frequently complicates haematological malignancies and small-cell lung cancer.

The clinical manifestations include neuromuscular cramps, tetany and arrhythmias. Oliguria and acute renal failure may develop from uric acid precipitation in the renal tubules.

Management

1 Initial treatment is hydration with normal saline and treatment of hyperkalaemia.
2 Urinary alkalinisation (50–100 mg $NaHCO_3$/L fluid, urine pH > 7) is of benefit in hyperuricaemia; however, in the presence of hyperphosphataemia and hypocalcaemia, alkali therapy can exacerbate symptoms.
3 Once adequate hydration has been established, diuretics may be added to maintain a high urine output.
4 Severe cases complicated by acute renal failure may require dialysis.

HYPERVISCOSITY

Very high white blood cell (WBC) counts (> 100 × 10^9/L) associated with haematological malignancies (acute leukaemias, chronic myeloid leukaemia (CML)) cause increased blood viscosity, which impairs flow in the microcirculation. The cerebral and pulmonary circulations are particularly susceptible. Hyperviscosity syndrome also occurs with high levels of paraproteinaemia, especially with immunoglobulin M (IgM) paraproteins, such as in Waldenstrom's macroglobulinaemia.

- Impaired cerebral circulation causes headache, dizziness, confusion, seizures and visual disturbance. The fundi show venous engorgement and haemorrhages.
- Cardiopulmonary consequences include angina, dyspnoea, myocardial infarction and cardiac failure.
- There may be bleeding from mucosal surfaces.

Management

1 Treatment begins with hydration.
2 Patients should be referred for leukapheresis or plasmapheresis.

HIV infection

Patients with HIV infection most commonly present with complications of immunosuppression and its treatment. With the improved prognosis of HIV in the era of highly active antiretroviral treatment (HAART), patients increasingly present with medical or surgical conditions unrelated to HIV and, while their treatment may be complicated by their HIV, their outcome and survival may be excellent.

PRIMARY HIV INFECTION

Within 1–6 weeks of infection (sometimes up to 12 weeks), 50–70% of patients develop a symptomatic illness. In most cases this is mild to moderate in severity and does not usually present to the ED.

- The seroconversion illness can resemble infectious mononucleosis.
- Patients develop fever, fatigue, anorexia, headache, nausea and vomiting.
- Myalgias and arthralgias, a non-exudative pharyngitis, rashes and diarrhoea are common.
- Severe cases may develop meningism or encephalitis.

Investigations

The differential diagnosis is wide, so investigations should include FBC, UEC, LFTs and monospot, along with serology for CMV, EBV, hepatitis and syphilis. In those with a recent high-risk exposure it is important to think of the diagnosis. In more severe cases, immunosuppression may be profound and the seroconversion illness may be complicated by an opportunistic infection. Not uncommonly, other sexually transmitted infections (STIs) may occur at the same time and should be screened for.

Current HIV-1 antibody tests are usually positive by 2 weeks after the onset of symptoms (4 weeks after exposure), but earlier-generation enzyme immunoassay (EIA) tests may be negative or give indeterminate results.

Prior to antibody responses the virus can be detected by direct detection of viral p24 antigen or, in some centres, by nucleic acid amplification tests such as proviral DNA tests. Assays of plasma HIV-1 RNA used for monitoring HIV infection may pick up the presence of virus prior to the production of antibodies in this early stage of the infection; however, they have a substantial false positive rate in low seroprevalence settings and can give a false negative result with certain strains of the virus. Therefore this test should not be used diagnostically.

Management

During the first 6 months of HIV infection, there is uncontrolled viral replication and destruction of CD4+ T-cells. Presentation with a severe seroconversion illness is associated with faster disease progression. There are ongoing trials of antiretroviral treatment in early HIV infection with the goal of controlling viral replication and slowing T-cell decline; however, antiretroviral therapy in primary HIV infection is not routinely recommended. Patients should be referred to a specialist in HIV medicine early, particularly those with symptomatic seroconversion.

Patients should also receive risk-reduction counselling as, with the high levels of virus circulating in these patients, they are highly infectious and likely to pass on the infection to others.

OPPORTUNISTIC INFECTIONS (OIs)

- A wide range of OIs affect HIV patients once their CD4+ cell counts decline. Information that helps narrow the differential diagnosis includes a recent CD4+ count and viral load, use of antiretrovirals and prophylaxis.
- The knowledge of previous serology for infections such as CMV and toxoplasmosis is very useful, as presentations with OIs most often represent recrudescence of previously controlled latent infections.
- Patients presenting for the first time with late-stage disease, or those that have not sought medical care, may present with multiple opportunistic infections simultaneously. This should be considered in the diagnostic work-up.
- Bacterial infections are common in HIV patients, and bacterial sepsis is a more frequent cause of ICU admission than *Pneumocystis jiroveci (carinii)* pneumonia (PCP; see below). Sources include pneumonia, catheter-related infections, orthopaedic and soft-tissue infections, urinary tract infections (UTIs) and bacteraemia of unknown aetiology.

PULMONARY INFECTIONS

The incidence of HIV-associated pneumonia changed with the use of HAART, with bacterial pneumonia becoming increasingly common. Pneumonia in HIV patients is more often bacterial than due to an opportunistic agent, and is 10 times more common in HIV patients than in non-HIV patients. The common community-acquired bacteria are the usual culprits, with most pneumonia being caused by *S. pneumoniae*, *H. influenzae* and *S. aureus*.

PCP (*Pneumocystis jiroveci (carinii)* pneumonia)

Since the introduction of HAART in 1996, the incidence of PCP as an AIDS-defining illness has declined, although it remains the most frequent serious opportunistic infection. The disease occurs in patients with a CD4+ count below 200 cells/microL, particularly when antibiotics prophylaxis has not been used.

Fever, cough and shortness of breath are the usual presenting symptoms of PCP. The respiratory examination may reveal few signs other than tachypnoea and accessory muscle use. Oxygen saturations are often reduced and severe cases may be cyanosed at presentation.

Investigations

- Chest X-ray typically reveals bilateral diffuse reticular or granular opacities. The extent of these changes may be less than expected by the degree of hypoxaemia.
- Arterial blood gas analysis assists in grading severity and planning treatment.
  - Mild to moderate cases have an arterial partial oxygen pressure (PaO_2) of > 70 mmHg on room air (A–a gradient < 35 mmHg, or O_2 saturations > 94% on room air)
  - Severe cases have a PaO_2 of < 70 mmHg on room air (A–a gradient > 35 mmHg, or O_2 saturations < 94% on room air).

Diagnosis

A provisional diagnosis is made on clinical findings and chest X-ray. Definitive diagnosis requires direct visualisation of *Pneumocystis* cysts or trophic forms from respiratory specimens (induced sputum or broncho-alveolar lavage).

Management

1. Trimethoprim-sulfamethoxazole is the treatment of choice for mild to moderate PCP, in oral doses of 5 mg/kg + 25 mg/kg to 7 mg/kg + 35 mg/kg 8-hourly for 21 days.
   - If sulfamethoxazole is contraindicated, clindamycin 450 mg 8-hourly plus primaquine 15 mg daily may be used.
   - Dapsone 100 mg PO daily with trimethoprim 300 mg PO 8-hourly is a further alternative.
   - Patients who are also intolerant of trimethoprim or clindamycin can be treated with atovaquone 750 mg PO 12-hourly.
2. Severe disease is treated with intravenous trimethoprim-sulfamethoxazole 5 mg/kg + 25 mg/kg IV 6-hourly for 21 days.
   - Patients who are intolerant of or unresponsive to this may be treated with IV pentamidine 4 mg/kg up to 300 mg daily, or clindamycin 900 mg IV 8-hourly with primaquine 30 mg PO daily.
3. Pulmonary inflammation contributes to lung injury in PCP, so corticosteroids are given in severe disease. Prednisolone is

given at 40 mg PO 12-hourly for 5 days, then 40 mg daily for 5 days, then 20 mg daily for 11 days.

4 Antibiotic cover for community-acquired pneumonia may be added, particularly when the patient has purulent sputum.
5 Non-invasive positive-pressure ventilation is indicated in the non-obtunded patient with hypoxaemic respiratory failure, and it may avert the need for mechanical ventilation. Unless there are clear contraindications to intubation, such as end-stage malignancy or dementia, intubation and ventilation are appropriate in the patient with severe respiratory failure, as the prognosis from a first episode of PCP is good. Recurrent episodes may be complicated by cyst formation and pneumothorax.

TUBERCULOSIS (TB)

Worldwide, this is the most important HIV-associated opportunistic pneumonia. Reactivation or primary infection can occur at high CD4+ counts (> 400 cells/microL) and the disease becomes more common with declining counts. In the severely immunocompromised, extrapulmonary sites of infection are more frequent.

Presenting symptoms are cough, haemoptysis, fever, shortness of breath, sweats and weight loss. The onset is typically insidious. The diagnosis is more likely in patients from countries where *Mycobacterium tuberculosis* is endemic.

Investigations and diagnosis

Chest X-ray shows upper lobe cavitation or hilar adenopathy with diffuse infiltrates. Pleural effusions may be present. Miliary TB is uncommon in patients with poor cell-mediated immunity. Extrapulmonary manifestations or presentations are more common in patients with HIV infection.

Diagnosis remains difficult, as sputum microscopy is often negative, but PCR assays may be useful, though a negative result does not exclude the diagnosis. Fine-needle aspiration of extrapulmonary sites is often diagnostic.

Management

Treatment is specialised, involving multiple agents and complicated by interactions between antiretrovirals and antitubercular drugs. Early specialist referral is essential. If the diagnosis of open TB is considered likely, the patient must be isolated.

CENTRAL NERVOUS SYSTEM (CNS) INFECTIONS

A number of agents infect the CNS, causing the acute or subacute onset of seizures, headache, fever, neck stiffness, confusion or focal deficits. However, symptoms may be non-specific and space-occupying lesions may be present in the absence of clinical signs. Therefore, there should be a low threshold for the performance of a CT scan and/or lumbar puncture in patients with late-stage HIV infection. With the increasing longevity of these patients and the increased risk of vascular complications, cerebrovascular accident (CVA) should be included in the differential diagnosis of CNS presentations.

Cryptococcus neoformans

This fungus causes meningitis in patients with CD4+ counts below 100 cells/microL. Cryptococcal meningitis presents with the subacute onset of fever, headache, nausea and cranial nerve palsies.

Investigations

Lumbar puncture is diagnostic, with demonstration of the organism on India-ink staining or antigen testing. The CSF opening pressure is usually elevated.

Management

1. Treatment is with amphotericin B and flucytosine (seek expert consultation).
2. In cases with very high CSF pressures, urgent ophthalmology review is needed, as vision may be threatened.
3. Patients may need repeated lumbar punctures for CSF drainage.
4. Long-term prophylaxis is given with fluconazole (seek expert consultation).

Toxoplasma gondii

This protozoon is widespread in the community, but it rarely causes disease until CD4+ counts drop below 100 cells/microL. The incidence is decreased with prophylaxis with trimethoprim and sulfamethoxazole.

Presenting features are altered mental state, focal signs, headache, fever and seizures.

Investigations

The diagnosis is made by contrast CT, which shows ring-enhancing lesions.

Toxoplasma serology is supportive, and cerebral toxoplasmosis is very unlikely in a patient with negative serology. In this case the diagnosis is likely to be primary CNS lymphoma.

Management

1 Treatment is with sulfadiazine 1 g PO or IV 6-hourly *plus* oral pyrimethamine 50 mg loading dose then 25 mg daily, for 6 weeks.
   - Clindamycin 600 mg PO 8-hourly is used if the patient is hypersensitive to sulfonamides.
   - If sulfadiazine is used, folinic acid 20–25 mg/day should be added to reduce marrow toxicity.

2 Anticonvulsants should be started to prevent seizures.

3 The use of steroids is not recommended, unless the lesions are associated with substantial oedema and exerting significant mass effect.

AIDS dementia

Patients with the AIDS dementia complex exhibit a gradual decline in memory and/or psychomotor function, ataxia and personality changes. It may also present with signs of spinal cord myelopathy. The syndrome usually affects patients with CD4+ counts below 200 cells/microL but may occur earlier. Drugs, infections and metabolic derangements can exacerbate dementia in affected patients. CT scans of the brain show atrophy.

There is no specific treatment, although HAART may improve symptoms.

Progressive multifocal leucoencephalopathy (PML)

Progressive CNS infection with John Cunningham virus (JC virus) usually occurs in patients with CD4+ counts below 100 cells/microL. PML presents with seizures, focal weakness, cranial nerve palsies, visual field deficits, cerebellar signs and confusion.

Investigations

- CT scans are relatively insensitive and, while these may reveal focal hypodensities, they are often non-contributory.
- MRI usually shows characteristic white-matter changes with cortical sparing; the absence of these changes does not exclude the diagnosis, however.
- JC virus can be identified in CSF by PCR, but this test is offered only in specialist laboratories.

Management

HAART may improve symptoms; however, there is no specific treatment.

GASTROINTESTINAL (GI) TRACT INFECTIONS

Candidiasis

Candida albicans frequently affects the oropharynx and/or the oesophagus, to an extent that is unusual in immunocompetent patients. Oesophageal candidiasis presents with oropharyngeal or retrosternal pain, dysphagia or odynophagia. There may be bleeding. White plaques with underlying erythema cover the affected areas.

Management

1 While simple oral candida will respond to topical treatment with amphotericin or nystatin solutions or lozenges, oesophageal involvement requires systemic treatment with fluconazole 200–400 mg PO daily for 14–21 days or, occasionally, itraconazole 200 mg PO daily for 14 days.
2 Resistant cases may be treated with voriconazole or posaconazole.
3 Fluconazole may be used for secondary prophylaxis or maintenance therapy.

Cyclospora, Isospora, Cryptosporidium parvum

These may all cause chronic diarrhoea. *Cryptosporidium* is less common since the advent of HAART. These infections should be considered in those presenting with chronic gastrointestinal symptoms, especially if resistant to therapy. The disease is often refractory to treatment.

Bacterial infections

Campylobacter jejuni, Salmonella or *Shigella* infections occur with increased frequency and severity of manifestations compared with the non-HIV-infected population. They may be more resistant to treatment than the uninfected population.

Viral hepatitis

A significant number of HIV patients, particularly those who are intravenous drug users, are also infected with hepatitis B or C. Antiretroviral drugs may worsen hepatic dysfunction and fluctuating immune function may be associated with flares of viral hepatitis. The treatment of hepatitis in the HIV patient is complex, and early specialist referral is essential.

SYSTEMIC INFECTIONS

Herpes simplex

Severe mucocutaneous infections occur more frequently than disseminated infection. These may be in the form of chronic, aggressive, poorly healing perianal ulcers.

Management

Treatment is with:

- famciclovir 1500 mg PO as a single dose
  OR
- valaciclovir 2 g PO 12-hourly for 1 day
  OR
- aciclovir 400 mg PO 5 times daily for 5 days.

These drugs may be used as suppressive therapy to prevent frequent recurrences.

Herpes zoster virus (HZV)

Recurrent HZV infections are often an early indicator of progressive CD4+ T-cell depletion. Infections remain dermatomal despite severe immunosuppression, though the extent of blistering may be severe and haemorrhagic. CNS infections with herpes viruses should be considered in the differential diagnosis of an encephalitic picture.

Cytomegalovirus (CMV)

Opportunistic CMV infection affects patients with CD4+ counts below 50 cells/microL.

- CMV retinitis presents with floaters, decreasing acuity and field loss. Fundoscopy reveals peripheral flame haemorrhages and exudates. However, the retinal lesions are often very peripheral and so can be missed. Dilation of the pupil and ophthalmological review are required to exclude diagnosis.
- Any part of the GI tract may be involved, with colitis, oesophagitis and gastritis being common presentations.
- CNS involvement causes encephalopathy and a polyradiculopathy.
- Interstitial pneumonitis is rare in HIV, in contrast to solid-organ transplant recipients.
- CMV adrenalitis presents with symptomatic adrenal insufficiency, hyponatraemia or hyperkalaemia.

Investigations

Detection of CMV RNA or DNA by nucleic acid testing in plasma or CSF is an aid to diagnosis. The presence of the classical inclusion bodies on biopsy of involved tissue is required for a definitive diagnosis of GI tract disease or pneumonitis.

Management

CMV is usually treated with valganciclovir, ganciclovir and, in problematical or resistant cases, foscarnet or cidofovir with probenecid. A specialist in HIV medicine should be consulted, along with urgent ophthalmology review in cases of suspected retinitis.

Mycobacterium avium–intracellulare complex (MAC)

This occurs in patients with CD4+ counts below 50 cells/microL. The incidence has decreased with the use of HAART and azithromycin prophylaxis. It presents as a systemic infection with fever, weight loss, night sweats, neutropenia, anaemia and lymphadenopathy. The diagnosis is made by blood culture.

Management

Treatment is with ethambutol plus either clarithromycin or azithromycin, with consideration of the addition of rifabutin in severely immunocompromised patients.

Malignancy in HIV/AIDS

HAART has changed the epidemiology of AIDS-related malignancies.

- The incidence of **non-Hodgkin's lymphoma** has declined, especially primary CNS lymphoma (seen in patients with profound immunosuppression and CD4+ counts below 50 cells/microL). Most still present with advanced disease (extranodal, meningeal, GI tract and bone marrow disease are common) and B symptoms (fever, night sweats, weight loss). There has been improved survival with combination chemotherapy and HAART.
- **Kaposi's sarcoma** has also become much less common over the last decade. This malignancy is associated with infection with human herpes virus 8 and occurs with CD4+ counts less than 300 cells/microL.
  - Skin involvement usually presents as painless, hyperpigmented purple nodules or plaques, but in pressure areas these may become painful and/or ulcerate. Especially in later disease, lesions may be more systemic, and be associated with lymphatic obstruction in the limbs and also involve the

oropharynx, GI tract (causing pain, ulceration, obstruction, bleeding or perforation).
- Involvement of the lung (with pleural effusion, pulmonary infiltrates or hilar adenopathy) is a poor prognostic sign.
- Treatment consists of antiretrovirals in early stage disease, with chemotherapy in advanced disease. Systemic involvement, especially of the lung, is resistant to intervention.

Cervical cancer remains a common problem in HIV-infected women, with no impact on the disease from antiretrovirals. Treatment is as for the immunocompetent patient.

Human papilloma virus (HPV) infection may also cause premalignant and malignant changes in the rectum of HIV-infected men who have sex with men (MSM).

Non-AIDS-defining malignancies are becoming more common with increasing longevity.

Immune reconstitution inflammatory syndrome (IRIS)

With the widespread use of HAART in HIV/AIDS, complications arise from the recovering immune system directing an inflammatory response against antigens associated with infectious agents.

IRIS presents as worsening signs or symptoms of infection in late-stage patients (< 100 CD4+ cells/microL at commencement of therapy) who have recently commenced antiretroviral therapy (ART). It usually manifests within 4 weeks, and may begin within days, although occasionally it develops after months of treatment. Patients with very low CD4+ cell counts (< 50/microL) and high pathogen loads are at highest risk.

The opportunistic infections most commonly associated with IRIS are MAC, CMV, HZV and fungi such as *Cryptococcus*. Worldwide, TB is the most common cause, with up to one-third of late-stage patients developing IRIS after starting ART. It occurs more frequently when HAART is given in the presence of an untreated infection. For this reason ART is usually not commenced in the presence of a known opportunistic infection. Commencement of ART is usually delayed until the active infection is cleared or the patient has commenced maintenance suppressive or prophylactic therapy.

IRIS often represents a diagnostic dilemma, as the presentation is often non-specific and atypical. The differential diagnosis includes a new opportunistic infection or drug toxicity. The diagnosis is essentially one of exclusion.

PCP-associated IRIS presents with a worsening of respiratory status and occasionally unmasks clinically silent PCP. MAC- or CMV-associated IRIS presents with fevers, lymphadenopathy and systemic symptoms. CMV may present with worsening of retinitis which may result in the permanent loss of sight.

MANAGEMENT

- Prevention of IRIS by commencing ART before CD4+ T-cell counts are very low, and screening for infection with treatment before initiating ART, is preferable.
- Treatment of IRIS involves supportive care with cessation of ART in severe cases. Corticosteroids may be used to blunt the inflammatory response.

Antiretroviral drugs

The introduction of HAART, combination therapy with 3 or 4 antiretroviral drugs, has led to improvements in morbidity and mortality in HIV/AIDS, decreased transmission and increased quality of life. Patients often have restoration of their immune function and a fall in viral load to undetectable levels.

The main classes of antiretrovirals are nucleoside reverse transcriptase inhibitors, non-nucleoside reverse transcriptase inhibitors and protease inhibitors. More recently, 2 types of entry inhibitors (fusion inhibitors and chemokine (C–C motif) receptor 5 (CCR5)-blockers) have been licensed. In addition, the first drug in a potent new class of antiretrovirals, the integrase inhibitors, has been licensed for use. Specific inhibitors include:

- nucleoside reverse transcriptase inhibitors: abacavir, didanosine, emtricitabine, lamivudine, stavudine, tenofovir, zidovudine
- non-nucleoside reverse transcriptase inhibitors: efavirenz, nevirapine
- protease inhibitors: atazanavir, fosamprenavir, indinavir, lopinavir, ritonavir, saquinavir, darunavir, tipranavir
- fusion inhibitor: T20/enfuvirtide which is given as an injection
- CCR5 inhibitors: maraviroc
- integrase inhibitors: raltegravir.

Indinavir is now rarely used. The others are usually used in combination with low-dose ritonavir (which is a protease inhibitor) and also a cytochrome P450 inhibitor which increases drug levels of the protease inhibitors. It allows the doses of the protease inhibitors to be reduced.

DRUG TOXICITIES

Lactic acidosis

- Nucleoside/nucleotide reverse transcriptase inhibitors (notably didanosine and stavudine) can cause lactic acidosis via mitochondrial toxicity. Patients with a reduced creatinine clearance and lower CD4+ counts are at higher risk.
- The severity ranges from asymptomatic acidaemia to a life-threatening syndrome. Abdominal pain and distension, nausea and vomiting are common, along with myalgias, peripheral neuropathy, dyspnoea and hepatic steatosis with raised transaminases.
- Cessation of drugs may lead to resolution, or there may be progressive multisystem involvement and respiratory and circulatory failure.
- Initial lactate levels higher than 5 mmol/L may be life-threatening.

Management

1. Treatment involves cessation of ART and supportive care.
2. Riboflavin, L-carnitine and thiamine may reverse toxicity.
3. In severe cases, bicarbonate therapy and haemodialysis may be needed.

Hypersensitivity reactions

Rashes are common in HIV patients, and are often minor and self-limiting and do not mandate cessation of therapy. Non-nucleoside reverse transcriptase inhibitors and antibiotics (especially trimethoprim-sulfamethoxazole) are frequent causes. The more serious Stevens–Johnson syndrome is also associated with these drugs, with widespread rash and blistering, mucosal involvement and fever.

Abacavir is associated with a life-threatening hypersensitivity syndrome, usually beginning in the first 10–14 days of treatment, with rash, fever, nausea, vomiting and abdominal pain. Patients may develop interstitial pneumonitis, hypotension and respiratory failure. The cause of this is now known to be strongly linked to the carriage of HLA-B5701. All patients being considered for abacavir therapy should be screened for the carriage of this HLA allele prior to commencement.

Nevirapine is a cause of fulminant hepatitis upon initiation of therapy, particularly in men with a CD4+ count > 400 cells/microL or women with a CD4+ T-cell count > 200 cells/microL.

Management

For severe hypersensitivity reactions, all antiretrovirals (and other potential causes such as antibiotics or anticonvulsants) should be stopped and supportive care instituted.

Other toxicities

Many other antiretrovirals (particularly protease inhibitors) can cause hepatitis.

- Pancreatitis occurs with stavudine, didanosine and lopinavir/ritonavir.
- Renal colic and haematuria may occur with indinavir.
- Peripheral neuropathy, which is often painful, is associated with stavudine and didanosine.
- Myelosuppression occurs with zidovudine.

DRUG INTERACTIONS

Many drug interactions occur due to inhibition of the induction of the hepatic cytochrome P450 system. Of particular note are:

- increased sedative effects from midazolam (lorazepam is unaffected)
- decreased levels of methadone, causing narcotic withdrawal
- increased levels of norpethidine, the toxic metabolite of pethidine
- a disulfiram-like reaction with metronidazole
- increased cardiovascular effects of amiodarone, diltiazem, nifedipine and sildenafil.

Systemic levels of the more potent long-acting inhaled corticosteroids can be driven high enough to induce Cushing's syndrome. Short-acting low-dose inhaled steroids should be used in patients on ritonavir-boosted protease inhibitors.

CARDIOVASCULAR COMPLICATIONS

- Long-term ART is associated with metabolic and cardiovascular toxicities, dyslipidaemia, atherosclerosis, endothelial dysfunction and glucose intolerance with insulin resistance.
- Age-adjusted rates of coronary artery disease and myocardial infarction are elevated in HIV-positive men. The treatment of acute coronary syndromes is the same as in HIV-negative patients.

Post-exposure prophylaxis in HIV

Post-exposure prophylaxis (PEP) is the use of antiretrovirals to prevent seroconversion after potential exposure to HIV. PEP is effective when given less than 72 hours after exposure, although there is declining efficacy after 36 hours.

- In non-occupational exposures, the HIV status of the source is often unknown. Assessment of the risk of HIV transmission requires knowledge of the risk of transmission from the method of exposure and the risk of the source being HIV-positive.
- High-risk exposures include receptive anal intercourse (1/120), sharing contaminated injecting equipment (1/50), occupational needle-stick (1/333), receptive vaginal intercourse (1/1000) and insertive anal or vaginal intercourse (1/1000).
- Although case reports of transmission exist, the risk of transmission by oral intercourse, bites, exposure to intact mucous membranes or skin and community-acquired needle-stick is so low it is not measurable.
- The risk of the source of exposure being HIV-positive varies between populations.
  - In MSM (men who have sex with men), the estimated HIV rates are 14% in Sydney, 9% in Melbourne, 6% in Brisbane and 5% in Perth.
  - Australian intravenous drug users (IVDUs) have lower rates of infection than overseas cohorts, with an estimated prevalence of 1%. However, IVDUs who are also MSM have a 17% rate of HIV infection.
  - The HIV rate among heterosexuals (including sex workers) is 0.1%, unless the source is from sub-saharan Africa, where the estimated rate is 7%.

PROPHYLACTIC REGIMENS

- Choice of regimen:
  - If the risk of transmission equals or exceeds 1/1000, PEP with three drugs is indicated.
  - If the risk of transmission is between 1/1000 and 1/10,000, two-drug PEP is indicated.
  - PEP with two drugs is considered when the risk is between 1/10,000 and 1/15,000. PEP is not recommended in lower-risk exposures.
- Two-drug regimens use two nucleoside reverse transcriptase inhibitors, such as emtricitabine + tenofovir.
- Three-drug regimens use either two nucleoside reverse transcriptase inhibitors and a protease inhibitor, or three nucleoside reverse transcriptase inhibitors. An example of a three-drug regimen is tenofovir + emtricitabine + efavirenz.

- Treatment duration is 28 days.
- Baseline blood testing should be performed, including FBC, LFTs, and serology for HIV and hepatitis B and C. Screening for other sexually transmitted diseases may be undertaken at the first follow-up appointment, which should be within the next few days.
- Some patients require emergency contraception, immunisation for hepatitis B and tetanus immunisation.
- The need for safe behaviour to avoid further exposure and potential transmission should be emphasised.
- Repeat courses of PEP are safe and should be given as indicated.
- The use of PEP does not increase the rate of high-risk exposures.

Solid-organ transplants

The immunosuppression required for the survival of transplanted organs leaves the recipient prone to infections, which are a leading cause of mortality.

- Infections are caused by a broad spectrum of pathogens and there may be minimal signs and symptoms at presentation, followed by rapid deterioration.
- Non-infectious causes of fever (rejection, malignancy and drugs) are common in the transplant population.
- The likely cause of infection varies with the length and intensity of immunosuppression.
- The likely exposures to infection vary with the time post-transplant, with donor- or hospital-acquired infections common in the early postoperative period, and opportunistic and community-acquired infections emerging later. Patients may have had vaccinations and chemoprophylaxis.
- The unwell transplant patient may present with non-specific symptoms or fever alone.

EXAMINATION AND INVESTIGATIONS

- Examination should include a thorough search for sites of infection, including the skin, mouth and retina. A specific diagnosis may be elusive.
- Urine, sputum and blood should be sent for culture, along with blood for serology.
- Any lesions should be swabbed.
- A chest X-ray is indicated in most cases.

MANAGEMENT

It is vital that the transplant team be involved in the patient's management as early as possible. Antibiotic therapy should be broad-spectrum; however, there are multiple potential interactions with immunosuppressive drugs. Macrolides are generally contraindicated.

INFECTIONS IN THE EARLY POST-TRANSPLANT PERIOD

Within the 1st month after transplant, most infections are not opportunistic. Subclinical infections suffered by the donor can be transmitted to the patient (this is uncommon and is most often a viral infection). The patient is often colonised with microbes such as MRSA, *Pseudomonas* and fungi preoperatively, and the induction of immunosuppression can precipitate clinical disease.

Injury to the transplanted organ from ischaemia and reperfusion can give rise to a site for infection, such as in the bile ducts or lung. Wounds, intravascular catheters and drains provide further sites of potential infection. The transplanted kidney is prone to pyelonephritis, the liver to abscesses, wound infections and cholangitis and the heart/lung to mediastinitis and pneumonia. These postoperative infections are mostly bacterial and may be resistant to antibiotics.

INTERMEDIATE PERIOD INFECTIONS

Unusual and opportunistic infections emerge in the 2nd to 6th months following transplantation.

- CMV can present as a systemic infection or as a pneumonitis. Nucleic acid testing (NAT) for CMV is used to detect CMV replication, allowing the diagnosis of subclinical infection and commencement of pre-emptive treatment according to standard protocols.
- Pneumonia may be caused by a wide range of pathogens. Most cases are bacterial, but *Pneumocystis, Legionella, Aspergillus, Nocardia* and viruses also occur.
- Reactivation of latent tuberculosis can occur, often leading to disseminated disease.
- HSV is the most frequent cause of CNS disease. *Listeria, Cryptococcus, Toxoplasma* and JC virus are other causes.
- The GI tract may be infected with CMV or *Clostridium difficile.*
- It is important to note that graft rejection also presents with fever, as do some drug reactions.

Prophylaxis has led to decreasing incidences of PCP, HSV, CMV, *Listeria, Nocardia* and toxoplasmosis. The duration of prophylaxis varies between centres.

Management

- Trimethoprim-sulfamethoxazole is used to prevent PCP, *Toxoplasma, Nocardia, Listeria* and common urinary, respiratory and gastrointestinal pathogens.
- Oral antiviral agents are used against CMV and HSV.

LATE INFECTIONS

After 6 months post-transplant, the risk of infection declines as immunosuppression is tapered off. Patients with rejection requiring ongoing high levels of immunosuppression will remain at risk of opportunistic infections; however, the majority of infections will be community-acquired diseases such as pneumonia. Patients are at increased risk from intracellular pathogens like *Listeria, Nocardia* and fungi.

Chronic viral infection may cause insidious graft injury. Recurrent disease may occur in patients who have received transplants for HCV. Renal transplants may become infected by the BK polyomavirus, causing declining graft function.

Long-term immunosuppression increases the risk of malignancy. Skin and anogenital cancers are the most common. Post-transplant lymphoproliferative disease can also develop. This has a spectrum of presentations, from an infectious mononucleosis-like illness to lymphoma.

GRAFT-SPECIFIC PROBLEMS

Acute rejection presents with systemic symptoms, including fever, along with signs of organ insufficiency. Chronic rejection develops over years, with gradual organ failure.

Heart

- The transplanted heart is denervated, the loss of vagal stimulation leading to a baseline tachycardia of 100–110 bpm. Catecholamines and antihypertensive drugs are effective in these patients, although atropine will be ineffective.
- Myocardial ischaemia is painless, presenting as chronic cardiac failure (CCF), arrhythmias, hypotension or syncope.
- Atherosclerosis is accelerated in organs with chronic rejection.
- Routine biopsy detects most cases of rejection at an early, asymptomatic phase. More-advanced rejection manifests as CCF, arrhythmias and low QRS voltages on the ECG.

Liver

- Rejection presents with fever, right upper quadrant pain and tenderness, jaundice and elevations in transaminases.
- Biliary obstruction, wound infections and cholangitis are common postoperative complications.

Kidney

- Rejection presents with fever, pelvic swelling, pain and tenderness and decreased urine output.
- Chronic rejection takes the form of nephrosclerosis, with hypertension and declining renal function.
- The kidney may be injured in trauma to the pelvis.

Lung

- Rejection presents in a similar way to infection, with fever, shortness of breath, cough and hypoxia, with infiltrates on chest X-ray.
- Chronic rejection causes bronchiolitis obliterans.

Pancreas

Drainage of exocrine secretions into the bladder predisposes to UTI, haematuria and chronic non-anion-gap acidosis (due to bicarbonate loss).

DRUG TOXICITY

Newer immunosuppression regimens using sirolimus, mycophenolate mofetil, T-cell and B-cell depletion and co-stimulatory blockade have largely replaced high-dose steroids and azathioprine.

- Corticosteroids cause decreased mobilisation and function of neutrophils, monocytes and lymphocytes.
  - There is increased susceptibility to pyogenic bacteria due to depressed leucocyte activity at sites of inflammation. These patients may have diminished clinical signs of peritonitis.
  - Patients are also at higher risk of severe infections with HSV and varicella zoster virus (VZV). The risk of infection increases with lengthy treatment and doses of > 20 mg/day (e.g. of prednisone).
  - Corticosteroids may mask fever and chronic use causes adrenal suppression. Consideration should be given to Addisonian symptoms in those on chronic corticosteroids and to increasing doses of corticosteroids in acute deterioration to ensure sufficient coverage.

- Cyclosporin suppresses cellular and humoral immunity. It has a number of adverse effects including nephrotoxicity, hypertension, hyperuricaemia and seizures, along with multiple interactions with drugs and food.
- Azathioprine is associated with neutropenia.
- Mycophenolate generally has few side effects. It may cause gastrointestinal disturbance, leucopenia and thrombocytopenia.
- Sirolimus causes an idiosyncratic non-infectious pneumonitis which resembles PCP or viral pneumonia.
- Tacrolimus may lead to nephrotoxicity, neurotoxicity, hyperglycaemia or hyperkalaemia.
- T-cell-depleting antibodies can cause fever, hypotension and pulmonary oedema, along with reactivation of viruses such as CMV and EBV.

Early discussion with the specialist caring for the patient is recommended in cases of suspected drug reactions.

Immunosuppression for non-malignant disease

Newer immunosuppressive agents with lower toxicities have led to an expansion in the use of immunosuppression for non-malignant disease, widening the population at risk of opportunistic infection. Patients with autoimmune disease, multiple sclerosis and inflammatory bowel disease may be sufficiently immunocompromised to present with similar infections to the patient with HIV, malignancy or solid-organ transplant.

Rituximab is a monoclonal antibody that depletes B cells and is used in the treatment of autoimmune diseases and haematological malignancies. Patients are susceptible to infections related to poor humoral immunity. Rituximab can cause infusional reactions due to antibodies to monoclonal components. These may be acute or delayed. The delayed reaction is a serum sickness-like illness, with fever, arthritis and rash, which is treated with steroids.

Tumour necrosis factor inhibitors, infliximab and etanercept, are used in rheumatoid arthritis and inflammatory bowel disease. There is increased susceptibility to tuberculosis and bacterial sepsis.

In addition to these agents, corticosteroids, cyclosporin, azathioprine, mycophenolate and cytotoxic drugs such as cyclophosphamide and methotrexate are used in the treatment of autoimmune diseases.

Asplenia

Asplenia may result from trauma, splenectomy for idiopathic thrombocytopenia (ITP), lymphoma or haematological malignancy, autosplenectomy in sickle-cell disease or functional asplenia in haematological disease, sarcoid, amyloid or autoimmune disease.

Patients without a functioning spleen are predisposed to overwhelming sepsis with pneumococcus and other encapsulated bacteria. The risk is highest in the first few years after splenectomy. Early intervention in any septic presentation is essential.

Pneumococcal vaccine is routinely given; however response may be diminished in patients with severe underlying disease. Vaccinations for *Haemophilus influenzae* type B, influenza and meningococcus are also given, and patients take penicillin or macrolide prophylaxis for 2–5 years.

Chapter 43
Emergency department haematology

F X Luis Winoto, Rebecca Walsh
and Anthony J Dodds

Common haematological emergencies
NEUTROPENIC SEPSIS

(Also see Chapter 42, 'The immunocompromised patient'.)
Severe neutropenia is defined as a neutrophil count of $< 0.5 \times 10^9$/L, but severe sepsis is unusual until the neutrophil count is $< 0.2 \times 10^9$/L.

Causes for severe neutropenia include cancer chemotherapy drugs, agranulocytosis (an idiosyncratic reaction to an otherwise non-marrow-suppressive drug) and haematological disorders causing marrow failure (acute and chronic leukaemias, myeloma, lymphoma, aplastic anaemia, etc).

Patients presenting with a fever above 38°C require urgent investigation and therapy.

Investigations

- Investigations should be directed to possible sites of infection; however, local sites are detected in fewer than 50% of such patients.
- Suggested investigations include chest X-ray, blood cultures and urine culture.
- If there is a central line, cultures through this line are also important.

Management

- Therapy with broad-spectrum antibiotics should not be withheld while investigations are being performed.
- Gram-negative infections usually arising from the gut are the commonest causes but, in the presence of a central venous catheter, treatment of possible Gram-positive skin organisms should also be considered.
- Most institutions have an approved protocol to treat such patients:

— Usually a broad-spectrum 3rd-generation cephalosporin or piperacillin and tazobactam is combined with gentamicin until *Pseudomonas* has been excluded.
— If the fever does not respond to this after 48 hours or a central venous catheter is present, then additional anti-staphylococcal therapy is added.

SEVERE THROMBOCYTOPENIA AND BLEEDING

Severe spontaneous bleeding with thrombocytopenia is not usually a problem until the platelet count is less than 10×10^9/L. When patients present with bleeding secondary to thrombocytopenia, an urgent assessment of the cause of the thrombocytopenia is necessary.

Differential diagnosis

1 Marrow failure, e.g. chemotherapy drugs, haematological malignancy, etc. Such patients usually have a pancytopenia and a history of being given marrow-suppressive therapy. Urgent platelet transfusion is indicated.
2 Peripheral destruction of platelets.
  — This may be an autoimmune disorder (immune thrombocytopenic purpura, ITP) or less commonly an immune drug-related disorder. Heparin is a common drug cause for immune thrombocytopenia.
  — Patients presenting with ITP may have no preceding history and have isolated thrombocytopenia.
  — The disorder may be post-viral and reversible in children but commonly chronic in adults.
  — If there is any doubt about the diagnosis, a marrow biopsy is indicated. This will show a normal marrow with plentiful megakaryocytes.
  — **Treatment:** urgent corticosteroids (prednisolone 1 mg/kg PO daily) are indicated for ITP with severe thrombocytopenia, especially with bleeding. Platelet transfusion is usually not given in immune thrombocytopenia unless in the presence of bleeding and is contraindicated in heparin-induced thrombocytopenia.
3 Disseminated intravascular coagulation (DIC). DIC can occur with malignancy or severe sepsis. Treatment is aimed at the underlying cause rather than treating by platelet transfusion alone.

SICKLE-CELL DISEASE

Sickle-cell disease (SCD) is an inherited disorder due to homozygosity for abnormal haemoglobin. SCD can produce a wide spectrum of manifestations and patients may present with life-threatening complications such as vaso-occlusive crisis, stroke, aplastic crisis, acute chest syndrome and sepsis.

Acute painful crisis

This is the most common manifestation of SCD requiring hospitalisation. It is caused by vaso-occlusion of the vasculature by the abnormal sickled red cells. This can be spontaneous or precipitated by infection, stressors or dehydration. The mainstay of management is adequate analgesia including opiates and adjuvant non-opiate analgesia.

The anaemic patient

Anaemia is defined as a reduced haemoglobin (Hb) concentration in the blood. The red cell mass and the plasma volume can affect this value, so both these factors must be considered when interpreting a single value. Thus, severe dehydration can produce an elevated Hb and increased plasma volume, such as in pregnancy, can produce a falsely low Hb.

The symptoms and signs of anaemia (pallor, fainting, lethargy and anorexia) are unreliable. Anaemia may be asymptomatic and detected only on a routine blood count. The cause of anaemia can be ascertained by a logical sequence of investigations as follows. This is based on the mean corpuscular volume (MCV), which is part of an automated blood count.

MICROCYTIC (NORMAL MCV)

Common causes:

- Iron deficiency—serum ferritin low
- Thalassaemia trait—serum ferritin normal or raised

NORMOCYTIC (NORMAL MCV)

Common causes:

- Anaemia of chronic disease—
  - — serum ferritin normal or raised
  - — serum iron low
  - — serum transferrin normal or low
  - — positive inflammatory markers (erythrocyte sedimentation rate (ESR), C-reactive protein (CRP)), e.g. chronic infection, neoplasm, renal failure

- Bone marrow disease—(usually pancytopenia), e.g. aplastic anaemia, marrow infiltration, marrow malignancy
  - acute blood loss
  - haemolysis—raised reticulocyte count, positive direct antiglobulin test in immune haemolytic anaemia, low serum haptoglobin level, raised serum bilirubin and lactate dehydrogenase (LDH) levels.

MACROCYTIC (RAISED MCV)

Common causes:

- Megaloblastosis—low serum B_{12} or red cell folate levels
- Secondary macrocytic anaemia, e.g. alcohol, liver disease, hypothyroidism, some marrow disorders, marked reticulocytosis

PRINCIPLES OF THERAPY

1. Establish the cause and treat.
2. Blood transfusion only indicated for:
   - acute anaemia with hypovolaemia
   - refractory anaemias (Hb < 80 g/L)
   - severe symptoms of anaemia, e.g. angina.
3. Most patients with anaemia do not need blood transfusion unless the Hb is < 80 g/L. Transfusion can be risky with severe compensated anaemia, especially in the elderly and those with cardiac disease.

The patient with abnormal bleeding

Screening haemostasis tests are not warranted or cost-effective in the absence of clinical signs or history to suggest a bleeding diathesis. The following are suggestive:

- family history of bleeding disorder
- past history of excessive bleeding with minor haemostatic insults, e.g. tooth extraction, minor surgery, minor trauma, childbirth
- excessive local bleeding without an obvious cause
- generalised bleeding or bruising.

The usual screening tests are:

- vascular or platelet disorder—platelet count (PC), platelet function tests
- coagulation disorder—prothrombin time (PT), activated partial thromboplastin time (APTT), thrombin time (TT).

The following is a guide to the interpretation of these tests.

PLATELET AND VASCULAR DEFECTS

Platelet count low

- Marrow failure, e.g. aplastic anaemia, malignancy
  or
- Peripheral destruction or sequestration, e.g. ITP, drug-induced immune thrombocytopenia, hypersplenism (splenomegaly), DIC.

Platelet count normal

- Primary platelet dysfunction
- Secondary platelet dysfunction, e.g. aspirin, uraemia

Table 43.1 Summary of the coagulation abnormalities seen in the commonly encountered acute conditions

Condition	PT	APTT	TT	PC	FDP
Severe liver disease	↑	↑	N or ↑	N or ↓	N or ↑
Heparin therapy	N	↑	↑	N	N
Coumarin (warfarin) therapy	↑	N	N	N	N
DIC	↑	↑	↑	↓	↑
Massive blood transfusion	↑	↑	N or ↑	↓	N

↑, prolonged/increased; ↓, decreased; APTT, activated partial thromboplastin time; DIC, disseminated intravascular coagulation; FDP, fibrin degradation products; N, normal; PC, platelet count; PT, prothrombin time; TT, thrombin time

COAGULATION DEFECTS

- PT prolonged, APTT prolonged, TT prolonged
  - Dissemination intravascular coagulation
  - Deficiency of fibrinogen (rarely)
  - New oral anticoagulation therapy—direct thrombin inhibitors (dabigatran etexilate)
- PT prolonged, APTT prolonged, TT normal
  - Severe liver disease
  - Lupus inhibitor
  - Congenital factor deficiencies (factor X, V, II or multiple)
  - New oral anticoagulation therapy—direct factor Xa inhibitors (rivaroxaban, apixaban)
- PT prolonged, APTT normal or slightly prolonged, TT normal
  - Oral anticoagulant (warfarin) therapy
  - Vitamin K deficiency
- PT normal, APTT prolonged, TT normal
  - Lupus inhibitor
  - Haemophilia (factor VIII or IX deficiency)
  - Other intrinsic pathway factor deficiency

Therapy

Specific therapy is usually only required if the patient is bleeding or an operative procedure is contemplated. Components available include:

1. fresh frozen plasma (FFP)—DIC, massive transfusion, liver disease
2. platelet concentrates—thrombocytopenia due to marrow failure
3. factor concentrates—Prothrombinex (freeze-dried concentrate of human blood coagulation factors II, IX and X) for reversal of warfarin therapy or specific factor concentrates for factor deficiencies.

Anticoagulant therapy

UNFRACTIONATED HEPARIN

Heparin inhibits coagulation at a number of sites, mainly via activation of antithrombin-III. Administration is usually via constant IV infusion.

- Monitoring: the APTT is the usual method. A baseline APTT should be established, repeated 4 hours after commencing heparin, then therapeutic interval checked with laboratory. A platelet count should be done every 2nd day.
- Reversal: for overdose or serious bleeding, stop the heparin and give protamine sulfate slowly IV (1 mg/100 units of heparin).
- Side effects: bleeding; thrombocytopenia–thrombosis (heparin-induced thrombotic thrombocytopenia syndrome (HITTS)).

LOW-MOLECULAR-WEIGHT HEPARINS

- These are often used for prophylaxis but are also commonly given for ambulatory full-dose therapy. They are usually given by subcutaneous injection.
- They have a much longer half-life than unfractionated heparin.
- They cannot be monitored by APTT testing and cannot be reversed by protamine sulfate.
- They cause less bleeding and less thrombocytopenia.

VITAMIN K ANTAGONISTS (E.G. WARFARIN)

- These are oral anticoagulants that inhibit synthesis of vitamin-K-dependent clotting factors (II, VII, IX, X plus protein C and protein S).
- International normalised ratio (INR) is a standardised prothrombin ratio and is used to monitor side effects: bleeding; rash; teratogenesis.

Surgery in patients receiving vitamin K antagonists

What to do will depend on the type of surgery and the reason for administering anticoagulants.

- For minor procedures (e.g. tooth extraction), therapy may not need to be ceased (see institutional protocols).
- For major procedures, it may be necessary to change to heparin if continuing anticoagulation is required (e.g. artificial heart valve).

Changing from heparin to vitamin K antagonists

When commencing vitamin K antagonists, the INR will begin to fall within 36 hours, but this only reflects factor VII levels. It is necessary to continue heparin at lower doses for at least a 3-day overlap when commencing oral anticoagulants.

Reversal

Fresh frozen plasma or Prothrombinex will acutely reverse the effect in bleeding patients. Vitamin K will act more slowly and permanently reverse the effect, but in large doses may make it more difficult to anticoagulate the patient again.

A protocol for the management of an elevated INR is shown in Figure 43.1.

NEW ORAL ANTICOAGULANTS

Recently several new oral anticoagulants have become available. These are dabigatran etexilate, a direct thrombin inhibitor, and rivaroxaban and apixaban, both direct factor Xa inhibitors.

In routine situations these agents don't need monitoring or dose adjusting. As yet, there are no standardised assays to monitor and assess these agents, which may be useful in an emergency situation when a patient is bleeding or there is suspicion of overdose. The APTT and ecarin clotting time may be useful in assessing dabigatran; and the PT, APTT and anti-Xa assays for assessing rivaroxaban and apixaban.

Reversal

A specific antidote to reverse these agents in a bleeding patient is not available. In the event of haemorrhagic complications with dabigatran, consideration may be given to the use of FFP, Prothrombinex, recombinant factor VIIa and dialysis. Prothrombinex may be useful in reversal of rivaroxaban. Consultation with a haematologist is also advisable in this situation.

St Vincent's Hospital
GUIDELINES FOR THE MANAGEMENT OF AN ELEVATED INTERNATIONAL NORMALISED RATIO (INR) IN ADULT PATIENTS WITH OR WITHOUT BLEEDING

Note:

- ***Prothrombinex-HT* can only be prescribed after consultation with a haematologist.**
- The anticoagulant effect of warfarin may be difficult to re-establish for some time after vitamin K is used. Use the lowest dose possible and, if possible, consult the treating specialist prior to using vitamin K.
- Small oral doses of vitamin K are obtained by measuring the dose from the injectable formulation and administering orally. Vitamin K effect on INR can be expected within 6–12 hours; however, the full effect of vitamin K in reducing the INR can take up to 24 hours.

Table 1 Guidelines for the management of an elevated international normalised ratio (INR) in adult patients with or without bleeding

Clinical setting	Action
INR higher than the therapeutic range but < 5; bleeding absent	Lower the dose or omit the next dose of warfarin. Resume therapy at a lower dose when the INR approaches therapeutic range. If the INR is only minimally above therapeutic range (up to 10%), dose reduction may not be necessary.
INR 5–9; bleeding absent	Cease warfarin therapy; consider reasons for elevated INR and patient-specific factors. Bleeding risk increases exponentially from INR 5 to 9; INR ≥ 6 should be monitored closely. If bleeding risk is high (see Table 2), give vitamin K (1–2 mg orally or 0.5–1 mg intravenously). See the notes above for further information about vitamin K. Measure INR within 24 hours and resume warfarin at a reduced dose once INR is in therapeutic range.
INR > 9; bleeding absent	Where there is a low risk of bleeding, cease warfarin therapy, give 2.5–5 mg vitamin K orally or 1 mg intravenously. Measure INR in 6–12 hours, resume warfarin therapy at a reduced dose once INR < 5.0. Where there is high risk of bleeding (see Table 2), cease warfarin therapy, give 1 mg vitamin K intravenously. Consider Prothrombinex-HT (25–50 IU/kg) and fresh frozen plasma (150–300 mL), measure INR in 6–12 hours, resume warfarin therapy at a reduced dose once INR < 5. ***Prothrombinex-HT* can only be prescribed after consultation with a haematologist.** See the notes above for further information about vitamin K.

Figure 43.1 St Vincent's Hospital guidelines for the management of an elevated INR in adult patients with or without bleeding (continues)
FFP, fresh frozen plasma; INR, international normalised ratio; PTX, Prothrombinex
Based on Tran HA, Chunilal SD, Harper PL et al, on behalf of the Australasian Society of Thrombosis and Haemostasis. An update of consensus guidelines for warfarin reversal. Med J Aust 2013;198(4):198–9

Clinical setting	Action
Any clinically significant bleeding where warfarin-induced coagulopathy is considered a contributing factor	Cease warfarin therapy, give 5–10 mg vitamin K intravenously, as well as Prothrombinex-HT (25–50 IU/kg) and fresh frozen plasma (150–300 mL), assess patient continuously until INR < 5, and bleeding stops. OR If fresh frozen plasma is unavailable, cease warfarin therapy, give 5–10 mg vitamin K intravenously, and Prothrombinex-HT (25–50 IU/kg), assess patient continuously until INR < 5, and bleeding stops. OR If Prothrombinex-HT is unavailable, cease warfarin therapy, give 5–10 mg vitamin K intravenously, and 10–15 mL/kg of fresh frozen plasma, assess patient continuously until INR < 5, and bleeding stops. Prothrombinex-HT can only be prescribed after consultation with a haematologist. In all situations carefully reassess the need for ongoing warfarin therapy.

Table 2 Risk factors for bleeding complications of anticoagulation therapy

Risk factor category	Specific risk factors
Age	> 65 years
Cardiac	Uncontrolled hypertension
Gastrointestinal	History of gastrointestinal haemorrhage, active peptic ulcer, hepatic insufficiency
Haematological/oncological	Thrombocytopenia (platelet count < 50 × 10^9/L), platelet dysfunction, coagulation defect, underlying malignancy
Neurological	History of stroke, cognitive or psychological impairment
Renal	Renal insufficiency
Trauma	Recent trauma, history of falls (> 3 within previous treatment year, or recurrent, injurious falls)
Alcohol	Excessive alcohol intake
Medications	Aspirin, non-specific non-steroidal anti-inflammatory drugs (COX-II inhibitors do not impair platelet function, but can influence warfarin effect), 'natural remedies' that interfere with haemostasis. Careful monitoring of warfarin effect is critical to minimise risk in patients taking multiple medications.

Figure 43.1 Continued

Blood transfusion

TRANSFUSION REACTIONS

Haemolytic

Immediate (haemolysis of donor cells usually due to ABO incompatibility). It is recognised that the majority of haemolytic reactions to red cells are due to clerical errors in transfusion practice.

- The following are manifestations of an acute haemolytic reaction: flushing, backache, chest pain, rigors, haemoglobinuria.

- **Treatment:**
  - Stop blood.
  - Take urine and blood samples for investigation by the blood bank.
  - Watch urine output and give frusemide or 20% mannitol, depending on the intravascular volume.
  - If oliguria persists, treat as acute renal failure.
  - Watch for shock and DIC.
- Differential diagnosis: already haemolysed blood from freezing or heating.

Delayed (1–2 weeks after transfusion). This is due to a secondary antibody response and there is often no incompatibility at initial cross-match. The following suggest a delayed haemolytic transfusion reaction:

- fall in haemoglobin or late jaundice
- positive Coombs' test and antibody screen.

Reactions to white cell antibodies—occur after previous transfusion or pregnancy ('febrile reactions'). This is now very infrequent, if red cell and platelet products are leucodepleted.

- Such reactions are delayed by 0.5–3 hours after start of transfusion.
- There is a brisk rise in temperature to 38–40°C with chills and headache.
- Diagnosis is by the presence of white cell antibodies.
- Give paracetamol orally or antihistamine IV, and slow rate of transfusion.

Urticarial and anaphylactic reactions

- Anaphylaxis is rare—due to allergy to donor plasma.
- Occasionally occurs in IgA-deficient individuals.
- Shock—bronchospasm, laryngeal oedema, severe urticaria.
- Stop blood, treat with adrenaline, antihistamines and occasionally corticosteroids.

Urticarial reaction

(Occasionally accompanied by asthma.)

- Response to antihistamines usually.
- Washed red cells may be used.

Table 43.2 Commonly used blood products in emergency medicine

Product	Emergency indications
Fresh whole blood	Massive blood loss
Red cell concentrate	Severe or refractory anaemia Moderate blood loss
Platelet concentrate	Thrombocytopenia with bleeding Platelet dysfunctional bleeding
Fresh frozen plasma (FFP)	Massive transfusion Severe liver disease with bleeding Reversal of warfarin therapy
Prothrombinex	Reversal of warfarin therapy

Reactions to bacterial pyrogens and bacteria

- Pyrogenic reaction:
  - Extremely rare.
  - Clinical picture resembles leucocyte and platelet antibody reaction.
- Infected blood or platelets:
  - Causes shock, fever, coma, convulsions, sudden death. Beware blood removed prematurely from blood bank or heavily haemolysed supernatant or previously punctured top.
  - Take blood for cultures.
  - Treat shock and give large doses of appropriate antibiotics.

It is recognised that platelet transfusions carry an increased risk of bacterial infection because platelet donations are stored at room temperature. Central blood banks have introduced screening of platelet concentrates for infections that has reduced the risk of bacterial contamination.

Circulatory overload

- Slow or stop transfusion, treat as for cardiac or pulmonary oedema.
- May need venesection.

Transfusion-related acute lung injury (TRALI)

- TRALI is a serious pulmonary complication of transfusion. It is an immune-mediated reaction caused by donor leucocyte antibodies causing non-cardiogenic pulmonary oedema.
- Manifestation includes dyspnoea and bilateral pulmonary oedema without signs of circulatory overload within 6 hours of transfusion.
- Respiratory supportive therapy.

Air embolism

- Raised jugular venous pulse (JVP), cyanosis, hypotension, praecordial murmur.
- Treat with head down, feet up and patient on left side.
- Administer 100% oxygen.

Citrate intoxication

- Usually only in neonates, impaired liver function and massive blood transfusion.
- Muscles twitching, hypotension, ECG changes, bleeding.
- Give calcium gluconate, 10 mL of 10% by IV injection.

Massive transfusion

(See Figure 14.2, 'Massive transfusion guideline'.)

- Hypothermia (use blood warmer).
- Deficiency of coagulation factors. Check coagulation profile (use fresh frozen plasma).
- Thrombocytopenia (use platelet transfusion).
- Acidosis.
- Hypocalcaemia.

Infectious complications

Possible risk with nucleic acid testing (NAT):

- HIV, < 1:920,000
- Hepatitis B, < 1:100,000
- Hepatitis C, < 1:10,000
- human T-lymphotropic virus type 1 (HTLV-I), < 1:100,000
- others, e.g. syphilis, malaria, cytomegalovirus (CMV). CMV has the highest incidence but the lowest risk to the patient unless they are immunocompromised.

Inappropriate use of blood components

There is considerable evidence of inappropriate use of blood components. Various strategies have been developed to reduce this, including guidelines, consensus conferences, monitoring, education and self-audit by clinicians. Informed consent, including the potential risks and benefits of transfusion, is a vital part of any transfusion.

Online resources

Australian clinical practice guidelines on the use of blood components. www.nhmrc.gov.au/guidelines/publications/cp78

Australian Red Cross Blood Service www.transfusion.com.au

Australasian Society of Thrombosis and Haemostasis www.asth.org.au/resources/publications

Consensus guidelines for warfarin therapy (updated) www.mja.com.au/journal/2013/198/4/update-consensus-guidelines-warfarin-reversal

National Blood Authority of Australia www.nba.gov.au

Royal College of Pathologists of Australasia, online pathology test manual www.rcpamanual.edu.au

Chapter 44
Rural and Indigenous emergencies

Mark Byrne and Bonita Byrne

Rural and remote Australia

A doctor providing medical services in a rural or remote area requires a broad skill-set with the ability to work independently in a setting with limited or no immediate access to specialist care.

The rural practitioner provides holistic care within a setting that often has unique socio-cultural issues.

Every community is different, and local knowledge is essential. What works in location A may not work in location B, so working closely with the community is important.

Australia is a vast country with a relatively small population of 23 million. One-third of Australians live outside urban areas, many in remote, isolated locations. There are recognised differences in health status among rural Australians, compared with their urban counterparts. Despite efforts to bridge these inequalities, access to health services and health professionals for rural Australians is generally poorer.

Approach to the rural patient

The initial approach to the undifferentiated rural patient is the same as if the patient presented to a major tertiary centre. For example, the principle of 'airway, breathing, circulation' is fundamental. The provision of services may require adaptation as resources may be limited.

Modern technology does provide many rural sites with video conference facilities which link the rural practitioner with a tertiary hospital and can provide real-time, interactive specialist assistance. Ringing for advice and utilising the internet to gain opinion on ECGs (etc) is worthwhile.

Patient travel, transport and retrieval

(This has been covered in detail in Chapter 21, 'Patient transport and retrieval.')

Developing an understanding of who is responsible for the transport and retrieval of patients is essential. Area health services will have a local protocol.

Early planning for patients is important and, if unsure, it is better to discuss the patient early if there are any doubts or perceived management dilemmas.

Each state has provision for financial assistance for people who need to travel long distances to obtain specialist medical or dental treatment that is not available locally. Medical staff have a responsibility to complete documentation associated with travel assistance.

Indigenous patients

EPIDEMIOLOGY

Indigenous Australians are the most disadvantaged across all socio-economic denominators. These disadvantages stem from colonisation and land dispossession.

Aboriginal health not only includes physical health but also encompasses social, emotional and cultural wellbeing.

Aboriginal and Torres Strait Islanders comprise 2.4% of the total Australian population. Most (69%) live outside the major urban centres, with 1 in 4 Indigenous Australians living in remote areas compared with only 1 in 50 non-Indigenous Australians.

Over 50% of Indigenous Australians live in New South Wales (29%) and Queensland (27%). Although only 12% of all Indigenous Australians live in the Northern Territory (NT), they represent 29% of the total population of the NT.

HEALTH STATUS

Aboriginal history has continued implications for health care, and the health status of Indigenous Australians is worse than that of other Australians. Life expectancy is worse than in many underdeveloped nations: 53% of men and 41% of women die before the age of 50.

Aboriginal patients may have chronic conditions at a younger age and, therefore, age-based risk stratification is often not applicable among Indigenous Australians.

Cardiovascular disease is the leading cause of death for Indigenous Australians, with respiratory, endocrine and external causes the other major causes.

Indigenous Australians also have higher rates of mortality from all major causes of death. Mortality rates for Indigenous males and females for endocrine, nutritional and metabolic diseases are around 7-fold and 11-fold higher than those for non-Indigenous males and females.

CULTURAL ISSUES

Providing affordable, culturally appropriate facilities and transport will improve access and attendance.

Mandatory training should be available so that all health staff can be educated in Aboriginal culture, with emphasis on the local community.

Treating Indigenous patients as individuals and avoiding cultural stereotyping is essential.

Cultural and communication barriers can affect the patient–doctor interaction. Finding a balance between medical priorities and social needs is essential.

ABORIGINAL HEALTH WORKERS

An Aboriginal health worker or Aboriginal liaison officer is an invaluable resource and should be consulted when appropriate.

There are over 130 Aboriginal community-controlled health services and Aboriginal medical services throughout Australia that are also excellent local resources.

Communication

Many Indigenous Australians have difficulty in understanding and/or being understood by a health provider. Therefore, culturally appropriate communication is essential for effective patient management.

For example, in the Northern Territory, 70% of the Aboriginal population speaks a language other than English at home. This has implications in relation to providing information on appropriate care, obtaining informed consent, explaining diagnosis and treatment and reinforcing compliance.

Eye contact is often avoided and should be understood within its cultural context.

Aboriginal people have strong family ties and kinships, and the inclusion of the extended family in decisions is appropriate.

Many Aboriginal people have a fear of hospitals, which they may associate with death. Be patient, and make allowances if compliance is to be achieved. Further, consider alternatives to admission such as daily reviews and ambulatory IV antibiotics.

Where possible, a doctor of the same gender should see an Indigenous patient, as there is men's business and women's business. This includes not placing men and women in the same room.

Provide written information and instructions each and every time, prior to discharging. Use everyday language, without jargon, and take the time to make sure the patient understands the information. Arrange prompt follow-up and provide written information to the referral service.

Allow time and space for the extended family during grieving and when a death has occurred.

Alcohol and substance abuse

Indigenous Australians are less likely to drink alcohol than other Australian people. However, there is a higher prevalence of dangerous drinking levels among Aboriginal people.

Alcohol and substance abuse is a major contributing factor to the poor health and wellbeing status of many Aboriginal people. It has a causal and a non-causal relationship with domestic violence, mental health, suicide, road deaths, imprisonment, sexually transmitted infections and sexual abuse.

Alcohol abuse has a major impact on Indigenous communities. The immediate management of alcohol-related ED presentations is no different than in the wider community.

Illicit drug use, including marijuana, amphetamines, heroin and inhalants such as glues, aerosols and petrol, is also a major problem in many communities.

Proactive and opportunistic provision of culturally appropriate intervention is the role of all primary-care medical staff, as even small reductions in alcohol consumption have benefits for both the individual and the wider community.

Despite widespread alcohol and substance abuse, a non-judgmental, non-stereotypical attitude is essential. Individual assessment is paramount, and making assumptions based on Aboriginality is inappropriate.

Editorial Comment

Especially for those emergency doctors working in the many city or rural hospitals that see and treat these groups, it is important and rewarding to actively become familiar with and good at caring for these patients (e.g. by doing courses, rural rotations, locum work); there are simple but important differences of engagement and communication that are not intuitive and are important to be aware of. We all know that there are health challenges to improve many aspects of Indigenous health, thus leading to decreased morbidity and mortality. There should be access for the health professional to involve liaison workers who can support, work and follow up with family, elders and other agencies. Care must not end with only an ED visit.

Online resources

Australian Indigenous HealthInfoNet
www.healthinfonet.ecu.edu.au
Australian Institute of Health and Welfare: Indigenous health
www.aihw.gov.au/indigenous-health

Chapter 45
Advanced nursing roles

Barbara Daly, Sarah Hoy, Gordian W O Fulde,
Wayne Varndell and Kirsty McLeod

Advancing nursing practice is a global phenomenon: in the context of the Australian experience, this has evolved over the past three and a half decades. The evolution of advance nursing practice is an ongoing process, moving nursing practice forward for the benefit of the patient.[1] This change of practice is directly related to changes in the delivery of healthcare services and the implementation of new models of patient-focused care. An important driver in the development of the advanced practice nurse is the political demand to meet government-set performance indicators and benchmarks aimed to reduce emergency department waiting times and patient length of stay and to increase patient satisfaction.[2] Another factor that has contributed to evolving advanced practice is medical and nursing workforce shortages and skill-mix problems. These developments have provided the impetus for emergency nurses to take on new opportunities to develop and increase their scope and complexity of practice in the field of emergency medicine. These advanced nursing roles are now core roles that work with and support the medical and clerical staff to expedite the patient's journey through the ED.

The triage nurse

The patient's journey in the ED begins at triage. Triage is an essential function in the delivery of care in all ED. It is the point at which emergency care begins. Triage is a brief clinical assessment that determines the urgency of treatment and the time sequence in which patients should be seen in the ED. The purpose of the triage system is to ensure safe quality of care and equity of access to health services. In all healthcare environments, the triage process is underpinned by the premise that a reduction in the time taken to access definitive medical care will improve patient outcomes.[3]

Most importantly, triage is a dynamic and ongoing process in which patients are continually reassessed. Their clinical urgency and triage category may be changed as a result, depending on parameters such as changes in level of pain and haemodynamic stability. For example, if a patient's level of pain increases compared with initial triage assessment, or they become tachycardic or hypotensive, the patient will be re-triaged to a higher category.

In Australasian EDs a standardised triage system known as the Australasian Triage Scale (ATS) is the primary clinical tool for ensuring that patients are seen in a timely manner, commensurate with their clinical urgency. The practical application of the ATS is the process by which the triage nurse assesses a patient's presenting complaint, which is identified by a brief history of the presenting illness or injury. Triage decisions using the scale are made on the basis of observation of general appearance, focused clinical history and physiological data.[3] This decision-making process may also require consultation and discussion with medical staff.

In practical terms triage refers to two domains, which are:

Domain 1. The ATS has five levels of acuity that categorise patients according to a rating scale from 1 to 5. (Also see Chapter 39, 'Psychiatric presentations', Table 39.1 on mental health triage.)

Domain 2. Time-to-treatment criteria attached to the ATS categories identify the maximum time a patient can safely wait for medical assessment and treatment.

Please refer to Table 45.1 for triage examples.

There are 5 core components for a nurse undertaking the role of triage nurse:

1. patient assessment
2. initiation of first-aid treatment
3. delegation of reassessment and management of waiting-room patients to appropriate nursing staff
4. provision of public education
5. acting as a liaison for members of the public and other healthcare professionals.[4]

The ability to undertake effective and efficient triage is dependent on extensive knowledge of and experience with a wide range of illness and injury patterns. Therefore, it is essential that the triage nurse is appropriately prepared through education and experience.

The triage nurse will perform a 7-step triage assessment, which identifies the following key points as physiological predicators underpinning the allocation of urgency using the ATS.

Step 1. Identify and manage risks to self, patients and the environment is the first principle of a safe triage practice.

Table 45.1 ATS categories for treatment acuity, performance thresholds and examples of possible presenting problems

ATS category	Treatment acuity (maximum waiting times)	Performance indicator (% compliance)	Examples of possible presenting complaints
Category 1 *Immediately life-threatening*	Immediate	100	Respiratory/cardiac arrest, multi-trauma, ruptured AAA, unconscious (GCS < 9), burns to > 20% BSA
Category 2 *Imminently life-threatening*	10 minutes	80	Cardiac chest pain, acute CVA, acute severe pain, anaphylaxis, headache with symptoms of meningitis, fracture/dislocation with neurovascular compromise, sepsis, violent/aggressive patients (danger to self/others)
Category 3 *Potentially life-threatening or important time-critical treatment*	30 minutes	75	Moderate dyspnoea (chest infection, moderate asthma), seizure/post-ictal, complicated lacerations/avulsions, abdominal pain, acute psychosis or manic behaviour
Category 4 *Potentially life-threatening, serious or situational urgency or significant complexity*	60 minutes	70	Minor trauma (soft-tissue distal limb injury), PV bleeding, uncomplicated lacerations, suspected DVT/cellulitis
Category 5 *Less urgent*	120 minutes	70	Immunisations, rash, medical certificates, dressings, referral requests, DOA

AAA, abdominal aortic aneurysm; ATS, Australasian Triage Scale; BSA, body surface area; CVA, cerebrovascular accident; DOA, dead on arrival; DVT, deep venous thrombosis; GCS, Glasgow Coma Scale; PV, peripheral vein.

Step 2. First impressions of general appearance should always be considered when making a triage decision.

Step 3. Always ask the question: 'Does this person look sick?'

Step 4. The primary survey approach is used to identify and correct life-threatening conditions at triage.

Step 5. Other conditions in which timely intervention may significantly influence outcomes (such as thrombolysis, an antidote or management of acid or alkali splash to eye) must also be detected at triage.

Step 6. Timely access to emergency care can improve patient outcomes.

Step 7. Early identification of physiological abnormality at triage can inform focused ongoing medical assessment and investigation.[3]

Once the triage assessment is complete, the patient may follow a variety of treatment paths and interact with any of the following ED staff and teams:

- clinical initiatives nurse (CIN)
- aged service emergency team (ASET)
- rapid assessment team (RAT)/immediate initiation of care (IIOC)
- nurse practitioner (NP).

All of these advanced practice roles assist in expediting treatment and initiation of care and will now be discussed in terms of how they interact with the patient during their ED journey.

Clinical initiatives nurse (CIN)

The CIN role works as an adjunct to the triage position. The primary purpose of the CIN role is to provide nursing care to patients in the waiting room. The care delivered by the CIN is prioritised in the following way.

- Maintenance of an ED nursing presence in the waiting room to facilitate a safe clinical environment.
- Communication with patients and carers regarding emergency processes, waiting times and provision of relevant education on their health issues.
- The assessment of patients following triage with a view to:
  - initiation of diagnostics or treatment
  - escalation of care where required
  - appropriate referral of patients to suitable services, which may be external to the ED as per locally agreed protocols (e.g.

medical assessment units (MAUs) or inpatient teams. The CIN is not able to discharge patients, and hands over care of the patient to another nurse once treatment has been initiated.

Nurses working at CIN level should have:

- significant triage experience
- confidence
- high-level clinical skills
- advanced practice skills, or ready to be trained to an advanced practice level
- well-developed conflict resolution and negotiation skills with focus on customer satisfaction.

Initiated care may include:

- ordering radiological tests
- insertion of peripheral intravenous cannulae
- withdrawal of venous blood for pathology
- initiation of medication such as oral analgesia, antiemetic agents and intravenous narcotic analgesics
- fracture management such as application of 'back slab' plaster
- wound management, including suturing
- referral to other hospital services, for example outpatient clinics or social worker.[5]

The CIN role enables the nurse to commence patient treatment via pre-approved standing orders for specific presentations under the supervision of an ED registrar or consultant. See example in Box 45.1.

Aged service emergency team (ASET)

ASET is led by a clinical nurse consultant specialising in aged care. ASET is a multidisciplinary team including a nurse, a physiotherapist, a social worker and, in some areas, an occupational therapist.

The specific objectives of this team include:

- undertaking a comprehensive assessment of elderly patients over 70 years of age presenting to the ED
- aiming to prevent avoidable admissions by setting up services or accessing respite care
- identifying potential admission for patients who are considered at risk
- commencing treatment for patients being admitted by providing physiotherapy and social work input while in the ED
- encouraging health promotion by providing information on social and educational activities available for older people in the community

Box 45.1 Example 1. Patient presenting with an ankle fracture

- Patient presents to ED with painful left ankle following a simple trip and fall.
- Triage assessment indicates pain and tenderness at posterior edge of lateral malleolus, ankle is swollen and deformed and the patient is unable to weightbear. The left ankle is neurovascularly intact, and the patient describes pain severity as 6/10. Vital signs are within normal limits, Glasgow Coma Scale score is 15, there are no known allergies.
- Triage category 3 is allocated by triage nurse.
- Patient is referred to CIN nurse who orders left ankle X-ray according to Ottawa ankle rules, application of rest/ice/elevation. Due to level of pain, CIN inserts IV cannula, places patient on oxygen saturation monitoring and initiates administration of IV morphine 2.5 mg bolus as per nurse-initiated protocol.
- Patient's ankle X-ray attended.
- CIN nurse views X-ray with ED registrar. X-ray shows fracture to left lateral malleolus.
- CIN applies back slab plaster as per standing order.
- Ongoing medical treatment by ED registrar as required.
- Patient is referred to orthopaedic team.

- improving communication between hospital and community workers, and hospital and residential care staff, regarding patients presenting to the ED.

An example of how the ASET functions is described in Box 45.2.

Rapid assessment team (RAT) or immediate initiation of care (IIOC)

There are various names and abbreviations, such as RAT and IIOC, which describe models of rapid assessment and treatment within the emergency department. These models involve having a team of a senior doctor and nurse meeting patients as they arrive. What they actually do for each patient will depend on the nature and seriousness of the problem, as well as the prevailing patient flow constraints at the time.

This is so that:

- Senior ED medical decision-making is moved to the earliest point in the patient's ED care, so as to streamline subsequent processes.
- Senior ED nurse involvement ensures the availability of advanced nursing skills, and streamlining of subsequent nursing care.

Box 45.2 Example 2. 80-year-old female presenting with recurrent falls

- Patient presents via ambulance to the ED with recurrent falls. Patient found on the floor by neighbour with painful right hip, unable to weightbear.
- Triage assessment indicates painful right hip, shortening and external rotation of right leg. Patient is confused regarding day/date/time. Unable to confirm past medical history. Vital signs within normal limits. Triage category 3 is allocated. Referral made to CIN and ASET nurse.
- CIN orders right hip X-ray, chest X-ray, IV cannula is inserted, bloods taken for pathology (FBC, renal profile, group-and-hold), analgesia given as per nurse-initiated narcotic protocol, ECG, intravenous fluids, pressure risk assessment, patient remains nil by mouth.
- ASET nurse undertakes comprehensive assessment including:
  - Pre-morbid mobility assessment to identify level of independence. This also includes history of falls and potential causes. This may lead to a referral to other specialty teams, e.g. dizziness may require investigation by neurology team.
  - Ability to perform activities of daily living (ADLs).
  - Community services usage and frequency of services.
  - Current home support, e.g. family, contact numbers, need for respite care.
  - Mental status is assessed via Abbreviated Mental Test Score (AMTS) and Confusion Assessment Method (CAM) diagnostic algorithm. Both these tests are performed with involvement of the patient's family.
- Early linkage to community care packages is made to ensure safe and timely discharge of the patient back to the community after acute admission. Early involvement of the GP is an important aspect of the discharge planning process.
- Medical staff continue treatment and management of the patient in conjunction with ED nurses and the ASET.
- Once clinical work-up is complete, referral to orthogeriatric team for admission for fractured right neck of femur.
- Medical officer decides the need for further investigations in ED—e.g. if head injury present or if the patient is on warfarin, need to consider CT of brain.

- Working in partnership, the team will leverage each other's skills, making each more effective than working alone.

The concept for all these models is the same in that they move experienced medical and nursing staff to the front door so that the patient's journey starts with them rather than ends with them, as is currently the case.

The specific objectives of these teams are to:

- provide senior medical decision-making at the earliest point in the patient's ED care, so as to streamline ED processes for the patient and for the department
- triage patients to the appropriate area for care
- organise appropriate investigations
- minimise unnecessary interventions
- initiate analgesia early
- provide a quick assessment, referral, fix and discharge from the front if appropriate.

All members of the team are capable of multitasking, according to their skills. Doctors and nurses will triage according to current guidelines. Nurses will provide definitive treatment using written guidelines, as well as being under the direct supervision of senior medical staff.

The two biggest dangers of these models are:

1. Trying to do too much at the front door. The senior doctors and nurses must be resolute in their efforts to avoid this.
2. Errors of omission or duplication due to inadequate handover as the patient moves from one area of the department to another. A written form should be utilised to avoid this.

An example of how the RAT/IIOC works is set out in Box 45.3.

The nurse practitioner (NP)

In Australia, NPs are specifically authorised registered nurses with extensive specialist education and experience, who function autonomously and collaboratively in an advanced and extended clinical role.[6] The NP provides leadership, expertise, support and direction within a variety of clinical settings, assessing, diagnosing and initiating treatment within a specific scope of practice. Their role may include the direct referral of patients to other healthcare professionals, discharging patients with a range of conditions, prescribing medications and ordering diagnostic investigations. Each NP has an individual scope of practice that is endorsed at a local level, and is specific to their specialist clinical area of work (e.g. paediatric oncology). Patients that fall outside of the NP's scope of practice or expertise are referred on to the most appropriate medical officer.

Within the ED setting, the NP scope of practice has largely focused around primary care and/or minor injury presentations. However, NPs are increasingly managing complex patient-care needs across the life span in conjunction with emergency medical staff. The NP

Box 45.3 Example 3. Patient presenting with renal colic

- Patient presents to ED with a 1-hour history of severe loin pain radiating to the groin.
- Triage assessment indicates that patient is distressed and in severe pain, severity described as 10/10. The patient is observed to be diaphoretic, pale, hypertensive and feels nauseated. Nil past medical history, regular medications or allergies. Triage category 2 is allocated.
- Patient is referred to RAT for ongoing management.
- RAT doctor conducts a brief history and examination to confirm likelihood of diagnosis and then orders opioid and non-steroidal anti-inflammatory medication (e.g. morphine 5 mg IV and indomethacin 100 mg PR); nurse to perform basic pathology investigation, FBC, urea, electrolytes and creatinine (UEC) and midstream urine (MSU) and administer medications.
- History and clinical examination results reviewed by other ED staff to ascertain whether presentation is complicated or uncomplicated.

Uncomplicated:

- Pathology results for FBC, UEC: if all 'nothing abnormal detected' (NAD) and pain settles, discharge home with outpatient referral for CT KUB (kidneys–ureters–bladder) and urology consult

Complicated:

- Confirmed through pathology results, history of strictures, indwelling stents, abnormal urinary tract or evidence of fever or ongoing pain
- Investigation via CT KUB and inpatient consultation/admission with the urology team
- Ongoing analgesia as required

role has been shown to have a positive impact on ED waiting times[7,8] and has enhanced the collaborative clinical management of patients within the ED setting.[9,10]

Two examples of the NP scope of practice are given in Boxes 45.4 and 45.5. The first example outlines the assessment and management of an acute sore throat. The second outlines the assessment and management of a patient with central chest pain.

Box 45.4 Example 4. Patient presenting with acute sore throat

The management of an acute sore throat will depend on the severity of symptoms, the presence of other signs and symptoms and the patient's previous history.

Presenting complaint as stated by the patient or significant other:

- acute onset of a sore throat
- painful
- fever
- cervical lymphadenopathy.

Nurse practitioner assessment

The NP will be continually assessing and initiating:

A Airway
B Breathing
C Circulation: BP (manual and bilaterally if possible), total peripheral resistance (TPR), oxygen saturations (SpO_2)
D Differentials: a mildly sore throat may be a feature of most patient presentations with upper respiratory tract infections and may require no more than adequate pain relief
E Evaluation or escalation? Do we continue independently or is there a need for medical assistance? Can we use clinical directives to instigate blood sampling or morphine, etc?

The NP will also document the following as part of the clinical assessment:

- medications—current treatment, over-the-counter medications, recreational, missed medications
- allergies
- past medical history—past medical history, instructions from past attendances to GP/ED
- family medical history—in summary, gained from the above history taking
- social history—e.g. housing status, lifestyle, recreational activities or support services
- risk factors.

The general assessment will consist of:

- vital signs
- appearance of throat
- tonsillar exudate
- redness
- oedema
- petechiae at junction of hard and soft palate
- lymphadenopathy
- splenomegaly
- hepatomegaly
- ear examination.

Management will consist of either a medical pathway or an NP pathway.

Nurse practitioner management

- Paracetamol/aspirin (may be gargle)
- Adequate oral hydration
- Antibiotic therapy if there is:
  - tonsillar exudate
  - fever
  - bilateral cervical lymphadenopathy
  - history of documented Group A beta-haemolytic streptococcal infection in a person with whom there has been close contact.
- Review in 24–48 hours or at the request of the patient.

Refer to medical officer if:
- History of rheumatic heart disease
- History of prosthetic valve
- Immunocompromised patient
- Presence of hepatomegaly or splenomegaly
- Presence of peri-tonsillar abscess.[11]

Box 45.5 Example 5. Patient presenting with chest pain

The assessment of the patient presenting with central chest pain will vary according to the urgency of the situation, the experience of the NP and the resources available, e.g. whether a doctor is immediately available. However, an expedient, logical and systematic appraisal of the patient's condition is vital to patient safety and the timeliness of treatment.
- Presenting complaint: as stated by the patient or significant other.
- History of presenting complaint and assessment will include the following (mnemonic—CHEST PAIN):[12]
  - C *Commenced when?* Establish a timeframe and if there were any associated **events** such as exertion, activity, emotional distress.
  - H *History/risk factors?* Any previous heart conditions or unexplained shortness of breath on exertion, chest pain, etc. Any 1st-degree relatives (parents/siblings) with heart complaints, stroke or raised blood pressure. Risk factors may include smoking, high-fat diet, diabetes, hypertension, obesity or a sedentary lifestyle.
  - E *Extra symptoms?* Any complaints of feeling nervous, nauseated, sweating, palpitations, shortness of breath, dizzy or weakness? Also remember ethnicity-associated increases in cardiovascular disease.
  - S *Stays/radiates?* Does the pain stay in one place, or does it move? If the pain radiates, where does it go? Myocardial infarction pain can present as toothache and neck/jaw pain and, in the elderly or diabetic neuropathy patient, symptoms can be deranged and not clearly detectable.
  - T *Timing*? How long does the pain last? Any previous episodes, if so, how long did they last? When did the pain become continual?
  - P *Place?* Where is the pain? Check the point of tenderness with palpation.
  - A *Alleviating or aggravating factors?* What makes the pain worse, or better?
  - I *Intensity?* How intense is the pain, what does it stop you doing?
  - N *Nature?* Ask the patient to describe their pain; do not suggest descriptors. Listen for key symptoms.
- While going through the above, the NP will be continually assessing and initiating:
  - A Airway
  - B Breathing

C Circulation: BP (manual and bilaterally if possible), total peripheral resistance (TPR), SpO_2, signs of cyanosis

D Differentials: chest pain can present from myriad pathologies—indigestion, musculoskeletal chest pain or aortic arch dissection, for example. The NP should be familiar with the main differentials for chest pain and their symptomatology along with appropriate assessment or diagnostic strategies to, as far as possible, exclude these differentials.

E Evaluation or escalation? Do we continue independently or is there need for assistance? Can we use clinical directives to instigate GTN, blood sampling or morphine, etc?

- The NP will also document the following as part of their clinical assessment:
  - medications—current treatment, over-the-counter medications, recreational, missed medications
  - allergies
  - past medical history—past medical history, instructions from past attendances to local GP/ED
  - family medical history—in summary, gained from the above history taking
  - social history—e.g. housing status, lifestyle, recreational activities or support services
  - risk factors.
- The general management of chest pain will consist of diagnosis and risk stratification and management as per local protocols and pathways for high, intermediate and low risk. (See Chapter 7, 'Acute coronary syndromes'.)

Pearls

- The most crucial aspect of triage is effective communication to ensure accurate information to make well-informed decisions. That is why when triaging you must remain calm, listen to the patient, interpret and explain all your actions and check that the patient understands what you have said.
- Teamwork is crucial in the ED; everyone needs to communicate well, especially at hand-overs.
- Make sure you know where your resources are, or ask where to find ED protocols, drug protocols, clinical pathways.
- It is important to appreciate that approximately 75% of your diagnosis comes from information gained at history taking, leaving only approximately 25% originating from your physical examination, diagnostics tests etc.[13]
- *Remember:* Triage is the first point at which a patient enters the ED, and this experience will influence how the patient responds and evaluates the care and treatment they receive.
- *Remember to ask for help/advice readily if you need it*—the medical, nursing, allied health and clerical staff will assist you.

Editorial Comment

Future professional and career roles for nurses must continue to progress due to the enormous healthcare needs of the community. We are in a time of re-engineering the patient journey (e.g. the 4-hour rule) linked to funding and key performance indicators (KPIs). This affects EDs, all hospital clinical services, ambulance services and community GPs and health workers. Thus, the imperative to more efficiently but also safely process the patient must be met by many changes.

Core (apart from inpatient bed availability) to all of this is front-loading—senior doctors and nurses starting decisions and diagnosis soon after triage. Also, reorganising the ED into teams and areas (fast-track, etc) relies heavily on nurses having advanced skills, training and supervision.

With these measures, it is even more vital that the nursing, medical and administrative ED staff meet weekly to solve and improve issues to ensure that staff actually lead the changes and process.

References

1. Por J. A critical engagement with concept of advancing nursing practice. J Nurs Man 2008;16:84–90.
2. Hudson P, Marshall A. Extending the nursing role in emergency departments: challenges for Australia. Australas Emerg Nurs J 2008;11:39–48.
3. Australian Government Department of Health and Ageing. Emergency Triage Education Kit, 2009. Online. Available at www.health.gov.au/internet/main/publishing.nsf/Content/5E3156CFFF0A34B1CA2573D0007BB905/$File/Triage Education Kit.pdf
4. CENA. Position statement triage nurse. Australas Emerg Nurs J 2007;10:93–5.
5. NSW Health. Clinical initiatives nurse in emergency departments: educational program, 2011. Online. Available at www.ecinsw.com.au/sites/default/files/field/file/cin_resource_manual_final.pdf 20 Apr 2013.
6. Nursing and Midwifery Board of Australia, n.d. ANMC National competency standards for the nurse practitioner. Canberra: NMBA. Online. Available at www.nursingmidwiferyboard.gov.au/Codes-Guidelines-Statements/Codes-Guidelines.aspx 20 Apr 2013.
7. Considine J, Martin R, et al. Emergency nurse practitioner care and emergency department patient flow: case-control study. Emerg Med Australas 2006;18:385–90.

8. Jennings N, O'Reilly O, et al. Evaluating outcomes of the emergency nurse practitioner role in a major urban emergency department, Melbourne, Australia. J ClinNurs 2008;17:1044–50.
9. Lee G, Jennings N. A comparative study of patients who did not wait for treatment and those treated by emergency nurse practitioners. Australas Emerg Nurs J 2006;9:179–85.
10. Fry M, Rogers T. The transitional emergency nurse practitioner role: implementation study and preliminary evaluation. Australas Emerg Nurs J 2009;12(2):32–7.
11. Dennis M, Waters W, Shanahan M. Emergency department nurse practitioner clinical practice guidelines. Greater Southern Area Health Service, NSW Department of Health; 2006.
12. Newberry L, Barret GK, Ballard N. A new mnemonic for chest pain assessment. J Emerg Nurs 2005;31(1):84–5.
13. Peterson MC, Holbrook JH, von Vales D, et al. Contributions of the history, physical examination and laboratory investigations in the medical diagnosis. West J Med 1992;156:163–5.

Online resources

Australasian College for Emergency Medicine
www.acem.org.au

Australian Government Department of Health and Ageing, Emergency Triage Education Kit
www.health.gov.au/internet/main/publishing.nsf/Content/casemix-ED-Triage+Review+Fact+Sheet+Documents

College of Emergency Nursing Australasia
www.cena.org.au

Nursing and Midwifery Board of Australia. Nurse practitioner competency standards
www.nursingmidwiferyboard.gov.au/Codes-Guidelines-Statements/Codes-Guidelines.aspx

Chapter 46

The general practitioner; Working with IT

Michael J Golding

Editorial Comment

Although these two topics are disparate, they are, for nearly every patient, core relationships and resources—i.e. part of safe patient care.

The ED and the GP

The disciplines of general practice and emergency medicine may be thought of as two ends of the same spectrum of general medicalist practice. While emergency medicine focuses on the more acute end, the similarities between the specialties are greater than the differences—although the differences are sufficient to mean that working effectively in one field does not predict success working in the other.

Unfortunately there is often a poor relationship between doctors working in ED and GPs: emergency department staff too often reflect negatively on the work of the GP in the community. GPs generally deal with 1 patient every 15 minutes; many will work (much) faster than this. (ED doctors are rarely able to deal with more than 1 patient an hour.) In that time the GP takes a history, performs an examination, formulates a diagnosis and management plan, organises investigations and initiates treatment. The GP must provide feedback to the patient, address immediate concerns of both the patient and the family and document the encounter. Most importantly, the GP takes sole responsibility for these decisions: there is no 'team' to share responsibility in the event of an adverse outcome.

GPs will often try to avoid referral to the public health system. They are usually (only too) aware of the constraints of the system and the lengthy process the patient will be subject to. GPs have been affected, just like EDs, by the developing reluctance in health care generally to accept 'risk' and increasing expectations of service delivery. What many admitting officers do not understand is that GPs on the phone are not really 'asking' if a patient could be referred to the ED—they are, in a polite way, 'telling' you. The ED admitting officer's interaction with the GP is too often (futile) efforts to prevent a referral rather than recognition of a (very valuable) opportunity to maximise information that may greatly help in management of the patient. Equally frustrating to an experienced GP, who is aware of the complex medical and social history of a patient, is to refer a patient to the ED for admission only to have the patient assessed by a junior doctor and then sent home. The lack of value of this type of assessment has led to development of 'third-door' initiatives, by which GPs refer patients directly to inpatient teams when their patients require admission.

Patients being discharged from the ED are routinely told to follow-up with their GP 'in the next couple of days'. But, in many areas, patients find it hard to get an appointment with a GP in this timeframe, and EDs need to recognise the difficulties many people have in organising appropriate GP follow-up. Often, discharging a patient to a GP is equivalent to doing nothing at all, and discharge management plans should not depend on GP review in less than 3 days without prior agreement directly with the GP.

Patients who die in the ED will often have had recent contact with their GP; their GP may have been managing the illness prior to their death. The GP should be notified of the death as soon as possible, using dedicated forms or standard work practices. The GP can then contact the family, with whom they may have enjoyed a long-standing relationship. The GP may also be able to help with a death certificate and avoid a coroner's examination. Most importantly, the GP is often able to help the patient's family and friends through the grieving process and 'defuse' their fears and concerns about the treatment provided in the ED. The GP is much more likely to do this if they have been involved or notified by the ED beforehand.

The GP can be a useful colleague when dealing with the 'difficult patient'. He or she will often have an understanding of the patient developed through multiple interactions over a long period of time. Usually, the GP is quite aware of the 'difficulty' and has already developed a risk-management framework: if not, the GP will be an essential partner to prevent repeated presentations to the ED.

The ED registration process should include confirming who the patient's current GP is and whether the patient gives permission for details of this presentation to be discussed with the GP. Each emergency department should have a list of local GPs with their contact details. Divisions of general practice are usually very well organised and helpful: they can provide accurate lists of local GPs, their hours, availability and capacity for bulk billing. Some divisions offer a uniform referral form. Adverse events (and complaints) can be reduced by communicating directly with the GP about the outcome of a consultation: if possible, in the presence of the patient.

Communication is particularly important when the GP has asked to be notified of the outcome of an ED referral. Effective communication is a prized skill of GPs and is strongly emphasised during their training, so any failure of communication (verbal or written) by the ED (or other hospital department) to the GP following a referral is not only frustrating, but also an unnecessary barrier to smooth transfer of their medical care for the future. All patients should get a discharge letter for their GP. A copy of this discharge letter should be sent to the GP by fax or email. (Patients will only rarely take their copy of the letter to their GP.)

The discharge letter, better called a GP referral letter, should include:

- a courteous opening, e.g. 'Dear Doctor ... , Thank you for ...'
- the reason the patient presented to the ED
- the provisional diagnosis
- a list of pending investigations
- any changes to medications made during the visit
- any consultations organised for the patient
- any management plan for the patient, with clearly-defined responsibilities (for many GPs, this is probably the most important part of the discharge letter)
- a courteous ending, e.g. 'Grateful for your further management and care, With thanks and regards, ...'
- a legible name and designation below the signature.

Emergency departments who employ GPs part-time will be enriched by the knowledge and practicality of these experienced decision-makers. Such interaction also enables GPs to experience the complexity and difficulties of working in a modern ED.

Most of all, know this: if the GP system fails, their patients will be found waiting (and unhappy) in (a very long) line at your ED.

Pitfalls

- Sending home a patient referred by a GP who has not been reviewed by a senior ED doctor. (There will usually be a good reason for the GP's referral.)
- Writing a discharge letter to a GP that does not include a clear management plan.
- Expecting a GP to follow up an investigation through a discharge letter given to the patient: written letters rarely find their way to the GP.

Pearls

- GP divisions are generally very well-organised and effective at communicating with local GPs.
- GPs working short shifts on weekend evenings can provide surge capacity of the ED at peak activity periods.

The ED and IT

Few emergency departments have realised the futuristic vision of freely flowing information that has been tantalisingly invoked by IT in so many other areas. Even more disappointingly, many EDs feel that they have ended up with IT products that are less efficient than the paper-based systems they were intended to replace.

The objective is to use IT in the ED to improve patient flow and to support improvements in work efficiency and delivery of care to the patient. And, at the same time, to ensure that the record is private and secure, accurate, current, comprehensive, complete, safe, available over many years and accessible to all those who may require access to it even if they are in a different health system or network. (If all of this is to be expected of an electronic system, it is perhaps not surprising that such slow progress has been made.)

The major components of an ED electronic system are:

- patient registration and tracking
- Electronic Medical Record (EMR)
- investigation ordering and results
- data archiving and access
- reporting and (in some cases) invoicing.

More specifically this includes:

- Providing real-time patient electronic tracking with departmental mapping to show the beds and bays.
- Recording patient information and key performance indicators (arrival time, status of consults, triage information, referral to inpatient team time, discharge status).
- Providing results and orders without separate log-on.
- Facilitating use of protocols, guidelines and best clinical practice.
- Generating relevant patient information sheets.
- Facilitating communication between the ED and other service providers.
- Supporting intelligent prescribing practices.
- Seamlessly interacting with inpatient systems.
- Seamlessly communicating with monitoring and recording systems at the bedside.
- Allowing for paperless EMRs and using voice recognition technology.
- Generating a (useful and cogent) patient discharge letter with distribution to relevant medical providers listing outstanding results, changes to medications and management plans.

- Incorporating links to medical calculators and medical reference materials.
- Using proximity technology to reduce time-wasting and frustrating multiple log-on requests from the system and patient tracking within the department.
- Taking advantage of wireless technology to free the clinician from the chains of the desk.

The development of the Patient Archiving and Communication System (PACS) for radiology is an example of the efficiencies which can be obtained using IT in the emergency department. However, in other respects, most EDs have a long way to go. Many existing IT patient-management systems are unable to even uniquely identify a patient. Many continue to generate discharge letters that start with 'To Dr Other' and are signed by 'Dr LocLoc' (locum); and, worst of all, many EDs rely on an out-of-date, ragged, but much-loved drug-reference book, despite the widely available personal digital-assistant-friendly electronic versions.

IT is really useful for storage and transmission of data.

- Medical reference information, departmental policies, guidelines and protocols can be centrally managed and viewed on all departmental computers; and the information management systems to support the archiving and delivery of this information are highly advanced and easy to use (e.g. Microsoft SharePoint).
- A departmental intranet website can also replace the departmental communication book and offers the opportunity of a blog for departmental discussion.
- There have been some wonderful uses of IT for orientation (locums turning up to work for the first time on Sunday!): give every new arrival to the department an MP3 player and headphones and they can walk around the department at their own pace.
- There is enormous potential for patient feedback portals to be developed (e.g. Survey Monkey); and nobody has really thought about the potential of social networking sites or Twitter.
- Perhaps most exciting of all is the potential of IT in education: virtual learning environment (VLE) 'Moodle'-type educational platforms will increasingly play an important part in ED educational programs.

Below are some examples of medical reference websites useful in ED practice (if your IT system allows access to the internet—another major problem for many departments):

- *UpToDate,* www.uptodate.com—(expensive) subscription service that offers excellent practical advice regarding general medical and paediatric conditions.
- *eMedicine,* http://emedicine.medscape.com—free service offering streamed, high-quality emergency medicine information in a standardised format; American-biased.
- *Toxicology,* www.toxinz.com and www.hypertox.com—(cheap) subscription services with an excellent ED perspective.
- *MD Consult,* www.mdconsult.com—(expensive) subscription service with an excellent search engine for medical queries and extensive online journals and clinics.
- *Australian Medicines Handbook,* www.amh.net.au—(cheap) subscription service for prescribing information.
- *Paediatrics:* most children's hospitals have websites with open access, complete with drug protocols, patient information sheets, drug calculators and asthma plan generators.
- *Therapeutic Guidelines,* www.tg.org.au—updated treatment protocols for a variety of sub-specialties, including the iconic Antibiotic Guidelines; subscription-based.

It is difficult to find a useful electronic replacement for the illustrated anatomy book or orthopaedic reference text: many EDs continue to stock a small library.

IT promises clinicians efficiencies that will translate to better patient care, but there is a cost:

- *Hardware*—initial cost, followed by maintenance and replacement. Make sure to purchase COWs (Computers On Wheels) for ward rounds.
- *Software*—whether custom-made or off-the-shelf, all software will require updates and modifications; these are generally expensive and slow to be implemented. Allow plenty of lead time and ensure there is a budget for ongoing training. Talk to an ED that is using the product before signing the contract.
- *Security*—an EMR is vulnerable to unauthorised retrieval or corruption; there is a happy balance between tracking all interactions with patient data and death by a thousand mouse-clicks.
- *Downtime*—IT systems rarely fail, but when they do it is rarely during business hours. It does not take long for the old paper system that has been displaced by IT to fall into disrepair. Ensuring the maintenance of a workable back-up

plan is time-consuming and is rarely a high priority for busy departments. However, a loss of IT capability can result in an internal disaster, and a back-up paper-based system is an essential part of ED risk management.

- *Maintenance*—the pressure to centralise IT support to a Help desk has proved overwhelming for most health organisations. The result can be a loss of engagement of IT staff in the clinical management of the department. A dedicated ED data manager is one way of maintaining continuity between the department and the supporting IT department.

The very poor functionality of the current ED systems contrasts with the remarkable usability of IT systems developed for general practice. These routinely use EMRs, interface seamlessly with other providers (except hospitals), electronically order and review investigation results, contain clinical guidelines and patient information sheets and have intelligent prescribing capability. The success of GP data-management programs offers a framework for the development of systems to allow emergency medicine to live the dream promised to it by the IT revolution.

Pitfalls

- Failing to survey and develop the IT skills of the workforce before introducing a new IT system. (How many of the department's workforce can touch-type?)
- Agreeing to any software (or hardware) until you have spoken to an ED that is using it.
- Depending on a remote Help service when the printer fails on a Sunday evening.

Pearls

- PACS is terrific: make sure the computer is supplied with headphones.
- Doctors' handwriting is generally abysmal; anything that can be done to reduce the requirement for handwritten notes has the potential for improved clinical practice.
- A departmental intranet is an extremely effective way of communicating with the staff.

Chapter 47
Administration, legal matters, governance and quality care in the ED

S Lesley Forster, Gordian W O Fulde and Sally McCarthy

How the law affects the practice of emergency medicine

(S Lesley Forster)

There have been a number of recent changes in society and in the law which greatly affect the practice of medicine in general, and emergency medicine in particular. Those practising emergency medicine need to be aware of these changes and to ensure that their practice conforms to the legal requirements. In court, ignorance of the law is no excuse.

This chapter also considers ways of decreasing the likelihood of legal action, and what to do if you are sued.

CONFIDENTIALITY

The overriding ethical maxim in the treatment of patients is that the doctor must keep secret anything he or she hears about the patient. (This also applies to social media websites. Any identifiable patient details/pictures are in breach.) There are, of course, exceptions; for example, where a patient consents to the disclosure of information, or when giving evidence in court.

When faced with requests from police officers for information regarding a patient's condition, ideally the written consent of the patient should be obtained first. It is the doctor's duty to ensure that information is given only to those who are entitled to it.

It is accepted that, in some instances, public interest can override a doctor's duty of confidentiality. If, for example, a patient confides to a doctor an intention to commit a serious criminal offence such as homicide or sexual assault, then it would be in order for the doctor to provide a relevant third party with that information.

There are other circumstances where the situation is not quite so clear, and judgment must be made according to the circumstances at the time as to what constitutes a serious criminal offence. It seems to be fairly well accepted among the medical profession, for example, that a doctor should not notify police of a patient's involvement in minor criminal activities, such as personal use of illicit drugs or property offences.

Some occasions arise where there is no absolute answer to the problem; for example, if a patient who is known to be involved in drug trafficking presents to the ED. In such a case where doubt may exist, the advice of colleagues, medical administration and, even better, the advice of a medical defence organisation should be sought in order to assist the doctor to make the very serious decision as to whether to override the duty of confidentiality.

For guidance, the St Vincent's Hospital policy regarding internally concealed drugs is shown in Box 47.1, overleaf.

Telephone calls

The decision as to whether information about a patient should be given over the telephone is one that arises frequently in the ED.

As a general rule, unless the patient has given consent, specific information regarding any patient should not be given over the telephone where it is impossible to be sure of the identity of the caller.

Relatives of very ill patients should be asked where possible to come to the hospital, where any information can be thoughtfully and sympathetically given. As a general rule, the results of tests (e.g. pregnancy, HIV, sexually transmitted diseases, etc) which have been performed in the department should not be released by phone. The patient should return to the ED or receive the results from the local doctor. In this way, mistakes and even medicolegal complications can be avoided.

Legal issues in medicine

NOTIFIABLE DISEASES

Notification by medical practitioners of certain diseases is mandatory. See Box 47.2.

MORE LEGAL OBLIGATIONS

Blood alcohol

In Australia, as in many countries, the treating doctor in an ED must perform a venepuncture and obtain a blood alcohol sample (refer to your own state legislation), basically within 12 hours of an accident, if the patient was on a public road and could have directly contributed to that accident, i.e. pedestrian, driver, skateboarder.

Box 47.1 St Vincent's Hospital policy and procedure for management of patients with internally concealed drugs

- These patients may present of their own accord or may be brought in by the police.
- Some drugs, e.g. heroin and cocaine, may cause death if leakage occurs. This is much less likely with hashish. Mechanical problems such as obstruction may occur with any ingested packets.
- Medical management should proceed as appropriate. Drug screens and other investigations are performed if medically indicated. Abdominal and chest X-rays, CT may be required. Close observation and supportive therapy are indicated. Specific antidotes such as naloxone may be required. Decontamination may be needed if packet rupture and toxicity have occurred (toxicity may occur by diffusion without packet rupture). Glycoprep (or similar) may be used to hasten transit. Laparotomy may be indicated to relieve mechanical obstruction or to urgently remove leaking packets which cannot be otherwise retrieved.
- If, in the judgment of the treating doctor, the amount of substance is small, i.e. unlikely to be intended for large-scale trafficking but rather intended for individual use, and the patient was not brought in by the police, then it is not mandatory that the police be contacted. Where large quantities are involved, the following steps should be taken:
  - Contact the emergency department director.
  - Contact medical administration.
  - A decision will then be taken regarding the need to contact police. The police will be contacted where the patient has obviously been involved in drug trafficking.
  - Medical management should never be impeded and remains first priority.
  - Patients should not be forcibly restrained.
  - Consent issues for medical procedures and treatment apply in the same way as with all patients.
  - The safety of St Vincent's Hospital staff should not be compromised.
  - Packets recovered are the responsibility of the police, if they are present. If the police are not present, recovered packets should be placed in a signed sealed bag, labelled and locked in the S.8 cupboard (checked in by two registered nurses). A check should be made between shifts to ensure that the seals remain unbroken. This must be documented in the S.8 book and in the patient's medical record. The packets should then be passed on to the police when they arrive.
  - Ensure that the documentation in the medical record is comprehensive and precise, as the history may be called in evidence.

Box 47.2 Notifiable diseases for hospitals*

Notifiable diseases (from NSW Public Health Act 2010 No 127)

- Acquired immune deficiency syndrome (AIDS)
- Acute viral hepatitis
- Adverse event following immunisation
- Avian influenza in humans
- Botulism
- Cancer
- Cholera
- Congenital malformation (as described in the *International Statistical Classification of Diseases and Related Health Problems*) in a child under the age of 1 year
- Creutzfeldt–Jakob disease (CJD) and variant Creutzfeldt-Jakob disease (vCJD)
- Cystic fibrosis in a child under the age of 1 year
- Diphtheria
- Foodborne illness in 2 or more related cases
- Gastroenteritis among people of any age, in an institution (for example, among persons in educational or residential institutions)
- Haemolytic uraemic syndrome
- *Haemophilus influenzae* type b
- Hypothyroidism in a child under the age of 1 year
- Legionnaires' disease
- Leprosy
- Lyssavirus
- Measles
- Meningococcal disease
- Paratyphoid
- Pertussis (whooping cough)
- Phenylketonuria in a child under the age of 1 year
- Plague
- Poliomyelitis
- Pregnancy with a child having a congenital malformation, cystic fibrosis, hypothyroidism, thalassaemia major or phenylketonuria
- Rabies
- Severe acute respiratory syndrome (SARS)
- Smallpox
- Syphilis
- Tetanus
- Thalassaemia major in a child under the age of 1 year
- Tuberculosis (TB)
- Typhoid
- Typhus (epidemic)
- Viral haemorrhagic fevers
- Yellow fever

* Under Section 81 of the NSW Public Health Act 2010, Hospital CEOs (or their delegates) are required to notify these diseases to the local public health unit.

These blood samples must be taken with supplied police kits. There is also a special kit for public transport accident victims (e.g. a passenger in a bus who fell).

Drug testing

At times the police will bring someone to the ED for drug testing. Each state has its guidelines and strict conditions, along with kits, and supervision of the passing of urine is required. At times the test (e.g. DNA sampling) should be taken by police doctors instead of the ED.

Sexual assault forensic tests

Sexual assault forensic tests should be done at sexual assault crisis units with trained staff and protocols.

How do you avoid a law suit?

The usual assumption is that good doctors are not sued. Sadly, this is not true. Good doctors are sued even when they do everything right and, if we are honest, even good doctors have bad days.

In a study, the most common reasons given for beginning a malpractice suit against a doctor were:

- advice from a knowledgeable friend (*Comment:* Be careful what you say about your colleague's work.)
- anger at being manipulated by medical personnel
- belief that a 'cover up' was taking place
- outcome failed to meet expectations
- was not told what was happening.

Think about these reasons carefully—they show that the remedy is in your own hands, but it has very little to do with your medical knowledge.

If you do not want to be sued, treat your patients and their relatives the way you would want to be treated in the same circumstances. Be open and friendly, concerned and, above all, talk to them and tell them what is happening. The attitude of your other staff (nurses, clerks, etc) is equally important—if the department is rude and uncommunicative, the hospital and the doctor will be sued.

Make your patients and their relatives feel that you value them as people and that you will spend the time and thought needed to make them well. Patients do not expect to be cured, but they do expect that everyone will treat them courteously (G Stubbs, personal communication).

CONSENT

There has been a change in the legal definition of informed consent following the *Rogers v Whitaker*[1] decision. Courts now believe that, in giving informed consent, a patient must be informed of all material risks. A risk becomes 'material' if the judge believes that a reasonable person in the patient's position would be likely to attach significant importance to it in deciding whether or not to have treatment.

As a general rule, emergency doctors who do not plan to perform a patient's definitive surgical or medical procedure should not accept the responsibility of 'getting a consent'. The emergency doctor may not even know exactly what the procedure involves, and cannot possibly be aware of all the material risks. In such a situation, it is impossible to obtain an 'informed consent' from the patient. However, for any invasive procedure, e.g. lumbar puncture, central line insertion, chest tube insertion, etc, a consent should be obtained if possible and signed by the patient and a witness.

PROCEDURAL MISTAKES

As we often hand over patients, take care to avoid doing the wrong test or the wrong procedure on the patient we do not know, e.g. 'The patient in bed 5 needs a CT or an LP'. We should, as is now routine in operating theatres, use the 'Time out' routine (see Box 47.3).

Box 47.3 Emergency department pre-procedure 'Time out'

Immediately prior to the commencement of the procedure, the procedure team MUST STOP activity and verbally confirm:

- Presence of the correct patient and consent.
- The correct site has been marked (if applicable).
- Correct procedure to be undertaken is documented.
- Availability of any special equipment.

REPORTS AND RECORDS

Comprehensive records, written when you saw the patient, are the keystone of your defence if you are sued. The better the records, the better your chance of a successful defence.

- It does not matter what you did—if you did not write it down, you did not do it!
- Conversely, if you did write it down, you did do it!

(Many requested legal reports centre around trauma, including assaults and car crashes. It really helps clinical care—e.g. follow-up—as well as your report to include a diagram with even estimated measurements and description of the injuries.)

Whenever you are asked for a report by the police or by a lawyer acting for a patient:

- You should immediately make several copies of all the hospital records pertaining to that period. This includes your notes, inpatient notes, test and X-ray results. Do not alter the records; this is the surest way to ensure you will get into trouble.
- Read your notes and, for your own information, expand them—explaining them and adding extra information that you remember (it may be years before you get to court, and your memory will decline with time).
- Make sure that the person asking is entitled and has gone through the correct hospital procedures. Make sure that the patient has signed the relevant release.
- Make your report factual, comprehensive and comprehensible, and you may avoid going to court.
- Remember, you can only report on what you learned first-hand. Do not draw conclusions, just report the facts (e.g. you can say, 'the patient smelt of alcohol' or 'he was unsteady of gait', but you cannot say 'he was drunk').

GOING TO COURT

The important rules in court appearances are: talk to a senior colleague before you go, stay calm, pause before you answer, keep it simple.

- The best answers are 'yes' or 'no'. Do not attempt to expand answers or to explain. Do not 'second-guess' where the questioner is heading.
- If you do not understand a question, ask for an explanation.
- Do not try to beat the barristers at their own game—you cannot, any more than they can intubate someone.
- Do not get angry—if you do, you will look bad and the lawyer will have won.
- Tell the truth, but say no more than you have to.

DOCTORS OUT-OF-HOURS OR AWAY FROM THEIR WORKPLACE

The well-publicised law case *Woods v Lowns & Anor*[2] has potentially radically changed the practice of medicine. While the eventual legal principles will be established in future cases, the implications for emergency doctors include:

- If a doctor in hospital is about to leave at the end of a shift, the doctor has a common law duty to attend to an emergency.

- If a doctor is at a theatre or sports event etc, not as a doctor, and a call is made 'Is there a doctor here?', the doctor may or may not have a duty of care towards the patient (we are not discussing moral duty here, just legal duty).
- If a doctor is not working, but is somewhere where he/she is known to be a doctor (such as a favourite restaurant or an aeroplane seat) or can be identified as a doctor (e.g. by a sticker on the doctor's car), then is the doctor under a legal duty of care? The answer is not clear, but probably he/she does.

The obvious answer is not to let people know you are a doctor, even in simple ways such as when booking airline seats, unless you are prepared to act in a case of emergency.

DUTY OF CARE: PATIENTS WHO REFUSE TREATMENT

The practice of emergency medicine has been based on the principle that it is always desirable to preserve life, and that all individuals want their lives to be preserved.

This tenet is now being challenged. The Northern Territory's 'euthanasia law', for example, demonstrates clearly that there are individuals who do not wish to preserve their lives at all costs. This raises questions for doctors in an emergency setting, who must balance their own obligation to treat versus the patient's 'right' to decline.

In the situation where a patient who is believed to need life-saving medical intervention refuses treatment, the future legal questions would possibly revolve around the question of the patient's competence, at that time, to make such a decision. Unless there is previously written and witnessed evidence of a pre-existing refusal by the patient, it is necessary for the doctor to be convinced that the patient is capable of making such a momentous decision—the patient's mind may be clouded by drugs, depression, pain or the nature of his/her illness. While the outcome of a legal challenge would be by no means certain, the truth is that, unless the doctor is absolutely certain and can prove that a patient is mentally competent when refusing life-saving treatment, the doctor should err on the side of active management.

Some clinical administration issues

(Gordian W O Fulde)

THE BASIC LEGAL PREMISE

Unlike on overseas TV programs, our medicolegal laws only expect a medical practitioner to provide reasonable, peer-practised care—i.e. rather than being the world's best or most expert at your level, you must provide what is reasonably expected from an intern or any equivalent, e.g. CMO, registrar, GP, etc.

Also, management that is considered 'peer-practised' does not have to be universally practised to be considered reasonable care.

THE HAND-OVER PATIENT

These patients, i.e. the ones we have not personally assessed, feature highly in legal cases and hospital incident reporting systems. We must take special care to fully communicate when handing over. One widespread system is the ISBAR clinical hand-over tool—**I**ntroduction, **S**ituation, **B**ackground, **A**ssessment, **R**ecommendation (see Table 21.1).

THE DYING OR RESUSCITATION PATIENT

- Appoint a main spokesperson or communicator among the relatives.
- Keep them informed, preferably by you; be frank and honest.
- Consider their presence by the bedside.
- Get the cavalry in—social worker, priest, clinician who knows the patient, etc.

THE DECEASED PATIENT

- Is it a coroner's case? See Box 47.4.
- Looking after a grieving family appropriately is a top priority—it is hard, it hurts; but it is vital.

CODES

Know them! Especially red, blue and black (Figure 47.1).

MEDICAL CERTIFICATES

- These are legal documents. Never backdate them. Stick to facts you can defend.
- Prescriptions—you must know the patient medically.

Fire/Smoke	Code Red
Medical Emergency	Code Blue
Bomb Threat	Code Purple
Internal Emergency	Code Yellow
Personal Threat	Code Black
External Emergency	Code Brown
Evacuation	Code Orange

Figure 47.1 Emergency codes

Box 47.4 The circumstances which necessitate that a death be notified to the coroner*

A 'coroner's case' is clearly defined as follows:

1. Sudden death of unknown cause, i.e. unable to write death certificate.
2. Death from a violent or unnatural cause or in suspicious or unusual circumstances.
3. Death within 1 year and 1 day of an accident to which the death is or may be attributable.
   Note: If the patient is 65 years or more and the accident was attributable to their age, contributed substantially to their death, was in no way suspicious or unusual and was not caused by an act or omission of another person, a death certificate may be written. If, however, the accident occurred in a hospital or nursing home, the death is always a coroner's case, regardless of a patient's age.
4. Death of a patient within 24 hours of an anaesthetic, general *or* local, administered in the course of a medical, surgical or dental operation or procedure, other than a local anaesthetic administered solely for the purpose of facilitating a procedure of resuscitation from apparent or impending death.
5. Death of a patient who has not been attended by a medical practitioner within the period of 3 months immediately prior to the death.
6. Death in an admission centre, mental hospital, residential centre for handicapped persons or similar facility or while in the custody of a police officer or in other lawful custody.

* If there is any doubt whether or not a death is a coroner's case, medical administration should be contacted.

- Be careful: do not leave prescription pads lying around.
- Again, if in doubt, ask—look it up.

INSURANCE

As an employee of the hospital, technically you are covered at hospital. But you are not covered for:

- professional matters, conduct
- informal consultations or opinions, e.g. given to your neighbours
- technically, cross-suits initiated by the 'hospital' against you as an individual.

Therefore, it is advisable to have even minimal indemnity cover.

APPEARANCE

In the first instance, it is not about *you*—rather, that you do not offend the patient. Keep it neutral and tidy—no radical-message T-shirts.

(You can always cover your clothes with a hospital gown when on clinical duties.)

MEDIA

You are not permitted to talk to the media or represent the hospital unless given permission by hospital administration. Media can be curly—beware!

COMPLAINTS

These will always occur, and may even involve you; they are vital to running and improving a good service.

- Treat each complaint seriously and empathetically.
- Do not judge until you have all the facts.
- Be honest.
- Respond ASAP (even a phone call from you on receipt of the complaint may solve the issue; in any case it will definitely decrease the aggro).
- Be constructive; do not be punitive or play the blame game.
- At least generically admit to issues, problems etc, should these exist.
- Notify and check with administration before making any written response.

Data relating to quality, key performance indicators (KPIs), adverse events, etc are a part of life—use them to help your department:

- They reflect workload, problems.
- It is essential to have them, to bargain for resources—or defend them!
- They often show where to focus for improvement.
- They are never perfect—ensure that data going out of your department makes sense, e.g. include a briefing note or interpretation with the data.

THREATS TO RESOURCES

Staff, budget, etc—it is all about money!

Do not explode or take to drink—even if the threat is the most stupid thing imaginable!

- Register your objection IN WRITING.
- Gather data—why are they doing this? Who is driving it?
- Rally support, especially from top management (go and talk to them—don't only email).
- Create a multi-prong attack—enlist nursing staff, etc.

- Offer an alternative solution to the problem.
- Be prepared to lose and win.

A HAPPY DEPARTMENT

- Talk to all the staff—try to know their first names.
- Be friendly, listen and be quick to praise or say thank you.
- If a problem occurs:
  - Are you the one to sort it out, or a fellow manager (especially if a different craft group)?
  - Ensure that discussion is professional, and private (± third party).
  - Avoid punitive actions—in the first place.
  - Be prepared to apologise—none of us is perfect.
- Beware:
  - Do not grizzle all the time—too easy!
  - Do not fight (even if it is a just cause) with the rest of the hospital, ambulance crew, GPs, etc.
  - Look at it from their point of view!
  - Kill conflict.

Treat patients and staff as you or a loved one would want to be treated. We aim for good care, but reasonable has to be the minimum standard.

Quality and governance in the ED

(Sally McCarthy)

WHAT IS QUALITY?

Clinical quality

Much of the discussion concerning quality in health care has arisen from various reports and international studies which have found unacceptably high rates of adverse events in hospitalised patients, resulting in significant morbidity and mortality. Subsequent attention has been focused on clinical quality, with one definition of quality in health being: *doing the right thing, the first time, in the right way, and at the right time.* Clinical care and services must be safe, effective, appropriate, customer-focused, accessible and efficient.

Customer-defined quality

More broadly, quality is defined with reference to the customer: as the difference between what a customer wants from the ED service and the perception of the actual performance of the service.

A customer is anyone who comes into contact with our work. They may include internal customers—those within the organisation who will be affected by the ED (e.g. diagnostic services, inpatient team registrars, ward nursing staff) and external customers—those outside the organisation who are affected by our work (e.g. patients and their families, ambulance service, GPs, taxpayers, politicians).

Organisation-wide quality

Quality management in an organisation is an organisation-wide effort to achieve sustained, ongoing improvements in quality, based on a study of organisational processes, and with decisions and results based on, and measured by, data. The *management style* is emphasised as a key to success: a management style that is proactive and leading, rather than reactive and authoritarian. Management recognises that employees care about their work and will take initiatives to improve it, and that employees are empowered to perform to their full potential when supported with appropriate tools and training. Management also recognises that quality is ultimately the responsibility of top management.

Clinical governance, with its concept of managerial legal responsibility for patient mishap, and clinical quality as an equal partner to fiscal control at board level, is consistent with a quality management approach.

PATIENT SATISFACTION

In emergency medicine, the available body of knowledge suggests that most ED patients want the same things: promptness, courtesy, compassion, privacy and information. Providing high-quality ED care hinges on our ability to empathise and communicate—to understand and be sensitive to the feelings, thoughts and experiences of our patients.

Communication with patients

Introduce yourself by title and name. Establish eye contact at the beginning of the consultation (unless culturally inappropriate) and maintain it at reasonable intervals to show interest. Apologise for the wait if appropriate, and indicate by your manner that you are ready to give the patient your full attention.

Key tasks to be covered in your communication with patients are:

- eliciting the patient's main problems, their perceptions of these problems, and the physical, emotional and social impact on themselves and their families

- tailoring information to what the patient wants to know, and checking their understanding
- eliciting the patient's reactions to the information given, and concerns raised
- determining how much the patient wants to participate in decision-making (when treatment options are available)
- discussing treatment options so that the patient understands the implications
- maximising the chance that patients will follow agreed decisions and advice.

Patient expectations

Management of patient expectations is fundamental to satisfaction. Studies suggest that dissatisfaction increases as patients' triage acuity decreases. The actual time waiting to be seen by a doctor and the total length of stay in the ED are not significant predictors of patient satisfaction. Managing the perception of waiting time, by communicating an expected waiting time to patients, seems to be more important for satisfaction than the actual waiting time.

Complaints

Avoidance of complaints is facilitated by good communication with patients. Review of the reasons why patients complain or litigate demonstrates the main reasons for patient dissatisfaction: patients felt their opinion was 'devalued'; information was poorly delivered; their viewpoint was not understood by the doctor; their complaint was not acknowledged; or they felt an honest explanation for an adverse outcome was not given. Criticism of treatment by a second doctor also made patients more likely to take legal action.

Dealing with complaints successfully involves apologising and 'owning' the problem, doing it quickly, giving a factual explanation of what happened and what is being changed to prevent a recurrence and thanking the person for bringing the problem to your attention. It is advisable to involve a senior staff member in this process.

RISK MANAGEMENT AND HUMAN FACTORS

Risk is the exposure to the possibility of such things as economic or financial loss, physical damage, injury or delay, as a consequence of pursuing or not pursuing a particular course of action. Risks and their consequences in the ED include:

- an adverse event during the care process
- a failure of equipment or computer systems

- patient or family dissatisfaction
- a threat to physical safety
- a breach of legal or contractual responsibility
- unfavourable publicity
- a breach of patient privacy
- fraud
- loss of patient valuables.

Managing risk requires proactive attention to predictable risk areas and moving away from the traditional approach to error in medicine, with its emphasis on personal responsibility, autonomy and accountability.

Human factors engineering (or ergonomics) is the study of how human beings interact with their environment, or the study of factors that make work easy or hard. A 'human factors' approach emphasises:

- systems rather than people, e.g. rosters to be according to 'safe hours' practices (night shifts preferably 8 hours or less, no more than 3 consecutive nights, no shift exceeding 16 hours, avoid on-call shifts with frequent night calls followed by normal working days, roster adequate time off after nights) to prevent fatigue-induced poor performance
- a non-punitive approach to adverse events, viewing errors or near-misses as a chance to learn about the system
- the multifactorial nature of errors
- an assumption that errors will occur, so that systems of work should be designed to make it difficult for clinicians to act erroneously—errors should be obvious before they cause harm and there should be multiple buffers to minimise the effect of errors
- team interactions
- 'sharp end, blunt end'—considering not only the point where the actual error occurred but the organisational policies and resource allocation decisions that created the system.

Occupational health and safety obligations of employers include maintaining a safe workplace for all employees through reducing the risk of occupational illness and injury. Specific examples in the ED include infection-control measures *and* minimisation of aggression and violence in the ED through staff training and provision of environmental controls (controlled access points to ED, video surveillance, security personnel, personal duress alarms, safe observation rooms for potentially violent patients).

QUALITY ASSURANCE

Ongoing monitoring of aspects of clinical care, human resource management, adverse events, complaints and staff wellbeing occurs to demonstrate compliance with basic standards.

Indicators assess compliance across the dimensions of:

- access—e.g. waiting times; access block
- safety—e.g. staff absence due to work-related injury; needle-stick injury; patient falls; aggressive or violent incidents towards staff
- acceptability/customer focus—e.g. complaint rate; appreciation letters
- effectiveness—e.g. admission by triage category; time to thrombolysis or analgesia
- efficiency—e.g. waiting time by triage category; total treatment time
- appropriateness—e.g. rate of unnecessary testing; antibiotic choice.

Editorial Comment

Although these topics are not foremost in the hearts of health carers, they are ignored at your peril as they are essential parts of what we do.

The quality and length of time with the patient has been proven to be the main factor contributing to dissatisfaction (complaints, law suits).

EDs are undergoing re-engineering of patient flow—the '4-hour rule.' There will be definite improvements for patients but also definite negative aspects, especially during any change. As with any clinical system issue, identify it and use your governance system (e.g. clinical review issue reporting) to document it; this allows actions, improvements and responsibility to be logged.

References

1. *Rogers v Whitaker* (1992) 175 CLR 479.
2. *Woods v Lowns & Anor* (1995) 36 NSWLR 344; *Lowns v Woods* [1996] Australian Torts Reports 81-376 at 63,151.

Chapter 48
A guide for interns working in emergency medicine

Tiffany Fulde and Richard Sullivan

Introduction

As for many interns about to start work in emergency medicine, this may seem like the most daunting term in your year as an intern, but don't be alarmed—for most junior doctors it is one of the most rewarding periods, and the term where an intern feels most useful as a doctor. You will learn a lot during this term through the variety of people and presentations you see, and you will gain confidence in initiating management and recognising sick patients. You will improve your procedural skills and your communication with colleagues and patients, and you will work closely with a large team of health professionals. By the end of the term, ward and after-hours work will seem more manageable, and the term can be a big turning point for your year.

Emergency medicine does have a more rapid turnover than other parts of the hospital, and a greater focus on service provision, but with a good approach you should be able to balance this with your educational needs and enjoy your term.

Day 1—getting started

On your first day, make sure you take a moment to familiarise yourself with your surroundings. Introduce yourself to the team, including the registrars and consultants, other junior doctors, nurses, ward clerks, physiotherapists, social worker, pharmacists and anyone else who is part of your emergency department (ED) team. The more familiar you are with the team and the more familiar they are with you, the easier the transition to a new term will be.

Orientation to the ED is very important. Most hospitals arrange a formal session of orientation to the department, including its layout, preferred documentation, use of IT for orders and results, electronic medical records (EMRs) and triage, and any relevant policies and clinical protocols/pathways. If you haven't had any orientation, ask the most senior staff in the department how the department works—especially the layout, where to pick up patients and where to take them to be seen, how to click patients off on the computer or list, and with whom you should discuss patient care. Each ED is set up differently—some are divided into acute and subacute, or fast-track, areas; others have mental health or paediatric areas. It is important to familiarise yourself with the way your ED works each time you start a new rotation. This will make your job a lot easier.

Always remember that everyone knows how daunting it can be for a new intern in the ED. You should never be afraid to ask questions—the more questions you ask, the more you will learn and the better you will be at your job. So ask questions of everyone around you—there is no such thing as a stupid question.

Working up a patient

Once you have familiarised yourself with the department and who you will be working with, it will be time for you to dive in and start seeing a patient. If you are unsure, you can ask the registrar who they would like you to see first; otherwise, take the next patient on the list.

Generally, interns are expected to see the lower triage categories (categories 3–5). If you would like to see a higher-priority patient, tell the registrar or consultant before seeing the patient. You should try to see more-complex and higher-category patients as you progress through the term.

You should do the initial work-up and then report back to your registrar or consultant, and discuss further management. Prior to this discussion, try to formulate differential diagnoses and a potential management plan; this will be the best way to learn and gain confidence to work more independently. As you progress through the term, you may be able to initiate more investigations and management independently, but you should always discuss your patients with someone more senior. The timing of this discussion depends on how sick the patient is, and on your experience—the earlier the better if the patient is deteriorating, or if you are unsure. Some special cases will always require early involvement of senior doctors, for example paediatric presentations.

1 ASSESSING THE PATIENT

Once you have 'clicked off' your patient, take a look at the history on the triage sheet, and start thinking of likely differentials and what further information you will need from your history, examination and investigations. Make sure you have an appropriate environment in which to assess the patient:

- Do they need monitoring?
- Are they likely to be violent or abscond?
- How mobile are they?
- Will they need a bed?
- Will you need to perform any invasive investigations/ examinations? (e.g. internal or rectal examinations will need a private area)
- Do you need any special equipment (e.g. slit lamp)?

You can discuss these with the triage nurse and the nurse in charge to ascertain where you should see the patient. If you have to wait for an ideal environment, see if there is anything you can start doing in the meantime—e.g. initial history, bloods, X-rays or ECG.

In the ED, assessment and management of patients often occur simultaneously, and initial management may precede a full history. Some management and investigations may have been started at triage, for example analgesia and antiemetics or X-rays in suspected fractures. You should develop a systematic approach to identify the main complaint and start treatment as appropriate (e.g. bronchodilators in an asthma attack) before returning to take a full history and ensuring nothing gets missed. You will become more skilled at performing a multitude of tasks simultaneously during your ED term, but keep it simple at the start. Remember your training; and if you are stuck, go through the process of ABCDE and go back to the first principles of history, examination and investigations.

Also, think about possible sources for more information: old notes, notes from other hospitals, referral letters and family members and friends may all be useful sources. It may take you a while to get all this information, so the sooner you request it, the better.

It is very important that if you are ever worried about a patient at any stage during your work-up, do not hesitate to go immediately to a registrar or consultant and request help—they expect it, and welcome early recognition of a deteriorating patient. A key skill for junior doctors is to recognise your own limitations, and seniors will respect you for this. Ensuring your own safety and patient safety is particularly important as an ED doctor.

2 INVESTIGATIONS

- Most patients in the ED will require bloods, and many ED doctors and nurses will advise you to place a cannula while you are taking bloods—that way you have access if you need it, and you will save the patient having an extra needle later on. As a general rule, a 20G cannula should suffice. This is a great way to practise your cannulation skills.

- In most cases, if you are taking bloods you should take at least one purple tube, one lime or gold, and one blue. You may not need to order tests for all of these tubes, but this will enable you to add on most common tests if you need them and avoid the need for further venepuncture as you work through your likely differentials. Consider whether blood cultures may be necessary.
- Similarly, if the patient requires radiology, try to order all tests at the same time, e.g. chest X-ray and foot X-ray, to avoid multiple trips to radiology and unnecessary delay.
- As a general rule for a junior, you should talk to a senior doctor before arranging more-extensive investigations (i.e. other than bloods, X-rays, ECG, spirometry). Various departments will have different policies regarding the ordering of CT scans and this should be discussed with someone more senior. If a test is urgent, make sure you communicate this clearly, usually both on the order form and via phone.
- Make sure you chase results for each test you have ordered (or hand-over that they need to be chased) and discuss these results with a senior doctor.

3 DISCUSSION

Once you have taken your history and done your examination (± bloods and basic radiology), it is probably time to run over the case with a registrar or consultant (*remember to speak to someone earlier if you are worried about a patient, even if the history and examination is not complete*). The purpose of this conversation is to come to an agreed working diagnosis or problem list, and an agreed management plan.

Communication with the registrar and the consultant is a useful skill to develop and will help you when making referrals over the phone to other teams (which most doctors find more difficult than face-to-face).

- Practise being succinct, and present only the findings which are relevant to the diagnosis and management of your patient.
- It is very useful to start the conversation with an overarching statement which summarises the case and your thoughts on disposition and management, as this helps frame the

conversation for the listener (e.g. 'I have just seen a 49-year-old man with intermediate-risk chest pain who I think requires admission for stress testing and monitoring.' Then go into further detail of the history).

- It is important that you know the patient's vitals before you begin the conversation, and make sure you include what has already been done for the patient.
- You might try to finish your presentation with how you would like to manage the situation and ask if anything else needs to be done or if you have left anything important out.
- If you are really concerned, do not hesitate to ask for a senior review.

At all times, remember that *patient safety comes first.* If the senior doctor asks you something you do not know or forgot to ask, never pretend that you know the answer or make up information—the senior can usually tell, but more importantly this may give a false impression of how your patient is and what should be done. As an intern, you are still learning, and it is OK not to know all the answers.

4 FURTHER REFERRAL

Following the discussion with your senior, you should have a clear plan for the patient, whether it is further assessment, investigations or examination, or management. Make sure you continue to monitor your patient, and chase any outstanding investigations.

- If you think the patient is likely to be discharged, you might start your discharge planning, including letter, scripts and follow-up appointments or referrals to extra services. Liaise with social work and physiotherapy if necessary, and consider how the patient is going to get home: will they need transport or a family member to collect them, are they safe to go by themselves or will they need extra help? Try to arrange these things early so that there is no delay when the patient is ready for discharge. There is often an aged-care service in the emergency team which can assist with this process, so liaise closely with them. Some hospitals offer a 'Hospital in the Home' program; if so, consider whether the patient is suitable for this. If given the option of home- or hospital-based treatment, most patients would choose home.
- If you think the patient is likely to require admission, you might start to organise your referral to the appropriate team's registrar. It is a good idea to be prepared with the patient's notes and

investigation results easily accessible. Consider which team you are referring to, and why: What is the problem you think they should manage? Is the patient known to a particular doctor or team? Do you have all the relevant information? You may not need to wait for every investigation result before calling the registrar, unless it is integral to the diagnosis. For example, if the patient has appendicitis clinically, you don't necessarily need to wait for the WCC—but you would probably wait for a beta-hCG in a female patient.

As with your earlier discussion with your senior ED doctor, try to synthesise your **referral information** and keep your findings relevant to the problem and team you are speaking to. Think about what information that team cares about—it might be slightly different to what the ED thinks is the most important information. A concise opening sentence about the presentation, followed by an explanation of the diagnosis including relevant history, examination and investigations and the patient's current situation, is usually all that is required. Try using the principles of ISBAR to aid your communication (see Box 48.1).

Don't be rattled if you are asked questions or met with scepticism, as this can be quite common with ED referrals. Make sure you communicate clearly and calmly; if you run into serious obstruction, notify your senior who will advise you what to do.

Box 48.1 ISBAR model for clinical hand-over

I	Introduction *Identify yourself, your role and your location* *Identify the patient*
S	Situation *State the patient's diagnosis/reason for admission and current problem*
B	Background *What is the patient's history?*
A	Assessment *What are the most recent observations? What is your assessment?*
R	Recommendation *What do you want the person taking over care of the patient to do? When should this occur?*

Sometimes it may be appropriate to refer to a team for further assessment or management before the principal diagnosis has been decided. Do not be afraid to be upfront about this during your referral, but explain why you think the patient should be seen at this stage. For example, 'This 30-year-old man has presented with LLQ abdominal pain. I am not entirely sure of the cause, but the patient has required ongoing morphine and I am concerned about [*insert diagnosis*] and would like a medical/surgical opinion regarding admission and further investigation.' While such referrals may be met with resistance, medicine often requires doctors to be prepared to deal with uncertainty, and not all patients will fit a clear diagnosis. This is particularly true in the ED. Patients may often require admission to further investigate and observe the development of symptomatology.

Once you have made your referral, make sure you **document** any recommendations by the team, and arrange any investigations or management they have requested. It is also important to follow up on the patient to ensure their condition has not changed, that they have been seen by the registrar and to ensure that a plan is being implemented.

- If the patient is to be admitted, make sure they are ready for the ward, including charting all medications.
  - Some medications given in the ED are not able to be given on the ward (e.g. IV morphine), so make sure there are appropriate alternatives available.
  - Think about when the patient is likely to be reviewed next, and make sure they have everything they need arranged until then, e.g. IV fluids, cannula.
  - Order any necessary tests and make sure that anything that is time-critical is clearly handed over to the ward resident, e.g. serial troponins.
  - If the registrar has not already done so, notify the nurse in charge that the patient requires a bed.
- If the patient is to be discharged, ensure you have a clear plan for necessary follow-up from the registrar.
  - For all patients who are to be discharged, make sure you have cleared them with a senior doctor before discharge.
  - All patients will need a discharge letter, including a clear outline of any outstanding investigations you would like their GP to follow up, and any further follow-up arrangements.
  - If the patient requires medications on discharge, you should ensure that they have a prescription (script) and will be able to fill this within an appropriate time (e.g. if discharging after hours, are there any pharmacies open or do you need to provide a take-home pack? Can the script wait until

morning?). You should also have a care for whether patients are unable to fill their prescription, e.g. due to financial burden. Clarify your approach in these situations with someone senior.

— Make sure you advise the patient of any special instructions on discharge, including warning signs for re-presentation, medication and timing of follow-up. If something is particularly important to follow up, do not hesitate to call the GP as well as providing a letter.

5 PATIENTS AND PATIENCE

One of the most important parts of your job is to communicate to the patient and inform them about the hospital process. Try to keep the patient updated as regularly as possible on their progress. Often patients do not know how the hospital works, or do not understand the need to refer to an inpatient team and for another doctor to see them before a decision on admission is made. It is also useful to advise patients on expected delays before certain test results may be available. All these discussions go a long way in assisting the patient to have a better experience in the department.

Also remember that patients and their families are often in a stressful and unfamiliar environment. Try to be patient with demanding patients—they may not understand the multiple demands on your time or that they are a lower priority than patients who are more unwell. Try to explain and reassure and be empathetic to their concerns. If you do, these interactions can be the most rewarding part of your job.

Further into the term/learning opportunities

1 RESUSCITATION/TRAUMA

Early in the term, the resuscitation bay may seem an intimidating place. Throughout your term, try to get involved as much as you can when patients are brought through for resuscitation or trauma calls. Begin by observing the process and the teamwork; then, when you feel comfortable, ask the team leader if you can be involved. A good place to start is as the procedures team-member: your job will be to place a large cannula, usually 18G is sufficient, and take blood, including for blood gases. Often an extra set of hands—for log-rolls or cardiac compressions—is really useful as well. It is a very different experience to be involved in managing a high-acuity situation, and a great learning opportunity. Get involved however you can.

As you progress through your term, you should also be proactive in seeing the higher-triage-category patients that come into these areas. When you first pick up the high-acuity patients in the resuscitation bay you may feel anxious about being alone with a very sick patient, but you will be surprised how many consultants and registrars are looking over your shoulder and are ready to support you. Don't be afraid to call out for extra help if you need it.

These experiences are invaluable, and will give you confidence in handling a patient that is deteriorating, which will help you significantly in the future when you are the first to see a deteriorating patient on the wards. Touch base with a senior sooner than with lower-category patients, and remember 'ABCs' if stuck.

2 FORMAL TEACHING AND EDUCATIONAL OPPORTUNITIES

It is greatly recommended that you attend any educational opportunities available. Most EDs provide a formal teaching program for junior medical officers. You should be supported to attend these by other staff, and you should make an effort to attend as many of them as possible. Discuss with seniors if there are any topics in particular you would like more exposure to. These sessions will help to ensure that you are familiar with the main ED presentations and skills, as you are unlikely to see the full variety in one term, and will make your work easier when managing these presentations for the first time.

A lot of teaching in the ED occurs 'on the job'. This can provide a lot of learning and experience in a variety of areas, including clinical assessment, investigation interpretation and management options. Take every opportunity to further your procedural and clinical skills under supervision, then with increasing independence as appropriate. Wound closure and suturing, plastering and fracture management and use of special equipment such as slit lamps are common ED skills that you should become proficient in. If you have the opportunity, try to gain exposure and experience in more-complex procedures, such as lumbar punctures or chest drain insertion.

Always work within your experience level, and if you are unsure ask someone more senior to supervise you.

3 FOLLOW-UP

A great opportunity to consolidate your learning is by following up on the patients you have seen in the ED who get admitted. If you have time before or after your shift, check what happened to your patients after admission, what the ultimate diagnosis was, what further investigations were useful and what management was implemented. This will give you a longitudinal view of patient care and a broader context for patient care in the ED. It will also help you to reflect on and evaluate your assessment and management in the ED. This can improve your diagnostic skills, build your confidence by seeing the things you did effectively and improve your management of future presentations.

Miscellaneous

1 CHERRY-PICKING

Patients on the ED waiting list are ordered according to the priority in which they need to be seen. If you do not follow this order and choose instead to see only the patients who are interesting or easy for you, also known as 'cherry-picking', you are performing a very great disservice—not just to the patient, but to the other doctors on your team and, importantly, to yourself. It is really important for your learning that you take all opportunities for exposure to a wide range of presentations and management. The ED is a unique environment in which to see a variety of undifferentiated and multisystem presentations. Challenge yourself: this is the time in your career where you are most supported and supervised—it is the best time to learn. Also, look after your colleagues—*you* wouldn't appreciate being left to see all the complicated or less-desirable presentations!

2 HAND-OVER BETWEEN SHIFTS

Hand-over is essential for the continuity of patient care and for patient safety, and also has implications for your own welfare. Internship can be a very stressful period and it is important that you try to leave on time and have a life outside of the workplace. As you approach the end of your shift, you should start preparing to hand over the care of your patients. If you can do this well, it will help your patients, your colleagues and yourself.

There are multiple ways to perform clinical hand-over, and each department will differ in its procedures. In some departments patients may be reassigned by a senior doctor or during a ward round, but often you will have to seek someone out on the later shift to take your patients.

Ideally you would facilitate the other doctor's taking over care as much as possible by preparing as much as you can of the plan. For example, if the patient is likely to be discharged but needs to wait for a test result, try to write the discharge letter before you hand over so that the other doctor need only add the result; or, if the patient is likely to be admitted, chart the medications. If possible, it is usually preferable for the person who has assessed the patient to make the referral to the registrar, as they know the patient best. If the work-up is incomplete, you may need to clarify that you are handing over to a certain ED doctor and agree with the registrar that the ED doctor will call again with further information once available.

It is important to communicate to the person taking over care what has been done and what they need to do for the patient. Try to make hand-over brief, clear and simple. Emphasise what you would like the person to do. For example, 'This is a 65-year-old man who had a simple mechanical fall with nil evident injuries. He is on warfarin for AF, and has an INR in therapeutic range. Could you please chase the CT head and if normal can you please discharge this patient—the summary is already written but just needs updating with the CT result.' Take care not to hand over irrelevant details, as the plan may get lost in the intricacies of the story (which you have already gone over with the senior), and usually all the information the listener needs or wants is what they have to do. That message will be diluted if you delve too deeply into the story, so leave that to your discussion with the senior when you are working out a plan.

Sometimes it is not possible to have your patients 'parcelled up' neatly before your shift ends—the department could be very busy, or there might be too much uncertainty regarding the patient's diagnosis and plan. Try to help your colleague as much as possible, but it is important to recognise your own limits. Just do the best you can. With this in mind, try to be understanding when someone else hands you over a patient who is incompletely worked up. Also, if you see someone from the earlier shift struggling to get out or over their time, offer them a hand. This will come back to you next time you're trying to end your shift.

If there is reluctance to take over patients who are incompletely worked up, the flow-on effect is that ED doctors are often reluctant to pick up new patients in the last hour of their shift, especially patients who are more complex or who may have delays with investigation, keeping them at work after their shift has ended. If you find yourself in this situation, there is still a lot you can do to help the department and your colleagues. You can try to see a patient who you think will be quick, and likely to go home; or ask if anyone needs a hand, and help start the work-up for patients who are waiting—put in cannulas and take bloods, order X-rays or chart medications. You can apply this at any stage: if your patient-load prevents you picking up a new patient but you have time while you wait for results, see if there is any way to help out.

Remember that you are part of a team—try to support each other, and if you are consistently finding it difficult to leave close to time or having problems with patient hand-over, ask a senior for advice and support.

3 BREAKS AND DEBRIEFING

As your day in the ED will usually be less structured than during other terms, it is often difficult to schedule regular breaks. Periods when the department is busy with many patients waiting, and when you have many patients or patients who are unwell and slightly unstable, are particularly difficult times and ED interns often feel compelled to skip their breaks. You may actually reach the end of your shift and realise that you forgot to eat lunch or dinner if you have been particularly busy.

Make sure you take the time to eat, have a drink and sit down. You will actually perform better after your break, which can make you more efficient and effective and ultimately save you time—and, importantly, it will help prevent you burning out and getting tired later in the term.

If you are finding it hard to have a meal, some of the best times to take a break are around the time the new staff arrive for their shift, and also when you are waiting for pathology or radiology results. When you go for a break, let someone on your shift know, and give a quick update to the nurses looking after the same patient about the progress. If you are worried about a patient, consider where you take your break. Can you stay in a more accessible area?

During your ED term you will inevitably experience situations that will be challenging, emotional and possibly even confronting. If you feel you need to take some time out, do not hesitate to go to the coffee room and have a 10-minute break to have a tea or coffee. Let someone know before you go; you will find that most people in the department will understand.

If you do encounter such situations, it is important that you debrief with someone afterwards—even days later, if you need time to digest things. Talk to someone you feel comfortable with—either at work or outside—about any events that you found difficult; it will help you cope and learn. Listening to others talk about their experiences can also be very positive. Sharing your experiences through the term with other interns and residents can be particularly helpful in understanding common challenges and realising that others may be having a very similar experience to your own.

You may also like to discuss things with someone more senior in the department; gaining feedback on how you are going, and how you might approach things differently, can be very productive and a central component to your development.

4 PERSONAL SAFETY AND PPE

Your workplace should be a safe environment. Unfortunately, the ED—more than most parts of the hospital—is a place where you encounter more-frequent risks, and you will need to be alert to potential dangers and be proactive in taking precautions to minimise these.

Due to the nature of presentations in the ED, including wounds, patients who present with vomiting, bleeding, etc, as well as the nature of management which includes a greater number of procedures, you will be at an increased risk of exposure to body fluids.

- Familiarise yourself with the personal protective equipment (PPE) available, where to find it, and local PPE protocols, and adopt universal precautions—e.g. during procedures, treat every patient as though they had a known blood-borne pathogen (even if they appear low-risk).
- If you are exposed, notify a senior immediately. Your ED will have a protocol for management of post-exposure prophylaxis. Always err on the side of caution: even if you feel it was low-risk, make sure you discuss this with a senior colleague
- As always, hand hygiene is important and should be performed with all patients. It is often forgotten, however, that multi-resistant organisms can be present in the ED and you should continue to use additional precautions (e.g. gown and gloves) if seeing a patient with previous infection or colonisation, to minimise risk of cross-infection to other patients. Remember to ask about recent travel.

In the ED you will also see aggressive patients, patients under the influence of alcohol or other substances, and mental health patients. You will need to adjust your approach to these patients according to the risk they present.

- Many EDs keep a record of patients who have previously been aggressive, via an alert on the triage system or EMR. Ask someone how to access this, and before you go to assess the patient, check if they have any alerts registered. This can be a useful indicator of their behaviour.

- Assess every patient for risk, including changeability. Ask the triage staff how the patient behaved at assessment and in the waiting room. Be careful where you see these patients, and if you are uncomfortable ask a colleague to accompany you. You may need to consider calling security to search the patient for weapons before you assess them. The ED nursing staff are particularly valuable in advising you of patient risk. The nurses may well have already treated the patient and be familiar with their pattern of behaviour.
- Take whatever precautions are appropriate for the environment (some hospitals may offer personalised duress alarms, for example), and make sure you familiarise yourself with the hospital protocol for aggressive or violent patients, including physical and chemical sedation.
- Again, you should always err on the side of caution. If you are concerned, ask for advice and seek help early.

5 ONLINE RESOURCES AND EMRS

Electronic and online resources are incredibly useful tools, and will hopefully be readily available in your ED. Familiarise yourself with what's available and how to access these.

- These references are very handy while you are seeing patients, to refresh your knowledge of detailed management, such as medication regimens, and to provide advice and direction in cases you have not seen previously. This is particularly helpful in the ED due to the wide variety of presentations you will see—you will inevitably see things you are unfamiliar with or have forgotten. E-resources are also useful to reinforce your learning after you have seen a patient.
- Some useful resources include the online Therapeutic Guidelines, Australian Medicines Handbook, MIMS, UpToDate and BMJ Best Practice (see 'Online resources'; many hospitals have subscriptions where necessary). There are also videos of procedures you can access from various websites to consolidate your learning.

Electronic medical records (EMRs) can give you access to previous discharge summaries, medications and pathology, which can provide helpful information against which to compare a patient's current condition and establish a baseline. If you have access to these capabilities, try to take advantage of their use and also keep them as up-to-date and accurate as possible for future reference.

These tools will help you to maximise your own learning and efficiency and improve patient outcomes.

6 DOCUMENTATION

In a rushed environment, writing good notes might seem a lower priority than starting management and chasing investigations. It is actually equally—if not more—important to document what you have done and who you have discussed your patients with. If you are busy, it is easy to forget or confuse details, and documentation should be part of a consistent, systematic approach. Some find it useful to jot down some rough notes while taking the patient history, then write more-detailed notes away from the patient. This may be especially useful if your ED uses EMRs and the patient is not yet logged on to the system. Find a system that works for you.

Accurate and detailed notes are particularly important in the ED. You may be asked to complete legal documentation months after you have seen a patient if their injuries are part of a court case, e.g. if you have seen an assault victim. As the treating doctor, it is your notes and your opinion that will be used. Months later you will not remember each patient, so make sure that you document relevant details, e.g. size and depth of wounds, consider drawing the location. Ask for guidance on how to complete any requests for medicolegal documentation from senior doctors, medical records and your medical indemnity association as you see fit.

7 NIGHTS/AFTER-HOURS

Night shifts can be tiring, but also a lot of fun, allowing you to bond with the rest of the ED team. In some hospitals, interns do not do night shifts in the ED.

The main difference on a night shift, and some after-hours shifts, is that certain services may not be available. It is usually difficult to get some tests done after-hours, for example CT and ultrasound. Discuss with the senior whether these tests are urgent, and whether someone should be called in. If it can wait until morning, make sure you order the test and get everything ready (e.g. if the patient needs a cannula) so that the test can be performed as early as possible in the morning. Similarly, you may change your approach to referring patients to other teams at unsociable hours—can the phone call wait until early morning, or is it urgent?

During nights and after hours there are often fewer people around in the ED. While this can make the ED feel calmer, you should be aware of increased risk to your safety in isolated areas. Do not take patients into areas where they may be unsupervised, e.g. subacute areas, unless there are appropriate staff around. It could endanger you, and your patient could deteriorate unnoticed.

8 WORK–LIFE BALANCE

Your ED term may be the first time you've done shift work. Shift work can be tiring and the odd hours can be antisocial and even isolating, so it's important to take care of yourself. On the plus side you may well find you have more time away from work. In many hospitals, ED shifts are 10 hours long, meaning 4 shifts a week. You also won't be doing the ward overtime shifts, which will give you more free time.

Make the most of these opportunities—whether it's for study or extra courses, time away or catching up on things you've been putting off; enjoy the increased flexibility. If you are looking to go away, you might even be able to swap shifts with someone in order to have up to 5 days off in a row without taking any extra leave; look into this early.

Intern year is a great time to enjoy yourself, and to learn, without the pressures of medical school exams or assessments. Although there may be many challenges in your ED term, there will be many rewards and opportunities both within and outside the hospital.

All the best!

Quick/general tips

- If in doubt, ask someone.
- Try to order all the tests you may need at the start, e.g. take one of each tube you may need for bloods.
- Carry some extra gauze and some tape.
- Always discuss your patient with a registrar or consultant. If you are worried, make sure you speak to someone more senior sooner.
- Every female is assumed pregnant until a beta-hCG has proven otherwise. Order a beta-hCG.
- Use the resources available—Therapeutic Guidelines, MIMS, Australian Medicines Handbook and clinical protocols.
- Make the most of the nursing and allied health staff. Keep them informed and involved in the patient's plan and progress.
- Look after your own safety.

- Never discharge someone without clearing the patient with a registrar or consultant.
- Adopt universal precautions, and if in doubt err on the side of caution.
- Always follow up any investigation you have ordered, including ECGs.
- Triage is a guide—if you are concerned about a patient deteriorating, you may need to see them sooner.
- Don't be ashamed if you do not know something: be honest, and you will learn for next time.
- Try not to be disheartened if you meet any obstruction or criticism. Try to learn from the experience, and understand the multiple factors at play in the situation. Remember you are part of a team, and ask for help if needed.
- If you're stuck remember your ABCs, and go back to the basics of history and examination.
- Look after each other. You are part of a team: ask for help when you need it, and offer help to others when you can.
- Have fun!

Online resources

Australian Medicines Handbook
  https://shop.amh.net.au
BMJ Best Practice
  http://bestpractice.bmj.com/best-practice/welcome.html
MIMS
  www.mims.com.au
Therapeutic Guidelines
  www.tg.org.au
UpToDate
  www.uptodate.com

Chapter 49

Students' guide to the emergency department

Sascha Fulde and Tiffany Fulde

The emergency department can be the highlight of a student's day or the place where you feel most out of place, or both at the same time. Hopefully, this chapter will outline some practical tips for getting the most out of this wonderful resource.

Advantages of the ED

As the place where almost all patients enter the hospital, the ED is a short-case heaven. In addition, you can see patients before they've been overrun by a thousand other students and doctors. Just think: by the time a patient gets up to a ward, they've most likely had the same questions asked and been poked in the sore spot by the ED intern, ED registrar, the intern on the admitting team and then the registrar, plus at least one nurse. They've had a stressful time, feel unwell and, ultimately, probably just want to be left alone; whereas in the ED they haven't been examined that many times. They're prepared to be undressed, poked and prodded because they recognise that that is what happens when they come to an emergency department. A student can often be useful: either confirming examination findings, sometimes finding something someone missed, either on history or examination; or just alleviating some of the patient's worry by spending some time with them while they're waiting for the results of investigations. Even if you're only doing an examination, it makes the patient feel that something is happening and that they're being taken care of. The patient is also in the mind-set where they really want to talk about their story and those niggly details of symptoms as it's pretty much all they can think about. Thus the ED is a fantastic resource for a medical student.

When patients present to the ED, they're much more likely to present in a way that is useful to a student. First, as no one knows what is wrong with them, you actually get a chance to test your clinical and diagnostic skills. Second, they present in the same way that short and long cases are often presented in exams. The complaints are also often at a level which you will be expected to know. For example, you are much more likely to see a patient with chest pain than one with a phaeochromocytoma.

LEARN TO HANDLE EMERGENCIES

As a student my biggest fear was that I would actually kill someone! My second biggest fear was failing exams. And the third was, how do I actually save someone's life? I'm not just talking about the big trauma cases, but also the smaller practical procedures. This is one of the greatest things the ED can teach you. By spending time there and talking to the doctors, you learn how to actually prioritise management and the basic couple of things that you need to do *right now* before you stop and work out the clinical management guidelines. You can also learn how to actually *do* them.

FIND PATIENTS FOR TUTORIALS, CASE HISTORIES AND PRESENTATIONS

Although the hospital is full of patients, it can often be hard to find patients that fit the requirements of the task you're trying to do—for instance, finding an interesting surgical case to present in a surgical tutorial or even for a bedside tutorial. As staff in the ED have seen all the patients that have entered the hospital, they are wonderful at knowing what patients are around and worth chasing up.

FITS WELL WITH PROBLEM-BASED LEARNING (PBL) COURSES

At the beginning of a PBL course it can often be difficult to approach medicine on the wards, as you have only learnt information on certain specific disorders or systems. This can make it overwhelming to approach a general medical or surgical term. However, in the ED the patients present in the same way as a case in a scenario, and this allows you to approach things you haven't seen before.

One of the strengths of PBL, which is that you focus on individual areas, can sometimes be slightly frustrating. By only focusing on one clinical vignette, you can sometimes feel like you don't know much about broader medicine. By hanging around the ED for even only a short period of time, you can very quickly start to counteract that and learn a lot across a broad range of areas.

PROVIDES A PLACE TO INTEGRATE A LOT OF KNOWLEDGE

Whatever level you're at in your training, the ED provides a great place to pull both your clinical skills and your esoteric knowledge together and practise what you've been learning. It's always easier to remember something when you've seen a patient with it and seen how they were managed.

GET A WIDE RANGE OF CLINICAL MATERIAL

With increasing specialisation of medicine and increasing numbers of students, often you only get to experience a limited number of different departments. For instance, you may never have had the opportunity to do a cardiology term. The ED is the place where you can compensate for this deficit. All the acute cardiology patients will come through the ED, so you can see how they are managed.

SEE MILD PATIENTS THAT GET DISCHARGED

The ED also has a range of severity of patients, so you get to see the simple sprains, cuts and bruises before they are discharged.

SEE GREAT SIGNS BEFORE THEY ARE TREATED

Often you trail around the hospital trying to find a patient to practise your examination signs on, only to find that while many people are unwell, they've already been treated, e.g. 'Mrs X had shifting dullness but we tapped it last night.'

In the ED you can see these signs often when they are at their peak before the arrhythmia is treated or the blood pressure lowered.

AVOIDING BEING BARRED

As a student, you're always going to be refused by some patients. Even though you know it's not personal, this is often demoralising. In contrast, it's always exciting to go and visit a patient you saw when they first presented in the ED and have them recognise you and happily let you repeat your examination to see their improvement.

The ED also provides an excellent opportunity to learn about the unspoken professional etiquette between different doctors. At some stage all doctors, whether interns or the most senior consultants, come to and interact in the ED. This allows you to learn a lot about the finer negotiations, for instance of getting staff up late at night.

Use it as a light at the end of the tunnel

Little encounters that you can have in the ED allow you to pretend to be a real doctor, even if only for a few seconds—not just a nurse or a cannulating technician doing a cannula or a blood pressure, but a real doctor. This not only reminds you what you're working for, but why you're working so hard. It really allows you to put all the hard decisions you're making into perspective. It can be even more important to remind yourself that there is a light at the end of the tunnel. This can be really motivating, either because being a doctor is exciting or because it makes you realise you're not quite knowledgeable enough yet.

How do you get the most out of it?

SO HOW DO YOU ACCESS THIS GEM?

First you must get access either by your swipe card or the keypad access code. This is crucial. Emergency department staff are usually very happy to have you there, but it's much easier if you just appear at the doctor's desk. If you have to constantly ask to come and go, you're probably much less likely to be there regularly.

Go to the ED regularly. If you become a familiar face to staff, they very quickly go out of their way to help you meet your learning goals or just to be friendly. A good tip is to leave the hospital via the ED. This forces you to see whether there are any interesting patients when you know you've got nowhere better to be. Even if you only see 1 patient a day, you'll start to become part of the hospital team.

The ED can get very busy. When this happens, people often get stressed. If you are around, do not automatically skulk back to the student room or ask if you can intubate the patient! Ideally, find a way to be involved while getting in as few people's way as possible. This can involve standing at the outer edge as resuscitation is going on, or going and seeing one of the low-triage-category patients by yourself to start with.

ATTACH YOURSELF TO A REGISTRAR

As the ED is usually very busy, you can also get a lot out of it by attaching yourself to a consultant or registrar and becoming their assistant. By doing the little tasks like chasing results, you can really help them out. This often engenders a lot of goodwill, which means that you get good teaching along the way and opportunities to do practical procedures if you're interested.

FOLLOW YOUR PATIENTS UP

When you have seen a patient in the ED, make sure you take the opportunity to follow them to the next step in their treatment. For instance, watch their surgery or check on them in the medical ward in a few days' time. Most teams are more than happy for you to be included in care when you explain that you saw the patient in the ED. Thus, you get to see many aspects of medicine and surgery.

DON'T COME IN HORDES

Although it's often less confronting to come in a group or with a partner, it'll be easier to get accepted by staff and patients if you come by yourself. It's also better to come alone, as this is how you're ultimately going to be in exams and it really allows you to realise your strengths and weaknesses and work on them.

ASK THE NURSES *FIRST*

Before doing anything, first ask a nurse. This is *very* important. Even if you have a doctor's permission and the nurse is busy, wait until they are finished and then ask their permission. Nurses often end up coordinating care, so they know whether they've had time to give the pain relief that the doctor has prescribed so that the patient can handle talking to you.

FIND THE THINGS THAT ARE USEFUL TO YOU AS A STUDENT BUT THAT NO ONE ELSE CARES ABOUT

There are many things happening in a hospital that are commonplace, barely thought-about activities but that can be really useful to a student. For instance, most people who come into the ED get an ECG and some blood tests. If you regularly look up the results and try to interpret them, whether you know the patient's history or not, you can become very good at interpreting results. This is easy to do and doesn't need any doctor's or nurse's help—you simply look them up and then check how the doctor interpreted them.

Another useful skill you can learn is to practise writing up notes. After seeing a patient, if you practise putting the salient points down on paper you can then compare your notes with the registrar's and see how good you were at getting all the points and putting them down in a clear format.

ASK ABOUT TEACHING

Most EDs have compulsory teaching sessions for interns, RMOs (residents) and registrars. They are often more than happy for a few students to attend. These sessions are usually filled with teaching on diseases that are of interest to you and will often make it into exams. So just ask some of the registrars and interns who organise the tutorials, if and when they're on and whether you can attend.

PRACTISE PROCEDURES—ALWAYS TAKE A BLUEY

The ED is a really good place in which to practise the basic procedures that you're expected to be able to do as an intern. There is always someone who needs bloods taken or a cannula or catheter, and people are usually happy to oversee you doing one. One important thing is to always check that you have all the equipment you need before you start a procedure. When you're doing anything you're a bit unfamiliar with, always take a bluey (a plastic protective sheet) so you don't make a mess of the sheets—this alienates the patient and makes the nurses cross. Also, always take a set of cotton balls and tape just in case something goes wrong—you can patch almost anything up.

If you have the chance, practise procedures on models. Many EDs have simulation centres or plastic models to practise procedures on. These can be fantastic for your first couple of times or if it's been a while since you've done one.

HAVE A SLIGHTLY THICK SKIN

Unfortunately, at some point as a student you're likely to get in trouble for something. While it's important to be considerate and do your best to avoid it, at some point you will get on someone's bad side. When this happens, just apologise and try to make it right. Then don't let it get to you. It happens to everyone.

FIND A FRIENDLY FACE AND TAKE ADVANTAGE OF THEM!

In every department there are a few really incredibly nice people. When you find them, make friends and then ask them about all those niggly things you need help with. They understand how hard it can be to be a student and they're more than happy to help, but you need to ask them. The worst they can say is 'no'.

TAKE MORE RESPONSIBILITY

When you're in more senior years, take more responsibility. You can use time in the ED as a pre-intern term. Go in at nights and help out. You can see some of the most interesting, diverse patients after dark. Plus, people appreciate your dedication and usually try to help you get the most out of it. You can even clerk patients from beginning to investigations and then take the write-up, just needing a signature, to your supervising doctor. This will help you, and hopefully save them a little time even if they then go back and check it.

Summary

Ultimately, make sure you enjoy both being a medical student and your life outside of medicine. Don't let the stress of medicine or all the advice above distract you from enjoying your time as a student. We hope that you learn a lot from this book and that this chapter has helped to inspire you to head into the ED.

Editorial Comment

It is our responsibility, privilege and delight to help and supervise our future colleagues, especially senior students who quickly and enthusiastically take up a workload. A very good system is to 'buddy' them with a doctor—even nights and weekend shifts; they love it. Also remember that you will be asked questions and that demonstration and teaching really improves and keeps your practice up-to-date.

The ED is often the most desired term, as students sense the joy and terror of being the first to deal with unknown, unexpected and potentially very ill patients—all this among a great gang of healthcare professionals.

It is usually final-year students that are attached to the ED. They are going to be interns in months—maybe at your hospital! So, even more so, time spent teaching them intern skills is very worthwhile.

Index

➡

E

➡

➡

H

M

N

➡

➡

➡

T

➡

➡

➡

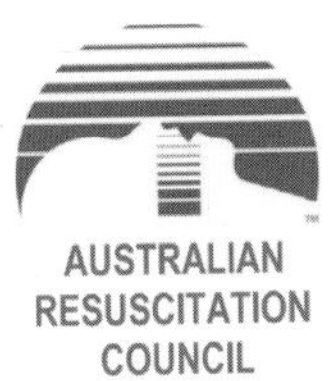

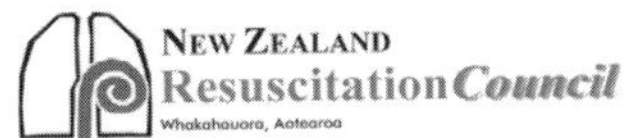

MANAGEMENT OF FOREIGN BODY AIRWAY OBSTRUCTION (CHOKING)

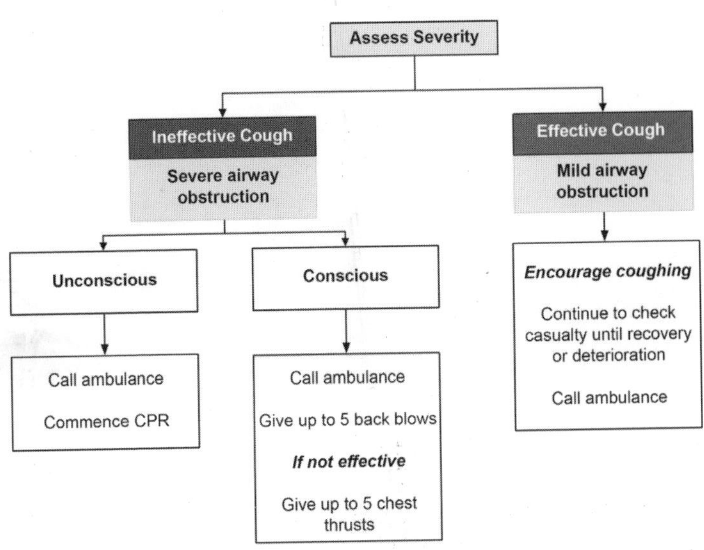

December 2010

Z

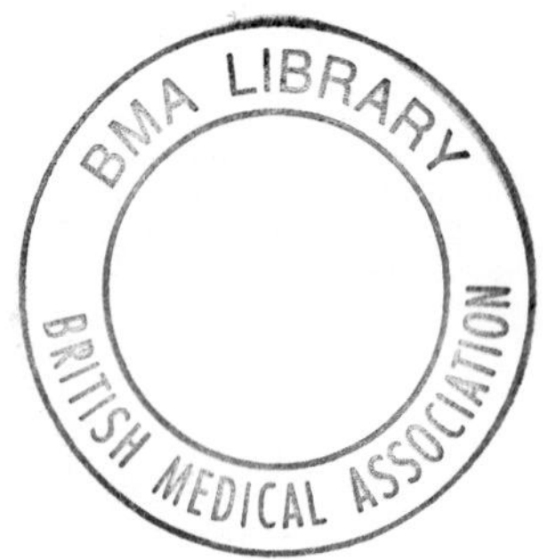